THE ATHLETE
AND HEART DISEASE

Diagnosis, Evaluation &
Management

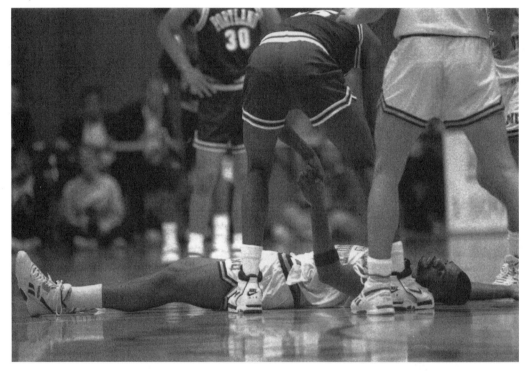

College basketball standout Hank Gathers, after he collapsed and later died of ventricular fibrillation due to cardiomyopathy during a game in Los Angeles, March 5, 1990. (Photograph by Gary Friedman. From *The Los Angeles Times* Syndicate, Los Angeles, CA, 1990, by permission.)

THE ATHLETE AND HEART DISEASE

Diagnosis, Evaluation & Management

Editor

Richard Allen Williams, M.D.
Clinical Professor of Medicine
University of California, Los Angeles
School of Medicine
Los Angeles, California
Chairman, Board of Directors
Minority Health Institute, Inc.
Beverly Hills, California

 LIPPINCOTT WILLIAMS & WILKINS
A **Wolters Kluwer** Company
Philadelphia · Baltimore · New York · London
Buenos Aires · Hong Kong · Sydney · Tokyo

Acquisitions Editor: Ruth W. Weinberg
Developmental Editor: Rebecca Irwin Diehl
Manufacturing Manager: Tim Reynolds
Production Manager: Kathleen Bubbeo
Production Editor: Michael Mallard
Cover Designer: Pinho Graphic Design
Indexer: Lynne Mahan
Compositor: Lippincott Williams & Wilkins Desktop Division
Printer: Maple Press

Printed in the United States of America

9   8   7   6   5   4   3   2   1

Library of Congress Cataloging-in-Publication Data
The athlete and heart disease: diagnosis, evaluation & management / editor,
  Richard Allen Williams.
        p.   cm.
     Includes bibliographical references and index.
     ISBN 0-316-88001-9 (pbk.)
     1. Heart–Disease.   2. Athletes—Diseases.   3. Cardiac arrest.
  4. Heart–Abnormalities.   I. Williams, Richard Allen, 1936–
     [DNLM: 1. Death, Sudden, Cardiac—prevention & control.   2. Death,
  Sudden, Cardiac–etiology.   3. Heart Diseases–complications.   4. Heart
  Diseases–diagnosis. 5. Sports Medicine, WG 205A869
     1998]
RC682.A815   1998
616.1′20088′796–dc21
DNLM/DLC
For Library of Congress   98-28127
     CIP

This book is dedicated most respectfully to three groups of people: First, to my mentors and professors who taught me so much about gaining strength in the face of adversity. These include Dr. George W. Thorn, the late Dr. Richard Gorlin, and Nobel Laureate Dr. Bernard Lown, all of Harvard Medical School. Second, to the athletes who have given their lives while making ours more enjoyable from their wondrous exploits, and to their surviving families who still experience the pain caused by the loss of their loved ones. Third, to my deceased parents, Walter S. and Mildred L. Williams, who made great sacrifices so that I could gain the education to produce this book in the first place. I owe a debt of gratitude to all of them.

Contents

Contributors

Craig R. Asher, M.D. *Staff Cardiologist, Department of Cardiology F-15, The Cleveland Clinic Foundation, 9500 Euclid Avenue, Cleveland, Ohio 44195*

Allen P. Burke, M.D. *Adjunct Professor, Department of Pathology, Georgetown University, 3800 Reservoir Road, NW; Pathologist, Department of Cardiovascular Pathology, Armed Forces Institute of Pathology, 6825 16th Street, NW, Washington, D.C. 20306-6000*

Bekir S. Cebeci, M.D. *Division of Cardiovascular Medicine, State University of New York Health Science Center at Brooklyn, 450 Clarkson Avenue, Brooklyn, New York 11203-2098*

Roseann M. Chesler, Ed.D. *Applied Physiologist, Division of Cardiovascular Medicine, State University of New York Health Science Center at Brooklyn, 450 Clarkson Avenue, Box 83, Brooklyn, New York 11203-2098*

Luther T. Clark, M.D. *Chief, Division of Cardiovascular Medicine, State University of New York Health Science Center at Brooklyn, 450 Clarkson Avenue, Box 1199, Brooklyn, New York 11203-2098*

Steven D. Colan, M.D. *Associate Professor, Department of Pediatrics, Harvard Medical School, 25 Shattuck Street; Director, Cardiac Noninvasive Laboratory, Children's Hospital, 300 Longwood Avenue, Boston, Massachusetts 02115*

Louis L. Cregler, M.D., F.A.C.P., F.A.C.C. *Professor of Medicine, Deputy Dean, Academic Affairs, City University of New York Medical School, 138th Street and Convent Avenue, New York, New York 10031; Attending Physician, Department of Medicine, Division of Cardiology, Maimonides Medical Center, 4802 Tenth Avenue, Brooklyn, New York 11219*

Nabil El-Sherif, M.D. *Professor of Medicine and Physiology, Director, Clinical Cardiovascular Medicine, Electrophysiology Program, State University of New York Health Science Center at Brooklyn, 450 Clarkson Avenue, Box 1199, Brooklyn, New York 11203-2098*

N. A. Mark Estes III, M.D. *Professor, Department of Medicine, Tufts University School of Medicine; Chief, Cardiac Arrhythmia Service, New England Medical Center, 750 Washington Street, Box 197, Boston, Massachusetts 02111*

Andrew Farb, M.D. *Department of Cardiovascular Pathology, Armed Forces Institute of Pathology, Alaska and 14th Street, NW, Room 2005, Washington, D.C. 20306-6000*

Gerald F. Fletcher, M.D. *Department of Medicine, Mayo Medical School, Mayo Clinic, 4500 San Pablo Road, Jacksonville, Florida 32224*

K. M. Gallagher, M.D. *Department of Integrative Physiology, University of North Texas Health Science Center, Fort Worth, Texas 76107*

Gary H. Gibbons, M.D. *Assistant Professor, Department of Medicine, Harvard Medical School; Brigham and Women's Hospital, Division of Cardiovascular Medicine, 75 Francis Street, Thorn-1326, Boston, Massachusetts 02115*

B. Waine Kong, Ph.D., J.D. *Chief Executive Officer, Association of Black Cardiologists, 225 Peachtree Street, NE, Suite 1420, Atlanta, Georgia 30303*

Stephanie H. Kong, M.D. *Senior Consultant, Coopers and Lybrand L.L.P., 1155 Peachtree Street, 1100 Campanile Building, Atlanta, Georgia 30309*

Harry M. Lever, M.D., F.A.C.C. *Department of Cardiology, Desk F-15, The Cleveland Clinic Foundation, 9500 Euclid Avenue, Cleveland, Ohio 44195*

Mark Steven Link, M.D. *Associate Professor, Department of Internal Medicine, Tufts University School of Medicine, 130 Harrison Avenue; Co-director, Electrophysiology Lab, Department of Cardiac Electrophysiology, New England Medical Center, 750 Washington Street, Boston, Massachusetts 02111*

Ali J. Marian, M.D. *Assistant Professor, Department of Medicine, Baylor College of Medicine, One Baylor Plaza, 543E; Staff Physician, Department of Medicine, The Methodist Hospital, 6550 Fannin, SM 677, Houston, Texas 77030*

Barry J. Maron, M.D. *Director, Cardiovascular Research Division, Minneapolis Heart Institute Foundation, 920 East 28th Street, Minneapolis, Minnesota 55407*

Jere H. Mitchell, M.D. *Harry S. Moss Heart Center, Departments of Internal Medicine and Physiology, University of Texas Southwestern Medical Center at Dallas, Dallas, Texas 75235*

Matthew J. Mitten, J.D. *Professor of Law, South Texas College of Law, affiliated with Texas A & M University, 1303 San Jacinto Street, Houston, Texas 77002-7000*

George Nseir, M.D. *Clinical Assistant Instructor of Medicine, State University of New York Health Science Center at Brooklyn, 450 Clarkson Avenue, Box 1199, Brooklyn, New York 11203-2098*

Marc Ovadia, M.D. *Division of Pediatric Cardiology, Cornell University College of Medicine/North Shore University; North Shore University Hospital, 300 Community Drive, Manhasset, New York 11030*

P. B. Raven, M.D. *Department of Integrative Physiology, University of North Texas Health Science Center, Fort Worth, Texas 76107*

Robert Roberts, M.D. *Don W. Chapman Professor of Medicine, Chief, Section of Cardiology, Baylor College of Medicine, 6550 Fannin, SM 677, Houston, Texas 77030*

Christine Seidman, M.D. *Professor, Department of Medicine, Harvard Medical School and Howard Hughes Medical Institute, 200 Longwood Avenue; Director, Cardiovascular Genetics Center, Department of Medicine, Cardiovascular Division, Brigham and Women's Hospital, 75 Francis Street, Boston, Massachusetts 02115*

Gioia Turitto, M.D. *Associate Professor, Department of Medicine, State University of New York Health Science Center at Brooklyn; Director, Coronary Care Unit, Electrophysiology Laboratory, State University of New York Health Science Center at Brooklyn, 450 Clarkson Avenue, Box 1199, Brooklyn, New York 11203-2098*

Renu Virmani, M.D. *Clinical Professor, Department of Pathology, Georgetown University, 3800 Reservoir Road, NW; Chairperson, Department of Cardiovascular Pathology, Armed Forces Institute of Pathology, Alaska and 14th Street, NW, Room 2005, Washington, D.C. 20306-6000*

Paul J. Wang, M.D. *Associate Professor, Department of Medicine, Tufts University School of Medicine, Associate Director, Cardiac Electrophysiology and Pacemaker Lab; Director, Adult Heart Station, Division of Cardiology, Department of Medicine, New England Medical Center, 750 Washington Street, Boston, Massachusetts 02111*

Richard Allen Williams, M.D. *Clinical Professor of Medicine, University of California, Los Angeles School of Medicine, Los Angeles, California 90024; Chairman, Board of Directors, Minority Health Institute, Inc., 8306 Wilshire Boulevard, Suite 288, Beverly Hills, California 90211*

Foreword

When Dr. Richard Allen Williams asked me to write the foreword for his book *The Athlete and Heart Disease: Diagnosis, Evaluation & Management,* I felt proud that he thought about me because of my interest in sports and sports medicine. However, before I accepted the task, I wanted to know the content of the book in depth, and I finished reading it yesterday. Today, I can write this foreword with great satisfaction.

The first question, in regard to a new book is, Is it really necessary? A recent editorial in *The New England Journal of Medicine* by its editors, Drs. J.P. Kassirer and M. Angell, calls for caution regarding redundant publications, while a simultaneous editorial in *Nature* by the editor, Dr. J. Maddox, points out that each new book or journal may offer something with a special focus which can be of wide general interest. Dr. Williams and other national and international experts who collaborated on *The Athlete and Heart Disease* fulfill this premise. They have put together an outstanding book in an era where exercise and sports are so much in the public eye. Diseases of the athlete or of the physically active individual have not been a major priority until recently, when several high-profile athletes died of various causes. It is shocking when a young, apparently healthy individual who is a regular participant in competitive and noncompetitive athletic exercises dies without warning. However, a large amount of information has been accumulated in the last few years that can help to identify such individuals or athletes at risk. Accordingly, there now seems to be a spirit of collaboration throughout the community between physicians, scientists, internists, ethicists, coaches, and sports organizations. In addition, during the last three years, the 24th Bethesda Conference, an expert report by the American Heart Association, and a recent report by *The Journal of The American Medical Association,* outline the importance of the topic. Because a comprehensive review on heart disease in the athlete is absent in most of the major textbooks, *The Athlete and Heart Disease* fills a very important void.

A second question in regard to this specific book is, Is it really necessary to address the athlete and heart disease in as many as 19 chapters? Indeed, the attractiveness of the book is in its wide approach addressing all aspects of importance for those who exercise on a competitive or noncompetitive basis, as well as those who do not exercise and should. The book begins with excellent general chapters, including The Historical Background of Sudden Cardiac Death in Athletes, Classification of Sports and the Athlete's Heart, Cardiovascular Genetic Disorders That Cause Sudden Death in Athletes, and The Molecular Biology of Cardiac Abnormalities in Athletes. The reader can then pursue specific disease entities in various chapters addressing problems such as hypertrophic cardiomyopathy, Marfan's syndrome, and congenital heart disease. In addition, a number of chapters address the clinical and technological advances for the screening and identification of the individuals at risk. Finally, it is quite rewarding to have specific chapters devoted to the important issues of Substance Abuse in Sports, Recreational and Competitive Athletics in the Older Adult with Cardiovascular Disease, Ethical, Economic, and Medicolegal Issues regarding Athletes in Heart Disease, and Race and Gender Considerations in Sudden Death in the Athlete.

The final question is, Can a book be comprehensive and unified with so many authors? I believe this is one of the few collaborated books that appears to have been written by a single author. Dr. Richard Allen Williams has put together an outstanding group of experts and assembled information that proceeds smoothly from the molecular biology of cardiac abnormalities in athletes to ethical, economical, and medicolegal issues. Dr. Williams and his collaborators are to be congratulated for what will become the standard book on the understanding of the athlete and heart disease. Such a well-integrated, didactic, and practical book will be invaluable to physicians, scientists, ethicists, coaches, and sports organizations.

Valentin Fuster, M.D., Ph.D.
The Richard Gorlin, M.D./Heart Research Foundation Professor of Cardiology
Director, The Zena and Michael A. Wiener Cardiovascular Institute
Dean For Academic Affairs, Mount Sinai Medical School of Medicine
President, American Heart Association

Preface

The time you won your town the race
We chaired you through the market place;
Man and boy stood cheering by
And home we brought you shoulder-high.
Today, the road all runners come,
Shoulder-high, we bring you home,
And set you at your threshold down,
Townsman of a stiller town.
—A.E. Housman, "To An Athlete Dying Young"

Death is an inevitable and accepted conclusion to life, but the sudden death of a young person, especially an athlete, is tragic and difficult to comprehend. It is, as *The Los Angeles Times* sports columnist Jim Murray calls it, "the most unwelcome spectator," terminating as it does the lives of those in our populace who are the most physically gifted and talented, often doing so while they are competing in front of us. We can cite several examples: Hank Gathers, Reggie Lewis, Flo Hyman, Sergei Grinkov, and Pete Maravich. There are many others who have been unmercifully cut down. They unwittingly sacrificed their very lives while innocently participating in sports.

Sports represent the major area of organized physical activity in the United States, involving millions of participants competing at diverse levels such as grade school, high school, college, and the professional ranks. The athletes may be recreational or elite, and they may participate through numerous clubs, leagues, associations, and myriad other organizations. There are millions of observers or spectators, and the amount of money spent on sports, invested in sports, and earned by athletes is in the multiple billions of dollars. The discipline of sports medicine has developed out of concern for the health problems and safety of the individuals who are at the center of this very intense activity, and hundreds of scientific studies have been performed relating to athletes and human performance. However, there has never been an in-depth book written on the cardiovascular problems that may afflict athletes.

It was over 20 years ago that I began to recognize that some of these wonderfully endowed individuals might appear healthy one minute, but might literally drop dead the next. At first, these appeared to be chance occurrences. On closer scrutiny, however, it became obvious that these deaths of mostly young athletes were not flukes or cardiovascular accidents any more than strokes are cerebrovascular accidents (CVAs). Specific causes could be identified, and a pattern could be noted in which certain types of athletes as well as particular sports were more likely to be associated with this phenomenon. In addition, it became evident later that the laws of genetics could be applied to several of the cardiovascular diseases found in the decedents. In the past several years, tremendous advances in molecular biology have led to an understanding of conditions such as hypertrophic cardiomyopathy (HCM), and today we are able in many cases to diagnosis and evaluate this most common cause of sudden cardiac death in young athletes. Other conditions may also be detected through the use of genetic techniques. Indeed, the prospect of genetic screening, for which there are pros and cons, is in the offing, and the era of genetic treatment and prevention of certain cardiac diseases seems not too far away.

In conceptualizing this book, it was my desire to assemble a group of the finest experts to present hard data on the theme of the athlete and heart disease, and to focus on sudden cardiac death in particular. I am confident that this goal has been achieved. This book is intended to provide authoritative information to a diverse readership consisting of physicians, sports medicine practitioners and other medical personnel, public health groups, officials in organized sports, coaches, trainers, and anyone who might be involved with and concerned about the health and safety of athletes. We have attempted to make it comprehensible for all, and we have tried to give the current best wisdom on diagnosis, investigation, and management. Our ultimate goal is to provide the information needed to allow the patient to make his or her own best decisions, with guidance from informed physicians and other advisors.

Finally, this book becomes especially pertinent because it is an attempt to give many athletes a better chance to perform their graceful routines and powerful programs without fear of disruption caused by a problem from deep within themselves. It also gives those athletes who should refrain from strenuous competition a warning that they may face the possibility of dying suddenly if they should continue. All of the answers are not here, and obviously there is still much to do scientifically before we can be certain which athletes fall into which of these two groups. We should not rest until we are able to prevent these devastating conditions from destroying what Dr. Bernard Lown called hearts too good to die.

Richard Allen Williams, M.D.

Acknowledgments

Producing a book is an effort involving input, advice, guidance, recommendations, and assistance from numerous individuals. Several people unselfishly aided me at different times in the development of *The Athlete and Heart Disease*, and I take this opportunity to thank them collectively for their contributions. They are Steve Van Camp, M.D., Ivor Benjamin, M.D., Nancy Landau, Paul Thompson, M.D., Ernestine Blue, Cheryl Martin, M.D., Fred Mueller, M.D., Garry Mendez, M.D., Maralynda West, and the editorial staff at Lippincott Williams & Wilkins, especially Ruth Weinberg, Tammerly Booth, Judith Hummel, Carol Field, Rebecca Irwin Diehl, and Michael Mallard. I would also like to express gratitude to all of my contributors who donated their expertise and time and who patiently tolerated my persistent urgings. I hope all of them share my deep sense of pride and satisfaction based on the fact that we have collaborated on a work that will bring a much-needed focus upon one of the most deadly covert health problems we face. Finally, my thanks to all of the unnamed coaches, trainers, college administrators, medical examiners, athletes, and many others who helped bring this project to a successful conclusion.

In Memoriam
Florence Griffith Joyner
(1959–1998)

The shocking news was delivered to me, while I was attending a medical conference, that former track superstar Florence Griffith Joyner, or FloJo, as she was affectionately called, had died suddenly at her California home on Monday, September 21, 1998 at the age of 38. The cause of death had not been determined at the time this was written, but it came, nonetheless, completely unexpected, with no reports of any recent health problems. While still reeling from the stunning surprise of this news, I was contacted by a reporter for *The New York Times* who was interested in exploring the various possibilities of the conditions which may have contributed to the death of such an outstanding, young, and apparently healthy woman. She had been at the pinnacle of her athletic prowess only ten years ago when she captured the attention and admiration of the entire world by winning four medals—three gold and one silver—during the 1988 Olympic Games in Seoul, South Korea, and in the process setting world records in the 100- and 200-meter dashes, marks which still endure to this day. Now suddenly, inexplicably, she is dead, and everyone wonders why.

While we await the results of the autopsy, there is a great deal of speculation as to what caused her death. There have been rumors circulating that she used performance-enhancing drugs to accomplish her incredible athletic feats. These ugly accusations persist despite the fact that FloJo was tested several times for illegal drugs during her athletic career, while never failing a test. Her performances and records have been accepted by all the governing bodies of track and field, and that is good enough for me. The results of the autopsy will surely come, but they do not really matter; anything that might be discovered now cannot be used to "prove" that she used drugs during her athletic career. By all of the rules of logic and evidence, she must be considered to have been "clean," and she therefore deserves the respect and reverence befitting her awesome accomplishments.

There was considerably more to FloJo than her victories on the track. She should also be remembered for being the poor African-American girl who rose out of a broken home in a Watts housing project to excel as a student athlete at UCLA, first to become an NCAA sprint champion and then an Olympic champion. I recall seeing her during practices at Drake Stadium, and she impressed me with her rare combination of speed, power, beauty, grace, and poise. Yet despite all of these assets, she was self-effacing, even shy, when I met her. A likeable young lady, indeed.

FloJo did much to demonstrate her strength of character as well. Several years ago, she established the Florence Griffith Joyner Youth Foundation to inspire disadvantaged youth to reach for the stars, as she herself had done. There were many other acts which established her as a humanitarian. She also showed her capacity for leadership by co-chairing the President's Council on Physical Fitness. Obviously, this was no mere one-dimensional athlete, but rather a sensitive, charitable woman who showed in concrete terms that she truly cared about the welfare of others.

Now FloJo is gone. What shall her legacy be? I believe that we should place her among the first rank of all-time great track athletes. Let us place her in the pantheon of those whose remarkable performances have rendered them immortal. And as far as the innuendoes, suspicions, and rumors are concerned, let us bury them as we bury her. May she rest in peace.

Richard Allen Williams, M.D.
Los Angeles, California

The Athlete and Heart Disease:
Diagnosis, Evaluation & Management,
edited by R. A. Williams.
Lippincott Williams & Wilkins, Philadelphia © 1999.

1

The Historical Background of Sudden Cardiac Death in Athletes

Richard Allen Williams

Department of Medicine, UCLA School of Medicine, Los Angeles, California 90024; Minority Health Institute, Inc., Beverly Hills, California 90211

The history of sudden death in humans is as old as history itself. The ancient Egyptians, according to Dr. Bernard Lown, made one of the first reports of a sudden death occurence (1). The Bible contains a reference that might be considered the first recorded instance of cardiopulmonary resuscitation (2):

> And he went up, and lay upon the child, and put his mouth upon his mouth, and his eyes upon his eyes, and his hands upon his hands; and he stretched himself upon the child, and the flesh of the child waxed warm.

The early Chinese may have unknowingly diagnosed cardiac arrhythmias and their association with sudden death when they spoke of a shortened life span correlated with irregularities of the pulse (3). In ancient Greece, Hippocrates of Cos (460–370 B.C.) was quoted as saying "Frequent recurrence of cardialgia in an elderly person announces sudden death," which was a reference to pain (presumably originating in the heart) and sudden death. He also antedated the findings of the Framingham study by announcing that there was a close correlation between obesity and dying suddenly (4). Leonardo da Vinci (1452–1519) made a clinical observation in Italy of an old man who died without warning while Leonardo was talking to him (5). Determined to find the reason for so gentle a death ("*la causa di si dolce morte*"), Leonardo da Vinci performed what was probably the first post-mortem examination, finding that the death proceeded from weakness through failure of blood and of the artery that feeds the heart and other members (6). Lusitania (1511–1568) described the differences between apoplexy (stroke) and sudden cardiac death, and in England, William Harvey (1578–1657), formerly a student at Padua under Fabricius and Casserius, described an episode of sudden death caused by ventricular rupture (7). He also wrote the epoch-making treatise, *De Motu Cordis et Sanguinis* (1628), which described the heart as a muscular force-pump responsible for the motion of the blood through the body. Also in England, the Earl of Clarendon gave what was probably the first written account of a case of angina pectoris in the person of his own father's disorder (1632), but William Heberden (1710–1801) provided the medical and scientific basis that linked this "disorder of the breast" to heart disease in 1772 (8).

Medical fascination with the phenomenon of sudden death regarding why, when, and how it occurred, and in whom, has continued for centuries. A number of techniques were developed to stimulate the arrested heart back to life (9,10). The assumption was that those persons who died suddenly were the victims of a heart seizure. Obstruction of the left anterior descending coronary artery was often found on autopsy, and this became known as the "artery of sudden death."

Most sudden cardiac death victims have been noted to be older individuals, many with a history of heart disease. It is unusual and surprising, therefore, when the stricken person is young, apparently healthy, and a regular participant in competitive athletic exercises.

The Olympic games may be regarded as an appropriate focus to initiate a historical review of sudden cardiac death in athletes. The ancient games began about 2,700 years ago in Olympia, Greece, as a religious festival held every 4 years and featuring athletic competition between neighboring communities on the Peloponnesian peninsula. Foot-races, chariot races, and other feats of physical skill were contested by kings as well as common soldiers and plebians competing absolutely nude for the simple honor of receiving an olive wreath, which was placed on the head of the victor in each event. The first victor recorded in history was a cook from the town of Elis named Coroebus, or Koroibus in Greek, who won a dash measuring about 200 meters, or one length of the stadium (*stade*). The first Olympiad in which records were kept occurred in 776 B.C., although the games may have been initiated as early as 820 B.C. on an edict jointly issued by Lycurgus of Sparta and Iphetus, King of Elis, and they continued for 1,200 years until they were banned as a pagan ceremony by Theodosius, emperor of Rome, in 394 A.D. (12).

Olympia was subsequently destroyed by earthquakes and floods. The ancient Olympiads had endured wars, political intrigues, and so many obstacles for centuries, and indeed, the most famous of the ancient Olympians, the legendary Pheidippedes, achieved his greatest moment during battle and became the first recorded victim of sudden cardiac death in an athlete. Pheidippedes, known variously as Phidippedes, Thersippus (Plutarch), and Philippedes (Lucian), had been an Olympic champion about 500 B.C. Ten years after his victorious exploits, in 490 B.C., the Persian army, dispatched by Darius and led by Hippias, landed at the Greek plain of Marathon with the intent of conquering Athens, about 25 miles away. Hearing of this threat, the Athenians sent courageous Pheidippedes to run quickly to Sparta to enlist the assistance of their army in repulsing the Persian attack, which was to come by sea. Running without rest for two nights, climbing mountains and swimming, he successfully recruited the Spartans, who joined the Athenians in outflanking the Persians and slaughtering them. During the battle, he also led troops against the invaders, and in a classic of military tactics, the Persians were defeated and Athens was saved (13).

But Pheidippedes' labors were not over; the Athenian generals sent their beleaguered, fatigued hero back to Athens from the battlefields of Marathon to tell the news of the victory. After running more than 25 miles, he reached Athens, announced to the citizens, "Rejoice, we conquer!" and then dropped dead. Thus originated the tradition of marathon running, the endurance race of more than 26 miles, which takes it name from the town in which the famous battle was fought—and won—by the Greeks, thanks to the brave exploits of Pheidippedes. Through his death, the spirit of the Olympic games was rekindled and sustained for centuries. No one else in history better exemplified the Olympic motto, *Citius, Altius, Fortius*—faster, higher, stronger—than did this great Greek athlete.

Pheidippedes' feats were more demanding than is generally recognized. Although he is remembered principally for his epic run from Marathon to Athens to bring the news of conquest over the Persians, he actually traveled *two* and possibly *three* long distances in a short space of time: first, as confirmed by Pliny the Elder, he ran from Athens to Sparta as a courier to enlist the military aid of the Spartans, a distance of 145 miles; next, he traveled probably by boat on the Aegean Sea with the Spartans, from Sparta to Marathon, where the great battle was joined; finally, he ran back to Athens from Marathon to deliver his dramatic message, another 25 miles. It is almost certain that such physical rigors have never been endured by any known athlete in history, and he must be accorded the full measure of credit for all of his mighty efforts. It would be a mistake to memorialize him only as the first known athlete to die of sudden cardiac death; indeed, he was the savior of his country, and without a doubt, he altered the course of history. Pheidippedes is the epitome of the athlete, a word derived from the Greek *athlios*, meaning like an athlete. Early Christian writers equated athletes with martyrs; the Greek term *agon,* from which the word *agony* is derived, means competition. The Apostle Paul describes his ordeals in the following passage from II Corinthians in the Bible:

> I have fought the good fight,. . .
> I have agonized the agon well,
> I have completed the run.
> I have kept the faith.
> What finally awaits me is
> The victor's wreath for righteousness.(14)

This quote indicates how highly esteemed athletics were in ancient times; mothers even took sick children to touch the hands of Olympic victors, believing that their magic was curative.

After the ancient games were abolished by Emperor Theodosius, it was not until 1,502 years later that they were restored in their modern version (14). This accomplishment was due largely to the efforts of Baron Pierre de Coubertin, who presided over the reconvening of the Olympics, fittingly in Athens, in 1896. They have continued every 4 years since, despite difficulties with terrorism, boycotts, wars, protests, demonstrations, and other problems, and in 1996 the centennial celebration of the modern Olympic games was held, involving 10,600 participants from 197 countries.

During our modern era, concerns have arisen about the safety of competitive athletes, especially regarding the use by some of performance-enhancing drugs such as stimulants, narcotics, and anabolic androgenic steroids. These concerns were increased when a British cyclist who was competing while under the influence of amphetamines died during the Tour de France in 1967 (15). The International Olympic Committee (IOC) has established a medical commission and has been conducting tests for banned substances since 1968. In the 1980s, the U.S. Olympic Committee joined with the National Football League (NFL) and the National Collegiate Athletic Association (NCAA) to conduct testing on their respective athletes in IOC-accredited laboratories at University of California at Los Angeles and Indiana University. This collaboration between major collegiate, Olympic, and professional sports organizations indicates the commitment that they have made not only to ensure fair play but also, and more importantly, to protect the hearts and lives of the competitors.

The sudden deaths of young athletes has not been a major health priority during this century until recently, when several high-profile athletes died of various causes. Previously, only an occasional anecdotal report would be presented or an unexpected death would be heard about and discussed among physicians, coaches, and others. However, in the past 30 years or so, media reports of the sudden death of well-known athletes such as Hank Gathers, Reggie Lewis, Flo Hyman, Len Bias, Don Rogers, Sergei Grinkov, and Pete Maravich have highlighted this phenomenon as a problem requiring attention and resolution. Historically, attention was focused on the problem of cardiovascular disorders in athletes when Dr. Paul Dudley White examined a young athlete with unexplained paroxysmal atrial fibrillation in 1928; the electrocardiogram revealed a short PR interval of 100 milliseconds and a wide QRS complex resembling bundle branch block (16). These abnormalities were seen at slow heart rates or after carotid sinus massage, but could be made to disappear with exercise or after an injection of atropine. Working with Louis Wolff, Dr. White combined this case and others with those of Sir John Parkinson in England, and in 1930 the trio published their classic paper on the Wolff-Parkinson-White (WPW) syndrome (17). It was determined many years later that the WPW syndrome occurs more frequently in athletes than in the general population, and in some instances has been the cause of sudden cardiac death. In the past several years, a number of reports have documented the fact that many other electrocardiographic abnormalities may be found in athletes more than in the general population;

these include sinus bradycardia, sinus pauses, sinus arrhythmia, wandering pacemaker, first-degree atrioventricular (AV) block, second-degree AV block of the Wenckebach type (seen in 10% of marathon runners), third-degree AV block, and atrial fibrillation. Ventricular tachyarrhythmias seen more commonly in athletes than in nonathletes include accelerated idioventricular rhythm, but ventricular arrhythmias emanating from ectopic foci are not found more frequently in athletes.

Interest in electrocardiographic changes and other cardiovascular alterations in athletes proliferated, and the concept of the athlete's heart was developed, in which it was theorized that cardiac enlargement ensued in highly trained young people and that deviations from normal, which were noted in the physical examination, chest x-ray examination, and other measurements, were due to physiologic adaptations to training (18). It was important to differentiate these benign changes from actual pathophysiologic aberrations caused by structural heart disease, which sometimes resulted in death. Pathologists became interested in what caused the sudden deaths of seemingly healthy, highly trained individuals. This development led to a pursuit of the culprit lesions, which paralleled the work of Wolff, Parkinson, and White. The dual clinical-pathologic approach culminated in the identification of the principal causes of sudden cardiac death in athletes. Hypertrophic cardiomyopathy (HCM) was found to be the main culprit in persons younger than 35 years of age, whereas coronary artery disease (CAD) was identified as the cause in three-fourths of the older population.

Although French and German investigators may have provided the first gross anatomic description of HCM around 1900 (19–21), it remained for Teare (22) to provide the most detailed report of this new disease in 1958. He elaborated on the pathologic findings in eight deceased patients with the disorder, of whom seven had died suddenly. Teare described the gross anatomic findings as demonstrating asymmetric hypertrophy of the left ventricle and septum without cavity dilation, with a

histologic pattern of myofiber disarray seen in the affected areas. Over the past 40 or so years, a number of studies have indicated the clinical, pathologic, and genetic details of the involvement of HCM in the sudden cardiac deaths of several athletes, and, as stated earlier, it has come to be recognized as the number one cause of sudden death in the young athlete (23). The historical sequence of studies of sudden cardiac deaths began with a report by James in 1967 on two subjects (24). Table 1 presents a chronology of several reports by various investigators. Dr. Barry J. Maron's contributions to the research on this malignant disorder have been the most important, most comprehensive, and most compellingly incisive. He has fairly well defined the parameters of the disease in particular and of sudden cardiac death in athletes in general, much more than any other investigator in history. Working at the National Heart, Lung and Blood Institute (NHLBI) of the National Institutes of Health (NIH) in Bethesda, MD, Maron also successfully led the way in settling the controversy regarding the nomenclature for the disorder, which has been known by at least 75 different named over the years; *hypertrophic cardiomyopathy* is the term that has come to be universally agreed upon as probably the most anatomically and physiologically correct one.

By the early 1980s there was sufficient concern about the safety of strenuous competition for individuals with cardiovascular abnormalities that a conference was organized to address this issue and to provide some guidelines for participants of affected athletes. The 16th Bethesda Conference on Cardiovascular Abnormalities in the Athlete was convened under the auspices of the American College of Cardiology (ACC) in October 1984, and from it evolved a number of recommendations regarding eligibility for competition (25). The holding of this conference was due mainly to Drs. Maron, Jere H. Mitchell, and Stephen E. Epstein, and it was a landmark meeting that gave official, scientific status to the concerns about athletic field deaths, which had been previously been ex-

TABLE 1. *Sudden cardiac death in athletes*

	James et al. Ann Intern Med 1967	Ople et al. Lancet 1975	Noakes et al. N Engl J Med 1979	Thompson et al. JAMA 1979	Morales et al. Circulation 1980	Maron et al. Circulation 1980	Waller et al. Am J Cardiol 1980	Virmani et al. Am J Med 1982	Northcote et al. Lancet 1984	Corrado et al. Am J Med 1990	Burke et al. Am Heart J 1991	Furianello et al. PACE 1992
No. of athletes	2	21	5	18	3	3	5	30	30	22	34	8
Age (yr)	15/18	17/58	27–44	42–60	17–54	17–54	40–53	18–57	35–60	11–35	14–40	14–40
Death during competition, training	++	++	++	++	++	++	++	(+)	++	18/22	++	7/8
Prodromal symptoms	1/2	9/21	1/5	6/18	—	—	1/5	?	22/30	12/22	?	?
Pathological findings	2	—	4	14	3	27	5	26	27	22	34	8
Organic changes	0	—	0	0	0	14	0	0	1	0	8	0
Hypertrophic cardiomyopathy	0	—	1	13	0	3	5	22	23	4	9	3
Coronary artery disease	0	—	0	0	3	3	5	0	0	2	6	0
Coronary anomaly/coronary artery bridging	0	—	0	0	0	5	0	3	0	0	3	0
Hypertrophy + + +	2	—	0	0	0	0	0	0	0	3	0	1
Abnormal conduction system	0	—	0	1	0	0	0	0	0	0	2	1
Myocarditis												
Compelling suspicion of CAD		18/21										

pressed largely in anecdotal terms. The 15th Bethesda Conference on Sudden Cardiac Death, chaired by Dr. Thomas N. James, was held earlier that year, but sudden cardiac death in sports was not specifically targeted as a subject for discussion (26). In January 1994, the 24th Bethesda Conference was held to revisit the issue of recommendations for athletes with cardiovascular abnormalities who plan to compete in competitive sports; it used more current information regarding assessment of individuals with suspected specific disorders, such as two-dimensional echocardiography and genetic testing in the evaluation of those with possible HCM (27). It also took into consideration more recently discovered conditions such as arrhythmogenic right ventricular dysplasia. In addition, the conferees expanded the ethical, legal, and practical considerations that affect the athlete and the doctor-patient relationship. The conference was sponsored again by the ACC and was cochaired by Drs. Maron and Mitchell. For the first time, it included representatives of college and professional sports organizations. Recommendations were updated for each of six task force areas of concern.

Meanwhile, efforts have been undertaken to focus more accurately on risk factors for sudden cardiac death in the athlete and to determine to what extent it is possible to prevent tragedies from occurring in participants in competitive sports. Identification of the person at high risk is a daunting task. An attempt to establish guidelines for preparticipation evaluation or screening was made with the selection of a panel of experts by the American Heart Association (AHA), which published its recommendations in 1996 (28). While deploring the current lack of adequate standards for retesting athletes, the panel acknowledged the difficulty of applying various noninvasive techniques, including genetic testing, and it also considered the economic impact in terms of cost that a sufficiently broad screening program would have. Nonetheless, the group was in favor of the establishment of some form of preparticipation cardiovascular screening for high school and college athletes, and it rec-

ommended the development of a national standard for such medical evaluations. These types of deliberations presumably will be ongoing.

Another factor of paramount significance concerns the collection of accurate data on individuals who suffer episodes of sudden cardiac death as a result of competitive exertion. At present, the main repositories of this type of data are the Armed Forces Institute of Pathology (AFIP) in Washington, D.C., and the National Center for Catastrophic Sports Injury Research (NCCSIR) at the University of North Carolina at Chapel Hill, as well as a registry maintained by Dr. Maron at the Minneapolis Heart Institute. Despite the excellent work by Dr. Maron, Dr. Renu Virmani at AFIP, and Dr. Fred Mueller at NCCSIR, however, a truly national registry of data on sudden cardiac deaths in athletes is a need that has not been met.

The past 20 years or so have seen the development of a growing interest and perhaps even a somewhat morbid fascination with this peculiar problem of sudden cardiac deaths in athletes. There is much to intrigue, as well as confuse, the investigator, and the cases of several elite athletes have been particularly perplexing. However, there seems to be a spirit of collaboration throughout the community such that physicians, scientists, attorneys, ethicists, coaches, and sports organizations are working to clarify the issues. For the first time, a well-read journal of medicine, the *Journal of the American Medical Association* (JAMA), devoted an entire issue (July 17, 1996) to health concerns of athletes, using the Centennial Olympiad as the backdrop. Thus, this discussion of some aspects of the history of sudden death in athletes has come full circle, from the earlier consideration of the ancient Olympic games and the heroic exploits of Pheidippedes to the present (29,30). The goal is to prevent many more modern-day sports heroes and heroines from collapsing on their fields of dreams, and, with a combined effort, to paraphrase Winston Churchill, to unravel this riddle embedded in a dilemma surrounded by mystery.

REFERENCES

1. Lown B. Sudden cardiac death: the major challenge confronting contemporary cardiology. *Am J Cardiol* 1979;43:313.
2. II Kings 4:34.
3. Major RH. *A history of medicine.* Springfield, IL: Charles C Thomas Publisher, 1954.
4. Leibowitz JO. *The history of coronary heart disease.* Los Angeles, CA: University of California Press, 1970.
5. Calder R. *Leonardo and the age of the eye.* New York: Simon and Schuster, 1970:173.
6. Warren JV. *Critical issues in the sudden death syndrome.* Princeton, NJ: Baylor College of Medicine Cardiology Series, 1982.
7. Garrison FH. *History of medicine.* Philadelphia: WB Saunders, 1929.
8. Heberden W. Some account of a disorder of the breast. *Med Trans Coll Physicians (Lond)* 1772;2:59.
9. Beck CS, Pritchard WJ, Feil H. Ventricular fibrillation of prolonged duration abolished by electric shock. *JAMA* 1947;135:985.
10. Kouwenhoven WB, Jude JR, Knickerbocker GC. Closed chest cardiac massage. *JAMA* 1960;137:1064.
11. Cantwell JD, Fontanarosa PB. An Olympic medical legacy. *JAMA* 1996;276:248.
12. Sweet WE. *Sport and recreation in ancient Greece.* New York: Oxford University Press, 1987.
13. Sweet WE. *Sport and recreation in ancient Greece.* New York: Oxford University Press, 1987, vi.
14. Henry B, Yeomans PH. *An approved history of the Olympic games.* Sherman Oaks, CA: Alfred Publishing, 1984:23.
15. Beckett AH, Cowan DA. Misuse of drugs in sport. *Br J Sports Med* 1979;12:185.
16. Shapiro E. The electrocardiogram and the arrhythmias: historical insights. In: Mandel WJ, ed. *Cardiac arrhythmias,* 3rd ed. Philadelphia: JB Lippincott, 1995:8.
17. Wolff L, Parkinson J, White PD. Bundle branch block with short PR interval in healthy young people prone to paroxysmal tachycardia. *Am Heart J* 1930;5:685.
18. Mukerji B, Alpert A, Mukerji V. Cardiovascular changes in athletes. *Am Fam Physician* 1989;40:169.
19. Schmincke A. Ueber linkseitige muskulose Connustenosen. *Dtsch Med Wochenschr* 1907;33:282.
20. Liouville H. Retrecissement cardiaque sous aortique. *Gazette Med Paris* 1869;24:161.
21. Hallopeau M. Retrecissement ventriculo-aortique. *Gazette Med Paris* 1869;24:683.
22. Teare D. Asymmetrical hypertrophy of the heart in young adults. *Br Heart J* 1958;20:1.
23. Maron BJ, Roberts WC, McAllister HA, Rosing DR, Epstein SE. Sudden death in young athletes. *Circulation* 1980;62:218.
24. James TN, Froggat P, Marshall TK. Sudden death in young athletes. *Ann Intern Med* 1967;67:1013.
25. Mitchell JH, Maron BJ, Epstein SE. 16th Bethesda Conference: Cardiovascular abnormalities in the athlete: Recommendations regarding eligibility for competition. *J Am Coll Cardiol* 1985;6:1189.
26. James TN. 15th Bethesda Conference Report: Sudden cardiac death. *J Am Coll Cardiol* 1985;5[Suppl]:5B.
27. Maron BJ, Mitchell JH. 26th Bethesda Conference: Revised eligibility recommendations for competitive athletes with cardiovascular abnormalities. *J Am Coll Cardiol* 1994;24:848.
28. Maron BJ, Thompson PD, Puffer JC, et al. Cardiovascular preparticipation screening of competitive athletes. *Circulation* 1996;94:850.
29. Hart HH. *Physical feats that made history.* New York: Hart Publishing, 1974:15.
30. Reinhold M. *Essentials of Greek and Roman classics.* Great Neck, NY: Barron's, 1946:136.

The Athlete and Heart Disease:
Diagnosis, Evaluation & Management,
edited by R. A. Williams.
Lippincott Williams & Wilkins, Philadelphia © 1999.

2

Classification of Sports and the Athlete's Heart

K. M. Gallagher, P. B. Raven, and *Jere H. Mitchell

*Department of Integrative Physiology, University of North Texas Health Science Center,
Fort Worth, Texas 76107; *Departments of Internal Medicine and Physiology, University of Texas
Southwestern Medical Center at Dallas, Dallas, Texas 75235*

CLASSIFICATION OF SPORTS

Sports can be classified according to the type and intensity of exercise performed and to the potential for bodily collision (1–4) (Table 1). The intensity of the exercise involved in the performance of sports is usually characterized as low, moderate, and high. Typically, sports are divided between two main types of exercise: dynamic and static. Dynamic exercise involves rhythmic contractions that change muscle length and joint angle and involves a relatively small development of intramuscular force. Static exercise involves a sustained contraction with relatively no change in muscle length and joint angle and a significantly large development of intramuscular force (3,4). Each sport can usually be classified into one of these types of exercise because each sport has a predominant type of activity. However, most sports activities contain aspects of both dynamic and static exercise.

CARDIOVASCULAR RESPONSES TO EXERCISE

Dynamic Exercise

The rhythmic contractions of dynamic exercise provide an immediate challenge to the cardiovascular system in that an adequate blood supply must be delivered to the active muscle while blood flow is maintained to the brain, heart, nonactive muscles, and other organs. The cardiovascular system accomplishes this by increasing cardiac output and redistributing blood flow to the active skeletal muscle via neural regulation of the hemodynamic responses and local regulation of the flow within the active muscle. Local blood flow regulation in the active skeletal muscle results in a decrease in total peripheral vascular resistance (increased vascular conductance). This increased conductance in the vascular bed is due to vasodilation and is proposed to be regulated by metabolic byproducts of the contractile process, such as nitric oxide (endothelium-relaxing factor), adenosine, and increased hydrogen ion (H^+). This local blood flow regulation can result in large increases in blood flow (250 to 400 mL/100 g/minute). Neural regulation of the cardiovascular system regulates hemodynamic responses by increasing heart rate, stroke volume, cardiac output, and oxygen extraction at the tissue level.

Local blood flow regulation in active skeletal muscle and neural regulation of cardiovascular hemodynamics together determine oxygen consumption, which can be expressed as follows:

$$\dot{V}O_2 = \dot{Q} \times \text{a-v } O_2\text{diff}$$

where $\dot{V}O_2$ is oxygen uptake, $\dot{Q}$ is cardiac output, and a-v O_2diff is the arteriovenous oxygen difference or the extraction of oxygen from the blood by the active tissue. Absolute oxygen consumption is usually measured in

TABLE 1. *Classification of sports: based on peak dynamic and static components during competition*

	A. Low dynamic	B. Moderate dynamic	C. High dynamic
I. Low static	Billiards Bowling Cricket Curling Golf Riflery	Baseball Softball Table tennis Tennis (doubles) Volleyball	Badminton Cross-country skiing (classic technique) Field hockey* Orienteering Race walking Racquetball Running (long-distance) Soccer* Squash Tennis (singles)
II. Moderate static	Archery Auto racing*† Diving*† Equestrian*† Motorcycling*†	Fencing Field events (jumping) Figure skating* Football (American) Rodeoing*† Rugby* Running (sprint) Surfing*† Synchronized swimming†	Basketball* Ice hockey* Cross-country skiing (skating technique) Football (Australian rules)* Lacrosse* Running (middle-distance) Swimming Team handball
III. High static	Bobsledding*† Field events (throwing) Gymnastics*† Karate/judo* Luge*† Sailing Rock climbing*† Water skiing*† Weight lifting*† Wind surfing*†	Body building*† Downhill skiing*† Wrestling*	Boxing* Canoeing/kayaking Cycling*† Decathlon Rowing Speed skating

*Danger of bodily collision.
†Increased risk if syncope occurs.
From ref. 4, with permission.

liters per minute (L/min); however, sometimes oxygen consumption is normalized with body weight and is measured in milliliters per minute per kilogram (mL/min/kg). Resting oxygen uptake is generally 0.25 L/min (3.6 mL/minute/kg).

Maximal oxygen consumption ($\dot{V}O_2$ max) is determined by the optimal ability to increase cardiac output, stroke volume, heart rate, and arteriovenous oxygen difference in order to increase oxygen delivery to the tissues of the body. Measures of maximal oxygen consumption ($\dot{V}O_2$ max) range from 2.0 L/min (28 mL/min/kg) for sedentary individuals, 3.0 L/min (43 mL/min/kg) for untrained average fit individuals, and 6.0 L/min (86 mL/min/kg) or more for endurance-trained athletes. Therefore, $\dot{V}O_2$ max is normally used as an index of

fitness level because it can be increased with endurance training. Oxygen consumption increases linearly with progressive increases in the intensity of exercise until $\dot{V}O_2$ max is achieved (Fig. 1).

Cardiac output is approximately 5 L/min at rest, and the cardiac output increases 5 to 6 L/min for every 1-L/min increase in oxygen uptake during dynamic exercise (Fig. 1). The increase in cardiac output is due to increases in heart rate and stroke volume. The product of heart rate and stroke volume equals cardiac output as follows:

$$\dot{Q} = HR \times SV$$

where $\dot{Q}$ is cardiac output, HR is heart rate, and SV is stroke volume. Maximal cardiac outputs ordinarily achieve 20 to 25 L/min in

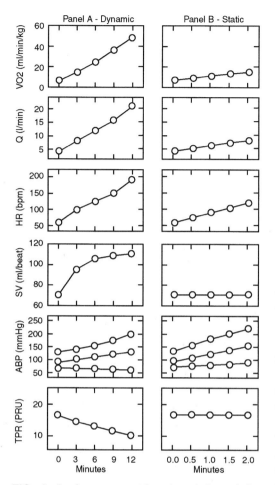

FIG. 1. A: A representative description of the cardiovascular responses to progressively increasing workload to $\dot{V}O_{2\,max}$: Q, cardiac output; SV, stroke volume; HR, heart rate; ABP, systolic (*top line*), mean (*middle line*), and diastolic (*bottom line*) arterial blood pressure; TPR, total peripheral resistance. **B:** A representative description of the cardiovascular responses to a sustained isometric contraction (30% MVC): Q, cardiac output; SV, stroke volume; HR, heart rate; ABP, systolic (*top line*), mean (*middle line*), and diastolic (*bottom line*) arterial blood pressure; TPR, total peripheral resistance. (From Mitchell JH, Raven PB. Cardiovascular response and adaptation to exercise. In: Bouchard C, Sheppard R, Stephens T, eds. *Physical activity, fitness and health: International Consensus Statement* (Chap. 17). Champaign, IL: Human Kinetics Publishers, 1994:286–298. Reprinted by permission.)

normally active boys and men but are capable of reaching 40 L/min in endurance-trained athletes.

Heart rate ranges between 60 and 70 beats/min at rest and increases linearly with oxygen uptake to a maximal heart rate of 190 to 200 beats/min (see Fig. 1). Unlike cardiac output and stroke volume, maximal heart rate tends to be set and cannot be altered with endurance training. It is generally considered that the initial increase in heart rate (up to 100 beats/min) is predominately due to the withdrawal of vagal influences on the control of heart rate. Additional increases, up to 150 beats/min, are due to an increasing sympathetic drive along with a decreasing amount of vagal activation. Heart rate changes of more than 150 beats/min to maximal heart rate are the result of further increases in sympathetic influence on the heart rate.

Stroke volume is approximately 70 to 80 mL/beat at rest in normally active men but can be as high as 130 to 150 mL/beat in endurance-trained athletes. The stroke volume of average fit individuals increases at the onset of exercise and continually increases until values of 120 to 140 mL/beat have been attained at 40% to 50% of maximal oxygen consumption (Fig. 1) (5). In contrast, recent evidence suggests that, in endurance-trained athletes, stroke volume can progressively increase until $\dot{V}O_{2\,max}$ has been attained (6), reaching amounts of 200 to 220 mL/beat.

As the intensity of exercise increases, the difference in the arterial oxygen content and the venous oxygen content increases, resulting in the widening of the arteriovenous oxygen difference. At rest and throughout exercise, arterial hemoglobin saturation remains at 97% and oxygen content remains at 200 mL/L. The body extracts approximately 23% of the oxygen at rest, resulting in a venous oxygen content of approximately 154 mL/L. During dynamic exercise to maximum, there exists an increased extraction of oxygen in the active muscles of approximately 85%. This results in a maximal extraction of approximately 170 mL O_2/L of blood (venous content 30 mL/L).

In general, systolic and diastolic blood pressure are 120 mm Hg and 80 mm Hg, respectively, with a calculated mean arterial pressure of 93 mm Hg. During exercise, systolic pressures increase because of the ejection of blood into the vascular system, resulting in pressures between 200 and 250 mm Hg at maximal workloads. As a result of local vasodilation in the active muscle during exercise, diastolic blood pressure can decrease to 60 mm Hg at maximal workloads. These changes in systolic and diastolic pressures lead to a slight increase in calculated mean arterial pressure to approximately 120 mm Hg (Fig. 1). This slight increase in mean arterial pressure occurs despite large increases (500% to 700%) in cardiac output and sympathetic vasoconstriction in the vasculature outside the active muscle beds and is a result of the reduction in peripheral vascular resistance of the active skeletal muscle.

During dynamic exercise, the increased demand for oxygen in the active muscle is efficiently met by increased vascular conductance in the exercising muscle and redistribution of an increased cardiac output by sympathetically induced vasoconstriction in nonexercising muscle and in the visceral organs. As exercise progresses in intensity, more muscle mass is activated to maintain the desired work. This increase in muscle mass leads to further increases in vascular conductance, which has the potential to increase flow demand in excess of the pumping capacity of the heart (7). However, the maintenance of adequate perfusion pressures is met by increases in active sympathetic vasoconstriction reducing blood flow to the working muscle (8).

Static Exercise

Static exercise is usually measured as a percent of maximal voluntary contraction (% MVC). During static or isometric exercise, muscles do not shorten to achieve the desired work. In contrast to dynamic exercise in which intramuscular pressures are only intermittently increased, large increases in intramuscular pressure do occur during static exercise. The large increases in intramuscular

pressure obtained with a static contraction are transferred to the muscle vasculature and tend to reduce blood flow by decreasing conductance. The decreases in blood flow are inversely proportional to increases in % MVC. Another difference between static and dynamic exercise is that the pumping action of the rhythmic contractions of the muscles during dynamic exercise increases blood flow, whereas the sustained contractions of static exercise fail to allow for an increase in blood flow in the muscle. The cardiovascular response to static exercise is an attempt to maintain adequate perfusion of the exercising muscle via large increases in sympathetic tone, resulting in systemic vasoconstriction and heart rate–induced increases in cardiac output. This response results in marked increases in blood pressure. The large increases in mean arterial pressure are surprisingly a result of the increased cardiac output, in that, despite sympathetic-induced vasoconstriction, systemic vascular resistance changes little during the contraction because of the local vasodilation in the active muscle (9) (Fig. 1). In addition, the increases in cardiac output are primarily the result of increases in heart rate because stroke volume varies little during static exercise. The increases in cardiac output do not enhance blood flow to the active muscle; rather, the majority of the increased cardiac output is redirected to the skin (hence, a person's face turns red when performing heavy resistance exercise) and nonactive muscle. The amount of muscle mass used and the intensity of the exercise both correlate directly with the cardiovascular response (10). The amount of force required to interfere with blood flow varies with each muscle group; however, once force exceeds 15% MVC, the cardiovascular response is activated to maintain adequate perfusion pressures (11,12).

CARDIOVASCULAR ADAPTATIONS TO EXERCISE TRAINING

Dynamic Training

Dynamic endurance exercise training results in several cardiovascular adaptations that are beneficial both at rest and during exercise. Maximal oxygen consumption or $\dot{V}O_{2\ max}$ is regularly used as an index of physical fitness. Mean $\dot{V}O_{2\ max}$ in normally active young male individuals approximates 45 mL/min/kg, whereas dynamic exercise training results in average $\dot{V}O_{2\ max}$ values of 55 to 60 mL/min/kg. However, $\dot{V}O_{2\ max}$ values of 80 mL/min/kg or more have been recorded in world class endurance-trained athletes (13). Oxygen uptake ($\dot{V}O_2$) and other cardiovascular adaptations to dynamic endurance exercise training are dependent on the intensity and the duration of training. In addition, sequence variations in mitochondrial DNA have been attributed to individual differences in $\dot{V}O_{2\ max}$ and the response of training, thus lending evidence that one's genetic propensity has an influence on training responses (14).

Resting and submaximal exercise cardiac outputs are not changed by exercise training; however, maximal cardiac output can be twice as much in elite athletes than in untrained individuals (Fig. 2). The changes in maximal cardiac output are primarily due to changes in

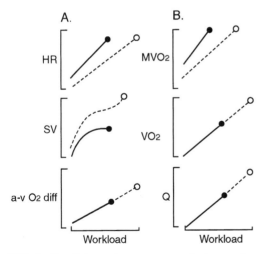

FIG. 2. Cardiovascular responses to increasing workloads to a maximum. Filled dot, untrained subject; open dot, endurance trained subject; solid line, submaximal responses in untrained subject; dashed line, submaximal responses in trained subject; Q, cardiac output; HR, heart rate; SV, stroke volume; a-v O_2, total body oxygen consumption; MVO₂, myocardial oxygen consumption. (From ref. 18, with permission.)

stroke volume because maximal heart rate is unaffected by training. Dynamic exercise training leads to a decrease in resting heart rate and a reduction in heart rate at any given submaximal workload or $\dot{V}O_2$ (Fig. 2). These reductions in heart rate are due to an increase in parasympathetic influence on the heart. It has also been proposed that there is an attenuation in the reflex heart rate response to myocardial stretch with exercise training (15). In summary, it appears that there are central nervous system, reflex, and peripheral adaptations to exercise training that influence the heart rate response to exercise (16). However, the change in stroke volume in response to exercise associated with exercise training is the main adaptation providing the impetus for increases in maximal cardiac output. In sedentary individuals, stroke volume plateaus at 40% of $\dot{V}O_{2\ max}$ (5), whereas endurance-trained athletes are capable of continuously increasing their stroke volume to maximum (Fig. 2) (6). In general, stroke volumes are increased at rest and at any given workload with exercise training. The increased stroke volumes associated with training are primarily the result of training-induced increases in blood volume or plasma volume. The changes in blood volume and plasma volume are related to increases in albumin concentrations, renin activity, and vasopressin secretion (17). Stroke volume adaptations also occur as a result of increases in cardiac dimensions occurring with endurance exercise training. Therefore, at any given $\dot{V}O_2$, endurance training results in a lower heart rate and an increase in stroke volume. Thus, there is an increased efficiency of the heart, resulting in a decreased double product (heart rate × systolic arterial pressure) at submaximal workloads. The double product is directly correlated with myocardial oxygen consumption and indicates that endurance training results in a reduced oxygen consumption of the heart at any given total body oxygen consumption (Fig. 2) (18).

Dynamic endurance training is accompanied by an increase in a-v O_2diff resulting from an increased oxidative capacity and vascular conductance (16). Training causes an increase in myoglobin (the oxygen-carrying protein complex in skeletal muscle) and hemoglobin (the oxygen-carrying protein complex in the circulation), which increases the oxygen-carrying capacity of the circulation and its oxygen delivery to the mitochondria (19,20). The increased oxygen delivery to the active muscle augments the diffusion capacity of oxygen in the muscle, allowing for an increased a-v O_2diff. In addition, the diffusion capacity is enhanced as a result of an elevated mitochondrial volume in the skeletal muscle, which further augments the oxygen extraction (21). Endurance training increases vascular conductance by increasing total systemic arterial compliance, which decreases total peripheral resistance (21,22). The mechanism for the increased vascular conductance is unknown but is postulated to be a result of an increased vascularity that occurs with exercise. It has been determined that dynamic exercise training results in an increase in capillary density and total number of capillaries in both skeletal and cardiac muscle (23,24). The increased vascular conductance decreases the total peripheral resistance, allowing for the increased cardiac output. Furthermore, the increased conductance increases the capillary diffusion surface area, which enhances capillary exchange between the vasculature and the tissue.

It is apparent that the ability to increase blood flow to active muscle tissue is not at its maximum during $\dot{V}O_{2\,max}$. There appears to be some level of tonic vasoconstriction of the vasculature that actually is augmented by increases in the amount of active muscle mass (8). It has been proposed that, if most of the skeletal muscle in the body were active, a cardiac output of 60 L/min would be required to maintain arterial blood pressure (7). These findings suggest that the pumping capacity of the heart is the primary limitation of $\dot{V}O_{2\,max}$ in the untrained and trained individuals. However, it has been demonstrated that there is significant arterial desaturation at maximal workloads in endurance-trained individuals, suggesting that the lungs also play a role in the limitations of $\dot{V}O_{2\,max}$ in endurance-trained individuals (25).

Static Training

Cardiovascular adaptations can occur with repetitive isometric (static) contraction training, commonly thought of as weight lifting. Isometric training results in an increase in lean body mass primarily by muscle fiber hypertrophy (26,27) and hyperplasia (5% to 15%) via stem cell activation (28). Because isometric training predominately involves anaerobic metabolism, there is little or no change in maximal oxygen consumption (29) and any increases that do occur in maximal oxygen consumption are probably due to the dynamic component of the training program. It has also been suggested that isometric training may result in reductions in resting heart rate and systolic blood pressure; however, this also could be due to the dynamic components involved in isometric training. Isometric training has also resulted in attenuated heart rate and pressor responses to absolute force of contraction resulting from the increase in MVC. However, when heart rate and pressor responses are compared to the same relative force (same % MVC), there is little change with isometric training. Most cardiovascular responses to isometric exercise remain unchanged with training.

Adaptations of the Heart to Exercise Training

Dynamic and static exercise present different types of stress on the heart of the individual. Dynamic exercise training increases stroke volume and cardiac output in the individual for extended periods of time. This type of training resembles the volume-overloaded stress of such pathologic states as aortic or mitral regurgitation. Static training, on the other hand, attempts to increase cardiac output against an increased afterload (arterial blood pressure). Arterial blood pressures have been recorded as high as 480/350 (systolic/diastolic) during static exercise of body builders (30). This type of training resembles the pressure-overloaded stress of such states as systemic hypertension and aortic stenosis. The heart attempts to overcome the stresses of dynamic or static training and maintain the wall tension within the four chambers of the heart. The Law of Laplace is represented by the equation:

$$T_{wall} = (P \times r) \div 2$$

where T_{wall} is wall tension, P is systolic pressure, and r is the internal radius of the heart chamber (i.e., the ventricle). Therefore, as the pressure is increased during exercise training, anatomic changes occur within the heart to maintain the normal wall tension per cross-sectional area. However, the anatomic changes that occur differ between the two types of training because of the different types of stresses that are introduced to the heart (volume versus pressure overload).

Both dynamic endurance training and static training result in a larger absolute left ventricular mass (21,31). This enlargement of the heart has been termed either *physiologic hypertrophy* or *athletes' heart*. This physiologic hypertrophy differs between the two types of exercise: dynamic or static. Dynamic exercise training results in a general eccentric hypertrophy, and static exercise training results primarily in concentric hypertrophy (31–33) (Fig. 3). The eccentric hypertrophy that occurs with dynamic exercise training is a result of increased volume returning to the heart (volume overload) because of the rhythmic

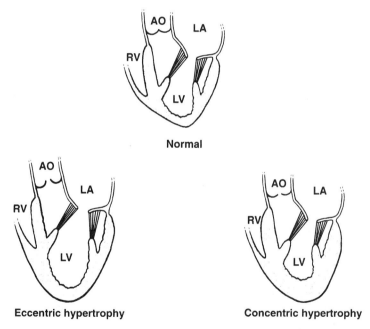

Normal

Eccentric hypertrophy   **Concentric hypertrophy**

FIG. 3. A representative picture of the heart in a normally active person and the cardiovascular adaptations that occur with either dynamic exercise training (eccentric hypertrophy) or with static exercise training (concentric hypertrophy). Dynamic exercise training results primarily in an increase in the end-diastolic dimensions in the ventricle, which is the result of the volume overloading associated with the rhythmic contractions (muscle pump) that occur during dynamic exercise. In addition, it has been determined that dynamic exercise training (eccentric hypertrophy) does result in a slight outward increase in wall thickness that is not represented in this figure. Static exercise training results primarily in an inward increase in wall thickness with little change in end-diastolic dimensions of the ventricle. The cardiac adaptation to static exercise, known as *concentric hypertrophy,* is due to the large increases in blood pressure that the heart must overcome (pressure overload) that occur with static exercise. AO, aorta; RV, right ventricle; LV, left ventricle; LA, left atrium.

contractions of the muscle pump, resulting primarily in an increase in the internal diameter of the ventricles along with a slight thickening of the walls of the ventricle. Static exercise training does not involve the rhythmic contractions that occur with dynamic exercise, thus there is no volume overloading. However, static exercise training results in higher generated blood pressures that the heart must contract against (pressure overload). This pressure overload results in little change in the internal diameter of the ventricle with thickening of the ventricular wall known as concentric hypertrophy (Fig. 3). Generally, most types of exercise or exercise training programs consist of both dynamic and static exercise; thus, the physiologic hypertrophy that occurs usually is a combination of different degrees of both concentric and eccentric hypertrophy. Furthermore, the amount of physiologic hypertrophy that occurs is related to the intensity and duration of the exercise or exercise training program and is directly related to the fitness level or $\dot{V}O_{2\ max}$ (21,31). Sometimes, the physiologic hypertrophy that occurs at the extremely high degrees of fitness resembles pathologic hypertrophy and can be incorrectly interpreted as pathologic. The introduction of M-mode echocardiography and magnetic resonance imaging has allowed for more accurate determinations of the dimensions and mass of the heart. These measurement techniques are reproducible within 1 to 2 mm and are the mainstay of determining anatomic changes that occur with exercise training.

Left ventricular mass is increased in endurance exercise–trained athletes. Even when normalized for lean body mass, body weight, and body surface area, the endurance-trained athletes still have significantly larger ratios than their matched nonathletic control groups (31). The range of increase in left ventricular mass in endurance-trained male athletes is between 23% and 80%, with an average of 45% to 50% (34,35). When left ventricular mass was normalized for body surface area, the increases ranged from 65 to 70 g/m^2 in normal sedentary men to 125 g/m^2 for the endurance-

exercise trained men. The greatest increases in left ventricular mass occur in competitive cyclists. Rodriquez et al. (36) demonstrated left ventricular mass indexes greater than 130 g/m^2 in 23 of 40 European competitive cyclists. This was attributed to the fact that total heart size has been strongly correlated with $\dot{V}O_{2\ max}$, maximal cardiac output, and maximal stroke volume (21,31). Furthermore, the cardiac hypertrophy occurred throughout the heart in these cyclists. Left atrial and right ventricular dimensions are consistently increased in both subjects and animals with left ventricular hypertrophy (21,37).

The increase in mass of the heart that occurs with dynamic endurance training is due to a combination of slightly increased wall thickness (septum and posterior wall) and increased dimensions within the heart cavities. End-diastolic dimensions in the left ventricle of endurance-trained athletes increase an average of 5.7 cm, even when normalized for body surface area or lean body mass. These changes remain within the clinically normal range (38). However, the greatest increases have been documented in cyclists, with measurements up to 7 cm (39). This suggests that the higher trained the athlete in dynamic exercise, the greater the increase in end-diastolic dimensions. In support of this postulate is echocardiographic evidence reporting an average increase in left ventricular end-diastolic dimensions of approximately 10%; however, because of the cube relationship of dimension to volume, this represents a total end-diastolic volume increase of 33% (38). Similar changes that occur in the left ventricle have been noted in the end-diastolic dimensions of the right ventricle (40) and left atrium; however, any increases in the transverse dimension of either the right ventricle or left atrium were within the clinically normal range (38). The end-systolic left ventricular cavity size was normal or slightly elevated in the endurance-trained athlete, but the differences were mild and were not always statistically significant from the sedentary individual (38). Because dynamically trained athletes exhibit increases in both left ventricular mass and end-diastolic volume, there was no significant increase in the left ventricular mass to volume ratio of endurance athletes when compared to normal sedentary individuals (33).

In endurance-trained athletes, volume overloading induces increases in end-diastolic dimensions. In order for the heart to maintain normal wall tension despite the increase in end-diastolic dimension (according to the Law of Laplace), there must be a compensatory increase in wall thickness. The increases in wall thickness occur primarily in the intraventricular septum and the posterior wall. The intraventricular septum on average increases from normal up to approximately 1.04 cm whereas the posterior wall on average increases up to approximately 1.06 cm (38). Thus, there occurs a 14% to 17% increase in the intraventricular septum and a 19% to 20% increase in the posterior wall of the ventricle in endurance-trained athletes (35,38). There have been greater increases noted, usually with the largest occurring in rowers and cyclists. Rodriquez et al. (36) in 1995 noted that 21 of 40 professional road cyclists in Europe exhibited posterior wall thicknesses of 1.3 cm or greater with a maximum of 1.9 cm. Echocardiographic studies have demonstrated that as many as 60% of endurance-trained athletes exhibit posterior wall thickness that exceeds the upper limit of the supposed normal value of 1.1 cm. The posterior wall thickness rarely exceeds 1.3 cm in endurance-trained athletes and does not begin to be considered pathologic until it reaches or exceeds 1.4 cm. Thus, the normal values for posterior diastolic wall thickness have been revised upward (41). Maron (42) noted intraventricular septum thicknesses of 1.3 to 1.5 cm in five rowers and one canoeist from Rome, Italy, who participated in the 1988 Seoul Olympic games. The normal ratio of intraventricular septal thickness to posterior wall thickness is less than 1.2. However, values for this ratio in endurance-trained athletes have been reported as high as 2.0 (41). Therefore, it is considered that only the intraventricular septum can increase to levels exceeding clinically normal limits when body mass

is taken into consideration (42). In endurance-trained athletes, there is an overall increase in cardiac mass, primarily resulting from increases in both the end-diastolic dimensions and wall thickness. However, the mass to volume ratio is not affected by endurance training despite the increase in wall thickness, which suggests endurance training results in primarily eccentric hypertrophy. The benefit of these anatomic changes in endurance-trained athletes is their ability to increase stroke volume during dynamic exercise, which allows for a greater maximal cardiac output and $\dot{V}O_{2\,max}$ while maintaining a constant wall tension.

The isometric or statically trained athlete demonstrates a concentric cardiac hypertrophy of the left ventricle (33). Isometric athletes exhibit thickened (unproportional) intraventricular septum and posterior walls without the left ventricular end-diastolic cavity enlargement (43). These changes in cardiac dimensions are due to the brief increases in cardiac output against a very high systemic vascular resistance, which somewhat resembles the pathologic condition of systemic hypertension. The isometric athlete exhibits increases in left ventricular mass when normalized for body weight compared to sedentary controls. However, when left ventricular mass was normalized for lean body mass, there was no significant difference between isometric athletes and sedentary controls (33). The increase in left ventricular mass or cardiac mass of isometric athletes was much less than that found in the endurance-trained athletes. Longhurst et al. (33) in 1980 determined that left ventricular hypertrophy, when normalized for body surface area, was approximately 90 g/m^2 in isometric athletes and approximately 105 g/m^2 in endurance-trained athletes. These comparisons were made in gender-, age-, and body configuration–matched control subjects, demonstrating a left ventricular hypertrophy/body surface area of approximately 65 to 70 g/m^2. Pellicia et al. (44) in 1993 compared 100 athletes who predominantly participated in strength-related sports (e.g., power lifting, weight lifting, wrestling) and compared them to normal sedentary controls. Their results indicated that the left ventricular mass index (left ventricular mass/body surface area) of the controls was 81 ± 8 g/m^2 while the left ventricular mass index of the isometric athletes was significantly higher at an average of 96 ± 12 g/m^2, with a range of 66 to 137 g/m^2. This increase was still less than what was normally documented in the endurance-trained athlete. It is suggested that weight lifters exhibit a range of increase in ventricular mass when normalized for weight or body surface area approximating 30% to 70% (45).

Unlike endurance-trained athletes, static-trained athletes fail to show any significant increases in left ventricular end-diastolic dimensions with (39) or without (44) normalization for body surface area. This results in an increase in left ventricular mass to left ventricular end-diastolic volume ratio in isometric athletes, which is not demonstrated in endurance-trained athletes. Both endurance-trained and static-trained athletes exhibit increases in intraventricular and posterior wall thickness in the left ventricle. Pellicia et al. (44) found the intraventricular septum and the posterior wall of the left ventricle to be significantly higher in isometric athletes (0.96 ± 0.08 cm and 0.88 ± 0.07 cm, respectively) than normal sedentary controls (0.9 ± 0.05 cm and 0.81 ± 0.04 cm, respectively). However, the average wall thicknesses in isometric athletes have been reported as high as 1.6 cm in shot putters and 1.7 cm in judo wrestlers. Therefore, the isometric athlete typically demonstrates an increase in wall thickness without an increase in left ventricular end-diastolic dimension, defined as concentric hypertrophy. Pellicia et al. (44) found that the isometric athlete has a significantly higher left ventricular wall thickness to left ventricular end-diastolic cavity dimension than the control subjects, which reinforces the concept of concentric hypertrophy.

There is an ever-increasing population of weight-trained individuals who use anabolic steroids to increase their muscle mass. In 1997, Dickerman et al. (46) determined that the use of anabolic steroids further increases the concentric hypertrophy that occurs in the isometrically trained athlete. The recruited subjects were nationally ranked heavyweight body builders who had a history of anabolic steroid use for 6 to 15 years. They were compared to nationally ranked body builders who were matched for size, strength, and length of exposure to resistance training and who did not use anabolic steroids. They found that there was no significant difference in the left ventricular end-diastolic dimensions between the two groups; however, the anabolic steroid users had significantly greater left ventricular posterior wall thickness (1.21 ± 0.1 cm) than the control group (1.03 ± 0.2 cm) and significantly greater ventricular septum thickness (1.12 ± 0.02 cm) than the control group (0.874 ± 0.25 cm). Therefore, the use of anabolic steroids appeared to further enhance the concentric hypertrophy in the isometric athlete.

It appears that there is an increase in left ventricular mass in athletes, with or without increases in volume, and that the absolute and relative magnitude of these changes is dependent on the type of exercise (45). These anatomic changes that occur in the myocardium appear to be load-induced. More specifically, the load-induced direct physiologic effects lead to cellular stress and strain, which in turn regulate gene expression and growth. When the amount of venous return (preload) is increased with dynamic exercise, the increase in diastolic stress results in the growth of fibers in series to increase diastolic volume and reduce the wall stress to normal. However, when the afterload (blood pressure) is increased with static exercise, the increase in systolic stress results in growth of fibers in parallel in order to reduce the systolic load per fiber until the stress is normalized (45).

Diastolic or systolic function appear to be unaffected by either dynamic or static exercise training. Estimates of diastolic and systolic function are difficult to analyze because training affects extracardiac performance variables, more specifically the autonomic state, preload, and afterload that alter cardiac function. These factors, therefore, must be taken into consideration when changes in cardiac function are analyzed. M-mode echocardiography has found normal peak rates of chamber enlargement and peak rates of wall thinning in endurance-trained and isometrically trained athletes even when normalized (45). In addition, peak early diastolic filling (E) and peak late diastolic filling (A) as well as their ratios (E/A) have been found to be normal in athletes regardless of training mode (45). Some groups have found increases in the ratio (E/A) and decreases in A (47), but this is probably due to an increase in chamber size and a decreased heart rate associated with the training bradycardia, which prolongs the diastolic filling time and reduces atrial filling. Regardless, diastolic function appears to be normal at rest for both dynamic and static exercise-trained individuals. It has been determined that endurance-trained individuals exhibit a greater ventricular diastolic chamber compliance and distensibility than nonathletes (48). This increased compliance results in an enlarged diastolic reserve, which leads to increased stroke volumes and cardiac outputs in response to elevated filling pressures during exercise (48). This raises the question of whether endurance training actually results in an enhanced diastolic function during dynamic exercise.

Contractility (systolic function) is extremely difficult to measure in humans, but it appears to be normal in both static and dynamically trained athletes. However, Rowell suggests that the increase in stroke volume in endurance-trained athletes is due to increases both in left ventricular end-diastolic dimensions and in contractility (12). There are reports of similar fractional shortening of the left ventricular internal dimension or ejection fraction and similar peak posterior wall velocity or peak velocity of the internal diameter change in both endurance-trained and isometric-trained athletes (35). Any increases or decreases in these indexes of systolic function were within normal limits. Therefore, cardiac function appears to be unaltered by the anatomic changes that occur with exercise training.

The increase in left ventricular mass and in left ventricular wall thickness could potentially endanger the myocardium of becoming stripped of its own blood supply and resulting in ischemia. However, experimental evidence indicates that there is an increase in the size of the coronary vascular bed with exercise training (23,38,49). Schaible and Scheuer have concluded that increases in coronary flow are proportional to the degree of training-induced increase in heart weight (50).

CONCLUSION

It is apparent that a long history of participation in various sports classified according to the dynamic or static exercise component (Table 1) along with the training for the various sports will result in significantly different normal variants in cardiac structure and function. Participation in the highly dynamic sports such as long distance running, road race bicycling, cross country skiing, and swimming results in eccentric hypertrophy and heart volumes of greater than 600 mL without pathologic condition. In addition, resting bradycardia of less than 40 beats/minute in sinus rhythm is not unusual. Because of the increased cardiac compliance, the dynamic exercise–trained athlete may be prone to orthostatic hypotension despite normal fluid and electrolyte balance.

In contrast to dynamic exercise sport participants, the heart of static exercise athletes such as wrestlers, weight lifters, body builders, and gymnasts, which is concentrically hypertrophied and dependent on whether steroids are used as part of the training regimen, may border on hypertrophic cardiomyopathy. Anatomic restriction of the aortic outflow tract has also been reported in some cases. Heart rate and rhythm are normal.

REFERENCES

1. Shaffer TE. The health examination for participation in sports. *Pediatr Ann* 1978;7:27–40.
2. Strong WB, Alpert BS. The child with heart disease: play, recreation and sports. *Curr Probl Cardiol* 1981;6: 1–38.

3. Mitchell JH, Blomqvist CG, Haskell WL, et al. Classification of sports. 16th Bethesda Conference. Cardiovascular abnormalities in the athlete: recommendations regarding eligibility for competition. *J Am Coll Cardiol* 1985;6:1198–1199.

4. Mitchell JH, Haskell WL, Raven PB. Classification of sports. *Med Sci Sports Exerc* 1994;26:S242–S245.

5. Astrand P-O, Rodahl K. *Textbook of work physiology. Physiological basis of exercise.* New York: McGraw-Hill, 1986:756.

6. Gledhill N, Cox D, Jamnik R. Endurance athletes' stroke volume does not plateau: major advantage is diastolic function. *Med Sci Sports Exerc* 1994;26:1116–1121.

7. Saltin B. Physiological adaptation to physical conditioning: old problems revisited. *Acta Med Scand* 1986;(Suppl)711:11–24.

8. Secher NH, Clausen JP, Klausen K, Noer I, Trap-Jensen J. Central and regional circulation effects of adding arm exercise to leg exercise. *Acta Physiol Scand* 1977;100:288–297.

9. Friedman DB, Peel C, Mitchell JH. Cardiovascular responses to voluntary and nonvoluntary static exercise in humans. *J Appl Physiol* 1992;73:1982–1985.

10. Mitchell JH, Schibye B, Payne FC III, Saltin B. Response of arterial blood pressure to static exercise in relation to muscle force, force development, and electromyographic activity. *Circ Res* 1981;48:I70–I75.

11. Hansen J, Jacobsen TN, Amtrop O. The exercise pressor response to sustained handgrip does not augment blood flow in the contracting forearm skeletal muscle. *Acta Physiol Scand* 1993;149:419–425.

12. Rowell LB. *Human cardiovascular control.* New York: Oxford University Press, 1993.

13. Mitchell JH, Blomqvist G. Maximal oxygen uptake. *N Engl J Med* 1971;284:1018–1022.

14. Dionne FT, Turcotte L, Thibault MC, et al. Mitochondrial DNA sequence polymorphism $\dot{V}O_{2\ max}$, and response to endurance training. *Med Sci Sports Exerc* 1991;23:177–185.

15. Walgenbach SC, Donald DE. Inhibition by carotid baroreflex of exercise-induced increases in atrial pressure. *Circ Res* 1983;52:253.

16. Crawford MH. Physiological consequences of systematic training. *Cardiol Clin* 1992;10:209–218.

17. Convertino VA, Brock PJ, Keil LC, Bernauer EM, Greenleaf JE. Exercise training-induced hypervolemia: role of plasma albumin, renin, and vasopressin. *J Appl Physiol* 1980;48:665–669.

18. Smith ML, Mitchell JH. Cardiorespiratory adaptations to training. In: American College of Sports Medicine, ed. *Resource manual for guidelines for exercise testing and prescription.* Philadelphia: Lea & Febiger, 1988:62–65.

19. Holloszy JO. Adaptation of skeletal muscle to endurance exercise. *Med Sci Sports Exerc* 1975;7:155.

20. Meldon JH. Theoretical role of myoglobin in steady-state oxygen transport to tissue and its impact upon cardiac output requirements. *Acta Physiol Scand* 1976;440:S93.

21. Blomqvist CG, Saltin B. Cardiovascular adaptations to physical training. *Ann Rev Physiol* 1983;45:169–189.

22. Cameron JD, Dart AM. Exercise training increases total systemic arterial compliance in humans. *Am J Physiol* 1994;266:H693–H701.

23. Hudlicka O. Growth of capillaries in skeletal and cardiac muscle. *Circ Res* 1982;50:451.

24. Ingjer J, Brodal P. Capillary supply of skeletal muscle fibers in untrained and endurance trained women. *Eur J Appl Physiol* 1978;38:291.

25. Dempsey JA. Is the lung built for exercise? *Med Sci Sports Exerc* 1986;18:143–155.

26. Gollnick PD, Tunson BF, Moore RL, Reidy M. Muscular enlargement and number of fibers in skeletal muscles in rats. *J Appl Physiol* 1981;50:936–943.

27. Borer KT, Edington DW, White TP, eds. *Frontiers of exercise biology.* Champaign, IL: Human Kinetics Publishers, 1983:27–50.

28. Mikesky AE, Giddings CJ, Matthews W, Gonyea WJ. Changes in muscle fiber size and composition in response to heavy-resistance exercise. *Med Sci Sports Exerc* 1991;23:1042–1049.

29. Saltin B, Astrand PO. Maximal oxygen uptake in athletes. *J Appl Physiol* 1967;23:353–358.

30. McDougall JD, Tuxen D, Sale DG, Moroz JR, Sutton JR. Arterial pressure response to heavy resistance exercise. *J Appl Physiol* 1985;58:785–789.

31. Milliken MC, Stray-Gunderson J, Peschock RM, et al. Left ventricular mass as determined by magnetic resonance imaging in male endurance athletes. *Am J Cardiol* 1988;62:301–305.

32. Riley-Hagan MR, Peschock M, Stray-Gunderson J, et al. Left ventricular dimensions and mass using magnetic resonance imaging in female endurance athletes. *Am J Cardiol* 1992;69:1067–1074.

33. Longhurst JC, Kelly AR, Gonyea WJ, Mitchell JH. Echocardiographic left ventricular masses in distance runners and weight lifters. *J Appl Physiol: Respirat, Environ Exercise Physiol* 1980;48:154–162.

34. Shapiro LM. Morphological consequences of systemic training. *Cardiol Clin* 1992;10:219–226.

35. Fagard RH. Impact of different sports and training on cardiac structure and function. *Cardiol Clin* 1992;10:241–256.

36. Rodriquez RJJ, Iglesias CG, Lopez J, et al. Prevalence and upper limit of cardiac hypertrophy in professional cyclists. *Eur J Appl Physiol Occup* 1995;70:375–378.

37. Muntz KW, Gonyea WJ, Mitchell JH. Cardiac hypertrophy in response to an isometric training program in cats. *Circ Res* 1981;49:1092–1101.

38. Maron BJ. Structural features of the athletic heart as defined by echocardiography. *J Am Coll Cardiol* 1986;7:190–203.

39. Rost R. The athletes heart. *Eur Heart J* 1982;3:193–198.

40. Bryan G, Ward A, Rippe JM. Athletic heart syndrome. *Clin Sports Med* 1992;11:259–272.

41. Shepard RJ. The athlete's heart: is big beautiful? *Br J Sports Med* 1996;30:5–10.

42. Maron BJ, Pelliccia A, Spataro A, Granata M. Reduction in left ventricular wall thickness after deconditioning in highly trained Olympic athletes. *Br Heart J* 1993;69:125–128.

43. Morganroth J, Maron BJ, Henry WL, Epstein SE. Comparative left ventricular dimensions in trained athletes. *Am Intern Med* 1975;82:521–529.

44. Pellicia A, Spataro A, Caselli G, Maron BJ. Absence of left ventricular wall thickening in athletes engaged in intense power training. *Am J Cardiol* 1993;72:1048–1054.

45. Colan SD. Mechanics of left ventricular systolic and di-

astolic function in physiological hypertrophy of the athlete heart. *Cardiol Clin* 1992;10:227–240.

46. Dickerman RD, Schaller F, Zachariah NY, McConathy WJ. Left ventricular size and function in elite bodybuilders using anabolic steroids. *Clin J Sport Med* 1997; 7:90–93.

47. Harrison MR, Clifton GD, Pennell AT, et al. Effect of heart rate on left ventricular diastolic transmitral flow velocity patterns assessed by Doppler echocardiography in normal subjects. *Am J Cardiol* 1991;67:622.

48. Levine BD, Lane LD, Buckey JC, Friedman DB, Blomqvist CG. Left ventricular pressure-volume and Frank-Starling relations in endurance athletes. *Circulation* 1991;84:1016–1023.

49. Wyatt HL, Mitchell JH. Influences of physical conditioning and deconditioning on coronary vasculature of dogs. *J Appl Physiol* 1978;45:619–625.

50. Schaible TF, Scheuer J. Cardiac function in hypertrophied hearts from chronically exercised female rats. *J Appl Physiol* 1981;50:1140–1145.

The Athlete and Heart Disease:
Diagnosis, Evaluation & Management,
edited by R. A. Williams.
Lippincott Williams & Wilkins, Philadelphia © 1999.

3

Sudden Cardiac Death due to Hypertrophic Cardiomyopathy in Young Athletes

Barry J. Maron

Cardiovascular Research Division, Minneapolis Heart Institute Foundation,
Minneapolis, Minnesota 55407

Over the past several years interest has heightened considerably in the medical community and with the lay public regarding the causes of sudden and unexpected deaths in young trained athletes (1). As a consequence, the underlying cardiovascular diseases responsible for these uncommon but devastating sudden events in trained athletes and others participating in sporting activities have been the subject of several reports and a large measure of clarification has resulted (2–10). Recognition that athletic field deaths may be due to a variety of detectable (but usually unsuspected) cardiovascular lesions has also stimulated intense interest in preparticipation screening (11), as well as in issues related to the criteria for eligibility and disqualification from competitive sports (12).

SUDDEN DEATH IN ATHLETES

Prevalence and Impact

The frequency of sudden unexpected death as a result of cardiovascular disease in young athletes participating in competitive sports appears to be low, in the range of 1:200,000 for high school competitors (13); lower estimates of the risk for sudden death have been calculated in marathon runners (i.e., 1:50,000) (13,14). Such estimates could suggest that the intense and persistent public interest in these tragic events is perhaps disproportionate to their overall significance in the population. However, the emotional and social impact of athletic field catastrophes remains high. To most of the lay public and physician community (and the news media), the competitive athlete symbolizes the healthiest segment of society, and the unexpected collapse of such a young person is a powerful event that inevitably strikes to the core of a person's sensibilities (1). For these reasons, and despite its low event rate, sudden death in young athletes will probably continue to represent an important medical issue. Indeed, it is an important responsibility of the medical community to create a fully informed public and, when prudent and practical, to pursue early detection of the causes of catastrophic events in young athletes, as well as to undertake preventive measures. On the other hand, because such events are uncommon relative to the vast numbers of athletes participating safely in sports, it is also an important concern that information about athletic field deaths not raise undue anxiety among youthful athletes and their families and, as a consequence, inhibit sports participation.

Causes

Several autopsy-based studies have documented the diseases responsible for sudden death in young competitive athletes or youthful asymptomatic individuals with active lifestyles (2–10). These structural abnormali-

TABLE 1. *Cardiovascular abnormalities in 134 competitive athletes with sudden death*

Primary cardiovascular lesions	No. (%) of athletes	Median age (range), years
Hypertrophic cardiomyopathy	48 (36.0)	17.0 (13–28)
Unexplained increase in cardiac mass ("possible hypertrophic cardiomyopathy")	14 (10.0)	17.0 (14–24)
Aberrant coronary arteries	17* (13.0)	15.0 (12–23)
Other coronary anomalies	8 (6.0)	17.5 (14–40)
Ruptured aortic aneurysm	6 (5.0)	17.0 (16–31)
Tunneled left anterior descending coronary artery	6 (5.0)	17.5 (14–20)
Aortic valve stenosis	6 (5.0)	14.0 (14–17)
Consistent with myocarditis	4 (3.0)	15.5 (13–16)
Idiopathic myocardial scarring	4 (3.0)	20.0 (14–27)
Idiopathic dilated cardiomyopathy	4 (3.0)	18.0 (18–21)
Arrhythmogenic right ventricular dysplasia	4 (3.0)	16.0 (15–17)
Mitral valve prolapse	3 (2.0)	16.0 (15–23)
Atherosclerotic coronary artery disease	3 (2.0)	19.0 (14–28)
Other congenital heart diseases	2 (1.5)	13.5 (12–15)
Long QT syndrome	1 (0.5)	...
Sarcoidosis	1 (0.5)	...
Sickle cell trait†	1 (0.5)	...
"Normal" heart‡	3 (2.0)	18.0 (16–21)

*Anomalous origin of left main coronary artery from right sinus of Valsalva in 13, anomalous origin of right coronary artery from left sinus of Valsalva in 2, anomalous origin of the left main (from between the left and posterior cusps) with acute-angled takeoff in 1, and origin of left anterior descending coronary from pulmonary trunk in 1.

†Judged to be the probable cause of death in the absence of any identifiable structural cardiovascular abnormality.

‡Absence of structural heart disease on standard autopsy examination.

ties are independent of the normal physiologic adaptations in cardiac dimensions evident in many trained athletes, and usually consist of increased left ventricular end-diastolic cavity dimension or, occasionally, wall thickness (15–18).

It is also important to be cautious in assigning strict prevalence figures for the occurrence of various cardiovascular diseases in studies of sudden death in athletes; patient selection biases and other issues unavoidably influence the acquisition of such data in the absence of an established systematic national registry. Indeed, studies differ with regard to the methods used to document cardiovascular diagnosis, and their data are derived from a variety of databases.

Even with these limitations, it has been possible to demonstrate convincingly that the vast majority of sudden deaths in young athletes (younger than age 35 years) are due to a variety of more than 20 primarily congenital cardiovascular diseases (Table 1; Fig. 1) (2). Indeed, virtually any disease capable of causing sudden death in young people may potentially do so in young competitive athletes (2). Also, the lesions responsible for sudden death do not occur with the same frequency, with many being responsible for only 5% or less of all deaths (2). Even though these diseases may be relatively common in young athletes dying suddenly, each is rather uncommon within the general population.

HYPERTROPHIC CARDIOMYOPATHY

Role in Sudden Death

The single most common cardiovascular abnormality among the causes of sudden death in young athletes is hypertrophic cardiomyopathy (HCM) (2,3,5–7,10,19–23), usually in the nonobstructive form and with a prevalence in the range of 35% (see Table 1; Fig. 2) (2). HCM is a primary and familial cardiac malformation with heterogeneous expression and diverse clinical course for which a large number of disease-causing mutations in five genes encoding proteins of the sarcomere have been reported. HCM is a rela-

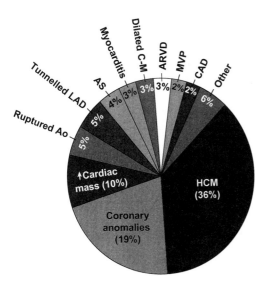

FIG. 1. Causes of sudden cardiac death in young competitive athletes (median age, 17 years) based on systematic tracking of 158 athletes in the United States, primarily 1985–1995. In an additional 2% of the athletes, no evidence of cardiovascular disease sufficient to explain death was found at necropsy. ↑, cardiac mass, hearts with increased weight and some morphologic features consistent with (but not diagnostic of) hypertrophic cardiomyopathy; LAD, left anterior descending coronary artery; AS, aortic stenosis; C-M, cardiomyopathy; ARVD, arrhythmogenic right ventricular dysplasia; MVP, mitral valve prolapse; CAD, coronary artery disease. (Adapted from ref. 2, with permission of the American Medical Association.)

for potentially lethal arrhythmias in some individuals, the stress of intense athletic training and competition (as well as associated alterations in blood volume, hydration, and electrolytes) undoubtedly increases risk to some degree.

Despite intense investigation, however, reliable identification of the individual HCM patient (or athlete) at high risk remains a major challenge. This is due, in part, to the fact that most data on risk stratification have been assembled at referral institutions and are based on selected patient populations already judged to be at increased risk. The multiplicity of mechanisms believed to cause sudden death in HCM and the uncertainties regarding their relative importance constitute other obstacles to risk stratification.

Nevertheless, disease variables that appear to identify young HCM patients at greatly increased risk include prior aborted cardiac arrest or sustained ventricular tachycardia; family history of multiple sudden or other premature HCM-related deaths or identification of a high-risk genotype; multiple-repetitive nonsustained ventricular tachycardia on serial ambulatory (Holter) electrocardiogram (ECG) recordings; recurrent syncope; and possibly a massive degree of left ventricular hypertrophy (22,23). Magnitude of the left ventricular outflow tract pressure gradient has not been associated with an increased risk for sudden death, which may occur both in patients with and in patients without subaortic obstruction.

Patients with HCM considered to be at particularly high risk for sudden death probably deserve aggressive preventive treatment, regardless of whether symptoms have intervened (22,23). The available therapeutic measures are the same as those used most frequently in coronary artery disease or dilated cardiomyopathy—that is, amiodarone administered in a relatively low maintenance dosage (200 to 300 mg per day) or use of the implantable cardioverter-defibrillator. The precise clinical criteria for choosing between these two treatment strategies have not been defined and randomized clinical data are not yet available.

tively uncommon cardiac malformation, recognizable clinically in approximately 0.2% (1 in 500) of the general population (24).

In referral hospital and outpatient-based patient populations, sudden death in HCM has shown a predilection for young and asymptomatic individuals, occurring frequently during moderate or severe exertion, similar to its demographic profile in athletic populations (25). This clinical profile is consistent with both the observation that HCM is a frequent cause of sudden death in athletes and the generally accepted and prudent recommendations of the 26th Bethesda Conference to disqualify young competitive athletes with HCM from intense competitive sports (12). Indeed, for a disease such as HCM in which there is a propensity

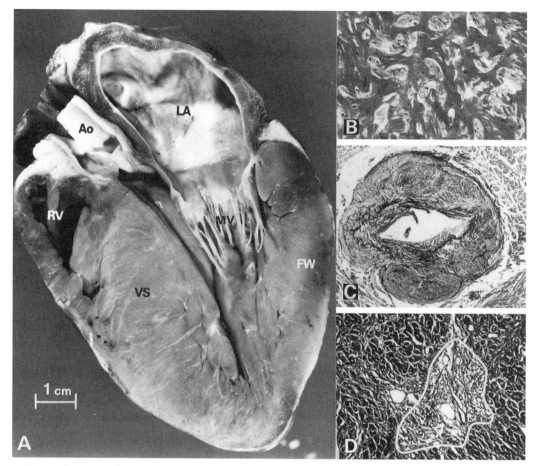

FIG. 2. Morphologic components of the disease process in hypertrophic cardiomyopathy, the most common cause of sudden death in young competitive athletes. **A:** Gross heart specimen sectioned in a cross-sectional plane similar to that of the echocardiographic (parasternal) long axis; left ventricular wall thickening shows an asymmetric pattern and is confined primarily to the ventricular septum (VS), which bulges prominently into the left ventricular outflow tract. Left ventricular cavity appears reduced in size. FW, left ventricular free wall. **B, C,** and **D:** Histologic features characteristic of left ventricular myocardium in HCM. **B:** Markedly disordered architecture with adjacent hypertrophied cardiac muscle cells arranged at perpendicular and oblique angles. **C:** An intramural coronary artery with thickened wall, resulting primarily from medial hypertrophy, and apparently narrowed lumen. **D:** Replacement fibrosis in an area of ventricular myocardium adjacent to an abnormal intramural coronary artery. Ao, aorta; LA, left atrium; RV, right ventricle. (From ref. 23, with permission of Lancet.)

Of note is the investigation of Corrado et al. (4) and associates (26), who reported arrhythmogenic right ventricular dysplasia (ARVD), rather than HCM, to be the most common cause of sudden death in athletes within the Veneto region in northeastern Italy. Although ARVD is also a component of the North American experience with athletic

field deaths, its frequency in North America is clearly in the range of less than 5% (2,5). The explanation for such discrepancies is uncertain, although it is possible that the relatively frequent occurrence of ARVD in a particular region of Italy reflects a unique genetic substrate. Furthermore, the relatively low frequency with which HCM is apparently responsible for sudden death in Italian athletes is an interesting but also a largely unresolved issue. Certainly, HCM appears to occur with reasonable frequency in Italy (27–30). It is possible that the longstanding and systematic Italian national program for the cardiovascular assessment of competitive athletes (31) has had the effect of identifying and disqualifying disproportionate numbers of trained athletes with HCM, because this cardiac malformation is much more easily identifiable clinically than ARVD (32–35).

Morphology and Diagnosis

Left ventricular hypertrophy has traditionally been regarded as the gross anatomic marker and likely the determinant of many of the clinical features and course in most patients with HCM (see Fig. 2) (19–23,36–38). Because the left ventricular cavity is usually small or normal in size, increased left ventricular mass is due almost entirely to an increase in wall thickness. Consequently, the clinical diagnosis of HCM has been based on the definition (by two-dimensional echocardiography) of the most characteristic morphologic feature of the disease—that is, left ventricular wall thickening associated with a nondilated cavity—and in the absence of another cardiac or systemic disease capable of producing the magnitude of hypertrophy present (e.g., systemic hypertension or aortic stenosis) (19–21, 23) (Fig. 3). Because the nonobstructive form of HCM is predominant (22,23), the well-described clinical features of dynamic obstruction to left ventricular outflow, such as a loud systolic ejection murmur, systolic anterior motion of the mitral valve, or partial premature closure of the aortic valve, are not required for diagnosis.

Based on both echocardiographic and necropsy analyses in large numbers of patients, it is apparent that the HCM disease spectrum is characterized by vast structural diversity with regard to the patterns and extent of left ventricular hypertrophy (21) (Figs. 4 and 5). While the anterior ventricular septum is usually the predominant region

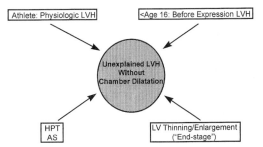

FIG. 3. Basic morphologic definition of hypertrophic cardiomyopathy showing those clinical conditions or cirucmstances that constitute exceptions that may obscure this diagnosis. AS, aortic stenosis; HPT, systemic hypertension; LV, left ventricular; LVH, left ventricular hypertrophy.

of hypertrophy, virtually all possible patterns of left ventricular hypertrophy occur in HCM, and no single phenotypic expression can be considered "classic" or typical of this disease. Although many patients show diffusely distributed hypertrophy, approximately 30% demonstrate localized wall thickening confined to only one segment of left ventricle.

Absolute thickness of the left ventricular wall varies greatly, although the average reported value is usually 21 to 22 mm (21). Wall thickness is profoundly increased in many patients, including some showing the most severe hypertrophy observed in any cardiac disease (with 60 mm being the most extreme wall thickness dimension reported to date) (38). On the other hand, the HCM phenotype is not invariably expressed as a greatly thickened left ventricle, and some patients show only a mild increase of less than or equal to 15 mm, including a few genetically affected individuals with normal thicknesses (less than or equal to 12 mm) (22,23, 37). Patterns of wall thickening in HCM are often strikingly heterogeneous, involving noncontiguous segments of the left ventricle (i.e., with areas of normal thickness evident in between), or demonstrating marked differences in wall thickness in contiguous segments. Transitions between thickened areas

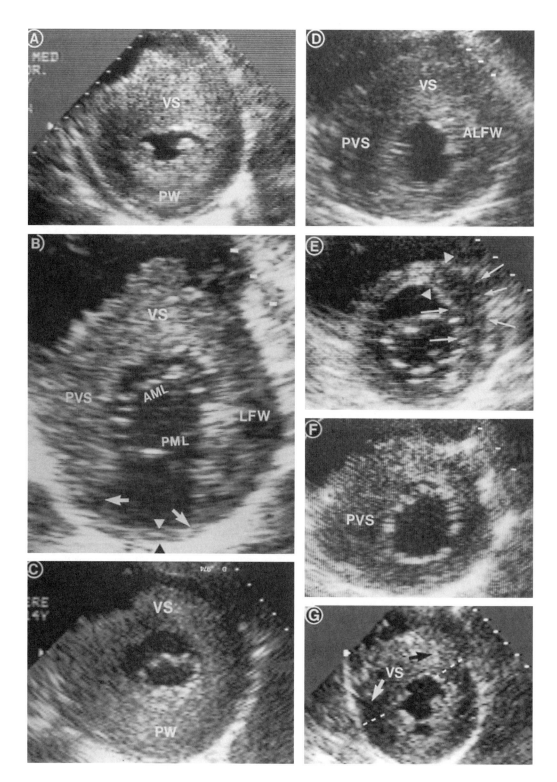

and regions of normal thickness are often sharp and abrupt, not infrequently creating right-angled contours of the wall. The variability in morphologic expression of HCM is underlined by the fact that even first-degree relatives with the disease usually show considerable dissimilarities in the pattern of left ventricular wall thickening (36).

Detection during Preparticipation Screening

Even though HCM may be suspected during preparticipation sports evaluations by the prior occurrence of exertional syncope, by family history of the disease or premature cardiac death, or by a loud heart murmur, such clinical features are relatively uncommon among all individuals affected by this disease. Most HCM patients have the nonobstructive form of this disease characteristically expressed by no murmur or only a soft heart murmur (19,20). Consequently, standard screening procedures with only history and physical examination cannot be expected to identify this disease in a reliable and consistent fashion (11). One retrospective study has shown that potentially lethal cardiovascular abnormalities, including HCM, were suspected by standard preparticipation history and physical in only 3% of 115 high school and collegiate athletes who ultimately died suddenly of such diseases (2) (Fig. 6).

Even when noninvasive testing (i.e., echocardiography) is used in screening athletes for HCM, false-negative results may occur by virtue of encountering individuals with this disease at a point of incomplete phenotypic expression during adolescence (39). In young individuals with HCM (younger than approximately age 13 to 15 years), left ventricular hypertrophy is often absent or mild; therefore, the echocardiographic findings (and phenotypic expression) may not be diagnostic at the time of the preparticipation screening.

Although educational institutions and professional sports organizations must use reasonable care in conducting their athletic programs, currently there is no clear legal precedent regarding their duty to require or conduct preparticipation screening of athletes to detect medically significant abnormalities (11). Also, a physician who has medically cleared an athlete to participate in competitive sports is not necessarily legally liable for an injury

---

FIG. 4. Variability of patterns of left ventricular hypertrophy in patients with hypertrophic cardiomyopathy, shown in a composite of diastolic stop-frame images in parasternal short-axis plane. **A, B,** and **D:** Wall thickening is diffuse, involving substantial portions of ventricular septum and free wall. In **(A),** at papillary muscle level, all segments of the left ventricular wall are hypertrophied, including posterior free wall (PW), but the pattern of thickening is asymmetric with the anterior portion of ventricular septum (AVS) predominant and massive (i.e., 50 mm). **B:** The hypertrophy is diffuse, involving three segments of left ventricle but with the posterior free wall spared and thin (less than 10 mm; arrowheads) and with particularly abrupt changes in wall thickness evident (arrows). **C:** Marked hypertrophy in a pattern distinctly different from **A, B,** and **D,** in which the thickening of posterior wall (PW) is predominant, and the ventricular septum is of near-normal thickness. **D:** Diffuse distribution of hypertrophy involving three segments of left ventricle similar to **(B),** but without sharp transitions in the contour of the wall. **E:** Hypertrophy predominantly involving lateral free wall and only a small portion of contiguous anterior septum (arrows). **F:** Hypertrophy predominantly of posterior ventricular septum (PVS) and to lesser extent the contiguous portion of anterior septum (AVS). **G:** Thickening involving anterior and posterior septum to a similar degree, but with sparing of the free wall. Calibration dots are 1 cm apart. AML, anterior mitral leaflet; LFW, lateral free wall; PML, posterior mitral leaflet. (From ref. 21, with permission of the American College of Cardiology.)

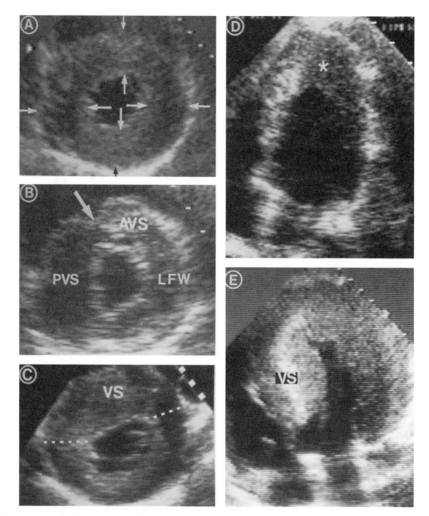

FIG. 5. Heterogeneity in patterns of left ventricular hypertrophy in five patients with hypertrophic cardiomyopathy, including examples of the uncommon concentric and apical forms. **A, B,** and **C:** Diastolic stop-frame images obtained in the parasternal short-axis plane. **D** and **E:** Apical four-chamber views. **A:** Relatively mild hypertrophy in a concentric (symmetric) pattern with each segment of septum and free wall having a similar thickness (paired arrows). **B:** "Butterfly" pattern with prominent indentation (arrow) and localized area of thinning interpositioned at the 11-o'clock position between adjacent thicker areas of ventricular septum. **C:** Hypertrophy of entire ventricular septum (VS) and sparing of free wall. **D:** Myocardial hypertrophy confined to left ventricular apex (asterisk). **E:** Image from another patient with hypertrophy involving the apex, but also diffusely involving the basal ventricular septum and free wall. Calibration marks are 1 cm apart. AVS, anterior ventricular septum; LA, left atrium; LFW, lateral free wall; LV, left ventricle; PVS, posterior ventriclar septum. (From ref. 21, with permission of American College of Cardiology.)

or death caused by an undiscovered cardiovascular condition. Malpractice liability for failure to discover a latent, asymptomatic cardiovascular condition requires proof that a physician deviated from customary or accepted medical practice in performing preparticipation screening of athletes and that the use of established diagnostic methods would have disclosed the specific medical abnormality (11).

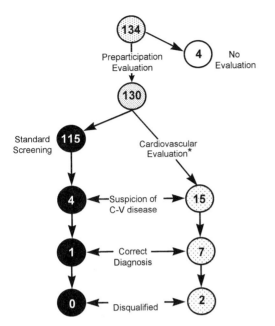

FIG. 6. Flow-diagram showing impact of preparticipation medical history and physical examinations on the detection of structural cardiovascular disease (and causes of sudden death), as well as subsequent disqualification from competitive athletics. Asterisk indicates cardiovascular evaluation with testing (independent of standard school or institutional preparticipation screening), performed in 15 athletes because of symptoms, family history, cardiac murmur, or other physical findings suggestive of heart disease. (From ref. 2, with permission of the American Medical Association.)

Differential Diagnosis of HCM and "Athlete's Heart"

Some young athletes with hypertrophy involving the anterior ventricular septum (wall thicknesses 13 to 15 mm), consistent with a relatively mild morphologic expression of HCM, may be difficult to distinguish from the physiologic form of left ventricular hypertrophy, which is an adaptation to athletic training (i.e., "athlete's heart") (40) (Fig. 7). This distinction between athlete's heart (15–18) and cardiac disease (19,20) has particularly important implications, because identification of cardiovascular disease in an athlete may be the basis for disqualification from competition in an effort to minimize risk (12). By the

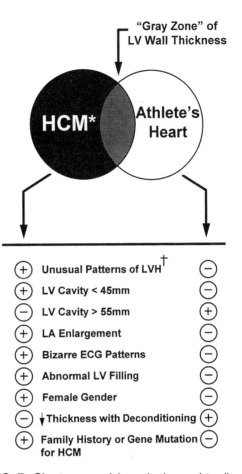

FIG. 7. Chart summarizing criteria used to distinguish hypertrophic cardiomyopathy (HCM) from athlete's heart when the left ventricular (LV) wall thickness is within the shaded gray zone of overlap (13 to 15 mm), consistent with both diagnoses. *Assumed to be the nonobstructive form of HCM, because the presence of substantial mitral valve systolic anterior motion would confirm, pere, the diagnosis of HCM in an athlete. [†]A variety of abnormalities may be involved, including heterogeneous distribution of left ventricular hypertrophy (LVH), in which asymmetry is prominent, and adjacent regions may be of greatly different thicknesses, with sharp transitions evident between segments; also, patterns in which the anterior ventricular septum is spared from the hypertrophic process and the region of predominant thickening may be in the posterior portion of septum or anterolateral or posterior free wall. ↓, decreased; LA, left atrial. (From ref. 40, with permission of the American Heart Association.)

same token, the improper diagnosis of cardiac disease in an athlete may lead to unnecessary withdrawal from athletics, thereby depriving that individual of the varied benefits of sports.

For asymptomatic individuals within this morphologic "gray zone," the differential diagnosis between athlete's heart and HCM can be approached by clinical assessment and noninvasive testing (40) (see Fig. 4). Although this distinction cannot be resolved with certainty in some athletes, careful analysis of several echocardiographic and clinical features permits this diagnostic differentiation in most instances (see Fig. 7).

Wall Thickness

In highly trained athletes, although the region of predominant left ventricular wall thickening always involves the anterior septum, the thicknesses of other segments of the wall are similar. In patients with HCM, whereas the anterior portion of the septum is also usually the region of maximal wall thickening, asymmetry is more prominent and areas other than the anterior septum may show the most marked thickening (21,41).

Cavity Dimension

An enlarged left ventricular end-diastolic cavity dimension (greater than 55 mm) is present in more than one-third of highly trained elite male athletes (16,42). Conversely, the diastolic cavity dimension in most patients with HCM is small, usually less than 45 mm, and is greater than 55 mm only in those who evolve to the end-stage phase of the disease with progressive heart failure and systolic dysfunction (43). Therefore, in some instances, it is possible to distinguish athlete's heart from HCM solely on the basis of left ventricular diastolic cavity dimension (40). For example, a cavity greater than 55 mm in an athlete with borderline wall thickness would constitute strong evidence against the presence of HCM; conversely, a cavity dimension less than 45 mm would be inconsistent with athlete's heart. However, in athletes in whom left ventricular cavity size falls between these extremes, this variable alone will not resolve the differential diagnosis.

Doppler Transmitral Waveform

Abnormalities of left ventricular diastolic filling have been identified noninvasively with pulsed Doppler echocardiography (40). Most patients with HCM, including those with relatively mild hypertrophy that could be confused with athlete's heart, show abnormal Doppler diastolic indexes of left ventricular filling and relaxation independently of whether symptoms or outflow obstruction are present (44,45).

On the other hand, trained athetes have invariably demonstrated normal left ventricular filling patterns (45–51). Consequently, in an athlete suspected of having HCM, a distinctly abnormal Doppler transmitral flow-velocity pattern strongly supports this diagnosis, whereas a normal Doppler study is compatible with either HCM or athlete's heart.

Gender

Sex differences with regard to cardiac dimensions and left ventricular mass have been identified in trained athletes (52–54). For example, female athletes rarely show left ventricular wall thicknesses greater than or equal to 12 mm (Fig. 8). Therefore, female athletes with wall thicknesses within the gray zone between athlete's heart and HCM (in the presence of normal cavity size) are most likely to have HCM (52).

Regression of Left Ventricular Hypertrophy with Deconditioning

Increased left ventricular cavity size or wall thickness can be shown to be a physiologic consequence of athletic training by serial echocardiographic examination, demonstrating a decrease in cardiac dimensions and mass after a short period of athletic deconditioning (17,55–57). For example, elite athletes with left ventricular hypertrophy may show reduction in wall thickness (of about 2 to 5 mm) with 3 months of deconditioning (57) (Fig. 9). However, identification of such changes in wall thickness requires compliance from highly motivated competitive athletes to interrupt training and requires serial echocardiographic studies of optimal techni-

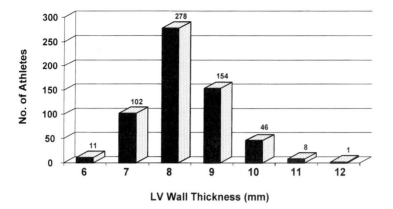

FIG. 8. Distribution of maximal left ventricular wall thickness of 600 highly trained competitive women athletes participating in a variety of sporting disciplines. Of note, wall thickness did exceed 12 mm and, therefore, did not fall into the equivocal "gray zone" of overlap between the physiologic athlete's heart and pathologic hypertrophic cardiomyopathy. (From ref. 52, with permission of the American Medical Association.)

cal quality. An unequivocal decrease in left ventricular wall thickness with deconditioning is inconsistent with the presence of pathologic hypertrophy and HCM.

Familial Transmission and Genetics

The most definitive evidence for the presence of HCM in an athlete with increased wall thickness comes from the demonstration of the disease in a relative (58–64). Therefore, in those athletes in whom the distinction between HCM

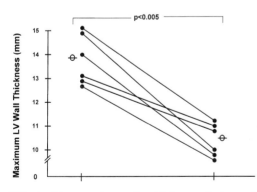

FIG. 9. Changes in maximal left ventricular wall thickness associated with deconditioning in Olympic level rowers. Cardiac dimensions were obtained with two-dimensional echocardiography at peak training and subsequently after 6 to 34 weeks of deconditioning following the 1988 Olympic games, with measurements made in a blinded fashion. (From ref. 57, with permission of Heart.)

and athlete's heart cannot be achieved definitively by other methods, one potential approach for resolving this diagnostic uncertainty is by the echocardiographic screening of family members. Absence of HCM in a family, however, does not exclude the diagnosis of HCM because the disease may be "sporadic" (i.e., absent in relatives other than the index case), presumably as a result of de novo mutation (61).

Recent advances in the understanding of the genetic alterations responsible for HCM raise the possibility of DNA-diagnosis in athletes suspected of having this disease (63,64). At present, mutations responsible for HCM have been identified in five genes located on chromosomes 14, 1, 9, 11, and 15; each of these genes encode proteins of the sarcomere: β-myosin heavy chain, cardiac troponin T, troponin-I, myosin-binding protein C, and α-tropomyosin, respectively (58–64). This substantial genetic heterogeneity and the expensive, time-intensive methodologies required, have made it difficult at present to use the techniques of molecular biology for the purpose of routinely resolving the differential diagnosis between athlete's heart and HCM in the clinical arena.

OTHER CAUSES OF SUDDEN DEATH IN YOUNG ATHLETES

Second in importance and frequency to HCM as a cause of sudden death on the athletic field is a spectrum of congenital vascular malformations of the coronary arterial tree, the most common of which appears to be anomalous origin of the left main coronary artery from the right (anterior) sinus of Valsalva (see Table 1; see Fig. 1). Less common causes of sudden death in young athletes (each accountable for 5% or fewer cases) (2,3,5,7) include myocarditis, dilated cardiomyopathy, Marfan syndrome with ruptured aorta, aortic valvular stenosis, atherosclerotic coronary artery disease, long QT syndrome, mitral valve prolapse, and ARVD (see Table 1; see Fig. 1). It has also been suggested that major coronary arteries tunneled within the left ventricular myocardium for part of their course (as an isolated finding) constitute a potentially lethal anatomic variant that may cause sudden unexpected death during exertion in otherwise healthy young individuals (2,65,66).

In addition, not infrequently at autopsy, hearts are seen with increased mass (and wall thickness) and nondilated left ventricular cavity suggestive of HCM, but the objective morphologic findings in these hearts are not sufficiently striking to permit a definitive diagnosis of this disease (2). It is uncertain whether some of these cases (often referred to as idiopathic left ventricular hypertrophy at autopsy) (6) represent a mild morphologic expression of HCM or possibly an unusual instance of athlete's heart with particularly marked physiologic left ventricular hypertrophy associated with deleterious consequences.

Occasionally, athletes dying suddenly demonstrate no evidence of structural cardiovascular disease, even after careful gross and microscopic examination of the heart. In such instances (approximately 2% in the series by Maron et al. [2]), it may not be possible to exclude with certainty noncardiac factors, such as drug abuse, or discern whether careful inspection of the specialized conducting system and associated vasculature with serial sectioning (which is not part of the standard medical examiner's protocol) would have revealed occult but clinically relevant abnormalities (67–69). It is also possible that such deaths are due to previously unidentified Wolff-Parkinson-White syndrome, rare conditions in which structural abnormalities of the heart are characteristically lacking at necropsy such as long QT syndrome, possibly exercise-induced coronary spasm, primary ventricular fibrillation (70), or undetected examples of segmental ARVD (26,71). There is no definitive evidence that systemic hypertension, per se, is associated with increased risk for sudden cardiac death in young athletes.

DEMOGRAPHICS OF SUDDEN DEATH IN YOUNG ATHLETES

Based primarily on data assembled from broad-based U.S. populations (2,3,5,6,10), a profile of young competitive athletes who die suddenly has emerged. Such athletes participated in a large number and variety of sports, with the most frequent being basketball and football (about 70%), probably reflecting the high participation level in (and intensity of) these popular team sports. Most athletic field deaths occur in male participants (approximately 90%); the relative infrequency in female participants probably reflects a lower participation level, sometimes less intense levels of training, and the fact that some diseases most commonly accounting for sudden death in athletes appear less frequently in female individuals (e.g., HCM). Most athletes are of high school age at the time of death (approximately 60%); however, other sudden deaths occur in young athletes who have achieved collegiate or even professional levels of competition.

Most athletes who incur sudden death (with HCM or other diseases) have been free of symptoms during their lives and were not suspected of harboring cardiovascular disease. Sudden collapse usually occurs associated with exercise, predominantly in the late afternoon and early evening hours, corresponding to peak periods of competition and training, particularly in organized team sports such as football and basketball (2) (Fig. 10). These observations substantiate that, in the presence of certain underlying structural cardiovascular diseases (including HCM), physical activity represents a trigger and an important precipitating factor for sudden collapse on the ath-

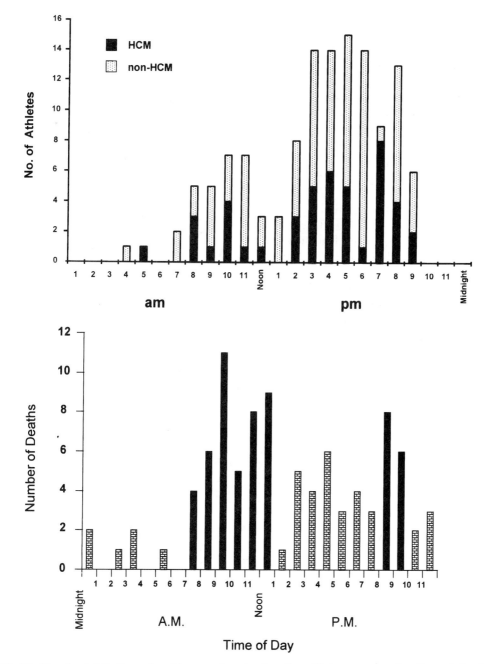

FIG. 10. Hourly distribution of sudden cardiac deaths. **Top:** Histogram showing time of death for 127 competitive athletes either with hypertrophic cardiomyopathy (HCM) (bold portion of bars) or a variety of other predominantly congenital cardiovascular malformations (lighter portions of bars). Death occurred predominantly in the late afternoon and early evening, corresponding largely to the time of training and competition. (From ref. 2, with permission of the American Medical Association.) **Bottom:** In contrast, histogram for 94 patients recognized as having HCM (who were not athletes) demonstrates a prominent early peak between 7 A.M. and 1 P.M. and a secondary peak in the early evening (most evident between 8 P.M. and 10 P.M.). (From ref. 72, with permission of the American College of Cardiology.)

letic field. The predilection for sudden death late in the day is similar in athletes with HCM and in athletes with other lesions. This observation for athletes with HCM contrasts strikingly with prior findings in patients with HCM for whom a bimodal pattern of circadian variability over the 24-hour day was evident, including a prominent early to mid-morning peak, similar to that described in patients with coronary artery disease (with sudden death, acute myocardial infarction, or angina) (see Fig. 4) (72).

Although most sudden deaths in competitive athletes have been in white males, a substantial proportion (greater than 40%) are African-American athletes (2,3,73). There is also evidence that HCM represents a common cause of sudden death in young African-American males (2,73) (Fig. 11). This substantial occurrence of HCM-related sudden death in young black male athletes contrasts sharply with the very infrequent identification of black patients with HCM in hospital-based populations. These data emphasize the disproportionate access to sub-specialty health care between the African-American and white communities in the United States that makes it less likely for

young black male individuals to receive a relatively sophisticated cardiovascular diagnosis, such as HCM, compared to their white counterparts. Consequently, young African-American athletes with HCM are also less likely to be disqualified from competition, in accordance with the recommendations of 26th Bethesda Conference (12), to reduce their risk for sudden death.

ELIGIBILITY CONSIDERATIONS FOR ATHLETES WITH KNOWN CARDIOVASCULAR DISEASES, INCLUDING HYPERTROPHIC CARDIOMYOPATHY

When a cardiovascular abnormality such as HCM is identified in a competitive athlete, the following considerations arise: (a) the magnitude of risk for sudden cardiac death associated with continued participation in competitive sports and (b) the criteria to be implemented for determining whether individual athletes should be withdrawn from sports competition. In this regard, the 26th Bethesda Conference sponsored by the American College of Cardiology (12) offers prospective and consensus recommendations for athletic eligi-

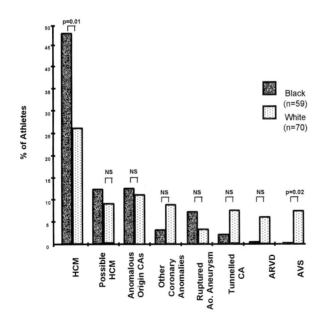

FIG. 11. Impact of race on cardiovascular causes of sudden death in competitive athletes. Ao, aorta; AVS, aortic valve stenosis; CA, coronary anomalies; HCM, hypertrophic cardiomyopathy. (From ref. 2, with permission of the American Medical Association.)

bility or disqualification, taking into account the severity of the cardiovascular abnormality as well as the nature of sports training and competition. The 26th Bethesda Conference recommendations are predicated on the likelihood that intense athletic training will increase the risk for sudden cardiac death (or disease progression) in trained athletes with HCM, although it is not yet possible to quantify that risk in precise terms.

Consequently, it is presumed that the temporary or permanent withdrawal of selected athletes from participation in certain sports is both prudent and beneficial by virtue of diminishing the perceived risk.

CONCLUSION

It is well recognized that all patients (or athletes) with HCM do not incur the same risk for sudden cardiac death (22,23). However, the differentiation of subgroups of young athletes and patients with differing risks has proved challenging and remains largely unresolved (22,23). Although electrophysiologic testing with programmed electrical stimulation has provided some measure of predictability with regard to outcome in high-risk patients with coronary artery disease, inferences from those data to patients with a different and heterogeneous disease such as HCM are frought with great uncertainty, particularly with regard to the highly selected subset of trained athletes with this disease. In a disease such as HCM in which there is a propensity for potentially lethal arrhythmias in some individuals, the stress of athletic training and competition as well as the associated alterations in blood volume, hydration, and electrolytes that may occur makes any extrapolation of risk assessment from nonathletes with HCM directly to highly trained competitive athletes with this condition very tenuous.

The fact that it is not possible to reliably stratify risk for individual young athletes with HCM is reflected by the homogeneous and conservative 26th Bethesda Conference recommendations for athletic eligibility:

Athletes with the unequivocal diagnosis of HCM should not participate in most competitive sports, with the possible exception of those of low intensity. This recommendation includes those athletes with or without symptoms and with or without left ventricular outflow obstruction (12).

DNA-based diagnosis has led to the identification of increasing numbers of children and adults with a preclinical diagnosis of HCM (59,60,74). These individuals have a disease-causing genetic mutation, but *without* clinical or phenotypic manifestations of HCM such as left ventricular wall thickening on echocardiogram or cardiac symptoms (a variety of alterations may, however, be evident on the 12-lead ECG) (75). Based on the available data, it is likely that most such genotype-positive, phenotype-negative children will develop left ventricular hypertrophy when achieving full body growth and maturation (39,74). Genetically affected adults without phenotypic expression of left ventricular hypertrophy appear to be relatively uncommon but largely confined to non-myosin mutations such as myosin-binding protein C (59) and cardiac troponin T (60). The clinical implications of a primary molecular diagnosis of HCM and the appropriate management of such individuals are largely unresolved issues. However, there is at present no evidence to justify precluding most such genetically affected individuals without the HCM phenotype from competitive athletics or most other life activities. A possible exception is in those individuals with a family history of frequent HCM-related death or the documentation of a particularly malignant genotype in which efforts at risk stratification and possible restriction from competitive sports may be justified.

REFERENCES

1. Maron BJ. Sudden death in young athletes: lessons from the Hank Gathers affair. *N Engl J Med* 1993;329:55–57.
2. Maron BJ, Shirani J, Poliac LC, et al. Sudden death in young competitive athletes: clinical, demographic and pathological profiles. *JAMA* 1996;276:199–204.
3. Burke AP, Farb A, Virmani R, Goodin J, Smialek JE. Sports-related and non-sports-related sudden cardiac death in young athletes. *Am Heart J* 1991;121:568–575.
4. Corrado D, Thiene G, Nava A, Rossi L, Pennelli N. Sudden death in young competitive athletes: clinicopatho-

logic correlations in 22 cases. *Am J Med* 1990;39:
588–596.

5. Van Camp SP, Bloor CM, Mueller FO, Cantu RC, Olson HG. Nontraumatic sports death in high school and college athletes. *Med Sci Sports Exerc* 1995;27:641–647.

6. Maron BJ, Roberts WC, McAllister HA, Rosing DR, Epstein SE. Sudden death in young athletes. *Circulation* 1980;62:218–229.

7. Liberthson RR. Sudden death from cardiac causes in children and young adults. *N Engl J Med* 1996;334: 1039–1044.

8. Thiene G, Pennelli N, Rossi L. Cardiac conduction system abnormalities as a possible cause of sudden death in young athletes. *Human Pathol* 1983;14:706–709.

9. James TN, Froggatt P, Marshall TK. Sudden death in young athletes. *Ann Intern Med* 1967;67:1013–1021.

10. Maron BJ, Epstein SE, Roberts WC. Causes of sudden death in the competitive athlete. *J Am Coll Cardiol* 1986; 7:204–214.

11. Maron BJ, Thompson PD, Puffer JC, et al. Cardiovascular preparticipation screening of competitive athletes. *Circulation* 1996;94:850-856.

12. Maron BJ, Mitchell JH. 26th Bethesda Conference. Recommendations for determining eligibility for competition in athletes with cardiovascular abnormalities. *J Am Coll Cardiol* 1994;24:845–899.

13. Maron BJ, Stead D, Aeppli D. Prevalence of sudden cardiac death during competitive sports activities in interscholastic athletes in Minnesota. *Circulation* 1996;I-388(abst).

14. Maron BJ, Poliac LC, Roberts WO. Risk for sudden cardiac death associated with marathon running. *J Am Coll Cardiol* 1996;28:428–431.

15. Maron BJ. Structural features of the athlete heart as defined by echocardiography. *J Am Coll Cardiol* 1986;7: 190–203.

16. Pelliccia A, Maron BJ, Spataro A, Proschan MA, Spirito P. The upper limit of physiologic cardiac hypertrophy in highly trained elite athletes. *N Engl J Med* 1991; 324:295–301.

17. Shapiro LM, Smith RG. Effect of training on left ventricular structure and function: an echocardiographic study. *Br Heart J* 1983;50:534–539.

18. Huston TP, Puffer JC, Rodney WM. The athletic heart syndrome. *N Engl J Med* 1985;313:24–32.

19. Maron BJ, Bonow RO, Cannon RO, Leon MB, Epstein SE. Hypertrophic cardiomyopathy: interrelation of clinical manifestations, pathophysiology, and therapy. *N Engl J Med* 1987;316:780–789 and 844–852.

20. Wigle ED, Sasson Z, Henderson MA, et al. Hypertrophic cardiomyopathy. The importance of the site and extent of hypertrophy. A review. *Prog Cardiovasc Dis* 1985;28:1–83.

21. Klues HG, Schiffers A, Maron BJ. Phenotypic spectrum and patterns of left ventricular hypertrophy in hypertrophic cardiomyopathy: morphologic observations and significance as assessed by two-dimensional echocardiography in 600 patients. *J Am Coll Cardiol* 1995;26: 1699–1708.

22. Spirito P, Seidman CE, McKenna SJ, Maron BJ. The management of hypertrophic cardiomyopathy. *N Engl J Med* 1997;36:775–785.

23. Maron BJ. Hypertrophic cardiomyopathy. *Lancet* 1997; 350:127–133.

24. Maron BJ, Gardin JM, Flack JM, Gidding SS, Bild D. Assessment of the prevalence of hypertrophic cardiomyopathy in a general population of young adults: echocardiographic analysis of 4111 subjects in the CARDIA study. *Circulation* 1995;92:785–789.

25. Maron BJ, Roberts WC, Epstein SE. Sudden death in hypertrophic cardiomyopathy: a profile of 78 patients. *Circulation* 1982;65:1388–1394.

26. Thiene G, Nava A, Corrado D, Rossi L, Pennelli N. Right ventricular cardiomyopathy and sudden death in young people. *N Engl J Med* 1988;318:129–133.

27. Spirito P, Rapezzi C, Autore C, et al. Prognosis of asymptomatic patients with hypertrophic cardiomyopathy and nonsustained ventricular tachycardia. *Circulation* 1994;90:2743–2747.

28. Cecchi F, Olivotto I, Montereggi A, Santoro G, Dolara A, Maron BJ. Hypertrophic cardiomyopathy in Tuscany: clinical course and outcome in an unselected regional population. *J Am Coll Cardiol* 1995;26:1529–1536.

29. Cecchi F, Montereggi A, Olivotto I, et al. Risk for atrial fibrillation in patients with hypertrophic cardiomyopathy assessed by signal-averaged P-wave duration. *Heart* 1997;78:44–49.

30. Spirito P, Chiarella F, Carratino L, Zoni-Berisso M, Bellotti P, Vecchio C. Clinical course and prognosis of hypertrophic cardiomyopathy in an outpatient population. *N Engl J Med* 1989;320:749–755.

31. Pelliccia A, Maron BJ. Preparticipation cardiovascular evaluation of the competitive athlete: perspectives from the 30 year Italian experience. *Am J Cardiol* 1995;75: 827–828.

32. Casolo GC, Rega L, Renzi PD. The diagnostic role of magnetic resonance imaging (MRI) in sports cardiology: MRI in right ventricular dysplasia. *Int J Sports Cardiol* 1995;4:59–73.

33. Ricci C, Longo R, Pagnan L, et al. Magnetic resonance imaging in right ventricular dysplasia. *Am J Cardiol* 1992;70:1589–1595.

34. Kisslo J. Two-dimensional echocardiography in arrhythmogenic right ventricular dysplasia. *Eur Heart J* 1989; 10:22–26.

35. McKenna WJ, Thiene G, Nava A, et al. Diagnosis of arrhythmogenic right ventricular dysplasia/cardiomyopathy. *Br Heart J* 1994;71:215–218.

36. Ciró E, Nichols PF, Maron BJ. Heterogeneous morphologic expression of genetically transmitted hypertrophic cardiomyopathy: two-dimensional echocardiographic analysis. *Circulation* 1983;67:1227–1233.

37. Solomon SD, Wolff S, Watkins H, et al. Left ventricular hypertrophy and morphology in familial hypertrophic cardiomyopathy associated with mutations of the beta-myosin heavy chain gene. *J Am Coll Cardiol* 1993;2: 498–505.

38. Maron BJ, Gross BW, Stark SI. Extreme left ventricular hypertrophy. *Circulation* 1995;92:2748.

39. Maron BJ, Spirito P, Wesley YE, Aroe J. Development and progression of left ventricular hypertrophy in children with hypertrophic cardiomyopathy. *N Engl J Med* 1986;315:610–614.

40. Maron BJ, Pelliccia A, Spirito P. Cardiac disease in young trained athletes: Insights into methods for distinguishing athlete's heart from structural heart disease with particular emphasis on hypertrophic cardiomyopathy. *Circulation* 1995;91:1596–1601.

41. Maron BJ, Gottdiener JS, Epstein SE. Patterns and significance of the distribution of left ventricular hypertro-

phy in hypertrophic cardiomyopathy: a wide-angle, two-dimensional echocardiographic study of 125 patients. *Am J Cardiol* 1981;48:418–428.

42. Spirito P, Pelliccia A, Proschan MA, et al. Morphology of the "athlete's heart" assessed by echocardiography in 947 elite athletes repreenting 27 sports. *Am J Cardiol* 1994;74:802–806.

43. Spirito P, Maron BJ, Bonow RO, Epstein SE. Occurrence and significance of progressive left ventricular wall thinning and relative cavity dilatation in patients with hypertrophic cardiomyopathy. *Am J Cardiol* 1987; 60:123–129.

44. Maron BJ, Spirito P, Green KJ, et al. Noninvasive assessment of left ventricular diastolic function by pulsed Doppler echocardiography in patients with hypertrophic cardiomyopathy. *J Am Coll Cardiol* 1987;10:733–742.

45. Lewis JF, Spirito P, Pelliccia A, Maron BJ. Usefulness of Doppler echocardiographic assessment of diastolic filling in distinguishing "athlete's heart" from hypertrophic cardiomyopathy. *Br Heart J* 1992;68:296–300.

46. Colan SD, Sanders SP, MacPherson D, Borow KM. Left ventricular diastolic function in elite athletes with physiologic cardiac hypertrophy. *J Am Coll Cardiol* 1985;6: 545–549.

47. Granger CB, Karuimeddini MK, Smith VE, et al. Rapid ventricular filling in left ventricular hypertrophy. I: physiologic hypertrophy. *J Am Coll Cardiol* 1985;5:862–868.

48. Pearson AC, Schiff M, Mrosek D, Labowitz AJ, Williams GA. Left ventricular diastolic function in weight lifters. *Am J Cardiol* 1986;58:1254–1259.

49. Fagard R, Van den Brocke C, Bielen E, Venhees L, Amery A. Assessment of stiffness of the hypertrophied left ventricle of bicyclists using left ventricular inflow Doppler velocimetry. *J Am Coll Cardiol* 1987;9: 1250–1254.

50. Finkelhor RS, Hanak IJ, Bahler RC. Left ventricular filling in endurance-trained subjects. *J Am Coll Cardiol* 1986;8:289–293.

51. Nixon JV, Wright AR, Porter TR, Roy V, Arrowhead JA. Effects of exercise on left ventricular diastolic performance in trained athletes. *Am J Cardiol* 1991;68: 945–949.

52. Pelliccia A, Maron BJ, Culasso F, Spataro A, Caselli G. Athlete's heart in women: echocardiographic characterization of highly trained elite female athletes. *JAMA* 1996;276:211–215.

53. Milliken MC, Stray-Gundersen J, Pesock RM, Katz J, Mitchell JH. Left ventricular mass as determined by magnetic resonance imaging in male endurance athletes. *Am J Cardiol* 1988;62:301–305.

54. Riley-Hagen M, Peshock RM, Stray-Gunersen J, et al. Left ventricular dimensions and mass using magnetic resonance imaging in female endurance athletes. *Am J Cardiol* 1992;69:1067–1074.

55. Ehsani AA, Hagberg JM, Hickson RC. Rapid changes in left ventricular dimensions and mass in response to physical conditioning and deconditioning. *Am J Cardiol* 1978;42:52–126.

56. Fagard R, Aubert A, Lysens R, et al. Noninvasive assessment of seasonal variations in cardiac structure and function in cyclists. *Circulation* 1983;67:896–901.

57. Maron BJ, Pelliccia A, Spataro A, Granata M. Reduction in left ventricular wall thickness after deconditioning in highly trained Olympic athletes. *Br Heart J* 1993; 69:125–128.

58. Maron BJ, Nichols PF, Pickle LW, Wesley YE, Mulvihill JJ. Patterns of inheritance in hypertrophic cardiomyopathy: assessment by M-mode and two-dimensional echocardiography. *Am J Cardiol* 1984;53:1087–1094.

59. Watkins H, Conner D, Thierfelder L, et al. Mutations in the cardiac myosin binding protein-C gene on chromosome 11 cause familial hypertrophic cardiomyopathy. *Nat Genet* 1995;11:434–437.

60. Watkins H, McKenna WJ, Thierfelder L, et al. Mutations in the genes for cardiac troponin T and α-tropomyosin in hypertrophic cardiomyopathy. *N Engl J Med* 1995;332:1058–1064.

61. Watkins H, Thierfelder L, Hwang DS, et al. Sporadic hypertrophic cardiomyopathy due to de novo myosin mutations. *J Clin Invest* 1992;90:1666–1671.

62. Watkins H, Rosenzweig A, Hwang D-S, et al. Characteristics and prognostic implications of myosin missense mutations in familial hypertrophic cardiomyopathy. *N Engl J Med* 1992;326:1108–1114.

63. Schwartz K, Carrier L, Guicheney P, Komajda M. Molecular basis of familial cardiomyopathies. *Circulation* 1995;91:532–540.

64. Marian AJ, Roberts R. Recent advances in the molecular genetics of hypertrophic cardiomyopathy. *Circulation* 1995;92:1336–1347.

65. Morales AR, Romanelli R, Boucek RJ. The mural left anterior descending coronary artery, strenuous exercise and sudden death. *Circulation* 1980;62:230–237.

66. Schwarz ER, Klues HG, vom Dahl J, et al. Functional, angiographic and intracoronary Doppler flow characteristics in symptomatic patients with myocardial bridging: effect of short-term intravenous beta-blocker medication. *J Am Coll Cardiol* 1996;27:1637–1645.

67. Bharti S, Lev M. Congenital abnormalities of the conduction system in sudden death in young adults. *J Am Coll Cardiol* 1986;8:1096–1104.

68. Burke AP, Subramanian R, Smialek J, Virmani R. Nonatherosclerotic narrowing of the atrioventricular node artery and sudden death. *J Am Coll Cardiol* 1993;21:117–122.

69. Corrado D, Thiene G, Cocco P, Frescura C. Non-atherosclerotic coronary artery disease and sudden death in the young. *Br Heart J* 1992;68:601–607.

70. Benson DW, Benditt DG, Anderson RW, et al. Cardiac arrest in young, ostensibly healthy patients: clinical, hemodynamic and electrophysiologic findings. *Am J Cardiol* 1983;52:65–69.

71. Basso C, Thiene G, Corrado D, et al. Arrhythmogenic right ventricular cardiomyopathy: dysplasia, dystrophy or myocarditis? *Circulation* 1996;94:983–991.

72. Maron BJ, Kogan J, Proschan MA, et al. Circadian variability in the occurrence of sudden cardiac death in patients with hypertrophic cardiomyopathy. *J Am Coll Cardiol* 1994;23:1405–1409.

73. Maron BJ, Poliac LC, Mathenge R. Hypertrophic cardiomyopathy as an important cause of sudden cardiac death on the athletic field in African-American athletes. *J Am Coll Cardiol* 1997;29[Suppl A]:462A(abst).

74. Rosenzweig A, Watkins H, Hwang D-S, et al. Preclinical diagnosis of familial hypertrophic cardiomyopathy by genetic analysis of blood lymphocytes. *N Engl J Med* 1991;325:1753–1760.

75. Panza JA, Maron BJ. Relation of electrocardiographic abnormalities to evolving left ventricular hypertrophy in hypertrophic cardiomyopathy. *Am J Cardiol* 1989;63: 1358–1365.

The Athlete and Heart Disease:
Diagnosis, Evaluation & Management,
edited by R. A. Williams.
Lippincott Williams & Wilkins, Philadelphia © 1999.

4

Cardiovascular Genetic Disorders that Cause Sudden Death in Athletes

Christine Seidman

Department of Medicine, Harvard Medical School and Howard Hughes Medical Institute;
Cardiovascular Genetics Center, Brigham and Women's Hospital, Boston, Massachusetts 02115

The prominence of sports in American life has increased dramatically over the past 25 years. Programs based in local communities, schools, and clubs enable boys and girls, men and women, to participate in team and individual sports as beginners, intermediate players, and highly trained amateur athletes. Regardless of whether this heightened athleticism reflects increased awareness of the benefits of exercise on health or a complex infrastructure that supports the business of professional athletics, sports has become an integral part of late twentieth century life. For most individuals, participation has both physical and social benefits; but for some, the consequence of participation is death. In addition to unforeseen traumatic events, substantive media coverage of professional (1,2) and amateur athletics (3,4) around the world has documented many unexpected nontraumatic deaths on athletic fields. Whereas sudden death is sometimes unexplainable, some of these devastating events occur secondary to well-defined cardiovascular disorders. Furthermore, sudden death in some instances is the consequence of an unrecognized heritable disease that has been transmitted from generation to generation in a family.

Application of molecular genetic techniques to the study of cardiovascular disorders has led to the elucidation of several gene defects that cause inherited heart conditions.

Disease-causing mutations that cause hypertrophic cardiomyopathy, prolonged QT syndrome, and Marfan syndrome have been and continue to be identified. Although disease genes have not yet been identified for other inherited disorders such as arrhythmogenic right ventricular dysplasia (ARVD), familial dilated cardiomyopathies, and some congenital heart disorders, the chromosomal locations of these disease genes are being reported at increasing speed. Each of these disorders is transmitted as a monogenic trait, and affected individuals transmit the disease gene to some of their offspring. Thus, the physician's role in caring for families with these disorders involves caring for affected patients in multiple generations, identifying those with undiagnosed disease, and counseling young family members at risk for disease development. Inevitably, this care involves not only treatment of disease symptoms but also giving advice regarding lifestyles and participation in sports. This chapter reviews the molecular genetics of inherited cardiovascular disorders that contribute to incidence of sudden death on the athletic field.

MODES OF INHERITANCE OF CARDIOVASCULAR DISEASE

Accurate diagnosis and risk assessment is often a substantive problem facing athletes, their families, and the physicians who care for them. The technologic improvements and widespread use of noninvasive cardiac imaging diagnosis have fostered both earlier diagnosis of structural and functional defects of the myocardium and great vessels. The sensitivity and specificity of advanced technologies are discussed elsewhere (5) and are summarized herein in the context of specific disorders. These advances in diagnosis have fostered greater awareness of the familial nature of many disorders, which has enabled molecular genetic studies aimed at defining causal genes. Familial or genetic disorders of the cardiovascular system can be classified by their patterns of inheritance (Fig. 1) as auto-

somal dominant, autosomal recessive, or matrilineal. For the researcher, patterns of transmission can direct strategies for identification of the responsible gene defect. For the clinician, understanding the mode of inheritance is essential for identifying individuals at risk of inheriting these disorders.

Genetic information is transmitted through genes contained in nuclear chromosomes (autosomes 1–22 and sex chromosomes, X and Y) as well as on a single mitochondrial chromosome. Family history, potentially combined with clinical evaluation of the first degree relatives of an individual with a heritable disorder, enables the physician to discern the mode of transmission of a disease gene. Im-

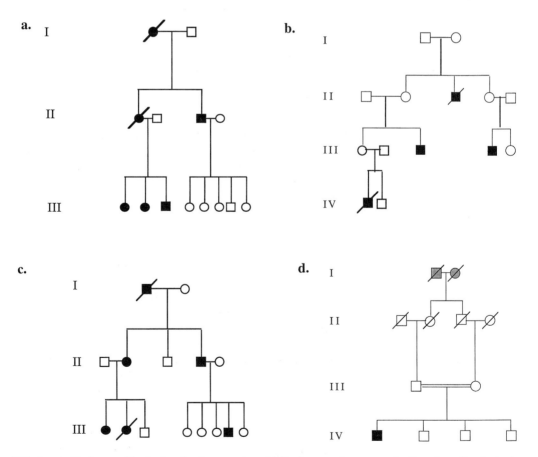

FIG. 1a–d. Pedigrees illustrating the four modes of inheritance of monogenic disorders. Symbols denoted men (squares), women (circles), and clinical affection status (solid, affected; clear, unaffected; speckled, unknown status.) Deceased individuals are denoted with slashes.

portantly, knowledge of the mode of transmission of a disease gene can guide the physician in identifying additional family members at risk for development of the inheritable disorders. Matrilineal transmission of a disorder (see Fig. 1a) should suggest a mitochondrial gene defect; hence, all of the offspring of affected women but none of the offspring of affected men are at risk of development of the inherited condition. A disorder that occurs only in male family members (see Fig. 1b) suggests an X-linked disorder; hence, the male offspring of affected men will not be affected, but the offspring of clinically unaffected women may be at risk. Autosomal dominant conditions occur in male and female family members in each generation (see Fig. 1c); each offspring of affected individuals has a 50% chance of inheriting the disorder. Autosomal recessive inheritance (see Fig. 1d) is recognized by "skip" generations; because both parents are unaffected carriers, approximately one-fourth of their children will be affected.

Recognition of the mode of transmission by which disease is inherited has enabled application of molecular genetic strategies that identify the chromosome location of disease genes, and, ultimately, definition of disease genes. Substantial progress in this arena has demonstrated multiple gene mutations that alter the structure and function of the myocardium and vasculature. This has provided preclinical recognition of individuals who have inherited gene defects, and, in some instances, provided insights to disease outcomes. These principles are illustrated in the subsequent review of four autosomal dominant disorders: familial hypertrophic cardiomyopathy, ARVD, long QT syndrome, and Marfan syndrome. Each disorder is recognized to cause sudden, unexpected cardiovascular death in asymptomatic individuals. These findings thus provide the reader with a preview of the growing relevance that genetic studies will have for aiding the physician in the evaluation, counseling, and management of individuals who participate in sports.

HERITABLE CARDIOVASCULAR DISORDERS ASSOCIATED WITH SUDDEN DEATH IN ATHLETES

Familial Hypertrophic Cardiomyopathy

Hypertrophic cardiomyopathy is a primary disorder of the myocardium characterized by increased mass with myocyte and myofibrillar disarray (6), which can be familial and transmitted as an autosomal dominant trait or as sporadic disease (7). There is neither a racial nor ethnic predisposition to the condition. Although the incidence of familial hypertrophic cardiomyopathy is unknown, a recent survey of more than 7,000 young adults demonstrated echocardiographic criteria for disease in 0.2% (8).

The pathologic features and natural history of hypertrophic cardiomyopathy is characterized by marked diversity (9). Cardiac hypertrophy can be subtle or massive, concentric or asymmetric, diffuse or focal. Similarly, the clinical manifestations and natural history of the disease vary considerably in affected individuals. Hypertrophic cardiomyopathy can occur without signs or symptoms; in these individuals, diagnosis occurs as part of a family screening. Most affected individuals typically experience dyspnea or angina, symptoms that often progress insidiously over time. Palpitations are common and may herald the development of atrial fibrillation or ventricular arrhythmias.

There is marked variability in the survival of individuals with hypertrophic cardiomyopathy. Life expectancy is normal or near-normal in most affected individuals. However, sudden death that occurs in minimally symptomatic or asymptomatic individuals is a recognized hallmark of the disease. Congestive heart failure and embolic events also contribute to the premature morbidity and mortality.

Genetic linkage studies in familial hypertrophic cardiomyopathy have demonstrated disease loci on chromosomes 1q31 (10), 3p (11), 7 (12), 11p13–q13 (13), 12q2 (11), 14q1 (14), and 15q2 (15). Except for the chromosome 7 locus, where the disease gene remains unknown, mutations in a contractile protein gene (cardiac troponin T, ventricular regulatory light chain, cardiac myosin-binding protein C, essential light chain, β cardiac myosin heavy chain, α tropomyosin) have been identified at each locus. These genetic data demonstrate that hypertrophic cardiomyopathy is a disease of the sarcomere (Fig. 2).

Definition of the gene mutations that cause hypertrophic cardiomyopathy has enabled preclinical identification of individuals who have inherited these defects. Clinical manifestations of disease are typically not present until the growth spurt that accompanies puberty (16); hence, genetic studies can often provide the most accurate diagnosis in children (Fig. 3). In families with a history of sudden death, identification of a gene defect that predisposes the person to this serious risk is particularly beneficial. However, because any one of many gene defects can cause familial hypertrophic cardiomyopathy, DNA testing of children at risk for this disease requires prior identification of the relevant mutation in family members.

The diverse genetic causes of familial hypertrophic cardiomyopathy (Fig. 4) contribute to the variable manifestations of the disease. Different hypertrophic responses and distinct patterns of survival appear related, in part, to the affected individual's genotype. As such, definition of the disease-causing mutation in a family can provide information that assists the clinician in assessing prognosis and in risk stratification.

The degree of myocardial hypertrophy found in adult individuals with familial hypertrophic cardiomyopathy caused by β cardiac myosin heavy chain mutations is typically substantial. A mean maximal left ventricular wall thickness equal to 23.7 ± 7.7 mm was found in affected individuals from families with different myosin mutations (17). In contrast, the mean maximal left ventricular wall thickness resulting from six different cardiac troponin T mutations was 16.7 ± 5.5 mm, and some adults with these mutations had normal cardiac wall thickness (18). Hypertrophic cardiomyopathy caused by cardiac myosin binding protein-C mutations is characterized by particularly late onset; echocardiographic studies of individuals with these

mutations may not demonstrate myocardial hypertrophy until middle age (19).

Identification of individuals at risk for premature death in familial hypertrophic cardiomyopathy has been a difficult clinical issue. In general, the degree of cardiac hypertrophy does not correlate with sudden death, although survival is diminished when ventricular wall thickness is greater than 30 mm (9). Noninvasive assessment of arrhythmias is frequently an insensitive technique for predicting sudden death (20). The consequences of specific gene mutations has recently been correlated with the incidence of death in familial hypertrophic cardiomyopathy and several intriguing observations have emerged. Survival in familial hypertrophic cardiomyopathy caused by cardiac troponin T gene mutations is typically poor (18). In contrast, near-normal life expectancy occurs with α tropomyosin mutations (21). β cardiac myosin heavy chain mutations have a variable effect on life expectancy; survival is diminished with the Arg403Gln mutation but normal with the Val606Met mutation (22).

Environment, lifestyles, and genetic background may further vary disease expression in hypertrophic cardiomyopathy. The development of murine models (23,24) that have been engineered to bear mutations identified in humans has helped address these issues. Because inbred mice share their genetic background, the influence of diet, exercise, and other nongenetic factors can be assessed. In one murine model (23) of a cardiac myosin (Arg403Gln) mutation, histopathologic study exhibited results comparable to those observed in human hypertrophic cardiomyopathy, including myocyte disarray, hypertrophy, and injury with replacement fibrosis. Surprisingly, male mutant mice exhibited more severe disease than female mutant litter mates. Sedentary mutant mice had normal survival, whereas vigorous swimming by mutant mice caused sudden death. These data provided evidence that male gender and exercise adversely influence the clinical manifestations of hypertrophic cardiomyopathy produced by myosin mutation Arg403Gln. The development and characterization of additional models with different human cardiovascular

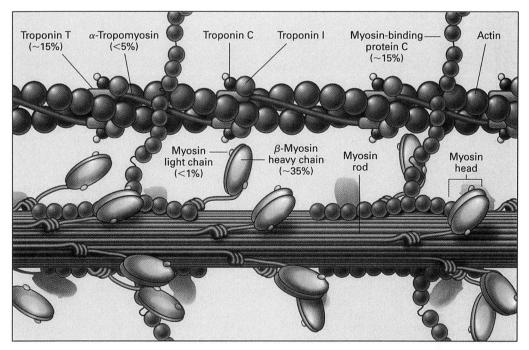

FIG. 2. Components of the Sarcomere. Cardiac contraction occurs when calcium binds the troponin complex (subunits C, I, and T) and α-tropomyosin, making possible the myosin-actin interaction. Actin stimulates ATPase activity in the globular myosin head and results in the production of force along actin filaments. Cardiac myosin-binding protein C, arrayed transversely along the sarcomere, binds myosin and, when phosphorylated, modulates contraction. In hypertrophic cardiomyopathy, mutations may impair these and other protein interactions, result in ineffectual contraction of the sarcomere, and produce hypertrophy and disarray of myocytes. Percentages represent the estimated frequency with which a mutation on the corresponding gene causes hypertrophic cardiomyopathy. (Modified from ref. Spirito and Seidman [9].)

Genotype versus Phenotype in Hypertrophic Cardiomyopathy

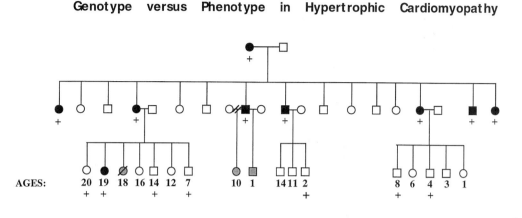

Clinical and Genetic Evaluation of Children

Individual	Age	2-D Echocardiogram	Electrocardiogram*	Genotype
III-1	20	Normal†	ABN Q; TWA	+
III-2	19	Septal / free wall hypertrophy	LVH; TWA	+
III-3	16	Normal	Normal	-
III-4	14	Normal†	LVH; TWA	+
III-5	12	Normal	Normal	-
III-6	7	Normal	TWA	+
III-7	14	Normal	Normal	-
III-8	11	Normal	Normal	-
III-9	2	Normal	Normal	+
III-10	8	Normal	QRS Δ	+
III-11	6	Normal	Normal	-
III-12	4	Normal	Normal	+
III-13	3	Normal	Normal	-
III-14	1	Normal	Normal	-

FIG. 3. Comparison of genotype and clinical manifestations of hypertrophic cardiomyopathy. Pedigree symbols are described in Fig. 1; plus sign denotes the presence of a missense mutation in the β cardiac myosin heavy chain gene. Note that clinical affection status and genotype are discordant in children, consistent with age-dependent penetrance of hypertrophic cardiomyopathy. (Adapted from ref. 16, with permission.)

mutations should aid the clinician in assessing the appropriateness of different lifestyles by individuals with these gene defects.

Arrhythmogenic Right Ventricular Dysplasia

ARVD is a primary disorder of the myocardium of unknown cause. This unusual cardiomyopathy produces progressive myocyte atrophy accompanied by fatty or fibrofatty tissue replacement, which typically involves the right ventricle more than the left ventricle (reviewed in reference 25). Pathologic features include marked thinning of the right ventricular wall and histologic features include myocardial necrosis with foci of inflammatory cells.

Familial Hypertrophic Cardiomyopathic Mutations

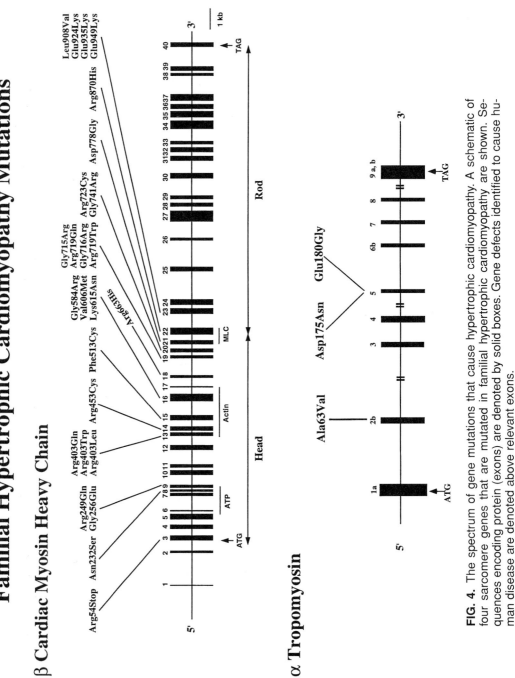

FIG. 4. The spectrum of gene mutations that cause hypertrophic cardiomyopathy. A schematic of four sarcomere genes that are mutated in familial hypertrophic cardiomyopathy are shown. Sequences encoding protein (exons) are denoted by solid boxes. Gene defects identified to cause human disease are denoted above relevant exons.

46

Cardiac Troponin T

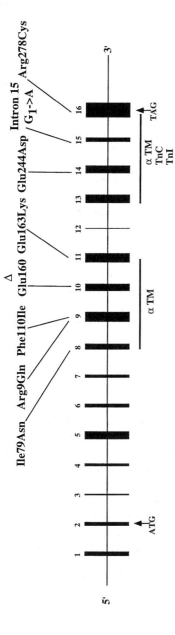

Cardiac Myosin Binding Protein-C

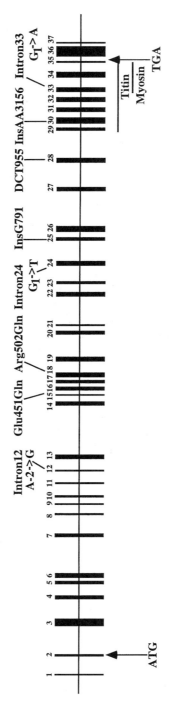

FIG. 4. *Continued.*

The clinical manifestations of ARVD result from the marked arrhythmogenicity, resulting from the right ventricular disease. Ventricular arrhythmias that cause syncope or sudden death are often the first indication of disease and typically occur late in childhood. Life-threatening arrhythmias often increase with disease duration (26). In some affected adults, symptoms of heart failure also develop (27).

Diagnosis of ARVD is often difficult. Non-invasive imaging of the right ventricle is often limited in transthoracic echocardiography, and magnetic resonance imaging may be more helpful in defining right ventricular dilatation or aneurysm (28). Endomyocardial biopsy can reveal the histopathologic features previously detailed, but focal involvement limits the sensitivity of this technique. Electrocardiographic findings may be absent or demonstrate right ventricular T wave inversion and conduction delays (29). The identification of tachyarrhythmias that originate from the right ventricle may help clarify the diagnosis.

ARVD is a familial disease transmitted as an autosomal dominant trait. Pedigree analyses demonstrate incomplete penetrance; that is, some obligate carriers lack clinical manifestation of disease. Molecular genetic studies of several large kindreds have localized the disorder to chromosomes 14q23–q24 (30), 14q12–q22 (31), and 1q42–q43 (32); however, neither genes nor mutations that cause this condition are known. Hence, ARVD remains an unsolved cause of sudden death in young individuals. Future research aimed at defining the molecular defect should improve understanding of this cardiomyopathy and help to define individuals at risk for the serious arrhythmias that characterize ARVD.

Long QT Syndrome

Cardiac arrhythmias occur secondary to underlying myocardial disease and as primary, often familial disorders. Wolff-Parkinson-White syndrome, atrial fibrillation, atrioventricular block, and long QT syndrome can be heritable autosomal dominant traits. Molecular genetic studies have defined the

chromosome location of familial Wolff-Parkinson-White syndrome and hypertrophic cardiomyopathy (chromosome 7;12) and familial atrial fibrillation (chromosome 1;33), but neither the genes nor the disease-causing mutations have been identified. Disease genes have been identified for prolonged QT syndrome on chromosomes 3p21 (34), 7q35 (34), and 11p15.5 (35), discoveries which have demonstrated this to be a disorder of the cardiac ion channel. Another as yet undefined gene has been localized to chromosome 4p25–27 (36). The advances made through molecular studies of long QT syndrome serve as a model for understanding other heritable and often life-threatening arrhythmias.

Autosomal dominant long QT syndrome occurs without physical findings. Affected individuals may experience symptoms of syncope, cardiac arrest, and sudden death (37). The predominant electrocardiographic finding is prolongation of the QT interval, which may be accompanied by dysmorphic ST-T waves and repolarization (aberrant T and U waves) abnormalities (38). The degree of QT prolongation can vary considerably in affected individuals, and because this interval varies in normal individuals (between 0.38 to 0.47 seconds) and is often prolonged by a variety of medications, including psychoactive and antiarrhythmic medications (39), diagnosis of this heritable syndrome can be difficult. Table 1 compares the duration of the QTc interval in affected and unaffected individuals from a multigeneration family with inherited long QT syndrome. In addition to autosomal dominant inheritance, long QT can also be transmitted as a recessive trait. However, this variant is easily distinguished by the coexistence of congenital neural deafness in affected individuals (40). The absence of physical findings, the often subtle (or absent) electrocardiographic manifestations of long QT syndrome, and the recognized predisposition to torsade de pointes can provide substantial diagnostic and management issues for clinicians caring for families with this disorder.

Mutations in a cardiac potassium ion channel gene (designated KVLQT1) (41), the human ether-a-go-go related gene (designated

TABLE 1. *Genotype and QT$_c$ Intervals in familial long QT syndrome*

Individual	Age, years	Sex	QT$_c$	HERG genotype
I-1	72	F	0.42	Normal
I-2	68	M	0.52	Ile593Arg
I-3	62	M	0.58	Ile593Arg
II-1	47	F	0.58	Ile593Arg
II-2	45	F	0.60	Ile593Arg
II-3	40	M	0.45	Ile593Arg
II-4	38	F	0.57	Ile593Arg
II-5	35	F	0.60	Ile593Arg
III-1	4	F	0.47	Ile593Arg
III-2	10	M	0.40	Normal
III-3	8	F	0.37	Normal
III-4	6	M	0.38	Normal
III-5	8	M	0.41	Normal

HERG, Human ether-a-go-go related gene.

HERG) (42), and a cardiac sodium channel gene (designated SCN5A) (43) cause long QT syndrome. Distinct types (missense, deletions, nonsense) of mutations have been identified in each gene, thereby suggesting that the consequence of a particular defect may uniquely alter a channel function. However, insights into the mechanisms by which these gene defects predispose to arrhythmia have been aided from characterizations of the electrophysiologic properties of ion channels in lower species. Analyses of HERG suggest that this channel is responsible for a delayed rectifier potassium current (44). HERG mutations may reduce channel function and consequently prolong action potentials (45). SCN5A mutations cause a gain of function that destabilizes inactivation of the channel, results in repetitive channel opening, and prolongs action potentials (46). Thus, a final common event may occur from a mutation in either of two distinct channels. Prolonged action potentials and delayed repolarization augment myocardial excitability, possibly through secondary early after-depolarizations, result in reentrant arrhythmias, and predispose to ventricular fibrillation.

Appropriate management of long QT syndrome first requires accurate diagnosis. With the identification of three disease genes and the identification of the chromosome locations of another, molecular diagnosis will become fea-sible. However, as with hypertrophic cardiomyopathy, there is significant complexity in gene-based diagnosis for long QT syndrome, and research is ongoing. Within families in which a mutation has been identified (47), DNA samples from children or adults can provide an accurate and efficient assessment of affection status. Therapeutics can then be directed to those at risk for life-threatening arrhythmias. The benefits of defining the genetic origin of long QT syndrome has also influenced therapeutic approaches. β-adrenergic antagonists, pacing devices, and automatic defibrillators have been the standard of care in long QT syndrome. Recognition of the distinct molecular origins of the disorder has suggested therapeutic strategies targeted to the mutated ion channel. Studies are underway to determine the efficacy of using sodium channel blockers to mitigate the gain of function mutations in SCN5A (48) or of increasing serum potassium to improve channel function altered by HERG mutations (49). The development of pharmacologic agents that selectively alter functions of other mutated ion channels may ultimately improve survival in long QT syndrome.

Marfan Syndrome

Unlike the disorders discussed previously, Marfan syndrome is a disorder affecting the connective tissue of multiple organ systems

(50). Recognition of the potential for underlying cardiovascular disease in these affected individuals can therefore be less problematic than with the disorders discussed previously. The alert physician may suspect the diagnosis based on skeletal manifestations including tall stature, arachnodactyly, pectus excavatum and carinatum, or kyphoscoliosis. These findings, however, are not uncommon in the general population. In the absence of genetic data or recognized disease in family members, diagnosis of Marfan syndrome therefore requires involvement of at least two organ systems. Marfan syndrome also frequently perturbs connective tissues of the eye and heart. Ocular manifestations include ectopia lentis, myopia, and a predisposition to retinal detachment. Fifty percent of affected individuals have cardiovascular involvement (51), including mitral or aortic valve deformation, accounting for valvular prolapse and regurgitation, and aortic dilation.

The most serious consequences of Marfan syndrome result from progressive dilation of the aorta, which is predisposed to rupture. Aortic aneurysm develops most commonly in the ascending thoracic aorta but may occur in any aortic segment. Marfan syndrome is the most common cause of aortic dissection in young individuals, and complications (most notably rupture) account for 80% of cardiovascular deaths in this disorder (52). Longitudinal studies of Marfan patients have demonstrated that the risk of aortic rupture increases with greater dilatation; prophylactic composite aortic valve replacement with ascending aortic conduit surgery in patients with an aortic root dimension greater than 5 cm improves survival (53). Long-term β-blockade in Marfan syndrome has documented significant attenuation in the progression of aortic root dilation (54), with a concomitant delay in the need for surgical intervention. Early and accurate diagnosis combined with serial assessment of aortic dimensions is therefore particularly important.

Molecular genetic studies have defined this autosomal dominant disorder to result from a mutation in the protein fibrillin, which is encoded on chromosome 15q (55). This micro-filament protein is widely expressed in connective tissue and appears to stabilize elastic fibers. Despite the variable clinical manifestations observed in affected individuals, Marfan syndrome is not genetically heterogeneous. Identification of disease-causing mutations is, however, still quite complex in part because of the large size of the fibrillin-1 gene (spanning 100 kilobases of DNA) and its complex organization into 65 exons (56). Twenty-five percent of affected individuals have no family history of Marfan syndrome; de novo mutations in the fibrillin-1 gene account for these sporadic cases (57).

More than 100 unique fibrillin-1 gene defects, including missense mutations that alter the encoded amino acid, small deletions, and defects in RNA splice signals have been identified in affected individuals. Analyses have failed to demonstrate a correlation between the type of mutation or location within the fibrillin-1 gene and the clinical manifestations of Marfan syndrome, suggesting that genotype may not predict phenotype in this disorder (58). The role of genetics in Marfan syndrome may be most important for accurate diagnosis. Clinical or gene-based diagnosis must be combined with serial assessment of an individual's cardiovascular status to ensure appropriate timing of surgical intervention.

CURRENT PERSPECTIVES AND FUTURE CONSIDERATIONS

Clinical evaluation of individuals at risk for genetic cardiovascular disorders currently requires careful history, examination, and selected testing. Molecular genetic studies have demonstrated the potential for improving these traditional approaches by providing accurate diagnosis and risk assessment, and by directing therapies. Why, then, has translation of genetic research into clinical applications remained limited? Technology, cost, education, and ethics all contribute to this answer. Molecular research has demonstrated that a single clinical disorder can be caused by one of a vast array of potential genetic bases. To identify the genetic basis for hypertrophic cardiomyopathy in one individual could require accurate determination of the sequence of more than 200,000 nucleotides encoding six disease genes. This task is further complicated because affected individuals are heterozygous for a disease-causing mutation; only one of the two copies of all human genes will contain the defect. The recent development of DNA-chip technologies promises to provide accurate and efficient sequences analyses that should accelerate the acquisition of genetic data. Associated costs of this and future technologies will certainly be an important factor in clinical use. The educated and ethical use of such testing is perhaps a more critical issue. Whether molecular genetics improves or threatens an individual's quality of life has already become a societal debate. Education of physicians as well as patients and their families in the relevance and limitations of human genetics may help to focus this dialogue toward improved health care delivery.

The identification of an individual at risk for sudden cardiac death remains a difficult task. An awareness of the causal role of heritable cardiovascular disorders is critical for reducing the incidence of these catastrophic events. Clinical evaluation complemented by genetic information should ultimately provide a comprehensive approach to diagnosis and management of these important disorders.

ACKNOWLEDGMENTS

This work was supported by grants from the Howard Hughes Medical Institute and the National Institutes of Health.

REFERENCES

1. Noonan D. Heart of the matter. *Sports Illustrated* 1996; 84(10):68–78.
2. Maron BJ. Sudden death in young athletes: lessons from the Hank Gathers affair. *N Engl J Med* 1993;329:55–57.
3. Rhoden WC. Deaths of teen-age athletes raise questions over testing. *The New York Times,* March 14, 1994;Sect A:1 (col 5).
4. Van Camp SP, Bloor CM, Mueller FO, Cantu RC, Olson HG. Nontraumatic sports death in high school and college athletes. *Med Sci Sports Exerc* 1995;27:641–647.
5. Skorton DJ, Brundage BH, Schelbert HR, Wolf GL. Relative merits of imaging techniques. In: Braunwald E, ed. *Heart disease, a textbook of cardiovascular medicine,* 5th ed. Philadelphia: WB Saunders 1997:349.
6. Maron BJ, Bonow RO, Cannon RO, Leon MB, Epstein SE. Hypertrophic cardiomyopathy: interrelations of clinical manifestations, pathophysiology, and therapy. *N Engl J Med* 1987;316(13):780–789.
7. Watkins H, Thierfelder L, Hwang D-S, et al. Sporadic hypertrophic cardiomyopathy due to a *de novo* mutation myosin mutations. *J Clin Invest* 1992;90:1666–1671.
8. Maron BJ, Gardin JM, Flack JM, et al. Prevalence of hypertrophic cardiomyopathy in a general population of young adults: echocardiographic analysis of 4111 subjects in the CARDIA study. *Circulation* 1995;92:785–789.
9. Spirito P, Seidman CE, McKenna WJ, Maron BJ. The management of hypertrophic cardiomyopathy. *N Engl J Med* 1997;336:775–785.
10. Watkins H, MacRae CA, Thierfelder L, et al. A disease locus for familial hypertrophic cardiomyopathy maps to chromosome 1q3. *Nat Genet* 1993;3:333–337.
11. Poetter K, Jiang H, Hassanzadeh S, et al. Mutations in either the essential or regulatory light chains of myosin are associated with a rare myopathy in human heart and skeletal muscle. *Nat Genet* 1996;13:63–69.
12. MacRae CA, Ghaisas N, Kass S, et al. Familial hypertrophic cardiomyopathy with Wolff-Parkinson-White syndrome maps to a locus on chromosome 7q3. *J Clin Invest* 1995;96:1216–1220.
13. Carrier L, Hengstemberg C, Beckmann JS, et al. Mapping of a novel gene for familial hypertrophic cardiomyopathy to chromosome 11. *Nat Genet* 1993;4:311–313.
14. Jarcho JA, McKenna WJ, Pare JAP, et al. Mapping a gene for familial hypertrophic cardiomyopathy to chromosome 14q1. *N Engl J Med* 1989;321:1372–1378.
15. Thierfelder L, MacRae CA, Watkins H, et al. A familial hypertrophic cardiomyopathy locus maps to chromosome 15q2. *Proc Natl Acad Sci USA* 1993;90:6270.
16. Rosenzweig A, Watkins H, Hwang D-S, et al. Preclinical diagnosis of familial hypertrophic cardiomyopathy by genetic analysis of blood lymphocytes. *N Engl J Med* 1991;325:1753–1760.
17. Solomon SD, Wolff S, Watkins H, et al. Left ventricular hypertrophy and morphology in familial hypertrophic cardiomyopathy associated with mutations in the β myosin heavy chain gene. *J Am Coll Cardiol* 1993;22:498–505.
18. Watkins H, McKenna WJ, Thierfelder L, et al. The role of cardiac troponin T and α-tropomyosin mutations in hypertrophic cardiomyopathy. *N Engl J Med* 1995;332:1058–1064.
19. Niimura H, Bachinski LL, Watkins H, et al. Human cardiac myosin binding protein C mutations cause late-onset familial hypertrophic cardiomyopathy. *N Engl J Med* 1998;338:1248–1257.
20. McKenna WJ, Deanfield J, Faruqui A, et al. Prognosis in hypertrophic cardiomyopathy: role of age and clinical, electrocardiographic and hemodynamic features. *Am J Cardiol* 1981;47:532–8.
21. Coviello DA, Maron BJ, Spirito P, et al. Clinical features of hypertrophic cardiomyopathy caused by mutation of a "hot spot" in the alpha-tropomyosin gene. *J Am Coll Cardiol* 1997;29:635–640.
22. Watkins H, Rosenzweig A, Hwang D-S, et al. Characteristics and prognostic implications of myosin missense mutations in familial hypertrophic cardiomyopathy. *N Engl J Med* 1992;326:1108–1114.
23. Geisterfer-Lowrance AAT, Christe M, Conner DA, et al. A murine model of familial hypertrophic cardiomyopathy. *Science* 1996;272:731–734.

24. Vikstrom KL, Factor SM, Leinwand LA. A murine model of hypertrophic cardiomyopathy. *Kardiol* 1995; 84:49–54.

25. Thiene G, Basso C, Danieli GA, et al. Arrhythmogenic right ventricular cardiomyopathy: a still underrecognized clinical entity. *Trends Cardiovasc Med* 1997;7(3): 84–90.

26. Corrado D, Thiene G, Nava A, et al. Sudden death in young competitive athletes: clinicopathologic correlation in 22 cases. *Am J Med* 1990;89:588–596.

27. Daliento L, Turrini P, Nava A, et al. Arrhythmogenic right ventricular cardiomyopathy in young versus adult patients: similarities and differences. *J Am Coll Cardiol* 1995;25:655–664.

28. Daliento L, Rizzoli G, Thiene G, et al. Diagnostic accuracy of right ventriculography in arrhythmogenic right ventricular cardiomyopathy. *Am J Cardiol* 1990;66: 741–745.

29. Nava A, Scognamiglio R, Thiene G, et al. A polymorphic form of familial arrhythmogenic right ventricular dysplasia. *Am J Cardiol* 1987;59:1405.

30. Rampazzo A, Nava A, Danieli GA, et al. The gene for arrhythmogenic right ventricular cardiomyopathy maps to chromosome 14q23–q24. *Hum Mol Genet* 1994;3: 959.

31. Severini GM, Krajiovic M, Pinamonti B, et al. A new locus for arrhythmogenic right ventricular dysplasia on the long arm of chromosome 14. *Genomics* 1996;31: 193.

32. Rampazzo A, Nava A, Erne P, et al. A new locus for arrhythmogenic right ventricular cardiomyopathy (ARVD2) maps to chromosome 1q42–q43. *Hum Mol Genet* 1995; 4:2151.

33. Brugada R, Tapscott T, Czernuszewicz GZ, et al. Identification of the first locus for familial atrial fibrillation utilizing a rapid novel pooled DNA strategy. *N Engl J Med* 1997;336(13):905–911.

34. Jiang C, Atkinson D, Towbin JA, et al. Two long QT loci map to chromosomes 3 and 7 with evidence for further heterogeneity. *Nat Genet* 1994;8:141–147.

35. Keating MT, Atkinson D, Dunn C, et al. Linkage of cardiac arrhythmia, the long QT syndrome, and the Harvey ras-1 gene. *Science* 1991;252:704–706.

36. Schott J, Charpentier F, Peltier S, et al. Mapping of a gene for LQT to chromosome 4p2527. *Am J Hum Genet* 1995;57:1114–1122.

37. Vincent GM, Timothy K, Leppert M, Keating MT. The spectrum of symptoms and QT intervals in carriers of the gene for the long QT syndrome. *N Engl J Med* 1992; 327:846–852.

38. Malfatto G, Beria G, Sala S, Bopnazzi O, Schwartz PJ. Quantitative analysis of T wave abnormalities and their prognostic implications in the idiopathic long QT syndrome. *J Am Coll Cardiol* 1994;23:296–301.

39. Kasanuki H, Ohnishi S, Tamura K, et al. Acquired long QT syndrome due to antiarrhythmic drugs and bradyarrhythmias. In: Hashiba K, Moss AJ, Schwartz PJ, eds. QT prolongation and ventricular arrhythmias. *Ann N Y Acad Sci.* 1992;664:57–73.

40. Splawski I, Timothy KW, Vincent GM, Atkinson DL, Keating MT. Molecular basis of the long-QT syndrome associated with deafness. *N Engl J Med* 1997;336: 1562–1567.

41. Wang Q, Curran ME, Splawski I, et al. Positional cloning of a novel potassium channel gene: KVLQT1 mutations cause cardiac arrhythmias. *Nat Genet* 1996; 12:17–23.

42. Wang Q, Shen J, Splawski I, et al. SCN5A mutations associated with an inherited cardiac arrhythmia, long QT syndrome. *Cell* 1995;80:805–811.

43. Curran ME, Splawski I, Timothy KW, et al. A molecular basis for cardiac arrhythmia: HERG mutations cause long QT syndrome. *Cell* 1995;80:795–803.

44. Keating MT, Sanguinetti MC. Molecular genetic insights into cardiovascular disease. *Science* 1996;272: 681–685.

45. Sanguinetti MC, Curran ME, Spector P, Keating MT. Spectrum of HERG K+ channel dysfunction in an inherited cardiac arrhythmia. *Proc Natl Acad Sci USA* 1996; 93:2208–2212.

46. Bennet PB, Yazawa K, Makita N, George AL. Molecular mechanisms for an inherited cardiac arrhythmia. *Nature* 1995;376;683–685.

47. Benson DW, MacRae CA, Vesely MR, et al. A missense mutation in the pore region of HERG causes familial long QT syndrome. *Circulation* 1996;93:1791–1795.

48. Schwartz PJ, Priori SG, Locati EH, et al. Long QT syndrome patients with mutations of the SCN5A and HERG genes have differential responses to Na+ channel blockage and to increases in heart rate. *Circulation* 1995;92:3381–3386.

49. Compton SJ, Lux RL, Ramsey MR, et al. Genetically defined therapy of inherited long QT syndrome: correction of abnormal repolarization by potassium. *Circulation* 1996;94(5):1018–1022.

50. Dietz HC. Molecular etiology, pathogenesis and diagnosis of the Marfan syndrome. *Progr Pediatr Cardiol* 1996;5:159–166.

51. Roberts WC, Honig HS. The spectrum of cardiovascular disease in the Marfan syndrome: a clinico-morphologic study of 18 necropsy patients and comparison to 151 previously reported necropsy patients. *Am Heart J* 1982;104:115–135.

52. Roman MJ, Rosen SS, Kramer-Fox R, Devereux RB. The prognostic significance of the pattern of aortic root dilatation in the Marfan syndrome. *J Am Coll Cardiol* 1993;22:1470–1476.

53. Pyeritz RE, McKusick VA. The Marfan syndrome: diagnosis and management. *N Engl J Med* 1979;300: 772–777.

54. Marsalese DL, Moodie DS, Vacante M, et al. Marfan's syndrome: natural history and long-term follow-up of cardiovascular involvement. *J Am Coll Cardiol* 1989; 14:422–428.

55. Nijbroek G, Sood S, McIntosh I, et al. Fifteen novel FBN1 mutations causing Marfan syndrome detected by heteroduplex analysis of genomic amplicons. *Am J Hum Genet* 1995;57:8–21.

56. Pereira L, D'Alessio M, Ramirez F, et al. Genomic organization of the sequence coding for fibrillin, the defective gene product in Marfan syndrome. *Hum Mol Genet* 1993;2:961–968.

57. Dietz HC, Cutting GR, Pyeritz RE, et al. Marfan syndrome caused by a recurrent de novo missense mutation in the fibrillin gene. *Nature* 1991;352:337–339.

58. Dietz HC, Pyeritz RE. Mutations in the human gene for fibrillin-1 (FBN1) in the Marfan syndrome and related disorders. *Hum Molec Genet* 1995;4:1799–1809.

The Athlete and Heart Disease:
Diagnosis, Evaluation & Management,
edited by R. A. Williams.
Lippincott Williams & Wilkins, Philadelphia © 1999.

5

The Molecular Biology of Cardiac Abnormalities in Athletes

A. J. Marian and Robert Roberts

Section of Cardiology, Department of Medicine, Baylor College of Medicine, Houston, Texas 77030

Advances in the techniques of molecular genetics and biology have led to elucidation of the molecular basis of a number of cardiovascular diseases such as hypertrophic cardiomyopathy (HCM) and the long QT syndrome. During the past few years, a number of genes and mutations for HCM, long QT, and many other cardiovascular diseases have been identified. In addition, functional studies have been performed to elucidate the molecular pathogenesis of these diseases. Furthermore, genotype-phenotype correlation studies in humans have been performed to determine the phenotypic correlates of the responsible mutations. These advances have set forth the possibility of genetic diagnosis, independent of and prior to development of the phenotype and genetic counseling, as well as genetic-based therapeutic interventions. Moreover, it has also become evident that the final phenotype in an intact organism is determined by the primary genetic defect, modifier genes, and their interplay with environmental factors. The rapid pace of progress in the field of molecular genetics is shifting the paradigm from gene mapping and mutation identification to functional studies and understanding the complex gene-to-gene interactions and the subsequent environmental interactions. This is well illustrated in the case of HCM. Whereas the underlying mutation in the sarcomeric proteins causes the HCM phenotypes, the extent and severity of phenotypes

are modulated not only by the underlying mutations but also by other modifier genes and probably by environmental factors such as exercise. The potential influence of exercise on the phenotypic expression of HCM, such as the risk of sudden cardiac death, is intriguing, in that HCM is the most common cause of death in young competitive athletes (1).

RESPONSES OF THE HEART TO STIMULI

The so-called "athlete's heart" represents a paradigm of the cardiac adaptive response to altered stress. Athlete's heart is characterized by an increase in left ventricular mass resulting from an increase in the left ventricular dimension and wall thickness (2). These changes are characteristic of the response of the heart to any form of altered stress. The heart, in response to any stimulus, undergoes hypertrophy, dilatation, or a combination thereof. Because adult cardiac myocytes are terminally differentiated, incapable of proliferation, the hypertrophic and dilatory responses of the heart to altered stress are restricted to enlargement of the myofibrils without cardiac myocyte hyperplasia. Despite their inability to proliferate, cardiac myocytes, however, exhibit remarkable plasticity in activation or suppression of a number of genes. Stimulus activates a cadre of so-called ubiquitous early genes such as c-*fos*, c-*myc*, and c-*jun*, followed by cardiac growth factors and genes specific for cardiac function. This occurs regardless of the nature of the underlying stimulus. Therefore, hypertrophy or dilatation could develop as a result of a physiologic stimulus such as exercise or a pathologic stimulus such as the presence of a mutation in the structural proteins. The latter is the case in patients with HCM, whereby mutations in sarcomeric proteins lead to myofibrillar hypertrophy (3). The primary purpose of the hypertrophic response of the heart to altered stress is adaptive, aiming to reduce the stress applied per unit of the working myofibril. However, despite the nondiscriminate response of the heart to stimuli as hypertrophy or dilatation, the physiologic consequences are likely to depend—in part—upon the underlying stimulus. Even though hypertrophy and dilatation resulting from a physiologic stimulus such as exercise are adaptive responses with salutary consequences, they are potentially maladaptive with detrimental consequences in pathologic conditions such as hypertrophic or dilated cardiomyopathy. Given the contrasting consequences, it is likely that different molecular mechanisms modulate the physiologic and pathologic hypertrophic and dilatory responses of the heart. Elucidation of the molecular basis of these responses is likely to provide opportunity to attenuate the maladaptive and promote the adaptive response of the heart to stimuli.

GENE EXPRESSION IN PHYSIOLOGIC CARDIAC HYPERTROPHY AND DILATATION

The human genome contains approximately 100,000 genes distributed in 23 pairs of chromosomes. Each nucleated cell in the body contains the entire genome and thus the entire 100,000 genes. However, only a fraction of the genes in the genome are expressed in each cell and in each organ. Expression refers to transcription of messenger RNA (mRNA) that encode for the synthesis of protein. Although humans have more than 20 trillion cells, only about 200 are uniquely different as defined by their function. This is

largely due to tissue-specific regulation of gene expression. Expression of many genes is also regulated developmentally. Although some are expressed exclusively in fetal life, others are expressed predominantly in adult life. A prototype example of such regulation is the expression of the myosin heavy chain (MyHC), the motor unit of the muscle cells. Myosin has two isoforms of α and β. Whereas the β-MyHC is the predominant myosin in the fetal heart, the α-MyHC comprises more than 90% of the myosin in postnatal and adult rat heart (4). In the adult human heart, the β-MyHC protein comprises approximately 95% of the total myosin (4,5).

Cardiac gene expression is regulated in response to physiologic as well as pathologic stimuli. Physical activity is an important regulator of expression of structural and metabolic proteins in the heart and skeletal muscle. Exercise could modulate cardiac gene expression through direct effects on cardiac loading conditions or indirectly through alteration in growth factors and catecholamines. The latter increases transiently during exercise and exerts significant influence on gene expression in the heart through adrenoreceptors. Daily physical exercise stimulates protein synthesis in the heart, leading to cardiac hypertrophy (6). Studies in animals have shown beneficial effects of exercise on cardiac gene expression. In particular, exercise has been shown to modify the altered cardiac gene expression in pathologic conditions (7–9). An example is the case of SERCA2a, which codes for the calcium adenosine triphosphate (ATP)ase of the sarcoplasmic reticulum. Expression of SERCA2a is diminished in heart failure as well as in aging. Physical exercise attenuates the decreased expression of SERCA2a gene in the myocardium of aged mice (7). Similarly, physical exercise also enhances expression of the mitochondrial genes such as cytochrome oxidase in the senescent rat heart (7). In the young rat heart, physical exercise increases the expression of the cardiac adenylate cyclase and attenuates the increase in guanine nucleotide-binding ($G_i\alpha$) proteins in the aged myocardium (8). Physical exercise also improves remodeling postmyocardial infarction through modulating expression of the myosin isoforms in the heart (9). It attenuates the abnormal expression of the α-MyHC gene in the rat heart following myocardial injury (9). Physical exercise not only modulates expression of the structural and contractile proteins in the heart, it also influences expression of the circulating growth factors such as insulin-like growth factor-1 (IGF-1) and its binding proteins (10). IGF-1 exerts direct effects on myocardial hypertrophy and function. IGF-1 increases expression of the contractile protein in the heart, leading to increased contractility and cardiac myocyte hypertrophy. Furthermore, expression of the circulating cytokines is also influenced by physical exercise. Modest changes in the plasma levels of interleukin (IL)-1, tumor necrosis factor (TNF)-α, IL-6, and IL-1ra have been observed following extraneous physical activity (11). However, the influence of chronic exercise on cytokine expression remains to be established.

Physical exercise not only provides beneficial effects on myocardial gene expression, it also modulates expression of nitric oxide in the coronary vasculature (12). Nitric oxide (NO) is an endothelial-derived relaxing factor that plays a major role in coronary circulation. NO is produced by nitric oxide synthase that converts the amino acid L-arginine into NO and citrulline. NO, through activating guanylate cyclase, induces vasodilatation. Upregulation of nitric oxide synthase during physical exercise is responsible for coronary vasodilatation and potentiates the vasodilatory response to acetylcholine (12). Overall, it is evident that the influence of physical exercise on cardiac gene expression provides salutary effects.

GENE EXPRESSION IN PATHOLOGIC CARDIAC HYPERTROPHY AND DILATATION

The terminally differentiated cardiac myocytes exhibit significant plasticity of gene expression in response to altered stress. A variety of genes that are not normally expressed in the adult heart are reexpressed in pathologic conditions. In addition, isoform switching is common in pathologic cardiac hypertrophy. The isoform switch in adult rat heart is characterized by the upregulation of the β-MyHC and downregulation of α-MyHC gene expression in response to an increased load (13). Such isoform switch in cardiac hypertrophy confers energy conservation to the working muscle, in that the β-MyHC is associated with a threefold to fivefold lower ATPase activity and a lower velocity of shortening as compared to α-MyHC (14).

Human myocardium is also capable of adapting to altered stress by reexpression of the fetal genes as well as isoform switch. Such isoform switch occurs in sarcomeric proteins such as the β-MyHC and cardiac troponin T (cTnT), known genes for HCM (5,15). In the human heart, the predominant isoform of the myosin is β-MyHC, comprising approximately 95% of the total expressed myosin (4). During cardiac hypertrophy, expression of β-MyHC increases to almost 100% and that of the α-MyHC almost disappears. Changes in the expression of other sarcomeric proteins such as cTnT isoforms also occur in cardiac hypertrophy and dilatation (15,16). Under normal conditions, only two isoforms of cTnT are expressed; under pathologic hypertrophy conditions, expression of four to six isoforms of cTnT have been demonstrated (15,16). More drastic changes occur in reexpression of other fetal genes such as atrial natriuretic factor, brain natriuretic factor, c-*fos*, c-*jun*, and c-*myc* in pathologic cardiac hypertrophy (17–19). Reexpression of these fetal genes has been demonstrated for pressure-overload hypertrophy as well as hypertrophic and dilated cardiomyopathies. However, it remains unknown as to whether reexpression of these genes also occurs in the human heart when subjected to a physiologic stimulus such as exercise. It is also intriguing to postulate that exercise could attenuate reexpression of the fetal genes in the pathologic conditions.

In addition to changes in the contractile proteins in response to altered stress, expression of genes involved in coupling excitation to contraction (e.g., SERCA, phospholamban, calsequestrin, and ryanodine receptor genes) is also altered in pathologic cardiac hypertrophy (20). The sarcoplasmic reticulum Ca^{2+}-ATPase is responsible for the active transport of the cytosolic calcium into the sarcoplasmic reticulum, resulting in a lowering of the cytosolic Ca^{2+} level. The latter induces myocardial relaxation. SERCA gene, through alternative splicing, produces two isoforms: SERCA2a and SERCA2b. SERCA2a is the primary isoform expressed in the heart. Expression of SERCA2a is decreased in advanced heart failure (20). Phospholamban is involved in regulation of Ca^{2+}-ATPase activity and myocardial contractility. A direct relation between phospholamban level and contractile state is present. Knockout deletion of phospholamban gene induces a hypercontractile state, and overexpression of phospholamban protein in transgenic mice results in decreased contractile state (21,22). In end-stage heart failure in humans, which is characterized by both hypertrophy and dilatation, expression levels of SERCA2a, phospholamban, and ryanodine receptor are decreased. In contrast, expression level of calsequestrin remains unchanged (20). A number of changes in the extracellular collagen matrix also occur in cardiac hypertrophy and dilatation in response to injury. These changes altogether probably provide an adaptive response in early stages. However, they subsequently lead to detrimental consequences.

MOLECULAR BIOLOGY OF HYPERTROPHIC CARDIOMYOPATHY

HCM, a paradigm of cardiac hypertrophic response, is characterized by left ventricular hypertrophy in the absence of an increased external load. HCM is caused by mutations in genes coding for sarcomeric proteins (3). A large number of mutations in seven genes—the β-MyHC, cTnT, myosin binding protein-C (MyβP-C), α-tropomyosin, essential light chain genes, and regulatory light chain genes, and cardiac troponin I—have been identified in patients with HCM (4,23–27). Mutations in the β-MyHC, cTnT, and MyBP-C genes account for approximately 30%, 15% to 20%, and 10% to 15% of HCM cases, respectively. Identification of mutations in seven different sarcomeric proteins has led to the notion that HCM is indeed a disease of the sarcomeric proteins. The molecular genetic aspects of this disease are discussed in Chapter 4. In this section, molecular biology of the sarcomeric proteins involved in HCM is discussed briefly.

Sarcomeric Proteins

Sarcomeres (see Fig. 2, Chapter 4) are the contractile units of the muscles. They are 2.2 μ in length and are attached to each other through the Z discs. Sarcomeres contain more than 15 different proteins that are arranged into thick, thin, and intermediary filaments. Thick filaments are comprised of several hundred MyHC molecules bound together in tail regions. A number of associated proteins such as MyBP-C, myosin light chain (MLC)-1, and MLC-2 are attached to MyHC in thick filaments. Thin filaments are comprised of actin, troponin complex, and α-tropomyosin. Other sarcomeric proteins (e.g., titin) span the entire length of the sarcomere and provide elasticity to the contractile units. Complex interactions between sarcomeric proteins lead to displacement of the MyHC globular head over the thin actin filaments, resulting in muscle contraction.

β-MyHC Protein

The β-MyHC protein is a 220-kD protein that forms the thick filaments of the sarcomeres. The β-MyHC is the predominant myosin in the human ventricles, comprising more than 95% of the myosin and 30% of the total myofibrillar protein (4,5). It is coded by a 6-kb mRNA transcribed from the β-MyHC gene on chromosome 14 (28). Mutations in the β-MyHC gene account for approximately one-third of HCM cases. The β-MyHC protein has three distinct components of globular (N-terminus), hinge, and tail (C-terminus) regions. The globular head of the β-MyHC contains the major active domains of the myosin molecule such as the actin and ATP-binding sites. The rod-shaped tail region is important in tail-to-tail interbinding of the myosin molecules. The hinge region is the site of flexion of the globular head over the rod-shaped tail. The rod regions of two myosin molecules are wound around each other in an α-helix, forming a homodimeric molecule with two globular heads. To each globular head, one essential myosin light chain (MLC-1) and one regulatory light chain (MLC-2) are attached in the hinge region, thus forming a hexameric molecule.

The three-dimensional structure of the globular head of the myosin molecule has been characterized, and the topography of ATP, actin, and light-chain binding sites have been delineated (29). Structure of the globular head of the myosin molecule is dominated by the presence of a number of α-helices, including a long (8.5 nm) α-helix that extends to the C-terminus and is the binding site for light chains. The NH_2-terminal region of the regulatory light chain (MLC-2) wraps around the COOH-terminus of the globular head, and its interaction with the MyHC is stabilized by a cluster of hydrophobic residues. The essential light chain also wraps around the MyHC long α-helix proximal toward the NH_2-terminal. Binding of the light chains to this long α-helix stabilizes the MyHC molecule. Removal of the light chain proteins from the MyHC eliminates the motility function of the myosin molecule (30). The head of the molecule is comprised of seven β sheets and contains the ATP and actin-binding sites, which are located in the opposite direction of the globular head. The central (fourth) sheet, along with a helix, forms part of the ATP-binding site. The actin-binding site is distal and in the opposite direction to the ATP-binding site. It is proposed that binding of an ATP molecule to the pocket leads to closure of the nucleotide binding pocket and produces a movement and rotation of the COOH-terminus of MyHC. The sequence of acto-myosin interaction leading to cardiac contraction and relax-

ation could be summarized as follows: Mg^{2+} ATP binds to the nucleotide binding pocket, leading to rotation of the MyHC COOH-terminus and rapid dissociation of the myosin from the actin filaments (31). The free MyHC hydrolyzes the ATP to adenosinde diphosphate (ADP) and Pi (inorganic phosphate). This is followed by binding of the actin molecule to MyHC–ADP complex. The latter results in release of the ADP from the nucleotide-binding pocket. The nucleotide binding pocket then becomes available for binding to another Mg^{2+} ATP and the cycle is reinitiated. Transduction of energy released from ATP hydrolysis into mechanical force occurs during binding of actin to myosin–ADP complex. Recently, new techniques have been developed that can accurately quantify the movement of a single myosin head over an actin filament during contraction (32,33). These data indicate that each myosin molecule generates forces of 3 to 4 picoNewtons that result in 4- to 11-nm displacement of the globular head of a single myosin molecule over thin filaments during each contraction.

Troponin T Protein

CTnT is a major protein of the thin filaments. It is coded by a 1.2-kb mRNA transcribed from the cTnT gene located on chromosome 1q3 (34, 35). Mutations in cTnT gene account for approximately 15% to 20% of the HCM cases. CTnT comprises approximately 5% of the total myofibrillar protein. The thin filaments are comprised of actin, α-tropomyosin, and troponin complex in a 7:1:1 molar ratio (36). CTnT in the thin filament exists as a ternary protein in complex with troponin I and troponin C. Together they play an important role in the Ca^{2+} responsive acto-myosin interaction. CTnT is responsible for positioning of the troponin complex on α-tropomyosin. Troponin T is the largest protein of the troponin complex with a molecular weight of approximately 35 kD. It is a highly polar molecule with acidic residues on the NH_2-terminus and basic residues on the COOH-terminus. Multiple isoforms of cTnT protein are expressed in human heart (15,16). Expression of the cTnT isoforms is regulated developmentally and is altered in pathologic conditions (15,16,37). It is generally believed that the function of cTnT is to increase the affinity of the troponin complex for the actin filament. However, cTnT also modulates the inhibitory effect of troponin I on actin filaments in the absence of Ca^{2+}. It is also involved in the removal of the inhibitory effect of troponin I as well as the ATPase activity of the acto-myosin complex (38). Overall, the interaction of cTnT with cTnI is important for intact organization of the troponin complex.

MyBP-C Protein

MyBP-C is a component of the thick filaments in the sarcomeres and is localized to the A bands. It binds to MyHC as well as titin (39). The latter is a giant sarcomeric protein that stretches between two M lines and provides elasticity to the heart muscle. The structure of the MyBP-C has been recently characterized (40). MyBP-C is a member of the intracellular immunoglobulin superfamily and has 10 distinct domains, named C1 through C10 (40). Seven domains are immunoglobulin I-set domains and three are fibronectin-III domains (40). Cardiac MyBP-C possesses a unique N-terminal motif between C1 and C2 domains, which is the phosphorylation site for cyclic adenosine monophosphate (cAMP)-dependent, as well as calcium/calmodulin-dependent protein kinases (41). Phosphorylation of this cardiac-specific motif could potentially modulate cardiac contractility. However, the exact function of the MyBP-C is not known. The MyHC binding site is comprised of the last 102 amino acids in the C-terminal C10 IgI domain of the MyBP-C protein. The C-terminal region is also the site of binding of the titin protein, which spans a large area between C8 through C10 IgI domains of the proteins (40).

The MyBP-C gene is located on chromosome 11 and has a complex structure containing 35 exons (40). The cardiac-specific motif comprised of nine amino acids is translated from exon 8 of the MyBP-C gene. Mutations in MyBP-C account for approximately 10% to 15% of HCM cases. These mutations are commonly frame-shift mutations or deletion mutations that affect the binding sites for MyHC and titin (25,26).

α-Tropomyosin Protein

α-Tropomyosin is a rod-shaped dimeric sarcomeric protein that is formed through coiled-coil α helices of two molecules. It comprises approximately 5% of the myofibrillar protein (42). Each tropomyosin coiled coil makes contact with seven actin monomers. In addition, it binds to adjacent tropomyosin molecules through head-to-tail interbindings. Thus, the function of tropomyosin is to bridge the binding of the troponin protein complex to actin filaments. The gene for tropomyosin is located on chromosome 15q2, and the mature tropomyosin mRNA is approximately 1 kb (42). Mutations in the tropomyosin gene account for less than 5% of HCM cases.

MLC-1 and MLC-2

Myosin light chain proteins are 18- to 28-kD proteins that bind to the long α-helix and provide stability to the MyHC molecule. Five different isoforms of MLC proteins are expressed in the human heart. Expression of MLC isoforms in the heart is developmentally regulated and is altered in response to stress (43,44). Both MLC-1 and MLC-2 are involved in regulation of cardiac muscle contraction (45–48). Removal of MLC proteins from the MyHC impairs acto-myosin interaction (30). Phosphorylation of MLC-2 modulates increased force production of the acto-myosin interaction (47). Mutation in the phosphorylation sites of MLC-2 reduces the power output of the striated muscles (48). In addition, switch in MLC isoforms has been shown to impair cardiac function (46). Mutations in ventricular isoforms of MLC-1 and MLC-2, coded by the *MYL3* and *MYL2* genes on chromosome 3p and 12q, respectively, are responsible for a small fraction of HCM cases (27).

INSIGHTS INTO THE MOLECULAR PATHOGENESIS OF HYPERTROPHIC CARDIOMYOPATHY

Identification of the responsible genes and mutations in a significant number of HCM cases has led to performing functional studies in order to elucidate the molecular pathogenesis of HCM. Given that the β-MyHC gene was the first and probably the most common responsible gene for HCM, it is not surprising that the majority of functional studies have been performed with the β-MyHC mutations. The first series of such functional studies addressed the acto-myosin interaction using an in vitro motility assay (49,50). This assay quantifies the displacement of the mobile labeled actin filaments by the fixed myosin molecules attached to a nitrocellulose membrane. Studies of human β-MyHC isolated from the skeletal muscles of patients with HCM carrying β-MyHC mutations and studies of expressed rat α myosin S1 subfragment carrying a corresponding β-MyHC mutation showed reduced ability of the mutant myosin to displace the actin filament (49,50). Stoichiometric studies conducted by mixing the different ratios of normal and mutant myosin proteins showed that the mutant myosin disproportionately reduced the velocity of actin displacement (50). Studies of the interaction of actin with the mutant β-MyHC were further corroborated in isolated single slow-twitch muscle fibers from patients with HCM (51). Lankford et al. (51) showed that slow-twitch muscle fibers carrying certain MyHC mutations exhibited reduced maximum velocity of shortening and isometric force generation. However, the heterogeneity of indices of acto-myosin interaction among different mutations both within in vitro motility assays as well as in isolated muscle fibers was observed. Nevertheless, these studies provided the first clue to the mechanism by which mutations in the β-MHC protein caused HCM.

The influence of HCM mutations on muscle contractile indices has also been studied for mutations in cTnT (52–54). Watkins et al. (52) expressed a truncated cTnT protein in cultured quail myotubes and showed that the truncated cTnT incorporated into myofilaments and impaired the contractile performance of the myotubes. In addition, focal disruption of the myofibrillar structure following expression of the truncated cTnT was observed. Lin et al. (53) measured the velocity of displacement of the thin filaments carrying a mutation in the 5′ end of cTnT by the heavy meromyosin in an in vitro motility assay and showed an increased velocity of contraction (53). We have used recombinant adenoviruses and expressed normal and mutant cTnT-Arg^{92}Gln proteins in adult cardiac myocytes (54). We showed the myofibrillar incorporation of the mutant cTnT in adult cardiac myocytes, which was associated with a significant decrease in the fractional and peak velocity of cell shortening (54). In addition, myofibrillar disarray was observed in a significant proportion of cardiac myocytes expressing the mutant cTnT protein.

Another set of functional studies involved analyzing the ATPase activity of the mutant MyHC. Sweeney et al. (50) showed that actin-activated ATPase activity of the mutant β-MyHC (Arg^{403}Gln) was reduced as evidenced by a reduced ATPase V_{max} and an increased ATPase K_m. Straceski et al. (55) studied the microfilament formation in COS cells following expression of normal and mutant rat α-MHC constructs (55). They showed that expression of the normal rat MyHC resulted in filamentous structure in COS cells. In contrast, approximately 25% of the transfected COS cells expressing the mutant rat MHC did not form filamentous structures. We addressed the impact of expression of a mutant β-MyHC protein on sarcomere assembly in adult cardiac myocytes and showed that expression of a mutant β-MyHC protein induced significant sarcomere disarray in approximately 50% of the adult cardiac myocytes (56).

An additional line of evidence regarding the pathogenesis of HCM was provided by development of a mouse model of human HCM, which was developed through gene targeting (57). Geisterfer-Lowrance introduced an $Arg^{403}Gln$ mutation into the mouse cardiac α-MyHC gene and induced a phenotype resembling that of HCM in man. Although the α-MyHC gene is not a responsible gene for human HCM and is expressed at low levels in the adult human heart, nevertheless, it is the predominant myosin in the mouse heart. In this model, cardiac morphologic findings were similar in mutant mice and their wild-type littermates at 5 weeks of age. However, by 15 weeks, left atrial enlargement and histologic evidence of disarray, hypertrophy, injury, and interstitial fibrosis developed in the mutant mice. Total heart weight and left ventricular weight did not differ between mice with the mutation and their normal littermates (57). Hemodynamic assessment showed impaired diastolic relaxation in mice with the $Arg^{403}Gln$ mutation in the α-MyHC gene.

Despite the limited number of functional studies and their shortcomings, it is generally agreed that primary abnormalities induced following expression of mutant sarcomeric proteins are impaired acto-myosin interaction and disruption of sarcomere structure. These abnormalities provide the impetus for a compensatory cardiac hypertrophy in HCM. The compensatory nature of hypertrophy in HCM is further corroborated by the observations that fetal isoforms of proteins such as nuclear protooncogenes c-*fos*, c-*jun*, and c-*myc* as well as atrial and brain natriuretic peptides are upregulated in the myocardium of patients with HCM as observed in conditions of compensatory pressure overload hypertrophy (17–19). Although the underlying mutations provide the impetus for a compensatory hypertrophy, the extent and magnitude of hypertrophy in HCM are also influenced by the genetic background and the environmental factors (58). Thus, as is the case for many genetic disorders, the final phenotype of HCM is determined by the underlying mutation, modifier genes, and their interaction with the environmental factors.

Despite the remarkable progress in the molecular genetics and biology of HCM, many intriguing questions remain to be addressed. How can the apparent dichotomy between the results of in vitro functional studies of mutant sarcomeric proteins and the clinical observation of preserved left ventricular systolic function be reconciled? Whereas in vitro functional studies show an impaired acto-myosin interaction or decreased cardiac myocyte contractility following expression of mutant sarcomeric proteins, the left ventricular ejection fraction, a measure of systolic function, is normal or increased in patients with HCM. Is an increased or preserved ejection fraction reflective of the cardiac contractile state in patients with HCM? Or is it (the increased ejection fraction) simply reflective of the left ventricular hypertrophy with a small cavity in the absence of an increased external load? Another intriguing aspect of HCM is the asymmetric nature of hypertrophy in approximately two-thirds of the patients with HCM. If, indeed, the hypertrophy in HCM is compensatory similar to the hypertrophy of pressure overload, then why does the hypertrophy in patients with HCM have an asymmetric nature? Is the asymmetric nature of hypertrophy modulated by the differential expression of local humoral factors or mechanical forces? The restriction of the phenotypic expression of HCM to the left ventricle, despite an equal level of expression of the sarcomeric proteins in the right and left ventricles, is also intriguing. Do the hemodynamic differences between the right and left ventricles account for the differential expression of the hypertrophy in the left ventricle? Do the loading conditions alter sarcomere and myofibril formation in patients with HCM? Unlike compensatory hypertrophy resulting from altered external load, which is not associated with myofibrillar disarray, the hypertrophy in HCM is characterized by the presence of myofibrillar disarray. The latter is probably reflective of altered sarcomere formation or stability of the formed sarcomeres in patients with HCM. Even though sarcomeric proteins are expressed to an equal level in the right and the left ventricle, it is intriguing that HCM is almost exclusively a disease of the left ventricle and involvement of the right ventricle is uncommon. Additionally, whereas hypertrophy is compensatory, disarray is the characteristic finding in HCM. Thus, despite a remarkable progress in understanding of the molecular pathogenesis of HCM, many issues and questions remain to be addressed.

MOLECULAR BIOLOGY OF DILATED CARDIOMYOPATHY

Dilated cardiomyopathy (DCM) is the primary cardiac muscle disease that is characterized by ventricular dilatation and decreased systolic function. It is the most common of the cardiomyopathies, accounting for approximately for 60% to 70% of all cardiomyopathies. Idiopathic or inherited forms are classically diagnosed by the presence of decreased left ventricular function, evidenced by a decreased left ventricular ejection fraction of 0.45 or less, left ventricular dilatation, evidenced by left ventricular end systolic diameter of greater than 2.7 cm/m^2 of body surface area, and, more importantly, absence of known causes of myocardial disease (59). The latter is important in that a significant portion of patients with so-called idiopathic dilated cardiomyopathy have known causes (60). Kaspar et al. (60), in a study of 673 referral patients, showed that approximately half of these cases had a known cause of heart failure such as coronary artery disease, myocarditis, and ethanol abuse. However, despite vigorous investigation, no cause was identified in the other half of these cases. Overall, it is estimated that 50% to 70% of DCM cases are idiopathic. The estimated prevalence of idiopathic DCM is approximately 36.5 per 100,000 population and the incidence of DCM is approximately 5 to 8 per 100,000 (61,62). Thus, in The United States alone, approximately 15,000 to 20,000 new cases of idiopathic DCM are identified annually.

Familial Dilated Cardiomyopathy

The familial nature of DCM was first recognized by Battersby and Glenner in 1961 (63). Since then, several reports have documented autosomal dominant, autosomal recessive, and X-linked modes of inheritance (64–66). However, the true incidence of the familial form of DCM remained unknown until recent years. Michels et al. (67), in a landmark prospective study, performed routine echocardiograms on the family members of 59 patients with DCM and showed that approximately 20% of DCM cases were familial. Subsequently, this group extended their study to 95 cases and showed that, in 25% of the cases, DCM was familial (68). An important observation in these studies was that approximately 10% to 20% of apparently healthy relatives of the index cases had significant left ventricular dysfunction on echocardiograms (67). This observation indicates that the true prevalence of familial DCM is higher than that estimated based on the presence of a family history of DCM alone.

Autosomal Dominant Dilated Cardiomyopathy

The most common form of familial DCM is the autosomal dominant form. Progress in the field of molecular genetic and linkage analysis has led to chromosomal mapping of five different responsible genes (69–73). The first locus identified for a familial form of dilated cardiomyopathy was in a large family in which dilated cardiomyopathy was associated with conduction disorder (69). The responsible gene in this family was mapped to the centromeric region of chromosome 1. Our group identified a pure form of familial DCM and, through linkage analysis, showed that the responsible gene was located on the long arm of chromosome 1q32 (70). In addition, loci on chromosomes 3p25, 9q13, and 10q21 have been identified (71–73). The responsible genes and mutations have yet to be identified. It is intriguing to postulate that the same class of genes located on five different chromosomes, as has been the case for HCM and the long QT syndrome, are responsible for DCM.

X-linked Dilated Cardiomyopathy

The molecular genetic basis of X-linked dilated cardiomyopathy has also been studied. The disease predominantly affects male individuals and, to a much lesser degree, female carriers. Two loci on Xp21 and Xq28 for X-linked DCM have been identified (74,75). The responsible gene on Xp21 is the dystrophin gene, which is also involved in Duchenne/Becker muscular dystrophy (74). Towbin et al. (74) showed that a mutation in the 5′ region of the dystrophin gene was responsible for the X-linked DCM. Muntoni et al. (76) showed cardiac-specific involvement in patients with mutation in the 5′ region of the dystrophin gene. Dystrophin is a large cytoskeleton protein that links the structural proteins such as actin to plasmalemma of the membrane through a number of dystrophin-associated proteins (77). Mutation in dystrophin are also responsible for the cases of Duchenne/Becker muscular dystrophy (78). It is generally accepted that this form of X-linked DCM is a form of Duchenne/Becker muscular dystrophy whereby the phenotypic expression of the disease is restricted to the heart. Indeed, cardiac involvement in Duchenne/Becker muscular dystrophy is common and cardiac failure is a common cause of death in these patients (79,80).

DCM is also observed in patients with Barth's syndrome (75). Barth's syndrome is a systemic disease that is associated with DCM, skeletal myopathy, neutropenia, and abnormal mitochondria. The responsible gene was initially mapped to Xq28 and subsequently was identified as the G4.5 gene. However, the function of the G4.5 gene remains unknown.

Dilated Cardiomyopathy and Triplet Repeat Syndromes

DCM also occurs in association with the so-called "triplet repeat" syndromes. These disorders affect primarily the neuromuscular system. The triplet repeat syndromes are due to expansion of the naturally occurring trinucleotide sequences that recur in tandem in the human genome (81). Under normal conditions, the number of triplet sequences repeated in tandem, although variable, seldom exceeds 50. Under pathologic conditions, the number of triplet repeats such as CTG (in myotonic dystrophy), GAA (in Friedreich's ataxia), and CAG (Huntington disease) expands several-fold and in certain disorders, up to 1,000 (81). Expansion of the triplet repeats results in unstable mRNA and is associated with clinical syndromes such as myotonic dystrophy or Friedreich's ataxia. The mechanism whereby expansion of triplet repeats induces mRNA instability is still not clear. This is most notable in syndromes such as myotonic dystrophy in which the triplet repeats are in the 3′ untranslated region of the gene, yet the disease is widespread, affecting multiple organs. Identification of a new family of proteins that specifically bind to the triplet repeats (82) and are responsible for the nucleocytoplasmic transport of the mRNAs containing triplet repeats has provided a new approach to the mechanism responsible for some of these disorders. Myotonic dystrophy is probably the most common form of triplet repeat syndromes and is due to expansion of the CTG repeats in the 3′ untranslated region of the myotonin protein kinase gene located on chromosome 19 (83). Cardiac involvement is common in triplet repeat syndromes and manifests as conduction defects and DCM or HCM. The extent of cardiac involvement correlates with the severity of trinucleotide repeat expansion (84,85).

Cardiac involvement also occurs in Friedreich's ataxia (85). The responsible gene is located on chromosome 19q33 and codes for a protein called frataxin (86). Expansion of the naturally occurring GAA in the frataxin gene results in Friedreich's ataxia. Cardiac involvement manifests as DCM or HCM and is common in this disorder. The severity of cardiac involvement correlates with the extent of triplet repeat expansion (85).

Mitochondrial DNA Mutations and Dilated Cardiomyopathy

Cardiac involvement in mitochondrial disease has been recognized for many years. Mitochondria are independent organisms inside the cell. Mitochondrial DNA are 16-kb circular DNA that replicate independently (87). Mutations commonly occur in mitochondrial DNA and the number of such mutations increases with aging. Mutations in mitochondrial DNA characteristically involve multiple organs such as heart, skeletal muscles, brain, eye, and others, as is the case in Kearne-Sayre syndrome (88). Cardiac involvement manifests as cardiomyopathies, both dilated and hypertrophic, as well as Wolff-Parkinson-White syndrome (89–91). DCM in the absence of other systemic disorders is unlikely to result from the mitochondrial DNA mutations. The principal characteristic of disease resulting from mitochondrial DNA mutations is maternal inheritance. This is due to inheritance of mitochondrial DNA from the ovum.

Metabolic Causes of Dilated Cardiomyopathy

Metabolic disorders such as glycogen storage diseases, mucoploysaccharidoses, and sphingolipidoses, as well as mutations in genes coding for the proteins involved in fatty acid oxidation, could also cause DCM (92). Mutations in medium-chain acyl-CoA dehydrogenase, as well as long-chain acyl-CoA dehydrogenase genes on chromosome 1 and 7, respectively, could lead to deficiency of these enzymes, resulting in DCM (92). Carnitine deficiency resulting from mutations in carnitine transporter or translocater genes impair β-oxidation of fatty acids and could also result in DCM (93). The interesting feature of DCM in this condition is its improvement following therapy with carnitine (94).

Genetic Susceptibility to Dilated Cardiomyopathy and Autoimmunity

The possibility of genetic predisposition to DCM and its phenotypic expression has been raised for many years. An intriguing candidate is the angiotensin-1 converting enzyme (ACE) gene that is known to play a major role in cardiovascular disease and cardiac remodeling (95). Recently, a polymorphism in the ACE gene has been described that is due to presence or absence of a 287-bp repeat sequence in intron 16 (96). This insertion (I)/deletion (D) polymorphism results in three genotypes: II, ID, and DD. The latter is associated with higher plasma levels of ACE and has been implicated in a number of cardiovascular diseases such as coronary artery disease, cardiac hypertrophy, and remodeling (58,97–99). An increased frequency of ACE genotype DD was also observed in patients with DCM (100). However, a subsequent study did not show an association between ACE I/D polymorphism and DCM (101). Given the significance of the ACE gene in modulating cardiac remodeling, it is likely that ACE genotypes could modify the phenotypic expression of familial DCM or DCM following myocardial injury such as myocarditis.

Immunologic factors have also been associated with DCM. Genes located within the major histocompatibility locus on chromosome 6 have also been implicated in predisposition to DCM. An increased frequency of human leukocyte antigens (HLAs) such as DR4 and Dqw4 has been reported in patients with DCM (102,103). Carlquist et al. (102) showed that five of 41 patients with DCM and zero of 53 normal individuals had the DR4-DQw4 haplotype. Another line of evidence that links the HLA class II antigens to autoimmunity in DCM is the presence of association between the HLA antigens and the anti-β receptor antibodies in patients with DCM (104). The latter, anti-β receptor antibodies, have been found more commonly in patients with DCM (104,105). In addition to anti-β receptor antibodies, a number of antibodies against cardiac structural proteins such the MyHC, MLC-1, α-tropomyosin, actin, heat-shock protein-60, and adenine nucleotide translocator have been identified in patients with DCM (106–108). The causality of these antibodies in DCM has not been established. It is likely that antibodies are produced secondarily as a result of the primary injury to the myocardium. The presence of antibodies against cardiac proteins, however, is likely to carry functional significance by impairing myocardial function and energy metabolism. Thus, it is likely that the presence of antibodies against cardiac proteins could influence the severity of the disease and carry prognostic significance. A recent study showed that immunoadsorption of anti–β-receptor antibodies in patients with DCM was associated with an improvement in hemodynamic parameters such as an increase in cardiac output and a decrease in left ventricular filling pressure (109).

REFERENCES

1. Maron BJ, Epstein SE, Roberts WC. Causes of sudden death in competitive athletes. *J Am Coll Cardiol* 1986; 7:204–214.
2. Pelliccia A, Maron BJ, Spataro A, Proschan MA, Spirito P. The upper limits of physiologic cardiac hypertrophy in highly trained elite athletes. *N Engl J Med* 1991;324:295–301.
3. Marian AJ, Roberts R. Recent advances in the molecular genetics of hypertrophic cardiomyopathy. *Circulation* 1995;92:1336–1347.
4. Swynghedauw B. Development and functional adaptation of contractile proteins in cardiac and skeletal muscles. *Physiol Rev* 1986;66:710–771.
5. Mercadier JJ, Bouveret P, Gorza L, et al. Myosin isoenzymes in normal and hypertrophied human ventricular myocardium. *Circ Res* 1983;53:52–62.
6. Katzeff HL, Ojamaa KM, Klein I. Effects of exercise on protein synthesis and myosin heavy chain gene expression in hypothyroid rats. *Am J Physiol* 1994;267: E63–E67.
7. Tate CA, Helgason T, Hyek MF, et al. SERCA2a and mitochondrial cytochromse oxidase expression are increased in hearts of exercise-trained old rats. *Am J Physiol* 1996;271:H68–H72.
8. Bohm M, Dorner H, Htun P, Lensche H, Platt D, Erdmann E. Effects of exercise on myocardial adenylate cyclase and G$_i$a expression in senescence. *Am J Physiol* 1993;264:H805–H814.
9. Orenstein TL, Parker TG, Butany JW, et al. Favorable left ventricular remodeling following large myocardial infarction by exercise training. *J Clin Invest* 1995;96: 858–866.
10. Koistinen H, Koistinen R, Selenius L, Ylikorkala O, Seppala M. Effect of marathon run on serum IGF-I and IGF-binding protein 1 and 3 levels. *J Appl Physiol* 1996;80(3):760–764.
11. Natelson BH, Zhou Z, Ottenweller JE, et al. Effect of acute exhausting exercise on cytokine gene expression in men. *Int J Sports Med* 1996;17:299–302.
12. Shen W, Zhang X, Zhao G, et al. Nitric oxide production and NO synthase gene expression contribute to vascular regulation during exercise. *Med Sci Sports Exerc* 1995;27:1125–1134.
13. Mercadier JJ, Lompre AM, Wisnewsky C, et al. Myosin isoenzyme changes in several models of rat cardiac hypertrophy. *Circ Res* 1981;49:525–532.
14. VanBuren P, Harris DE, Alpert N, Warshaw DM. Cardiac V$_1$ and V$_3$ myosins differ in their hydrolytic and mechanical activities in vitro. *Circ Res* 1995;77: 439–444.
15. Mesnard L, Logeart D, Taviaux S, et al. Human cardiac troponin T: cloning and expression of new isoforms in the normal and failing heart. *Circ Res* 1995;76: 687–692.
16. Anderson PAW, Greig A, Mark TM, et al. Molecular basis of human cardiac troponin T isoforms expressed in the developing, adult, and failing heart. *Circ Res* 1995;76:681–686.
17. Hengstenberg C, Maisch B. Increased nuclear proto-oncogene expression in hypertrophic cardiomyopathy. *Cardioscience* 1993;March 4 (1):15–20.
18. Derchi G, Bellone P, Chiarella F, et al. Plasma levels of atrial natriuretic peptide in hypertrophic cardiomyopathy. *Am J Cardiol* 1992;70:1502–1504.
19. Hasegawa K, Fujiwara H, Doyama K, et al. Ventricular expression of brain natriuretic peptide in hypertrophic cardiomyopathy. *Circulation* 1993;88:372–380.
20. Baker D, Arai M, Matsui H, et al. Regulation of sarcoplasmic reticulum gene expression during cardiac hypertrophy and heart failure. In: Dhalla NS, Pierce GN, Panagia V, Beamish RE, eds. *Heart hypertrophy and failure.* Boston, Kluwer Academic Publishers, 1995:139–154.
21. Kadambi VJ, Ponniah S, Harrer JM, et al. Cardiac-specific overexpression of phospholamban alters calcium kinetics and resultant cardiomyocyte mechanics in transgenic mice. *J Clin Invest* 1996;97:533–539.
22. Hoit BD, Khoury SF, Kranias EG, Ball N, Walsh RA. In vivo echocardiographic detection of enhanced left ventricular function in gene-targeted mice with phospholamban deficiency. *Circ Res* 1995;77:632–637.
23. Thierfelder L, Watkins H, MacRae C, et al. α-Tropomyosin and cardiac troponin T mutations cause familial hypertrophic cardiomyopathy: a disease of the sarcomere. *Cell* 1994;77:701–712.
24. Geisterfer-Lawrance AA, Kass S, Tanigawa G, et al. A molecular basis for familial hypertrophic cardiomyopathy: a β-cardiac myosin heavy chain gene missense mutation. *Cell* 1990;62:999–1006.
25. Watkins H, Conner D, Thierfelder L, et al. Mutations in the cardiac myosin binding protein-C gene on chromosome 11 cause familial hypertrophic cardiomyopathy. *Nat Genet* 1995;11:434–437.
26. Bonne G, Carrier L, Bercovici J, et al. Cardiac myosin binding protein-C gene splice acceptor site mutation is associated with familial hypertrophic cardiomyopathy. *Nat Genet* 1995;11:438–440.
27. Poetter K, Jiang H, Hassanzadeh S, et al. Mutations in either the essential or regulatory light chains of myosin are associated with a rate myopathy in human heart and skeletal muscle. *Nat Genet* 1996;13:63–69.
28. Saez LJ, Gianola KM, McNally EM, et al. Human cardiac myosin heavy chain genes and their linkage in the genome. *Nucl Acid Res* 1987;15:5443–5459.
29. Rayment I, Rypniewski RW, Schmidt-Base K, et al.

Three-dimensional structure of myosin subfragment-1: a molecular motor. *Science* 1993;261:50–58.

30. Lowey S, Waller GS, Trybus KM. Skeletal muscle myosin light chains are essential for physiological speeds of shortening. *Nature* 1993;365:454-456.

31. Rayment I, Holden HM, Whittaker M, et al. Structure of the actin-myosin complex and its implication for muscle contraction. *Science* 1993;261:58–65.

32. Finer JT, Simmons RM, Spudich JA. Single myosin mechanics: picoNewton forces and nanometer steps. *Nature* 1994;368:113–119.

33. Molloy JE, Burns JE, Kendrick-Jones J, Tregaer RT, White DCS. Movement and force produced by a single myosin head. *Nature* 1995;378:209–212.

34. Mesnard L, Samson F, Espinasse I, et al. Molecular cloning and developmental expression of human cardiac troponin T. *FEBS Lett* 1993;328:139–144.

35. Townsend PJ, Farza H, MacGeon C, et al. Human cardiac troponin T: identification of fetal isoforms and assignment of the TNNT2 locus to chromosome 1q. *Genomics* 1994;21:311–316.

36. Yates LD, Greaser ML. Troponin subunit stoichiometry and content in rabbit skeletal muscle and myofibrils. *J Biol Chem* 1983;258:5770–5774.

37. Anderson PAW, Greig A, Mark TM, et al. Troponin T isoform expression in humans. *Circ Res* 1991;69:1226–1233.

38. Farah CS, Reinach FC. The troponin complex and regulation of muscle contraction. *FASEB J* 1995;9:755–767.

39. Freiburg A, Gautel M. A molecular map of the interactions between titin and myosin-binding protein C: implications for sarcomeric assembly in familial hypertrophic cardiomyopathy. *Eur J Biochem* 1996;235:317–323.

40. Carrier L, Bonne G, Bahrend E, et al. Organization and sequence of human cardiac myosin binding protein C gene (MYBPC3) and identification of mutations predicted to produce truncated proteins in familial hypertrophic cardiomyopathy. *Circ Res* 1997;80:427–434.

41. Gautel M, Zuffardi O, Freiburg A, Labeit S. Phosphorylation switches specific for the cardiac isoform of myosin binding protein-C: a modulator of cardiac contraction? *EMBO J* 1995;14(9):1952–1960.

42. Zot AS, Potter JD. Structural aspects of troponin-tropomyosin regulation of skeletal muscle contraction. *Annu Rev Biophys Chem* 1987;16:535–559.

43. Hirzel HO, Tuchsmid CR, Schneider J, Krayenbuehl HP, Schaub MC. Relationship between myosin isoenzyme composition, hemodynamics, and myocardial structure in various forms of human cardiac hypertrophy. *Circ Res* 1985;57:729–740.

44. Whalen RG, Sell SM, Eriksson A, Thornell LE. Myosin subunit types in skeletal and cardiac tissues and their developmental distribution. *Dev Biol* 1982;91:478–484.

45. Morano M, Zacharzowski U, Maier M, et al. Regulation of human heart contractility by essential myosin light chain isoforms. *J Clin Invest* 1996;98(2):467–473.

46. Gulick J, Hewettt TE, Klevitsky R, et al. Transgenic remodeling of the regulatory light chains in the mammalian heart. *Circ Res* 1997;80:655–664.

47. Sweeney HL, Bowmann BF, Stull JT. Myosin light chain phosphorylation in vertebrate striated muscle: regulation and function. *Am J Physiol* 1993;264:C1085–C1095.

48. Tohtong R, Yamashita H, Graham M, et al. Impairment of muscle function caused by mutations of phosphorylation sites in myosin regulatory light chain. *Nature* 1995;374:650–653.

49. Cuda G, Fananapazir L, Zhu W, Sellers JR, Epstein ND: Skeletal muscle expression and abnormal function of beta myosin in hypertrophic cardiomyopathy. *J Clin Invest* 1993;91:2861–2865.

50. Sweeney HL, Straceski AJ, Leinwand LA, Tikunov BA, Faust L. Heterologous expression of a cardiomyopathic myosin that is defective in its actin interaction. *J Biol Chem* 1994;269:1603–1605.

51. Lankford EB, Epstein ND, Fananapazir L, Sweeney HL. Abnormal contractile properties of muscle fibers expressing β-myosin heavy chain gene mutations in patients with hypertrophic cardiomyopathy. *J Clin Invest* 1995;95:1409–1414.

52. Watkins H, Seidman CE, Seidman JG, Feng HS, Sweeney HL. Expression and functional assessment of a truncated cardiac troponin T that causes hypertrophic cardiomyopathy. Evidence for a dominant negative action. *J Clin Invest* 1996;98:2456–2461.

53. Lin D, Bobkova A, Homsher E, Tobacman LS. Altered cardiac troponin T in vitro function in the presence of a mutation implicated in familial hypertrophic cardiomyopathy. *J Clin Invest* 1996;97(12):2842–2848.

54. Marian AJ, Zhao G, Seta Y, Roberts R, Yu Q-T. Expression of a mutant (Arg[92]Gln) human cardiac troponin T, known to cause hypertrophic cardiomyopathy, impairs adult cardiac myocytes contractility. *Circ Res* 1997;81:76–85.

55. Straceski AJ, Geisterfer-Lowrance A, Seidman CE, Seidman JG, Leinwand LA. Functional analysis of myosin missense mutations in familial hypertrophic cardiomyopathy. *Proc Natl Acad Sci USA* 1994;91:589–593.

56. Marian AJ, Yu Q-T, Mann D, Graham F, Roberts R. Expression of the mutation causing hypertrophic cardiomyopathy disrupts sarcomere assembly in adult feline cardiac myocytes. *Circ Res* 1995;77:98–106.

57. Geisterfer-Lowrance AAT, Christe M, Conner DA, et al. A mouse model for familial hypertrophic cardiomyopathy. *Science* 1996;272:731–734.

58. Lechin M, Quinones M, Omran A, et al. Angiotensin 1 converting enzyme genotypes influence the phenotypic expression of hypertrophic cardiomyopathy. *Circulation* 1995;92:1808–1812.

59. WHO/ISFC Task Force. Report of the WHO/ISFC Task Force on the definition and classification of cardiomyopathies. *Br Heart J* 1980;44:672–673.

60. Kasper EK, Agema WRP, Hutchins GM, et al. The causes of dilated cardiomyopathy: a clinicopathologic review of 673 consecutive patients. *J Am Coll Cardiol* 1994;23:586–590.

61. Codd MB, Sugrue DD, Gersh BJ, Melton III LJ. Epidemiology of idiopathic and hypertrophic cardiomyopathy. A population-based study in Olmsted County, Minnesota. *Circulation* 1989;80:564–572.

62. Gillum RF. Idiopathic cardiomyopathy in the United States, 1970–1982. *Am Heart J* 1986;111:752–755.

63. Battersby EJ, Glenner GG. Familial cardiomyopathy. *Am J Med* 1961;30:382–391.

64. Graber HL, Unverferth DV, Baker PB, et al. Evolution

of a hereditary cardiac conduction and muscle disorder: a study involving a family with six generations affected. *Circulation* 1986;74:21–35.

65. Emauel R, Withers R, O'Brien K. Dominant and recessive modes of inheritance in idiopathic cardiomyopathy. *Lancet* 1971;2:1065–1067.

66. Berko BA, Swift M. X-linked dilated cardiomyopathy. *N Engl J Med* 1987;316:1186–1191.

67. Michels VV, Moll PP, Miller FA, et al. The frequency of familial dilated cardiomyopathy in a series of patients with idiopathic dilated cardiomyopathy. *N Engl J Med* 1992;326:77–82.

68. Goerss JB, Michels VV, Burnett J, et al. Frequency of familial dilated cardiomyopathy. *Eur Heart J* 1995; 16[Suppl 0]:2–4.

69. Kass S, MacRae C, Graber HL, et al. A gene defect that causes conduction system disease and dilated cardiomyopathy maps to chromosome 1p1-1q1. *Nat Genet* 1994;7:546–551.

70. Durand J-B, Bachinski LL, Bieling LC, et al. Localization of a gene responsible for familial dilated cardiomyopathy to chromosome 1q32. *Circulation* 1995; 92:3387–3389.

71. Olson TM, Keating MT. Mapping a cardiomyopathy locus to chromosome 3p22-p25. *J Clin Invest* 1996;97: 528–532.

72. Krajinovic M, Pinamonti B, Sinagra G, et al., and the Heart Muscle Disease Study Group. Linkage of familial dilated cardiomyopathy to chromosome 9. *Am J Hum Genet* 1995;57:846–852.

73. Bowles KR, Gajarski R, Porter P, et al. Gene mapping of familial autosomal dominant dilated cardiomyopathy to chromosome 10q21-23. *J Clin Invest* 1996;98: 1355–1360.

74. Towbin JA, Hejtmancik F, Brink P, et al. X-linked dilated cardiomyopathy: molecular genetic evidence of linkage to the Duchenne muscular dystrophy (dystrophin) gene at the Xp21 locus. *Circulation* 1993;87: 1854–1865.

75. Bolhuis PA, Hensels GW, Hulsebos JM, Baas F, Barth PG. Mapping of the locus for X-linked cardioskeletal myopathy with neutropenia and abnormal mitochondria (Barth syndrome) to Xq28. *Am J Hum Genet* 1991;48:481–485.

76. Muntoni F, Wilson L, Marrosu G, et al. A mutation in the dystrophin gene selectively affecting dystrophin expression in the heart. *J Clin Invest* 1995;96:693–699.

77. Ozawa E, Yoshida M, Suzuki A, et al. Dystrophin-associated proteins in muscular dystrophy. *Hum Mol Genet* 1995;4:1711–1716.

78. Matsuno M. Duchenne/Becker muscular dystrophy: from molecular diagnosis to gene therapy. *Brain Dev* 1996;18:167–172.

79. Melacini P, Fanin M, Danieli GA, et al. Myocardial involvement is very frequent among patients affected with subclinical Becker muscular dystrophy. *Circulation* 1996;94:3168–3175.

80. de Kermadec JM, Becane HM, Chenard A, Tertrain F, Weiss Y. Prevalence of left ventricular dysfunction in Duchenne muscular dystrophy: an echocardiographic study. *Am Heart J* 1994;127:618–623.

81. Monckton DG, Caskey CT. Unstable triplet repeat diseases. *Circulation* 1995;91:513–520.

82. Timchenko LT, Miller JW, Timchenko NA, et al. Identification of a $(CUG)_n$ triplet repeat RNA binding protein and its expression in myotonic dystrophy. *Nucl Acids Res* 1996;24:4407–4414.

83. Pizzuti A, Friedman DL, Caskey T. The myotonic dystrophy gene. *Arch Neurol* 1993;50:1173–1179.

84. Tokgozoglu LS, Ashizawa T, Pacifico A, et al. Cardiac involvement in a large kindred with myotonic dystrophy. Quantitative assessment and relation to the size of CTG repeat expansion. *JAMA* 1995;274:813–819.

85. Isnard R, Kalotka H, Durr A, et al. Correlation between left ventricular hypertrophy and GAA trinucleotide repeat length in Friedreich's ataxia. *Circulation* 1997;95:2247–2249.

86. Durr A, Cossee M, Agid Y, et al. Clinical and genetic abnormalities in patients with Friedreich's ataxia. *N Engl J Med* 1996;335:1169–1175.

87. Anderson S, Bankier AT, Barrell BG, et al. Sequence and organization of the human mitochondrial genome. *Nature* 1981;290:457–474.

88. Wallace DC. Diseases of mitochondrial DNA. *Annu Rev Biochem* 1992;61:1175–1212.

89. Remes AM, Hassinen IE, Ikaheimo MJ, et al. Mitochondrial DNA deletions in dilated cardiomyopathy: a clinical study employing endomyocardial sampling. *J Am Coll Cardiol* 1994;23:935–942.

90. Soumalainen A, Paetau A, Leinonen H, et al. Inherited dilated cardiomyopathy with multiple deletions of mitochondrial DNA. *Lancet* 1992;340:1319–1320.

91. Ozawa T, Tanaka M, Sugiyama S, et al. Multiple mitochondrial DNA deletions exist in cardiomyocytes of patients with hypertrophic or dilated cardiomyopathy. *Biochem Biophys Res Commun* 1990;170:830–836.

92. Kelly DP, Strauss AW. Inherited cardiomyopathies. *N Engl J Med* 1994;330:913–919.

93. Stanley CA, Hale DE, Berry GT, et al. A deficiency of carnitine-acylcarnitine translocase in the inner mitochondrial membrane. *N Engl J Med* 1992;327:19–23.

94. Winter S, Jue K, Prochazka J, et al. The role of L-carnitine in pediatric cardiomyopathy. *J Child Neurol* 1995;10:S45–S51.

95. Griendling KK, Murphy TJ, Wayne Alexander R. Molecular biology of the renin-angiotensin system. *Circulation* 1993;87:1816–1828.

96. Rigat B, Hubert C, Alhenc-Gelas F, et al. An insertion/deletion polymorphism in the angiotensin I-converting enzyme gene accounting for half of the variance of serum enzyme levels. *J Clin Invest* 1990;86: 1343–1346.

97. Cambien F, Poirier O, Lecerf L, et al. Deletion polymorphism in the gene for angiotensin-converting enzyme is a potent risk factor for myocardial infarction. *Nature* 1992;359:641–644.

98. Beohar N, Prather A, Yu Q-T, et al. Angiotensin converting enzyme genotype DD is a risk factor for coronary artery disease. *J Invest Med* 1995;43:275–280.

99. Pinto YM, van Gilst WH, Kingma JH, Schunkert H, for the Captopril and Thrombolysis Study Investigators. Deletion-type allele of the angiotensin-converting enzyme gene is associated with progressive ventricular dilatation after anterior myocardial infarction. *J Am Coll Cardiol* 1995;25:1622–1626.

100. Raynolds MV, Bristow MR, Bush EW, et al. Angiotensin-converting enzyme DD genotype in patients with ischaemic or idiopathic dilated cardiomyopathy. *Lancet* 1993;342:1073–1075.

101. Montgomery HE, Keeling PJ, Goldman JH, Humphries

SE, Talmud PJ, McKenna WJ. Lack of association between the insertion/deletion polymorphism of the angiotensin-converting enzyme gene and idiopathic dilated cardiomyopathy. *J Am Coll Cardiol* 1995;25:1627–1631.

102. Carlquist JF, Menlove RL, Murray MB, O'Connell JB, Anderson JL. HLA class II (DR and DQ) antigen associations in idiopathic dilated cardiomyopathy. *Circulation* 1991;83:515–522.
103. Lima CJ, Lima C. HLA antigens in idiopathic dilated cardiomyopathy. *Br Heart J* 1989;62:379–383.
104. Limas C, Limas CJ, Boudoulas H, et al. T-cell receptor gene polymorphisms in familial cardiomyopathy: correlation with anti-β-receptor autoantibodies. *Am Heart J* 1992;124:1258.
105. Limas CJ, Goldberg IF, Limas C. Autoantibodies against β-adrenoreceptor in human idiopathic dilated cardiomyopathy. *Circ Res* 1989;64:97–103.
106. Latif N, Baker CS, Dunn JM, et al. Frequency and specificity of antiheart antibodies in patients with dilated cardiomyopathy detected using SDS-PAGE and Western blotting. *J Am Coll Cardiol* 1993;22:1378–1384.
107. Obrador D, Ballester M, Carrio I, Berna L, Pons-llado G. High prevalence of myocardial monoclonal antimyosin antibody uptake in patients with chronic idiopathic dilated cardiomyopathy. *J Am Coll Cardiol* 1989;13:1289–1293.
108. Schultheiss HP, Bolte HD. Immunological analysis of auto-antibodies against the adenine nucleotide translocator in dilated cardiomyopathy. *J Mol Cell Cardiol* 1985;17:603–617.
109. Dorffel WV, Felix SB, Wallukat G, et al. Short-term hemodynamic effects of immunoadsorption in dilated cardiomyopathy. *Circulation* 1997;95:1994–1997.

The Athlete and Heart Disease:
Diagnosis, Evaluation & Management,
edited by R. A. Williams.
Lippincott Williams & Wilkins, Philadelphia © 1999.

6

The Marfan Syndrome: Implications for Athletes

Gary H. Gibbons

Department of Medicine, Harvard Medical School; Division of Cardiovascular Medicine,
Brigham and Women's Hospital, Boston, Massachusetts 02115

The Marfan syndrome is a heritable disorder of connective tissue with life-threatening manifestations among athletes. At a crudely estimated prevalence of about 1:10,000, it is a not a rare disease relative to other genetic disorders affecting the cardiovascular system. Moreover, it is speculated that the prevalence may be much higher among individuals participating in sports in which tall stature and long limbs are particular assets such as basketball and volleyball. Unlike some genetic disorders, the Marfan syndrome has been observed throughout the world in all races and ethnic groups and affects both genders equally. Given these epidemiologic considerations, the evaluation for Marfan syndrome must be a fundamental component of screening evaluations for individuals involved in competitive athletics.

The diagnosis of Marfan syndrome hinges upon the characteristic constellation of pleiotropic features that principally involve the cardiovascular, ocular, and musculoskeletal systems. A century has passed since Antoine-Bernard Marfan first described the striking musculoskeletal features of the case of a 5-year-old girl with disproportionately long, thin limbs and digits in whom thoracolumbar kyphoscoliosis and an anterior chest deformity later developed. Over the years, subsequent clinical studies recognized the ocular and cardiovascular features of this syndrome. More recent investigations have established the molecular basis of this disease. This chapter focuses on reviewing the pathobiologic basis of Marfan syndrome and its clinical manifestations with an emphasis on the diagnostic approach to detecting this condition in individuals involved in athletics.

PATHOBIOLOGY OF THE MARFAN SYNDROME

Although the molecular basis of Marfan syndrome remained to be defined, clinicians had speculated for many years that the disease reflected a defect in connective tissue structure. Indeed, recent molecular genetic studies have established that Marfan syndrome is caused by abnormalities in the fibrillin-1 gene. These genetic analyses confirmed earlier biochemical and morphologic experiments that indicated an abnormality within the elastic fibers of connective tissue. The clinical manifestations of the disease have come to be understood as an abnormality of elastic tissue structure. Fibrillin is abundantly expressed in the cardiovascular system within valvular and chordal structures in the heart and throughout the elastic components of the aorta. In the ocular system, fibrillin is a major component of the ligaments that hold the lens in place. In the musculoskeletal system and integument, fibrillin is found in cartilage and tendons, and within elastic fibers in the dermis. Thus, the pleiotropic nature of the syndrome reflects the widespread expression of fibrillin and its role in maintaining normal tissue structure.

Fibrillin is a large glycoprotein that is a major constituent of this highly organized, multimeric microfibrillar structure. Elastin, a major protein within the extracellular matrix that confers the elastic properties within tissues, is deposited on the scaffolding provided by the microfibrillar structure. Ultrastructural studies of elastic fibers have documented a perturbation in the structure of these protein complexes in patients with Marfan syndrome. Immunohistochemical analysis of skin obtained from Marfan syndrome patients exhibits marked reductions in fibrillin immunoreactivity as compared to that of normal subjects. Similarly, studies of fibroblasts from patients with Marfan syndrome have demonstrated an impaired capacity to incorporate fibrillin into the extracellular matrix. The impairment in elastic fiber structure may relate to the function of the mutant fibrillin allele as an endogenous inhibitor of normal microfibril assembly. Thus, the interplay between normal and abnormal microfibril proteins may determine the elastic properties of the connective tissue. The degree to which the abnormal microfibril proteins influence the elastic function of the tissue may explain some of the clinical variability of the Marfan syndrome. This working hypothesis implies that abnormalities in proteins within the microfibril structure other than fibrillin could exert a similar deleterious influence on connective tissue properties. Indeed, it is conceivable that the overlap between Marfan syndrome and other connective tissue abnormalities such as annuloaortic ectasia may be related to abnormal interactions between fibrillin and other microfibrillar proteins or mutations of other microfibrillar proteins that also influence elastic properties within certain tissue compartments. Further investigation of this area is likely to yield new insights into the pathogenesis and natural history of Marfan syndrome.

The elastic properties of the aorta appear to be essential to its role as a capacitor that stores the kinetic energy of ejected blood during ventricular systole and discharges this energy during diastole. The lamellar array of elastic fibers within the aorta is fundamental to this "shock absorber" function of this conduit vessel. The elastic fiber structure appears to become established relatively early in life. Indeed, much of the synthesis of elastin and fibrillin occurs in utero and appears to decrease dramatically after birth in animal models. These findings suggest that the elastic properties of the aorta manifest during adolescence and adulthood may reflect processes that occurred early in ontogeny. These observations in animal models are in accord with studies of the elastic properties of the aorta in patients with Marfan syndrome that have documented impaired aortic distensibility in children prior to any changes in overall vessel dimensions or aneurysm formation. Given the role of the aorta as a shock absorber, it can be inferred that an impairment in aortic distensibility may exacerbate the time-dependent "wear and tear" of the aorta that accompanies aging and results in "cystic medial necrosis" and aortic dilation. Thus, the defects in elastic fibers induced by mutations of the fibrillin gene appear to predispose to the principle cardiovascular complications of Marfan syndrome such as aortic aneurysms and dissection.

The precise link between genotype and phenotype in the Marfan syndrome remains to be further defined. A variety of mutations along the fibrillin gene appear to be sufficient to induce the syndrome. One would predict that different mutations would vary in their capacity to perturb elastic fiber structure and function and result in varying clinical manifestations of the disorder. However, the clinical variability within families that share the same mutation is often as striking as the variance between pedigrees with different mutations. Nevertheless, as more biochemical and genetic analyses are performed, it is anticipated that more precise genotype-phenotype correlations will be defined that will facilitate clinical diagnosis and prognostication.

CLINICAL FEATURES

In general, the clinical diagnosis of Marfan syndrome depends upon the fulfillment of at least three of four criteria: (a) a positive family history consistent with autosomal dominant inheritance of a connective tissue disorder, (b) cardiovascular features consistent with Marfan syndrome such as mitral valve prolapse or aortic pathology such as dilation, aneurysm, or dissection, (c) musculoskeletal features such as joint laxity, elongated limbs and digits, scoliosis, or pectus deformity, and (d) ocular manifestations such as lens dislocation.

The presence of various clinical manifestations listed in Table 1 differ in diagnostic sensitivity and specificity. For example, features such as mitral valve prolapse or scoliosis are common abnormalities that are prevalent among individuals without Marfan syndrome. Similarly, it is often difficult to distinguish variants of normal from pathologic abnormalities in the characterization of parameters such as joint laxity. In addition, it is estimated

TABLE 1. *Major physical findings in marfan syndrome*

Cardiovascular
    Ascending aorta dilation
    Aortic dissection
    Aortic regurgitation
    Mitral valve prolapse
    Myxomatous mitral valve
    Abdominal aortic aneurysm
    Peripheral vessel dissection
Ocular
    Ectopia lentis
    Flat cornea
    Elongated ocular globe
    Retinal detachment
    Myopia
Musculoskeletal
    Anterior chest deformity—pectus excavatum or
        pectus carinatum
    Disproportionately long limbs
    Flat feet
    Long, spider-like fingers
    Vertebral column deformity—scoliosis, thoracic
        lordosis, kyphosis
    Tall stature (disproportionate to other family
        members)
    High, narrow, gothic arch–like palate
    Dental crowding, malocclusion
    Joint laxity, hypermobility
Skin and fascia
    Stretch marks (striae)
    Hernias—recurrent, inguinal, incisional, umbilical
Pulmonary
    Spontaneous pneumothorax, apical blebs
Nervous system
    Dural ectasia

that 20% to 30% of cases involve spontaneous mutations and therefore have a negative family history. Moreover, the various manifestations of the syndrome may differ in the time course of expression. Hence, a child with a negative family history yet classical ocular and musculoskeletal features may not meet strict criteria for the diagnosis of Marfan syndrome because significant aortic dilation may not develop until after adolescence.

Clearly, the pleiotropic nature of the genetic defect combined with its clinical variability makes it difficult to create a rigidly consistent yet clinically useful nosologic definition of the syndrome. There is no single, definitive test for Marfan syndrome. In centers that screen large numbers of patients with heritable connective tissue disorders, there are inevitably many cases that remain uncharacterized within a phenotypic spectrum from classical cases of Marfan syndrome to variants of normal. Clinicians should use the criteria as a useful guide without undue rigidity, but recognize the crude and somewhat arbitrary nature of this nosology. It is hoped that the advances in diagnostic technologies coupled with the integration of genetic and biochemical testing will result in refined nosology based on relatively crude clinical criteria alone.

Cardiovascular

Classical natural history studies have documented that the life expectancy of Marfan syndrome patients was cut short by about one-third compared to matched controls. The most common cause of death was related to cardiovascular complications in more than 90% of patients. In general, the major causes of death involved aortic dissection, aortic regurgitation, and congestive heart failure secondary to valvular heart disease. The natural history of the disease has improved dramatically over the past 20 years owing to improvements in early diagnosis as well as advances in medical and surgical therapies.

The presence of fibrillin within the connective tissues of heart valves, chordae, and annulus combined with the mechanical stresses imposed on these structures results in the principal cardiac manifestations of Marfan syndrome. The connective tissue defect promotes the myxomatous, "floppy" nature of the leaflet tissue, elongation of the chordae tendineae, and dilation of the annulus that predisposes to the development of valvular prolapse, potential chordal rupture, and eventual incompetence. Mitral valve prolapse is notable in 50% to 75% of patients with Marfan syndrome. Although many of the features of mitral valve prolapse in Marfan syndrome patients are similar to those of the idiopathic variety, the disorder appears to have a far more malignant course in the context of Marfan syndrome. Deterioration in mitral valve function is often evident in Marfan syndrome patients early in childhood. Mitral valve replacement is the most common indication for cardiac surgery among Marfan syndrome patients in the pediatric population. Moreover, patients with Marfan syndrome are more likely to progress from mild prolapse of the valve to significant regurgitation. In addition, Marfan syndrome patients with mitral valve prolapse exhibit calcification of the annulus, as well as atrial and ventricular dysrhythmias, and they are are at increased risk for development of endocarditis.

During ontogeny, the primordium of the aortic annulus and valve arises from tissues common to the ascending aorta. The elastic properties of this proximal ascending root of the aorta are particularly critical given the biochemical forces imposed by ventricular ejection on this site. Accordingly, fibrillin is expressed throughout the elastic fibrils in this proximal component of the aortic root structure. It is therefore not surprising that thinning of the aortic leaflets, enlargement of the sinuses of Valsalva, dilation of the annulus, and aneurysm formation in the aortic root are prominent clinical manifestations of this genetic defect. These fundamental flaws in root structure have been noted even in affected neonates. Moreover, the intense mechanical stress imposed by the force of ventricular ejection further accelerates the deterioration

of these structures in a time-dependent manner. The connective tissue within these aortic root structures functions as a resilient scaffold that absorbs this mechanical stress yet maintains the integrity of normal tissue architecture. In patients with Marfan syndrome, it is postulated that the mechanical stress imposed on these aortic root structures promotes a "wear and tear" injury that leads to a deterioration of structural integrity. This altered tissue elasticity and loss of structural integrity promote thinning of the aortic leaflets, dilation of the sinuses of Valsalva and aortic annulus, fragmentation of the elastic laminae of the aorta, loss of medial smooth muscle cells within the aorta, and eventual aortic dilation with aneurysm formation and associated aortic regurgitation.

Recent studies suggest that these changes in tissue characteristics are the basis for functional changes such as the decline in vessel distensibility observed using either magnetic resonance imaging or ultrasound techniques. Studies of aortic dilation in Marfan syndrome patients have suggested a process of progressive distal dilation in which prominent sinuses of Valsalva and dilation of the annulus may precede the dilation of more proximal segments of the aortic root. The development of significant aortic regurgitation is often noted when the aortic annulus dilates beyond 4.5 to 5.0 cm. Similarly, the clinical complication of aortic dissection appears to be a function of aortic size. The greatest risk appears to be among patients with aortic dimensions beyond 5.0 cm. However, there are anecdotal reports of dissections in patients with aortic dimensions less than this value. Nevertheless, it is intriguing that among a population at relatively high risk for aortic dissection—pregnant Marfan patients—there is a relatively low incidence of complications among those with aortic dimensions less than 4.0 cm. Taken together, these data indicate that patients with Marfan syndrome are at increased risk for devastating complications such as aortic dissection compared to normal individuals, but that this risk is also a function of the size of the aorta. Aortic dimensions are clearly an important prognostic indicator that should be considered by clinicians in developing a management plan that includes an exercise prescription.

It is postulated that this loss of vessel distensibility initiates a pathologic vicious cycle in which the stiffness of the vessel accentuates the injury imposed by mechanical stress. This vascular injury promotes medial cell death (i.e., "cystic medial necrosis") and fragmentation of the elastic network. This compromise in vessel integrity promotes vessel dilation, aneurysm formation, and dissection. Dilation of the aorta further enhances the mechanical stress in accordance with the Law of Laplace and accelerates the vicious cycle. The increase in heart rate, blood pressure, and force of ventricular contraction that accompany strenuous exercise can further augment the mechanical stress imposed on the aorta. Thus, it is readily apparent why participation in competitive athletics may exacerbate the pathogenesis of aortic disease in these patients. Conversely, it has been hypothesized that reducing the mechanical stress imposed on aortic structures by reducing heart rate and the velocity of ejection by blockade of β-adrenergic receptors in patients with Marfan syndrome should have a salutary effect on the natural history of aortic dilation. Controlled clinical studies indicate that this management strategy significantly reduces the rate of expansion of the aorta in Marfan syndrome patients.

Taken together, these pathobiologic and clinical findings are consistent with the notion that mechanical forces imposed on the aortic root structures are an important etiologic parameter in promoting the clinical complications of Marfan syndrome. Thus, conditions that promote an increase in mechanical stress such as strenuous exercise may play an inciting role in triggering potentially lethal complications such as aortic dissection in Marfan patients who participate in competitive athletics.

Musculoskeletal

As discussed previously, the musculoskeletal features of classical Marfan syndrome are striking. The tall stature (often greater than the 95th percentile) is commonly associated with elongated limbs with a low upper body to lower body ratio (@0.85). The tall stature of these individuals is associated with a relative lack of muscle mass, resulting in a strikingly low weight to height ratio. The arm span may exceed the height by a proportion of 1.03:1.0.

Many patients with Marfan syndrome have a typical facial appearance characterized by a long, narrow skull and small jaw. This cranial structure is associated with a high, narrow "Gothic arch–like" palate and crowding of the dentition with resultant malocclusion. The thorax may be notable for apparent overgrowth of the rib cartilage and a pectus deformity—either concave or convex in shape. Scoliosis of the spine also is observed in many patients. In addition to these musculoskeletal features notable on physical examination, radiographic tests may also reveal protrusio acetabuli and spinal column changes related to dural ectasia. Research studies suggest that the bone density of patients with Marfan syndrome may be deficient. The maintenance of muscle bulk and tone, joint range of motion, and skeletal integrity over the long term may depend in part on an exercise prescription that balances the risks of strenuous exertion with fitness and sustained well-being.

The elongated, "spider-like" digits (arachnodactyly) is a particularly striking feature first noted by Antoine Marfan. A useful clinical marker is the positive wrist sign in which the combination of long digits and a thin wrist enables many of these patients to overlap the digits when the wrist is encircled by the fifth digit and thumb of the opposing hand. Although hand radiographs were proposed as a diagnostic modality, precise nomograms based on digit length have yet to be developed that are either sensitive or specific enough to provide data that warrant the radiation exposure.

The elongation of the limbs is typically associated with increased laxity of the joints. The phalanges, elbows, and knees may readily hyperextend beyond 180 degrees. Many patients are able to create a fist in which the thumb rests between the fingers and the palm yet protrudes beyond the ulnar aspect of the hand. This bedside test—a positive thumb sign—is a useful clinical marker of increased laxity within the hand joints. Similarly, the feet are often characterized by hammer toes and a flat arch resulting from digit elongation and joint laxity. In some individuals, the joint laxity predisposes to joint dislocation.

Ocular

Most of the characteristic features of the eye in Marfan syndrome are readily appreciated with optimal pupillary dilation and slit-lamp examination. One of the more definitive features of the disorder involves lens dislocation (ectopia lentis). However, a substantial proportion (perhaps 50%) do not have this manifestation. Nevertheless, a trained ophthalmologist with particular expertise in evaluating Marfan syndrome patients may detect more subtle features in the absence of frank lens dislocation. In its most readily apparent form, ectopia lentis may be detected by routine physical examination by assessing iridodonesis in which the iris of the eye flutters or shimmers like a shiny curtain when the eye accommodates. In addition, the shape of the cornea appears flatter, and overall the globe of the eye is more elongated in Marfan patients. Marfan patients are at risk of retinal detachment, particularly after intraocular surgery. This risk is a significant concern in individuals participating in athletics in which there is a potential for head trauma. The myopia often found in Marfan syndrome is due in part to the elongation of the globe of the eye and can often be corrected toward normal visual acuity with appropriate diagnosis and treatment.

Miscellaneous Features

In addition to the classical features involving the cardiovascular, musculoskeletal, and ocular systems, the Marfan syndrome affects several other body systems of significance. The protean manifestations of the Marfan syndrome are not surprising given the expression of fibrillin in the connective tissue underlying the skin and in fascial tissues of various structures. One of the most readily apparent manifestations is seen in the skin. Many patients with Marfan syndrome exhibit an alteration in skin texture that may relate to a thinner skin architecture, less subcutaneous fat, and a mild increase in elasticity. However, the presence of "stretch marks" in subjects who have never experienced substantial cycles of weight gain and loss is probably the most notable cutaneous feature of the Marfan syndrome. These striae are typically observed in areas of mechanical stress around the buttocks, shoulders, thighs, and abdomen. These cutaneous changes appear to be related to the loss of tissue integrity induced by relatively normal levels of mechanical stress imposed on the skin in these areas. Although wound healing is grossly intact, the surgical scars of these individuals often lack the taut appearance of normal subjects and may tend to stretch and spread over time without frank dehiscence.

Another malady among Marfan patients is the development of hernias. Similar to other clinical features, the manifestations of the syndrome in the fascia appear to reflect a deterioration in the integrity of the connective tissue. This may be of relevance to individuals involved in activities that involve dramatic changes in thoracic or intraabdominal pressures such as physical exercise. The process can be bilateral and may necessitate more aggressive surgical buttressing approaches to ensure effective prevention of recurrence. The weakness of tissue fascia may also relate to an abnormality that affects the nervous system. A common feature of the Marfan syndrome is the finding of aural ectasia. This appears to relate to a weakness in connective tissue that renders the dura ectatic, perhaps related to an inability to withstand the distending forces of the cerebrospinal fluid. In many cases, this is an incidental finding observed during computerized tomographic scanning or magnetic resonance imaging of the spine. However, in certain cases, this may present as a neurologic problem resulting from impingement of the dural sac on nerves or as a more subtle presentation as part of a pelvic pain syndrome.

Although not as common as cardiac or ocular features, patients with Marfan syndrome may also have problems related to the respiratory system. Perhaps one of the most important complications is the apparent predisposition to pneumothorax. These episodes appear to be related to a high density of apical blebs in these patients. The natural history is often more malignant with a high rate of spontaneous recurrence and a relatively low rate of spontaneous resolution without surgical interventions. In general, Marfan syndrome patients may require bilateral clipping of the blebs to avoid repeated episodes. Although Marfan syndrome patients appear to have a higher prevalence of pneumothoraces than the general population, this feature of the syndrome may not be directly related to a fibrillin defect within the lung parenchymal tissue. It is likely that this increased propensity is more directly related to the typical marfanoid habitus and the thin, elongated shape of the thorax. Other features of the syndrome such as pectus deformity and scoliosis may also have an indirect affect on the respiratory status. Similarly, the marfanoid facies in which the long thin face is coupled with the high-arched palate and lax fascial tissue of the upper airway can predispose to obstructive sleep apnea in a strikingly large proportion of patients with this disorder. Although there is little evidence of parenchymal disease in the lung, a number of features of the Marfan syndrome can compromise the respiratory system.

Taken together, the process of screening individuals for the Marfan syndrome must consider its pleiotropic nature in affecting various systems throughout the body. The comprehensive and definitive evaluation of these patients often entails a detailed analysis by an experienced clinical team with expertise in genetics, the diagnosis and evaluation of cardiovascular disease, and ophthalmology.

DIAGNOSTIC APPROACH

The evaluation of the patient with Marfan syndrome is fundamentally no different from the careful examination of any patient by a skilled and experienced clinician. One of the challenges is that, with a prevalence of 1:10,000 patients, it is likely that many physicians will practice for many years and not see a case. Nevertheless, it is also likely that no clinician would miss the striking features of a textbook case of Marfan syndrome. However, one of the intriguing aspects of this genetic disorder is its clinical variability. Although many patients can be identified in a crowd from across the room, other Marfan patients fail to fit the textbook picture and blend in imperceptibly with normal subjects. These are the individuals who fail to be diagnosed until after the aortic dissection or who die suddenly during an athletic event, such as in the case of Olympic volleyball star Flo Hyman.

The overall clinical approach to screening individuals for Marfan syndrome must be integrated with an understanding of the differential diagnosis of connective tissue disorders and other diseases that overlap with the manifestations of the Marfan syndrome (Table 2). In evaluating athletes as part of a general screening examination, one of the challenges is to define which individuals should be referred for more detailed diagnostic workup. No strict criteria exist for selecting these individuals. In the final analysis, this decision must be based on good clinical judgment derived from understanding the manifestations of Marfan syndrome, the differential diagnosis with other pathologic conditions, and the recognition that there is a spectrum of manifestations with variations of normal. The decision must be based

TABLE 2. *Differential diagnosis*

Homocysteinuria
Stickler syndrome
Ehlers-Danlos syndrome
Weill-Marchesani syndrome
Familial annuloaortic ectasia
Familial aortic dissection
Familial mitral valve prolapse
Takayasu's aortitis
Ankylosing spondylitis
Turner syndrome
Klinefelter syndrome
Beal's syndrome
Bicuspid aortic valve
Normal variant

on weighing the relative risk of competitive athletics in patients with connective tissue disorders versus cost effectiveness of extensive workups for relatively rare entities. As in many cases in clinical medicine, the most cost-effective strategy depends on the capacity of the clinician to use the clinical history and physical examination to identify normal subjects and to focus the more extensive workups on individuals who exhibit features compatible with a connective tissue disorder who are at high risk for sudden death induced by participation in competitive athletics.

In the general athletic screening process, any family history of an aortic aneurysm, dissection, rupture, or unexplained sudden death should warrant thorough investigation. In general, the analysis of any heritable connective tissue disorder is based on the construction of a detailed pedigree. This is useful in establishing the heritable nature of the condition and defining whether the condition follows a pattern consistent with an autosomal dominant genetic disorder such as Marfan syndrome as opposed to a recessive disorder such as homocysteinuria. My colleagues and I make it routine to analyze a family as a whole as a component of the evaluation of patients with a suspected connective tissue disorder. In some cases, the search for diagnostic features in a family member may be critical in firmly establishing the diagnosis in a proband. It is our routine to collect medical records and autopsy data to confirm the cause of death in deceased members of the family tree. Moreover, obtaining pictures of deceased family members is helpful as a means of further establishing the inheritance of certain morphologic features that may be diagnostic in retrospect. In addition to establishing the pattern of inheritance of certain traits, the history is also a means of obtaining information about the intellectual capacity of the patient that may help define features such as the retardation noted in some patients with homocysteinuria or Stickler syndrome. Similarly, a detailed past medical history may also help with distinctions from other disorders in the differential diagnosis such as Turner's syndrome. Finally,

a careful review of systems enables the clinician to gain insight into the manifestations of the Marfan syndrome that affect the patient such as the ocular, cutaneous, musculoskeletal, respiratory, and cardiac-related symptoms and signs.

In the physical examination, the facial features and elongated limbs often form a general gestalt that may be highly suggestive of the diagnosis. It is our practice to perform careful measurements of height, weight, and the span of digits and limbs as part of a detailed morphologic analysis. In children, tracking changes in these parameters may be particularly helpful in more equivocal cases in which changes may become more prominent with growth spurts. In adults, a careful morphologic analysis may be useful in the compilation of "the weight of evidence" in which the sum of many subtle signs may become highly suggestive of the diagnosis rather than the detection of a few striking features. It is hoped that the creation of detailed databases based on these morphologic analyses at centers that focus on patients with connective tissue disorders may foster the refinement of more objective criteria that are clinically useful for making the diagnosis.

As discussed previously, a detailed examination from head to toe is a critical aspect of the diagnostic approach. Changes in skin texture are a prominent feature of many forms of connective tissue disorders. Connective tissue disorders involving abnormal collagen structure such as the various subcategories of the Ehlers-Danlos syndromes may be manifest as soft, thin, nearly translucent skin with prominent veins and hypertrophic scars. Similarly, defects in collagen can also affect the elasticity of the skin. Although the differences in skin texture between the various connective tissue disorders may be subtle to detect, the presence of the striae of the Marfan syndrome is a more obvious and useful clinical sign. An athlete undergoing evaluation who exhibits a variance in skin texture in addition to suggestive morphologic features should be considered for more detailed assessment beyond the general screening examination.

As previously discussed, the structure of the face and palate are important points of the examination. In addition, it is useful to distinguish Marfan syndrome from other disorders that may influence the cartilage of the ears, such as those that promote floppiness, or involve a cleft in the palate as well as a high arch. Although the detection of iridodenesis can be performed at the bedside, it is of paramount importance that a dilated slit-lamp examination be performed by an experienced ophthalmologist who is knowledgeable about the Marfan syndrome in cases that raise the suspicion of a connective tissue disorder after the general screening examination. It is important to recognize that, although early onset myopia may be seen in many patients with Marfan syndrome, normal visual acuity does not exclude the possibility of more subtle ocular manifestations. In some cases, subtle changes such as furrowing can be seen before signs such as iridodenesis become manifest. Moreover, a careful examination by an experienced ophthalmologist can be helpful in the differential diagnosis by distinguishing the ocular manifestations of homocysteinuria from the Marfan syndrome. In short, if the Marfan syndrome is suspected based on cardiac or musculoskeletal features in a screening examination, the absence of ocular manifestations based on bedside assessment is inadequate for ruling out the diagnosis.

Careful assessment of the thorax is an important aspect of the screening examination. The finding of a pectus abnormality—either carinatum or excavatum—raises the suspicion of a potential connective tissue disorder. In some cases, patients with Marfan syndrome exhibit a more subtle elongation of rib cartilage with a perturbation in thorax structure without a definitive pectus deformation. Similarly, the thorax and spine examinations reveal scoliosis in many patients with the Marfan syndrome.

The physical examination of the heart is a central feature of the screening procedure and should involve careful inspection and palpation as well as auscultation. In particular, evaluation for aortic or mitral valve sounds consistent with valve incompetence or prolapse is critically important in defining lesions consistent with the Marfan syndrome. In addition, the cardiovascular examination of the thorax must be coupled with careful assessment of the peripheral pulses and blood pressure measurements in the limbs. These peripheral components of the examination may complement the assessment of the associated changes induced by aortic dissection or aortic valve incompetence consistent with Marfan syndrome or other entities in the differential diagnosis such as Takayasu's aortitis or congenital coarctation of the aorta with associated bicuspid aortic valve. In young individuals, it may be useful to use provocative maneuvers to facilitate auscultation of mitral valve prolapse. Some young individuals may exhibit another apparent syndrome in which there is a high co-incidence of pectus abnormality or joint laxity with mitral valve prolapse. These individuals may be difficult to distinguish from patients with definitive Marfan syndrome and warrant more extensive evaluations. The abdominal and pelvic examination should include a close assessment for hernias consistent with a connective tissue abnormality.

Overall, a careful history and physical examination should successfully identify the majority of individuals who are either at low or high probability for having a connective tissue disorder that confers an increased risk of death. Further workup with echocardiography or referral for ophthalmologic evaluation and consultation with a geneticist should be considered for those with (a) high probability of a connective tissue disorder such as Marfan syndrome based on examination or (b) equivocal findings in which the risk of competitive athletics is deemed high.

ACKNOWLEDGMENTS

I am deeply indebted to my former colleagues and patients at the Stanford University Center for Marfan Syndrome and Related Connective Tissue Disorders who taught me so much about this spectrum of disorders. This chapter would not have been possible without the great contributions of the doyens of Marfan syndrome—Reed Pyeritz and Victor McKusick.

SUGGESTED READING

Dietz HC, Cutting GR, Pyeritz RE, et al. Marfan syndrome caused by a recurrent de novo missense mutation in the fibrillin gene. *Nature* 1991;352:337–339.

Glesby MJ, Pyeritz RE. Association of mitral valve prolapse and systemic abnormalities of connective tissue. A phenotypic continuum. *JAMA* 1989;262(4):523–528.

Graham TP Jr, Bricker JT, James FW, Strong WB. 26th Bethesda Conference: Recommendations for determining eligibility for competition in athletes with cardiovascular abnormalities. Task Force 1: congenital heart disease. *J Am Coll Cardiol* 1994;24(4):867–873.

Hirst AE Jr, Gore I. Marfan's syndrome: a review. *Prog Cardiovasc Dis* 1973;16:187–198.

Jeresaty RM. Mitral valve prolapse: definition and implications in athletes. *J Am Coll Cardiol* 1986;7(1):231–236.

Pereira L, Levran O, Ramirez F, et al. A molecular approach to the stratification of cardiovascular risk in families with Marfan's syndrome. *N Engl J Med* 1994;331(3):148–153.

Pyeritz RE, McKusick VA. The Marfan syndrome: diagnosis and management. *N Engl J Med* 1979;300(14):772–777.

Pyeritz RE, Wappel MA. Mitral valve dysfunction in the Marfan syndrome. Clinical and echocardiographic study of prevalence and natural history. *Am J Med* 1983;74(5):797–807.

Tilstra DJ, Byers PH. Molecular basis of hereditary disorders of connective tissue. *Annu Rev Med* 1994;45:149–163.

The Athlete and Heart Disease:
Diagnosis, Evaluation & Management,
edited by R. A. Williams.
Lippincott Williams & Wilkins, Philadelphia © 1999.

7

The Adult Athlete with Congenital Heart Disease

Steven D. Colan

Department of Pediatrics, Harvard Medical School; Cardiac Noninvasive Laboratory,
Children's Hospital, Boston, Massachusetts 02115

Athletic participation is, to a large degree, the ultimate test of the adequacy of the cardiovascular system. As a result, the effort to detect heart disease in athletes is often well out of proportion to the frequency with which it is found. Congenital heart disease is rare in the adult athlete, both because of a low incidence in the general population and because many of these lesions, either with or without surgery, interfere with high-level exercise performance. The challenge to the clinician is to understand which of these disorders are compatible with extreme exertion and to design a cost-effective approach to their recognition and management. It is desirable to identify these individuals for several reasons. Sudden death during athletic participation is often the cardinal consideration in advising individuals with known or occult heart disease about participation in sports. This risk must be carefully weighed against the known benefits of regular exercise participation. In addition, in many patients with congenital cardiac malformations, exercise capacity can be considerably improved by interventions that reduce the hemodynamic load. Most cardiac procedures have been associated with a rapidly diminishing risk as experience is gained and methods improve. Patients with certain lesions, which are symptom-free at rest and which do not limit longevity but which do limit peak exercise capacity, may derive suffi-

cient improvement in their quality of life that a low-risk procedure with the primary goal of improving athletic performance is justified. In addition to the potential risks and benefits associated with regular exercise participation for all individuals, the issues that usually arise in advising the patient with congenital heart disease include assessing the additional risks of syncope and sudden death, the potential for myocardial injury secondary to exercise, the impact of the particular form of heart disease on maximal exercise performance, and whether therapies exist that may improve hemodynamic status and thereby enhance exercise performance. This review addresses these issues for those forms of congenital heart disease that are likely to be encountered in the adult athlete.

The types of congenital heart disease found in the adult athlete fall into several general categories (Table 1). Certain disorders may go unrecognized until adulthood. In part because of the subtle manifestations that can be associated with these diseases, these forms of occult heart disease include several of the most frequent causes of sudden, unexpected death during exercise. There are also a number of lesions such as valvar stenosis that may or may not have had previous interventions. In these instances, the severity of the physiologic abnormalities is the major determinant of whether intense athletic participation is possi-

TABLE 1. *Categories of congenital heart disease in the adult athlete*

Primary diagnoses
  Bicuspid aortic valve with mild stenosis or regurgitation
  Atrial septal defect
  Coarctation
  Dilated aortic root or ascending aorta
  Hypertrophic cardiomyopathy
  Familial dilated cardiomyopathy
  Right ventricular cardiomyopathy (arrythmogenic right ventricular dysplasia)
  Coronary artery anomalies
Unrepaired but previously diagnosed
  Valvar or subvalvar aortic stenosis
  Dilated aortic root or ascending aorta
  Aortic regurgitation
  Pulmonary stenosis
  Long QT syndrome
  Supraventricular tachycardia
Previously diagnosed and repaired
  Bicuspid aortic valve with residual stenosis or regurgitation
  Coarctation
  Tetralogy of Fallot
  Transposition of the great arteries
  Ventricular or atrial septal defect
  Totally anomalous pulmonary venous connection
  Pulmonary stenosis

---

ble. Finally, certain defects invariably have been previously recognized and surgically repaired. Table 1 does not include all forms of congenital heart disease because, in many instances, persistent physiologic abnormalities even after repair preclude high-level participation, even though moderate exercise may still be possible [e.g., in patients who have undergone right ventricular bypass type of surgery (the various modifications of the Fontan procedure)]. Numerous studies have documented a stable but reduced exercise capacity in these patients (1–4). The physiologic explanations for this are instructive of how cardiac performance can limit exercise performance, but it would be unusual to encounter an adult athlete with this type of heart disease. It is a testament to the continuing improvement in the surgery for many of these lesions that some conditions such as tetralogy of Fallot, which have previously been associated with limited exercise capacity (5), are no longer assumed to be invariably prohibitive of athletic success. Because of this, postopera-

tive patients comprise the most rapidly expanding population of adult athletes with congenital cardiac malformations. Because of the rapid rate of improvements and relatively short history of this degree of surgical success, these are also the patients for whom the least amount of relevant information is available. Certain surgical methods that represent a radical departure from earlier practice, such as the arterial switch operation for transposition of the great arteries (6), have become standard of care, but they are of such recent vintage that no patients have yet aged to adulthood.

PHYSIOLOGIC RESPONSE TO EXERCISE

Understanding of the normal physiologic response to exercise is particularly important in predicting the response of the diseased heart. The most fundamental cardiovascular response to exercise is an increase in cardiac output. Heart rate increases early in exercise and continues to increase linearly with respect to oxygen consumption until peak oxygen consumption is achieved (7,8). Initially, the predominant mechanism of cardioacceleration is vagal withdrawal, with sympathetic activity dominating during more intense exercise (9). During upright exercise, there is a 20% to 30% increase in stroke volume resulting from an increase in end-diastolic volume and a decrease in end-systolic volume (10–12). With supine exercise, the change in end-diastolic volume is attenuated or absent, resulting in little or no change in stroke volume, for both the left and the right ventricle (13). Thus, preload augmentation (Frank-Starling mechanism) plays a role in upright but not in supine exercise. The change in end-systolic volume reflects an increase in contractility caused by augmented sympathetic nerve activity and circulating catecholamines (11,12,14).

The net change in cardiac output is determined by the changes in heart rate and stroke volume; there may be as much as a fourfold to fivefold increase in trained individuals during exercise (from 5 to 25 L/minute). Because the ability of stroke volume to increase in response to increasing demand is so limited, rate increase is the principal mechanism of increasing systemic flow, accounting for 75% to 80% of the increase in cardiac output during upright exercise and 95% to 100% of the change during supine exercise. The dependence of exercise capacity on the ability to increase heart rate is exemplified by the age-associated decrease in the maximal attainable heart rate, which fully accounts for the age-related decrease in maximal cardiac output and maximal oxygen consumption (15,16). Impaired chronotropic competence is often the major factor limiting exercise capacity in patients after repair of congenital heart disease.

Simultaneous with muscle contraction, local metabolites induce dilation of the small (resistance) blood vessels. The increase in regional flow is proportional to the force of the local muscle contraction, a process which is predominantly under local control because it is not altered by sympathectomy. Despite vascular dilatation, flow is phasic as a result of the mechanical impedance imposed by muscular contraction, with the amplitude of the flow oscillations proportional to the strength of the muscular contraction (17). Overall, there is a net decrease in systemic vascular resistance, but the increase in flow is out of proportion to the decrease in resistance, causing blood pressure to increase. There is typically a 50% increase in systolic pressure with only a small or no increase in diastolic pressure (8). Functionally, this increase in pressure is necessary to provide an adequate driving force during the flow intervals and, therefore, is correspondingly greater when the flow interval is reduced at peak dynamic exercise and during the sustained contractions typical of isometric exercise.

Neurohumoral Changes

The autonomic nervous system acts to coordinate the systemic resistance and capacitance of vessels with changes in cardiac output demand. Failure of this system results in severe limitation of exercise because there is an inadequate increase in blood pressure, as is seen in patients with idiopathic orthostatic hypotension (18). Central neural mechanisms, along with reflex mechanisms involving skeletal muscle mechanoreceptors, are responsible for initiating the cardiovascular response to exercise. During exercise, vasodilation owing to local mechanisms in some regional beds must be balanced by centrally mediated vasoconstriction of other vascular beds to maintain adequate perfusion pressure. As exercise progresses, the need for dissipation of heat increases, eliciting cutaneous vasodilation, which is similarly balanced by centrally mediated regional vasoconstriction. Also, there is a powerful systemic neurohumoral response with tenfold increases in norepinephrine and epinephrine in plasma as well as smaller increases in renin activity and arginine vasopressin levels (14,19–21). It is believed that these neurohumoral factors contribute to the enhancement of myocardial contractility and improved delivery of blood to working muscle and heart, although this has not been proved. The net beneficial (19) or detrimental (22) impact of the neurohumoral response is an issue of some importance because many of the agents used in the therapy of heart disease (β-adrenergic blockers, angiotensin converting enzyme inhibitors, direct vasodilators) impede these control mechanisms.

Myocardial Oxygen Consumption

Cardiac response to exercise involves changes in preload (i.e., an increase in end-diastolic volume, as is seen with upright exercise), afterload (the force resisting muscle shortening, which increases because of the increase in blood pressure), contractility (in response to the rise in catecholamines), and heart rate. With increased heart rate and contractility, the velocity of contraction is more rapid, and systolic ejection time is shortened. The decrease in systolic time is proportional to the square root of the R-R interval; therefore, there is a proportionately greater decrease in diastolic time, resulting in a decrease in diastolic coronary perfusion time. This effect is particularly large in patients with abnormal ventricular conduction, a common problem in patients after repair of congenital heart disease, because prolongation of systolic activation further reduces the percent of time available for diastole. The compensating mechanisms that serve to maintain myocardial perfusion include coronary vasodilation ("coronary reserve") and the increase in arterial driving pressure. The demand side of this supply-demand equation is represented by the myocardial oxygen consumption, which depends on heart rate, the force of contraction (total systolic wall stress), and myocardial contractility (23). Wall stress, in turn, is directly dependent on intracavitary dimensions and pressure and inversely dependent on wall thickness (24). Because of the increase in diastolic volume and arterial blood pressure during exercise, wall stress increases dramatically. Thus, all the determinants of myocardial oxygen consumption (wall stress, heart rate, and contractility) are greatly increased during exercise. Two of the contributing factors (pressure and heart rate) are routinely measured during exercise testing, and their product (pressure × heart rate) provides a good estimate of the change in myocardial oxygen consumption during exercise (25). When arterial oxygen content is normal, coronary blood flow must increase from about 60 mL/100 g at rest to about 240 mL/100 g at peak exercise (26). These flow rates can be attained in the normal individual during progressive exercise, but there is some evidence that myocardial ischemia may develop in normal individuals involved in sudden, high-intensity exercise (27–29). This suggests that the healthy myocardial vasculature is capable of adapting to the high levels of coronary flow during vigorous exercise, but this adaptation may not occur rapidly enough to prevent ischemia during bursts of intense exercise.

Exercise-Induced Myocardial Dysfunction

There have been reports by several different groups of reduced ventricular function or contractility after intense and prolonged exercise (30–36). Impaired diastolic function after strenuous exertion has also been described (32,37). These findings are difficult to interpret because of the reduced state of hydration and electrolyte abnormalities that are typical after extreme exertion. Certainly the altered pattern of filling in this situation could well be entirely secondary to preload reduction. Nevertheless, the uncertain mechanisms and significance of these findings are intriguing. In pathologic hypertrophy, subendocardial ischemia is an important mechanism of exercise-induced myocardial dysfunction (38). However, there is abundant evidence to suggest that this mechanism is not operant in physiologic hypertrophy. A more compelling possibility has been suggested by the observed adverse impact of prolonged elevation in wall stress and myocardial oxygen consumption on the heart (39). Several reports suggest that prolonged exercise is associated with evidence of depleted cardiac antioxidant reserve (40,41) and augmentation of lipid peroxidation (40,42), an effect that is reduced by training (43) and by provision of antioxidants such as vitamin E (44,45) and coenzyme Q_{10} (46). Although little can be concluded from these early reports, this is a fascinating area of inquiry, particularly because of the possibility that dietary modification could play a modulating role.

Exercise Response of the Pulmonary Circulation

Table 2 lists cardiovascular parameters obtained in a group of normal volunteers during exercise. In both the systemic and pulmonary circulations, there is an increase in pressure with a decrease in resistance. Although the absolute increase in pulmonary pressure is small, the proportional increase is twice that of the systemic circulation (100% versus 40%). Because ventricular work is determined by the pressure-flow product, there is an overall 144% increase in right ventricular work compared with a 25% increase in left ventricular work during cardiovascular adaptation to this level of exercise. This excess demand on the

TABLE 2. *Systemic and pulmonary hemodynamic changes in response to exercise in 12 normal men*

	HR	CI	MAP	SVR	LVSWI	MPP	PVR	RVSWI
Rest	85	4.0	86	1640	59	15	260	9
Exercise	150	8.0	105	970	74	30	215	22
% change	76%	100%	41%	−40%	25%	100%	−17%	144%

HR, heart rate; CI, cardiac index; MAP, mean arterial pressure; SVR, systemic vascular resistance; LVSWI, left ventricular stroke work index; MPP, mean pulmonary pressure; PVR, pulmonary vascular resistance; RVSWI, right ventricular stroke work index.

right ventricle is demonstrated in chronically exercised animals in whom right ventricular hypertrophy exceeds that of the left ventricle (47). Thus, one would anticipate that the status of the right ventricle might be of particular importance with respect to exercise capacity. Indeed, right ventricular, but not left ventricular, function correlates with exercise capacity (48). This difference between the two circulations is of particular importance in subjects with congenital heart disease, in whom right ventricular overload is more common, than in subjects with acquired heart disease. Thus, in subjects who have undergone a right ventricular bypass procedure (Fontan operation), it is unlikely that a doubling of pulmonary pressures could be attained during exercise, thereby inherently limiting the potential increase in cardiac output. Further complicating this issue for subjects with congenital heart disease is the observation that, in the presence of pulmonary hypertension, the increase in pulmonary pressure during exercise is excessive, further augmenting the exercise burden of the pulmonary ventricle (49,50).

PHYSIOLOGIC HYPERTROPHY: CARDIAC EFFECTS OF CHRONIC EXERCISE PARTICIPATION

Cardiovascular adaptation to regular, intense exercise has been studied by many investigators. Frequent participation in aerobic exercise (isotonic) results in higher $\dot{V}O_{2\ max}$, higher anaerobic threshold, reduced heart rate, and a reduced blood pressure response to any given level of exercise, thereby reducing myocardial oxygen consumption for equivalent workload.

The preponderance of data is consistent with the understanding that left ventricular mass and volume are increased in athletes, even when adjusted for body size, although the magnitude of increase is rarely beyond what would be considered the upper limits of normal (51). Thus, the range of left ventricular mass and volume values in athletes is clustered at the high end of the normal range but does not represent a distinct group. When control and athlete groups are of comparable body mass or when volume and mass are appropriately normalized for body size, ventricular dimension and mass are higher in subjects who participate in endurance sports such as running, cycling, soccer, or swimming (52,53), usually by 35% to 45%. When adjusted for body size, weight lifters have normal left ventricular volume with a 30% to 70% increase in ventricular mass (52,54,55). Other "isometric" or strength activities such as wrestling are also associated with increased ventricular mass of nearly 50%, even though ventricular volume and body mass may not be increased (56). This difference in the pattern of hypertrophy in response to the type of exercise has been noted by many authors, with a pattern of commensurate increase in left ventricular mass and volume with a normal mass to volume ratio in athletes who participate in predominantly endurance-type exercise such as running (52), in contrast to a pattern of selective elevation of left ventricular mass and a secondary increase in the mass to volume ratio in athletes who participate in predominantly strength-type exercise such as weight lifting. The range for the reported mean thickness to dimension ratio in strength-type athletes is 0.25 to 0.28 (52,54,56) (normal is approximately 0.18) (52). Athletes whose training includes both types of exercise such as swimmers (52) and triathletes (57) typically have an intermediate pattern of hypertrophy. Studies performed in female athletes (53,58) have reported a quantitatively smaller but qualitatively similar response to that which has been noted in male athletes. Cardiovascular changes in older athletes are similar (59), but a higher blood pressure response to exercise has been associated with a greater magnitude of ventricular hypertrophy (60).

Control of Cardiac Hypertrophy

The mechanism for the structural alterations seen with chronic exercise participation is believed to be direct load-induced hypertrophy. It has been shown that mechanical load is a sufficient and perhaps primary factor responsible for growth regulation in adult mammalian myocardium (61,62). Load induction of growth appears to be mediated by regulation of gene expression in response to the direct physical effects of cellular stress and strain. The pattern of growth (Fig. 1) can be conceptually divided into addition of myofibrils in series (increase in chamber volume) and in parallel (increase in wall thickness) (63). In this paradigm, the stimulus for series growth appears to be preload (diastolic fiber length), whereas the stimulus for parallel growth appears to be afterload (systolic wall stress). These stimuli function as servo

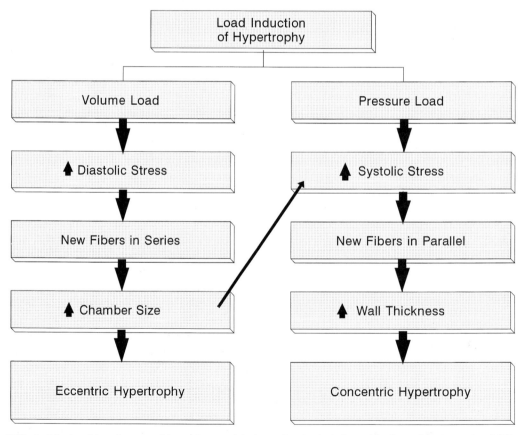

FIG. 1. Mechanism of concentric and eccentric hypertrophy in left ventricular volume overload. The mechanical control of hypertrophy is envisioned as illustrated. Note that eccentric hypertrophy must be accompanied by addition of fibers in parallel as well as in series if inadequate hypertrophy and afterload mismatch are to be avoided.

mechanisms whereby an increase in wall stress stimulates growth until stress is returned to normal. Athletes who experience a large increase in cardiac output without large pressure loads (endurance athletes) have a diastolic load and manifest a larger ventricular volume with normal mass to volume ratio. Athletes who experience a marked increase in blood pressure with a small or absent increase in cardiac output such as weight lifters (57) have a pattern of increased mass with little increase in volume and an increased mass to volume ratio. Most athletes fall between these two extremes.

Ventricular Systolic Function in Physiologic Hypertrophy

The functional consequences of the left ventricular structural changes observed in athletes have been evaluated in a number of studies. Many studies have reported left ventricular systolic function to be normal in athletes. However, occasional studies (52,64) have noted diminished or enhanced function in individual athletes or groups of athletes. The reason for this variability in observed systolic function appears to be the inability of ejection indices of systolic performance to distinguish between altered loading conditions and changes in contractility (24,65–68). Enhanced or depressed systolic function as has been occasionally noted in athletes has led to the conclusion that chronic exercise participation can lead to either an increase or a decrease in contractility. However, the substantial structural changes typical of these subjects results in altered afterload and preload, rendering these indices unreliable for assessing contractility. In those studies in which adjustment for load has been performed, resting contractility has been normal (32,33,52, 69). As recently reviewed by Moore and Korzick (70), there has also been a substantial body of data in small mammals (mice, rats, hamsters) in support of the concept that chronic exercise can result in adaptive alteration of intrinsic contractile function. However, there are also substantial data indicating

that control of gene expression in response to hemodynamic and hormonal influences in large mammals including humans does not parallel that which has been described in rodents. It therefore cannot be assumed that findings of enhanced contractility in response to exercise in small mammals are applicable to human athletes. Although there have been few investigations in humans that have assessed load-independent indices of contractility, those which have indicate that findings of enhanced resting systolic function can be explained by alterations in afterload and preload (32,33,52,69) without evidence of depressed or enhanced intrinsic contractility.

Ventricular Diastolic Function in Physiologic Hypertrophy

There is reason to assume that physiologic hypertrophy will adversely affect diastolic function. Pathologic hypertrophy is known to impair ventricular filling. The increased mass to volume ratio found in some athletes could reduce diastolic chamber compliance even if myocardial properties are undisturbed. Determining the contribution of myocardial factors (relaxation and elasticity) to diastolic function is problematic. Diastolic function is generally assessed in terms of filling parameters using any of several different indices. Early diastolic filling can be examined echocardiographically as the peak rate of chamber enlargement (dD/dt_{max}) or the peak rate of wall thinning (dh/dt_{min}), angiocardiographically as the peak rate of volume change (dV/dt_{max}), and by Doppler using a variety of indices including peak early velocity, peak or mean early acceleration, and deceleration rates. Late diastolic filling can also be quantified using imaging methods, but the majority of the data relevant to late diastolic filling and early versus late filling comes from Doppler techniques. In contrast to these chamber properties, myocardial diastolic properties can only be directly determined using diastolic pressure-volume analysis. The invasive nature of this type of data acquisition precludes measurement in normal athletes. Therefore, the data that are available consist of a number of studies examining diastolic filling parameters in athletes. Digitized m-mode echocardiograms have documented normal dD/dt_{max} and dD/dh_{min} in runners (69), swimmers (71), weight lifters (71), and triathletes (57). Because these indices depend on absolute chamber size and wall thickness, most studies have used some method of normalization. Nonetheless, in each case, early diastolic function was considered normal by these techniques, regardless of the degree or pattern of hypertrophy. More recently, Doppler echocardiography has been used to assess various indices of chamber diastolic function. Peak early (E) and late (A) flow velocities as well as their ratio (E/A) have been found to be normal in athletes (57,69,72–78). Some authors have noted increased early filling velocities in athletes (79), presumably related to the need to normalize for absolute volume flow. An increase in the E/A ratio has also been found (57,75,79), which can be explained by heart rate differences. Heart rate is known to have a direct effect on the E/A ratio, with a reduced atrial filling wave and higher E/A at lower heart rates (80). Thus, diastolic filling patterns have been found to be normal in athletes after consideration of the effects of ventricular chamber enlargement and bradycardia.

In contrast to the results in subjects with pathologic hypertrophy resulting from hypertension or aortic stenosis, the finding of normal diastolic function in physiologic hypertrophy as assessed using diastolic filling indices appears to indicate that diastolic myocardial properties are normal. There are several alternative explanations. The sensitivity of diastolic filling indices for detection of abnormalities may be inadequate because of the complex and variable relationship between myocardial properties and diastolic filling. The degree of hypertrophy may also be too mild to result in detectable changes. This interpretation is suggested by the finding that hypertensives with a similar degree of hypertrophy to athletes are also not different from control subjects with respect to diastolic filling indices (74).

PATHOLOGIC HYPERTROPHY: CARDIAC EFFECTS OF CHRONIC OVERLOAD

Increased hemodynamic load is one of the primary consequences of many forms of congenital heart disease. The more complex lesions involve pressure and volume loads that may affect both the right and left ventricles. Because these patients generally experience a level of compromise sufficient to preclude them from high-level athletic activities, this discussion focuses on the simpler examples of isolated left ventricular pressure or volume overload that are more relevant for the adult athlete.

Myocardial Response to Increased Pressure Load

The fate of the myocardium in aortic stenosis is primarily determined by a complex interplay between hypertrophy, wall stress, and function. Faced with an increased pressure load, compensatory hypertrophy successfully normalizes function and output, but there are several penalties. Chronic pressure overload myocardial hypertrophy is known to be associated with depressed ventricular function in animals and adult humans (81–85), although the mechanism is uncertain. The myocardium responds to a hemodynamic load by myocyte hypertrophy, although hyperplasia has been shown to occur in the first 3 to 6 months of life in some species (81,86,87) and may occur under severe stress even in mature myocardium (88). New formation of intracellular contractile material accounts for the expansion of myocytes. This hyperplasia of myofibrillar units results in an increase in oxygen utilization and requires a proportional growth of mitochondria responsible for oxygen consumption and energy supply. However, reduction of the mitochondrial to myofibrillar volume ratio has been found in pressure overload hypertrophy (89–91). Ventricular hypertrophy secondary to an acute pressure stimulus may also be associated with focal areas of necrosis with subsequent formation of collagenous connective tissue (92–97). Limitations in coronary vascular reserve have also been observed in adult animal and human models of pressure overload hypertrophy. This can be attributed to a disproportionate increase in ventricular mass compared to the microvascular growth, a rarefaction of the arteriolar bed, abnormal coronary vascular resistance, and extravascular compression by the ventricular mass (98–105). Finally, the cellular and biochemical changes engendered by pressure-overload hypertrophy may also influence ventricular function. Indeed, myocardial function can be modulated by synthesis of functionally different contractile proteins (106–110).

Cardiac function in congenital aortic stenosis has represented somewhat of an enigma. The inverse relation between myocardial shortening and afterload would seem to predict that ejection performance should be depressed by the elevated outflow impedance. However, ejection fraction is usually above normal with a direct correlation to the pressure gradient. This apparent paradox can be explained, in part, by considering the nature of myocardial afterload. Myocardial afterload is best represented by wall stress, the force per unit cross-sectional area. For a circular chamber such as the left ventricle, wall stress is proportional to (dimension × pressure)/thickness. For any constant

dimension and wall thickness, pressure elevation results in an elevation in wall stress. As discussed previously, the normal response to this mechanical stimulus is compensatory hypertrophy, which persists until the increase in wall thickness is sufficient to normalize wall stress. Conceptually, new fibers are added until the load per fiber is normalized, and systolic function is restored. This mechanism would predict that systolic function should be normal rather than enhanced. There are at least two explanations that have been put forward to explain this latter phenomenon.

First, there is evidence that elevated systolic function relates to alterations in the time course of wall stress during systole (111). Although peak systolic pressure is elevated in aortic stenosis, end-systolic pressure is normal, because, at the time of aortic valve closure, left ventricular pressure decreases below aortic pressure (Fig. 2). As shown by a number of investigators, peak systolic stress is the major determinant of hypertrophy. That is, it appears to be the peak load per fiber that serves as the feedback mechanism for formation of new fibers. In aortic stenosis, the proportionally lower end-systolic pressure compared with peak pressure results in a proportionally lower end-systolic pressure.

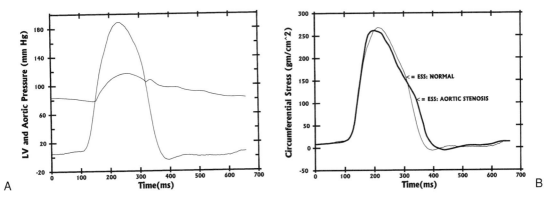

FIG. 2. Time course of left ventricular and aortic pressure in aortic stenosis (**A**) and time course of wall stress in aortic stenosis (*thick line*) compared with normal (*thin line*) (**B**). Although pressure is high in early systole, end-systolic pressure (pressure at the secondary crossover point) is normal or low. The hypertrophic response, which is controlled primarily by peak systolic stress, results in compensatory hypertrophy sufficient to normalize peak stress, so that peak stress is similar in the patient with aortic stenosis to the normal value. This hypertrophy results in "excess" muscle for the normal pressure load at end-systole, leading to end-systolic stress levels that are below normal.

Functionally, the marked hypertrophy that is required to normalize the elevated peak pressure results in "excess" muscle for the normal end-systolic pressure, and end-systolic stress is lower than normal. In contrast to control of hypertrophy, the force limiting the extent of shortening is end-systolic wall stress. Thus, normalization of peak stress leads to reduced end-systolic stress with consequent enhanced systolic performance. End-systolic stress represents the afterload that is relevant to systolic shortening, leading to the rather counterintuitive observation that myocardial afterload is reduced in aortic stenosis. Supranormal function is isolated to the affected ventricle, consistent with the hypothesis that local loading is the key determinant (112). Further support for this concept derives from the observation that relief of stenosis is followed by an increase in end-systolic stress toward normal with consequent reduction in function (113).

The second observation that has been proposed to explain the elevation in systolic performance is that there is an alteration in intrinsic myocardial trophic properties. This explanation is also based on excess hypertrophy leading to low afterload, but in this case the excess hypertrophy is proposed to be related to the age of onset of the pressure load. According to this hypothesis, pressure load early in life elicits a proportionally greater myocardial hypertrophic response, a property that persists if the aortic stenosis is not fully relieved. Supporting evidence includes reports of diminished wall stress throughout the cardiac cycle in children with aortic stenosis (114,115). This phenomenon may represent a persistence of the increased trophic response seen in normal infants (116), which is elicited by the presence of aortic stenosis from birth. Reduced total systolic stress also predicts that per-gram myocardial oxygen consumption should be reduced, a finding that has also been confirmed (117). This pattern of supranormal function with low end-systolic stress is less often seen in patients in whom stenosis develops later in life, although it appears to be more common in women than in men (118).

Systolic dysfunction is rarely encountered beyond the neonatal period in children with congenital aortic stenosis. When systolic dysfunction is present in adults with aortic stenosis, both afterload mismatch and contractile dysfunction may be responsible. However, in contrast to aortic regurgitation, in which afterload mismatch seems invariably to precede depressed contractility, patients with aortic stenosis may have either abnormality in isolation, with depressed contractility having the worse prognosis (119–123). Advanced myocardial hypertrophy in adult patients represents a significant risk factor for contractile failure (122,123) and postoperative mortality after aortic valve replacement for aortic stenosis (124). Morphologically and functionally, coronary abnormalities are found in these patients in proportion to the magnitude of hypertrophy, and they are believed to play a causative role in the adverse impact of hypertrophy on outcome (103,125). In animals (126,127) and humans (128), young age appears to provide considerable protection from these coronary abnormalities, with normal myocardial vascularity and coronary flow reserve present in young animals with pressure overload hypertrophy. Similarly, immature animals do not manifest contractile dysfunction or abnormal diastolic relaxation when exposed to pressure-load hypertrophy sufficient to elicit these abnormalities in mature animals (129,130). This age modulation of myocardial neovascularization may well contribute to the resistance to myocardial dysfunction in patients with aortic stenosis present from early in life.

For the athlete with left ventricular outflow tract obstruction, pathologic hypertrophy is compounded by the physiologic hypertrophic response to chronic exercise. There is little information concerning these combined effects. Studies in exercised rodents have indicated a beneficial coronary microvascular response to moderate levels of chronic exercise, although strenuous exercise may have the opposite effect (47). When exercise effects are superimposed on hypertension-induced hypertrophy, the impaired capillarization associated with pathologic hypertrophy is not alleviated, but it also does not appear to be exacerbated (131).

Myocardial Response to Increased Volume Load

In contrast to acquired heart disease, volume overload lesions are much more common in congenital heart disease than pressure overload. Valvar aortic regurgitation is not the most common of these disorders, but represents a relatively "pure" form of increased diastolic load without the complicating issues of left-to-right shunts, pulmonary hypertension, and biventricular overload. It therefore serves as a reasonable model in which to consider the impact of volume overload on the myocardium. Numerous studies have permitted the natural history of myocardial mechanics in aortic regurgitation to be described in some detail. The sequence of events in chronic aortic regurgitation can be divided into four stages of variable duration (Fig. 3). During the first and most prolonged period, ventricular dilation is accompanied by compensatory hypertrophy, maintaining normal mass to volume ratio, wall stress, and ventricular performance. The second phase is characterized by relative failure of the hypertrophic response, manifested as a decrease in the mass to volume ratio with secondary elevation in wall stress and reduction in function. At least for some period of time after the appearance of inadequate hypertrophy, contractility may remain normal (132). Adequate hypertrophy is also a critical factor for maintenance of normal left ventricular geometry, because the configuration of the ventricle is initially normal but tends to become more spherical as mass to volume ratio decreases (133,134). In the third phase, afterload mismatch increases with a further increase in wall stress and decrease in function, but at this stage the ventricular dysfunction is exacerbated by reduced myocardial contractility. Over the short term, the impaired contractility may be fully reversible, and valve replacement results in complete recovery of function and contractility. After an unpredictable period of time, the stage of irreversible myocardial damage is reached (135). At this stage in the disease, valve replacement may still be tolerated but does not restore myocardial mechanics to normal.

Although the sequence of events involved in the transition between compensated and inadequate hypertrophy and between reversible and irreversibly impaired contractility has been observed, the cause or causes are not fully understood. In both aortic stenosis and regurgitation, the afterload mismatch that results from inadequate hypertrophy appears to be a critical aspect of the myocardial damage. Aoyagi and colleagues have shown that experimentally sustained elevation of wall stress in animals results in the rapid appearance of impaired contractility (39). Wall stress is a major determinant of myocardial oxygen consumption, myocardial blood flow is impeded by elevated wall stress (particularly in diastole), and myocardial neovascularization is generally reduced in hypertrophy, all of which could contribute to a chronic substrate deficit. Afterload reduction has been shown to slow the rate of progression of myocardial dysfunction (136,137), supporting the concept that inadequate hypertrophy plays an important primary role. The factors that control hypertrophy and may determine this transition from compensated to inadequate hypertrophy are therefore of primary importance to understanding the pathophysiology of this disease.

It is uncertain why the normal feedback control mechanism for hypertrophy fails, but abnormalities of diastolic function provide a potential mechanism. The mechanical coupling between load and induction of hypertrophy is stretch-induced distortion of the cell membrane. Therefore, if the tissue becomes less stretchable and the increase in load does not result in the expected distortion of the cell membrane, then the normal compensatory hypertrophy mechanism fails. This is the mechanism for myocardial atrophy in patients with constrictive pericarditis. Patients with severe aortic regurgitation manifest depressed compliance in the more advanced stages of the disease, and impaired compliance appears to precede inadequate hypertrophy and de-

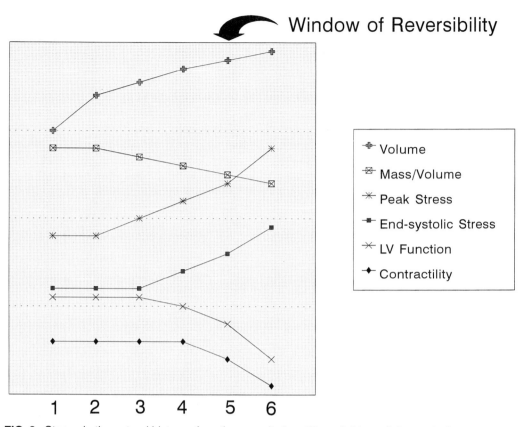

Window of Reversibility

Volume
Mass/Volume
Peak Stress
End-systolic Stress
LV Function
Contractility

1 2 3 4 5 6

FIG. 3. Stages in the natural history of aortic regurgitation. **Stage 1:** Normal. **Stage 2:** Compensated hypertrophy. When the volume load is imposed on the left ventricle, dilation is accompanied by proportional increase in wall thickness, maintaining a normal mass:volume ratio and afterload. The hypertrophy maintains peak and end–systolic wall stress in the normal range, and function and contractility are preserved. **Stage 3:** Inadequate hypertrophy. During this stage, dilation is no longer accompanied by commensurate hypertrophy, and the mass:volume ratio decreases. Peak stress increases, indicating less than full compensatory hypertrophy. This earliest stage of decompensation usually precedes the onset of elevated end–systolic stress, resulting in normal function and contractility. **Stage 4:** Afterload mismatch. Progressively inadequate hypertrophy leads to further decrease in the mass:volume ratio and increase in peak wall stress. End–systolic stress is elevated, and the afterload mismatch results in reduced function. Contractility remains normal during this phase. **Stage 5:** Reversible contractile failure. The process continues with further inadequate hypertrophy, reduction in the mass:volume ratio, and increase in peak and end–systolic stress. Systolic dysfunction worsens because of the combined influences of afterload mismatch and reduced contractility. There is a variable period of time during which the contractile abnormality appears reversible upon elimination of the hemodynamic overload. **Stage 6:** Irreversible contractile dysfunction. At this stage, each of the processes continues and they compound each other. Surgery at this stage can reduce the hemodynamic overload and lead to clinical improvement, but contractility will no longer normalize.

pressed myocardial contractility (138). It is therefore possible that the sequence of events is cumulative impaired diastolic compliance, which interferes with the normal transduction of myocardial hypertrophy and consequent inadequate hypertrophy.

Similar to the situation for the athlete with a pressure overload lesion, there are few data concerning the cumulative impact of increased physiologic demands in the face of an already volume-loaded ventricle. It is generally presumed that, in the presence of a volume load that is of sufficient magnitude to place the patient at risk of progressive myocardial dysfunction, the rate of progression may be augmented by superimposition of the additional volume load associated with exercise. As is discussed later, the physiology of exercise in patients with aortic regurgitation is actually more complex than this. Few data are directly relevant to this issue, forcing the clinician to base decisions on clinical judgment (the medical term for "an educated guess").

RISKS AND BENEFITS OF EXERCISE PARTICIPATION IN CONGENITAL CARDIAC DISEASE

The recognized benefits of aerobic exercise (improved peripheral vascular responsiveness, improved cardiac preload and afterload reserve) have prompted widespread recommendations in favor of exercise rehabilitation programs for patients recovering from myocardial infarction. Even patients with chronic congestive heart failure are able to benefit from a controlled exercise program. There is ample documentation that exercise performance in patients with congenital heart disease can be improved by training programs, although maximal heart rate and oxygen consumption may not increase (139–142). In comparison, there is relatively little information available concerning the impact of chronic exercise participation on risk of sudden death in patients with congenital heart disease and virtually none in patients who participate at a highly competitive level. Recommendations with regard to exercise participation by patients with congenital heart disease have been developed by several groups (143–146). Generally, the purpose of these recommendations is to prevent exercise-related injury, syncope, or sudden death. The data on which these recommendations are based are drawn from population studies of the relative frequency of the particular disease in autopsy studies of sudden death in athletes, sudden death in the general population or in patients with known congenital heart disease, and in some instances from "natural history" studies for particular lesions.

The cardiovascular causes of sudden death in athletes have been reviewed previously (147–149). The major causes in persons younger than age 35 years are hypertrophic cardiomyopathy, congenital coronary artery anomalies, and aortic dissection in Marfan disease, with numerous other less common disorders occasionally being recognized, including right ventricular dysplasia, myocarditis, coronary aneurysms after Kawasaki disease, and atherosclerotic heart disease. After age 35 years, coronary heart disease is the predominant etiologic factor. Certain cardiac malformations such as congenital valvar stenosis are striking in their absence from these reports, despite their known risk of sudden death. Although it is tempting to conclude from this observation that exercise does not increase risk of sudden death in patients with aortic stenosis, it is likely that the patients at highest risk have been excluded from athletics based on medical advice or inability to compete. Thus, these series indicate that, for some disorders such as congenital coronary artery anomalies, a high risk can be assumed because (a) the frequency in these series is high compared to the extremely low population incidence (150) and (b) premorbid recognition with resultant exclusion from athletic participation is unlikely. However, for the more common lesions such as valvar stenosis, these reports provide little help in assessing risk.

Turning next to reports examining the relative incidence of various congenital cardiac malformations resulting in sudden death in individuals with or without the heart disease previously having been diagnosed, results from several reports are summarized in Table 3. The results of older and more recent studies are quite different. The majority of cases in early studies were related to aortic stenosis, hypertrophic cardiomyopathy, and congenital lesions associated with pulmonary vascular obstructive disease or cyanosis with pulmonary stenosis. The later reports no longer include this bias toward structural defects with significant hemodynamic disturbances; instead, they have a distribution not dissimilar to the findings in studies of athletes with sud-

TABLE 3. *Cardiac causes of sudden death in children and young adults*

Reference	(190)	(237)	(238)	(208)	(239)
Year	1974	1985	1985	1995	1996
Age range, years	1–21	>1	1–21	1–35	1–21
Total deaths	254	101	51	58	40
Exercise related	10%	22%			
Aortic stenosis	18%	2%		5%	
Aortic regurgitation		3%			
Hypertrophic cardiomyopathy	16%	4%	7%	21%	15%
Eisenmenger's syndrome	15%	11%			
Cyanotic heart disease with pulmonary stenosis	10%	30%			
Endocardial fibroelastosis	7%				
Ebstein's disease	6%		4%		
Dilated cardiomyopathy	5%	8%	27%	35%	
Conduction system disorders	4%		12%	28%	
Primary pulmonary hypertension		2%	4%		
Coronary artery anomaly	1%	1%	6%	26%	30%
Aortic rupture	1%	1%	6%	12%	
Miscellaneous	15%	36%	32%	8%	20%

den death, except there is a higher incidence of dilated cardiomyopathies. The causes that dominate in the more recent studies are those for which insubstantial progress in diagnosis (coronary artery anomalies) or treatment (hypertrophic and dilated cardiomyopathies) has occurred, whereas those diseases for which good or excellent surgical palliation have come into common use have ceased to be a common cause of sudden death. Among patients with postoperative congenital heart disease, the distribution of those at risk includes patients with pulmonary hypertension, repaired tetralogy of Fallot, and transposition of the great arteries after Mustard or Senning operation (151). These patients nearly always have significant cardiovascular limitations of exercise participation.

Population studies have documented the apparent paradox that, although there is a transient increase in the risk for sudden death during intense exercise in patients with coronary artery disease who regularly participate in low and high level exertion, these individuals experience an overall reduction in their risk for sudden death (Fig. 4) (152–156). Additionally, individuals who do not exercise regularly have an exaggerated risk of sudden death during in-

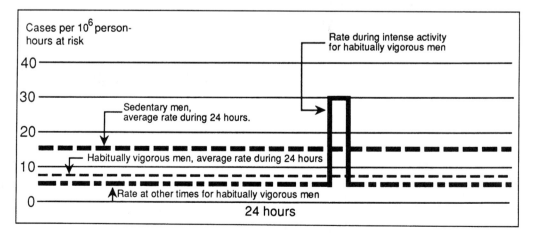

FIG. 4. Risk of primary cardiac arrest during vigorous physical activity and at other times, stratified according to level of habitual physical activity. (From ref. 153, with permission.)

tense exercise (155). Whether these statistics apply to other forms of heart disease is not known. However, excluding the few, well-defined patient categories such as myocarditis and acute ischemia in which exercise may cause direct myocardial injury, the recommendation of exercise avoidance in patients with congenital heart disease is generally based on clinical assumptions rather than proven benefits. The burden for the clinician caring for the athlete with congenital heart disease is to balance the known and quantifiable benefits of exercise participation against the usually unknown additional risk imposed by high-intensity, competitive athletic participation.

APPROACH TO RECOGNITION AND DIAGNOSIS OF CONGENITAL CARDIAC DISEASE IN ATHLETES

Family and medical history play a particularly important role in recognition of heart disease in the athlete. Many of the most dangerous forms of heart disease can be familial in nature, including hypertrophic cardiomyopathy and long QT syndrome. A family history of sudden death, syncope, or arrhythmias can provide important clues. The medical history should include prior experience with anesthesia, history of prolonged febrile illnesses suggestive of Kawasaki syndrome, and prior diagnostic evaluations. Many adolescents and young adults are surprisingly uninformed concerning their prior medical history, even to the point of not knowing the type of heart disease they have or what prior surgery has been performed. Relatively good health, a sense of immortality typical of adolescence, an affectation of invulnerability that seems common in athletes, and the extreme geographic mobility of modern society often lead patients with significant cardiac disease to lose touch with their cardiologists. In the Second Natural History Study of Congenital Heart Defects, 26% of patients with congenital aortic stenosis had not had a cardiac evaluation for at least 10 years (157). Collecting the details about earlier care can be challenging under these circumstances. Surgical de-

tails (e.g., closure of a ventricular septal defect through a right ventriculotomy rather than by a transatrial approach) carry significant implications concerning risk for syncope and sudden death but are usually not known to the patient. Pulmonary hypertension has been identified as an important risk factor for sudden death, indicating the importance of access to details such as pulmonary artery pressure at catheterization and postoperatively in the intensive care unit. Specific inquiry should be made concerning syncope or near syncope, dizziness, palpitations, bradyarrhythmias or tachyarrhythmias, and chest pain. In addition to the conduct of the usual cardiac examination, manifestations of Marfan syndrome should certainly be sought. Further testing is usually justified if abnormalities are suggested by the history or physical examination with the correct diagnostic approach being dictated by the individual history and findings. Diagnoses such as hypertrophic cardiomyopathy can be surprisingly vague in presentation, similar to congenital coronary anomalies and dilated ascending aorta, which may have no manifestations prior to specific diagnostic studies. These obstacles to diagnosis suggest the potential utility of electrocardiography, exercise testing, or echocardiographic screening programs. The rarity of the disorders results in an excessively high incidence of false-positive electrocardiograms (158,159) and exercise examinations (160, 161), and preparticipation echocardiographic screening programs in otherwise healthy athletes have not proven cost effective (162–165). Only in the presence of other clinical findings that increase the pretest probability of the disease are further tests indicated. On the other hand, once the disease is suspected, the clinician should not hesitate to obtain the appropriate tests. Echocardiography is accurate for most of the suspect lesions. For example, it is possible to document coronary artery origin and proximal course on most adolescents and young adults, and the anomalous course of the proximal coronaries can be prospectively diagnosed. With increasing body size and with age, acoustic access does become more difficult, and transesophageal imaging may become necessary. Although it is a more difficult procedure, it is still a nearly risk-free procedure in the healthy individual. Magnetic resonance imaging is less widely available but has also become a useful diagnostic tool that does not have the same limitations as echocardiography. Cardiac catheterization is rarely needed for diagnosis, but has become a valuable therapeutic modality with an ever expanding range of options, as is discussed in the next section.

SPECIFIC FORMS OF CONGENITAL CARDIAC MALFORMATIONS IN THE ADULT ATHLETE

Certain forms of congenital heart disease are of sufficient interest and are associated with such unique issues that individual chapters of this book have been devoted to them. These include familial hypertrophic cardiomyopathy, congenital coronary artery malformations, long QT syndromes, the Marfan syndrome, arrhythmogenic right ventricular dysplasia, and primary arrhythmias. This discussion focuses on some of the more common structural defects with an emphasis on the physiologic consequences of the disease or its repair.

Aortic Valve Disease

Bicommissural aortic valve (BAV) is one of the most common congenital cardiac lesions in the general population, being noted in up to 1% to 2% of autopsy studies, although the incidence is lower in clinical studies (166). The valve dysfunction is often associated with stenosis or regurgitation in childhood, and its magnitude is highly variable. The natural history is a tendency toward progression, although valve dysfunction may be absent in some instances into the seventh decade. Patients with moderate or severe valve dysfunction generally have been previously diagnosed, but individuals with mild or no stenosis or regurgitation may well not be detected during childhood. Severity of valvar stenosis represents the primary risk factor for

progression (157,166). In contrast, subvalvar stenosis may progress early in life but seldom worsens after adolescence. Aortic regurgitation as a primary disorder is far less common in the young, more often occurring after aortic valvotomy for aortic stenosis, in association with other forms of congenital heart disease such as subvalvar aortic stenosis or ventricular septal defect with prolapse of aortic valve leaflet, or as a consequence of bacterial endocarditis. Even in those individuals diagnosed early in life, good health and absence of negative impact on exercise capacity often result in failure to maintain regular medical care. The high incidence of the malformation, the apparent propensity of these individuals toward athletic participation, and the relatively preserved exercise capacity in patients with less than severe valve dysfunction combine to make aortic valve disease the mostly likely congenital cardiac disorder to be encountered in the athlete. Diagnosis is generally made by echocardiography, which can provide a morphologic description of the valve and the severity of valve dysfunction as well as an assessment of myocardial mechanics in the majority of individuals.

Exercise Response to Left Ventricular Outflow Obstruction

The physiologic response to exercise in valvar and subvalvar aortic stenosis is highly dependent on the severity of stenosis. Exercise leads to a disproportionate increase in ventricular pressure and transvalvar pressure difference despite a stable or reduced outflow resistance. The systolic gradient across the aortic valve depends on a number of factors, including valve area, stroke volume, and rate of ejection. The effect of flow on valve area is controversial, but exercise has not been found significantly to increase valve area (167). In normal subjects, there is typically a 5% to 10% increase in stroke volume, which may be as high as 25% in some athletes. However, augmentation of stroke volume does not contribute substantially to the increased gradient in congenital aortic stenosis because the change in stroke volume is normal in patients with mild stenosis but stroke volume remains the same or decreases in patients with severe obstruction even though they demonstrate the greatest increase in gradient (167–169). The failure of stroke volume to increase during exercise is secondary to reduced preload reserve (170), a manifestation of impaired diastolic myocardial properties that escalate during exercise (171,172). The higher velocity of flow and flow acceleration secondary to the increase in myocardial contractility, which normally results in a small increase in the instantaneous transvalvar pressure gradient (173), causes a marked increase in gradient with aortic stenosis (167,173), which is proportional to the severity of obstruction. This trend toward normal hemodynamics in patients with mild and moderate valve stenosis is noted also in the increase in blood pressure and cardiac output, which are progressively blunted in patients with more severe stenosis (169, 174–176). Inadequate increase in cardiac output limits O_2 transport capability, reducing maximum aerobic power. Exercise tolerance is normal in mild to moderate stenosis but is often impaired in patients with severe obstruction (176–179). Patients who have previously had valvotomy performed tend to have exercise physiologic responses proportional to the severity of residual obstruction (177, 180).

Exercise Response to Aortic Regurgitation

Exercise capacity is generally normal in well compensated aortic regurgitation although it is often diminished in patients with severe regurgitation and marked ventricular dilatation (181). The ability to increase cardiac output appropriately is usually normal in less than severe regurgitation, although the mechanisms by which this is achieved are not the same as in the normal heart. Ejection fraction response to exercise is quite variable in patients with mild to moderate regurgitation, but tends to decrease during exercise in those with severe regurgitation (182). A number of studies have documented that a decrease in

ejection fraction during exercise reliably identifies patients with severe regurgitation. In contrast to the 5% to 10% increase in end-diastolic volume typically seen during upright exercise in normal subjects, moderate to severe aortic regurgitation is often associated with a decrease in end-diastolic volume (183) resulting from a reduction in diastolic time and systemic vascular resistance leading to a reduced regurgitant volume (184,185). In contrast, isometric exercise leads to an increase in regurgitant volume (186). Overall, the change in systemic vascular resistance appears to be the most important factor in the ejection fraction response to exercise (185). This interpretation is further strengthened by the increase in exercise stroke volume and ejection fraction response to both isometric (187) and dynamic (188) exercise with afterload reduction therapy. Aortic regurgitation does not appear to represent a significant risk for exercise-induced sudden death. However, the natural history of severe aortic regurgitation almost always includes progressive myocardial injury and eventual failure. Most reviews have therefore recommended that patients with severe aortic regurgitation not participate in competitive sports (189).

Sudden Death in Aortic Stenosis

A number of studies have attempted to address the risk of sudden death in patients with congenital aortic stenosis. However, because of the changing nature of medical diagnostic capability and management options in these patients, it remains difficult to determine risk for individual patients. The large multicenter series reported by Lambert et al. (190) exemplifies the problem with interpreting these data. There were 33 instances of sudden death in medically managed aortic stenosis. Among these, 10 had a clinical diagnosis only, never having been catheterized. No details of the severity of stenosis in the others were provided, except that all 33 had severe obstruction in the form of angina, syncope, or electrocardiographic evidence of strain pattern. The study by Thornback et al. (191) reported a 1%

incidence of sudden cardiac death in aortic stenosis, all in patients after surgery for severe stenosis. Doyle et al. (192) reported a 4% (4 of 92) incidence of sudden death in patients with congenital aortic stenosis. All four had evidence of severe obstruction, three of the four were symptomatic, and the asymptomatic child had severe obstruction of both the left and right ventricular outflow tracts at cardiac catheterization. Keane et al. (157) reported a 5% total incidence of sudden death among a large cohort of 462 patients with congenital valvar aortic stenosis. More severe obstruction was noted to be a risk factor for death, but the severity of obstruction in those who died was not reported. It is likely that the outcome is in fact now better than these early reports indicated. Kitchiner et al. (166) reported the outcome of 239 patients with congenital aortic stenosis evaluated over a 30-year period. With the exception of neonates with critical aortic stenosis, no instances of sudden death were encountered.

Although some authors have stated that sudden death has occurred in cases of mild to moderate stenosis, leading them to conclude that the cause of sudden death does not seem to relate to the degree of stenosis (193), documentation of such morbid events in patients who do not have severe stenosis is difficult to find. The view of Arnold and Kitchiner (194) is better supported by published reports, namely, that sudden death has been reported exclusively with severe aortic stenosis. Under these circumstances, it is reasonable to conclude that cause for exercise restriction is limited to this group, which also defines the group for whom valvotomy or valve replacement is indicated. These observations also account for the changing recommendations for exercise participation in patients with aortic stenosis. There is little disagreement that severe aortic stenosis places the patient at significant risk during competitive sports. The recommendations for lesser degrees of stenosis are more controversial and have been evolving over time. Older recommendations (143–145) advised limits to exertion in patients with even mild aortic stenosis, whereas

more recent recommendations (146) do not limit subjects with mild stenosis and recommend against only the most demanding activities in patients with moderate stenosis. The latter recommendations were put together by the American College of Cardiology and the American College of Sports Medicine, but their recommendations were not liberalized to the same level as those of Arnold and Kitchiner (194), who recommend against any restrictions in patients with less than severe stenosis. As methods for noninvasive evaluation continue to improve and further data accumulate in the more modern era of management, it will hopefully become possible to decide more rationally between the alternatives of restriction or intervention. Until then, the patient with moderate aortic stenosis remains a focus of controversy as to when and how to intervene.

Mechanism of Syncope and Sudden Death in Aortic Stenosis

Several potential mechanisms have been proposed for acute morbid events in left ventricular outflow obstruction. These include ischemia, primary arrhythmias, and reflex-mediated autonomic phenomena. Each has accumulated a body of supporting evidence. Pathologic hypertrophy is associated with impaired coronary reserve and subendocardial dysfunction (38). In this setting, the repolarization abnormalities commonly observed in patients at risk for sudden death have been interpreted as indicating ischemia as a precipitating event. Exercise-induced repolarization abnormalities have been noted frequently in patients with aortic stenosis. The ST wave changes manifest more commonly and are more marked in direct proportion to the gradient in patients without prior surgery (176, 177,180,195–197), a relationship which is less reliable in postoperative patients (177). The QT interval has also been noted to become prolonged during exercise in patients with aortic stenosis, even in the absence of resting abnormalities (193). It is possible that this change contributes to the risk of exercise-associated sudden death. Ventricular arrhythmias are more common and higher grade in patients with aortic stenosis, possibly resulting from hypertrophy and subendocardial fibrosis (198,199). However, case reports of observed sudden death have cited hypotension (200–202) as the initial pathologic event, with arrhythmias appearing later. This decrease in blood pressure could be triggered by peripheral vasodilation as a reflex response to activation of left ventricular baroreceptors (Bezold-Jarisch reflex) (203). Alternatively, the decrease in blood pressure could be mediated by impaired contractility in response to acute ischemia. In either case, recognition of exercise-induced hypotension during treadmill testing is generally regarded as an ominous finding justifying intervention for the aortic stenosis, regardless of other indications of the severity of stenosis or level of myocardial compensation.

Bicommissural Aortic Valve with Dilated Ascending Aorta

The combination of dissecting aortic aneurysm and BAV has been recognized for some time as an occasional cause of sudden death based on autopsy studies (204–208). Hypertension is the chief risk factor for aortic dissection, but cystic medial necrosis, either in association with Marfan syndrome or aortic valvular disease, or as an isolated condition is less commonly present. Of 125 autopsy specimens with dissecting aortic aneurysm, Edwards et al. (204) described 17 with congenital BAV. In six, the valve was stenotic and the dissection occurred in the setting of endocarditis (205). Among the other 11 patients with no valvar stenosis, five were younger than age 29 years at the time of death. Coarctation was noted in three, and hypertension was inferred from cardiac weight in eight. Among 186 autopsy specimens with aortic dissection, Roberts et al. (206) found 14 with BAV, four of which were stenotic, one with associated coarctation. It remains unclear whether the association of aortic aneurysm and BAV relates to hemodynamic disturbances or excess fragility of the aortic wall. In subjects with BAV and no significant stenosis, the aortic root sinus diameter is larger than in control subjects (207). Fibrillin mutations have been described in patients with thoracic aortic aneurysms who did not have Marfan syndrome (209). These findings, in conjunction with ascending aortic aneurysms in subjects without significant valvar stenosis, may indicate deficient structural integrity as the primary cause. However, despite the absence of significant stenosis, flow in the ascending aorta can be quite disturbed in these patients as a result of the eccentric orifice. For example, magnetic resonance images obtained in a patient with aneurysm of the ascending aorta associated with a nonstenotic BAV are displayed in Fig. 5. Flow is diverted eccentrically against the anterior wall of the ascending aorta, with the largest diameter coinciding with the point of impact. Thus, altered vascular structure in response to endothelial shear stress may also play a role.

Diagnosis of this disorder is problematic. Hypertension and Marfan syndrome provide other diagnostic evidence of their presence, frequently but not always leading to the premorbid diagnosis. It is more difficult to recognize aortic aneurysm in association with BAV, because stenosis may be minimal or absent and the constant systolic click and hence the diagnosis may easily be unrecognized during childhood. With the increased availability and utilization of echocardiography, this combination has been increasingly recognized at my institution, although published reports remain few. Once diagnosed, management is based on information derived from patients with Marfan syndrome because there are so few data available for this disease. Patients with dilation of the ascending aorta in the Marfan syndrome are known to be at increased risk of dissection and sudden death, with exercise representing an additive risk. Exercise restriction, beta-blocker therapy, and surgery are therefore advised at arbitrary degrees of dilation. Although it is presently unknown whether similar risks ap-

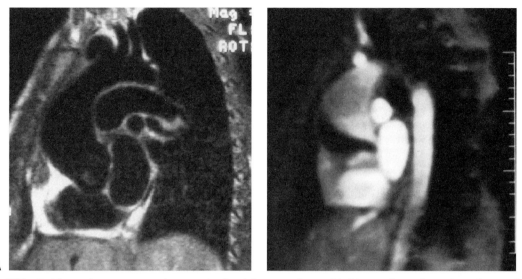

A   B

FIG. 5. Magnetic resonance image obtained in a patient with bicommissural aortic valve and aneurysm of the ascending aorta. The aneurysm (**A**) is largest at the point of impact of the eccentric jet (visualized as the black, negative signal in the proximal root; **B**).

ply to patients without Marfan syndrome, it appears prudent to assume so until further information is available.

Coarctation of the Aorta

If associated with only a modest increase in blood pressure, coarctation of the aorta commonly passes undetected through childhood. Even though the diagnosis is relatively easily made on physical examination based on the combination of murmur, hypertension, and femoral pulse transmission delay, it remains one of the most common forms of congenital heart disease repaired in adults. BAV may be found in more than 50% of cases, with the additional attendant risks associated with aortic valve disease. The primary risks represented by the aortic restriction relate to secondary hypertension and a risk for aortic aneurysm or dissection. Aneurysm and dissection of the aorta are not exclusively related to the effects of hypertension, because they can be seen in the segment of aorta distal to the coarctation (205). The myocardial hypertrophic response to the pressure load of coarctation appears to carry a worse prognosis than that of aortic

stenosis (111). In adult onset hypertension (210–213), left ventricular hypertrophy is commonly associated with a gradual deterioration in left ventricular function and contractility. Similarly, myocardial failure is seen in the natural history of unrepaired coarctation, usually in the third or fourth decade. For all of these reasons, surgical repair of coarctation is virtually always warranted.

Surgery eliminates resting hypertension in most patients who have surgery in childhood, but when surgery is delayed, persistent fixed hypertension is more common and long-term survival remains abnormal (214). Late death relates to rupture of aortic or cerebral aneurysms, myocardial failure, and myocardial infarction. Persistent hypertension at rest or with exercise appears to be a major factor in most cases. Even after successful surgical repair of coarctation, cardiovascular physiology is often not normal. Numerous persistent abnormalities of myocardial mechanics have been reported, including increased left ventricular mass (215–218). The cause of these persistent changes of myocardial structure and mechanics remains unclear. Minor residual gradients across the aortic arch and proximal descending aorta (215,216), abnormal small and large vessel function (219–222), labile hypertension (218), or endocrine abnormalities (217) may contribute to the persistent elevation in left ventricular mass. There are also numerous reports of exercise-induced upper limb hypertension (223,224), which does not appear to be explained adequately by a residual resting gradient. Once recognized, the excess pressure increase with exercise can generally be controlled pharmacologically with minimal impact on exercise tolerance. Consequently, aggressive diagnosis and treatment of residual arch obstruction as well as resting or exercise-induced hypertension should be pursued and should permit nearly all of these patients full exercise participation.

Valvar Pulmonary Stenosis

Pulmonary valve stenosis warrants particular mention not because it represents a threat to the patient, but because of the potential for benefit from treatment. The murmur and variable ejection click usually lead to diagnosis during childhood. Mild stenosis is at low risk of progression and has not previously been thought to warrant valvotomy. Consequently, some of these patients do not have long-term follow-up and may, at times, be seen as young adults without prior knowledge of the valve lesion. In general, surgical intervention has been advised for patients with a gradient of 50 mm Hg or more. Although not associated with diminished longevity or increased risk of sudden death, it is clear that even mild pulmonary stenosis (<40 mm Hg) is associated with reduced exercise tolerance (178,179). When surgical valvotomy was the only therapeutic alternative, limiting intervention to the more severe degrees of stenosis was justified on the basis of a small but measurable risk of surgery. However, transcatheter balloon dilation has been shown to be an effective form of therapy that often provides complete relief of stenosis at nearly zero risk with an insignificant risk of recurrence (225). This success has led to intervention at lower gradients, but improved exercise capacity in response to this intervention has, as yet, been inferred, not documented.

Atrial Septal Defect

Secundum atrial septal defects remain one of the most common forms of congenital heart disease diagnosed in the adult. The physical findings are often minimal early in life and may remain quite subtle throughout childhood. In addition, freedom from symptoms and minimum impact on exercise capacity combine to allow these children to escape recognition. However, exercise capacity is subnormal in these patients (178,179) and athletic success may well be impaired. The risk of sudden death is increased if pulmonary hypertension is present, but this is rarely the case in small to moderate defects diagnosed in the young adult. Diagnosis in the adult is more difficult than in the child because adequate transthoracic echocardiographic interrogation of the atrial septum is often not possible. Secondary signs of right ventricular volume overload can usually be noted, even if the atrial septum cannot be directly imaged, and should prompt transesophageal echocardiography or magnetic resonance imaging. Repair is indicated because of the risk of paradoxical embolism, right ventricular failure, and progressive pulmonary hypertension, but may not restore exercise tolerance to normal (226,227). Reduced exercise capacity late after repair of atrial septal defect appears related to chronotropic incompetence. A similar reduction in maximal heart rate response to exercise has been noted in many patients after repair of congenital heart disease (226), leading to the suggestion that surgery itself is responsible. If so, the recent advent of transcatheter delivery of devices (228) designed to eliminate the atrial level shunt nonsurgically may allow a greater restoration of physiologic capacity for these patients.

Postoperative Congenital Heart Disease

A thorough presentation of the topic of exercise participation in the adult with repaired congenital heart disease is beyond the scope of this discussion, but several issues warrant consideration. This is a field that is unfolding as more of these patients are surviving into adulthood and as the quality of surgical outcome improves. Exercise capacity has been reported to be diminished after repair of most of the common malformations, including after atrial-level repair of transposition of the great arteries (229,230), ventricular septal defect (226), tetralogy of Fallot (231), atrial septal defect (226,227), and totally anomalous pulmonary venous connection (232). Consequently, exercise capacity sufficient to permit a high level of athletic success is unusual in these patients. However, whereas the physiology after Fontan-type of right ventricular bypass operation may preclude a normal increase in cardiac output with exercise, some of these other patients may not experience such limitations. In particular, repair at an earlier age has demonstrably improved outcome for several of these diseases, including tetralogy of Fallot and atrial septal defect (227). Repair in infancy gained prominence in the late 1970s and became common practice in the early 1980s. Therefore, prior data are not likely to be relevant to the current generation of children who are entering young adulthood. New operations such as the arterial switch procedure for transposition of the great arteries have come into standard practice during this same time period and carry a completely new set of complications and risks (233,234). Current knowledge about the potential for athletic success among these patients is about to undergo a radical expansion.

The understanding of exercise-related risks faced by these patients is also based on data collected in patients repaired in an earlier surgical era and is similarly subject to revision. There have been particular groups of patients such as those with tetralogy of Fallot who appear to be at increased risk of sudden death late after repair (235,236). Even in this reasonably well-defined subgroup with a relatively greater risk of adverse events, it remains unclear whether exercise represents a significant risk factor. Patients considered at

higher risk for sudden death (residual right ventricular hypertension, significant pulmonary regurgitation, rhythm abnormalities) are advised to avoid high-intensity competitive sports (146). These recommendations are based on the observation that most patients at risk for sudden death are at highest risk during intense physical activity. Although seemingly prudent, this advice does not take into consideration the previously discussed paradoxical reduction in overall risk for individuals who participate in intense exercise despite the transient elevation in risk during exercise. There remains an enormous amount of work to be done before the relative risk and benefit of exercise for these patients is understood.

REFERENCES

1. Peterson RJ, Franch RH, Fajman WA, Jennings JG, Jones RH. Noninvasive determination of exercise cardiac function following Fontan operation. *J Thorac Cardiovasc Surg* 1984;88:263–272.
2. Mertens L, Rogers R, Reybrouck T, et al. Cardiopulmonary response to exercise after the Fontan operation—a cross-sectional and longitudinal evaluation. *Cardiol Young* 1996;6:136–142.
3. Cortes RG, Satomi G, Yoshigi M, Momma K. Maximal hemodynamic response after the Fontan procedure: Doppler evaluation during the treadmill test. *Pediatr Cardiol* 1994;15:170–177.
4. Harrison DA, Liu P, Walters JE, et al. Cardiopulmonary function in adult patients late after Fontan repair. *J Am Coll Cardiol* 1995;26:1016–1021.
5. Hirschfeld S, Tuboku Metzger AJ, Borkat G, et al. Comparison of exercise and catheterization results following total surgical correction of tetralogy of Fallot. *J Thorac Cardiovasc Surg* 1978;75:446–451.
6. Colan SD, Boutin C, Castañeda AR, Wernovsky G. Status of the left ventricle after arterial switch operation for transposition of the great arteries: hemodynamic and echocardiographic evaluation. *J Thorac Cardiovasc Surg* 1995;109:311–321.
7. McElroy PA, Janicki JS, Weber KT. Physiologic correlates of the heart rate response to upright isotonic exercise—relevance to rate-responsive pacemakers. *J Am Coll Cardiol* 1988;11:94–100.
8. Francis GS, Goldsmith SR, Ziesche S, Nakajima H, Cohn JN. Relative attenuation of sympathetic drive during exercise in patients with congestive heart failure. *J Am Coll Cardiol* 1982;5:832–839.
9. Robinson BF, Epstein SE, Beiser GD, Braunwald E. Control of heart rate by the autonomic nervous system. Studies in man on the interrelation between baroreceptor mechanisms and exercise. *Circ Res* 1966;19:400–411.
10. Manyari DE, Kostuk WV, Purves PP. Left and right ventricular function at rest and during bicycle exercise in the supine and sitting position in normal subjects and patients with coronary artery disease: assessment

and radionuclide ventriculography. *Am J Cardiol* 1983;51:36–42.

11. Steingart RM, Wexler J, Slagle S, Scheuer J. Radionu-clide ventriculographic responses to graded supine and upright exercise: critical role of the Frank-Starling mechanism at submaximal exercise. *Am J Cardiol* 1984;53:1671–1677.

12. Poliner LR, Dehmer GJ, Lewis SE, et al. Left ventric-ular performance in normal subjects: a comparison of the responses to exercise in the upright and supine po-sitions. *Circulation* 1980;62:528–534.

13. Mols P, Huynh CH, Naeije N, Ham HR. Volumetric re-sponse of right ventricle during progressive supine ex-ercise in men. *Am J Physiol Heart Circ Physiol* 1991; 261:H751–H754.

14. Francis GS, Goldsmith SR, Ziesche SM, Cohn JN. Re-sponse of plasma norepinephrine and epinephrine to dynamic exercise in patients with congestive heart failure. *Am J Cardiol* 1982;49:1152–1156.

15. Rodeheffer RJ, Gerstenblith G, Becker LC, et al. Exer-cise cardiac output is maintained with advancing age in healthy human subjects: cardiac dilation and in-creased stroke volume compensate for a diminished heart rate. *Circulation* 1984;69:203–213.

16. Higginbotham MB, Morris KG, Williams RS, Cole-man RE, Cobb FR. Physiologic basis for the age-re-lated decline in aerobic work capacity. *Am J Cardiol* 1986;57:1374–1379.

17. Andersen P, Saltin B. Maximal perfusion of skeletal muscles in man. *J Physiol (Lond)* 1985;366:233–249.

18. Marshall RJ, Schirger A, Shepherd JT. Blood pressure during supine exercise in idiopathic orthostatic hy-potension. *Circulation* 1961;24:76–81.

19. Huang AH, Feigl EO. Adrenergic coronary vasocon-striction helps maintain uniform transmural blood flow distribution during exercise. *Circ Res* 1988;62:286–289.

20. Covertino VA, Keil LC, Bernauer EM, Greenleaf JE. Plasma volume, osmolality, vasopressin, and renin ac-tivity during graded exercise in man. *J Appl Physiol* 1981;50:123–128.

21. Kotchen TA, Hartley LH, Rice TW, et al. Renin, nor-epinephrine, and epinephrine response to graded exer-cise. *J Appl Physiol* 1971;31:178–184.

22. Seitelberger R, Guth BD, Heusch G, et al. Intracoro-nary alpha-adrenergic receptor blockade attenuates is-chemia in conscious dogs during exercise. *Circ Res* 1988;62:436–442.

23. Weber KT, Janicki JS. Myocardial oxygen consump-tion—the role of wall force and shortening. *Am J Physiol* 1977;233:H421–H477.

24. Colan SD, Borow KM, Neumann A. Left ventricular end-systolic wall stress—velocity of fiber shortening relation: a load-independent index of myocardial con-tractility. *J Am Coll Cardiol* 1984;4:715–724.

25. Globel FL, Nordstrom LA, Nelson RR, Jorgensen CR, Wang Y. The rate-pressure product as an index of my-ocardial oxygen consumption during exercise in patients with angina pectoris. *Circulation* 1978;57:549–556.

26. Cannon PJ, Weiss MB, Sciacca RR. Myocardial blood flow in coronary artery disease: studies at rest and dur-ing stress with inert gas washout techniques. *Prog Cardiovasc Dis* 1977;20:95–120.

27. Foster C, Dymond DS, Carpenter J, Schmidt DH. Ef-fect of warm-up on left ventricular response to sudden strenuous exercise. *J Appl Physiol* 1982;53:380–383.

28. Barnard RJ, MacAlpn JR, Kattus AA, Buckberg GD. Ischemic response to sudden strenuous exercise in healthy men. *Circulation* 1973;34:833–837.

29. Foster C, Anholm JD, Hellman CK, et al. Left ventric-ular function during sudden strenuous exercise. *Circu-lation* 1981;63:592–596.

30. Carrió I, Serra-Grima R, Berna L, et al. Transient al-terations in cardiac performance after a six-hour race. *Am J Cardiol* 1990;65:1471–1474.

31. Douglas PS, O'Toole ML, Woolard J. Regional wall motion abnormalities after prolonged exercise in the normal left ventricle. *Circulation* 1990;82:2108–2114.

32. Douglas PS, O'Toole ML, Hiller WDB, Hackney K, Reichek N. Cardiac fatigue after prolonged exercise. *Circulation* 1987;76:1206–1213.

33. Yamazaki H, Onishi S, Sekihara T, et al. [Left ventric-ular function after prolonged exercise]. *Kokyu to Junkan* 1990;38:1241–1245.

34. Vanoverschelde J-LJ, Younis LT, Melin JA, et al. Pro-longed exercise induces left ventricular dysfunction in healthy subjects. *J Appl Physiol* 1991;70:1356–1363.

35. Ketelhut R, Losem CJ, Messerli FH. Is a decrease in arterial pressure during long-term aerobic exercise caused by a fall in cardiac pump function. *Am Heart J* 1994;127:567–571.

36. Seals DR, Rogers MA, Hagberg JM, et al. Left ven-tricular dysfunction after prolonged strenuous exercise in healthy subjects. *Am J Cardiol* 1988;61:875–879.

37. Niemela K, Palatsi I, Ikaheimo M, Airaksinen J, Takkunen J. Impaired left ventricular diastolic function in athletes after utterly strenuous prolonged exercise. *Int J Sports Med* 1987;8:61–65.

38. Hittinger L, Shen YT, Patrick TA, et al. Mechanisms of subendocardial dysfunction in response to exercise in dogs with severe left ventricular hypertrophy. *Circ Res* 1992;71:423–434.

39. Aoyagi T, Fujii AM, Flanagan MF, et al. Transition from compensated hypertrophy to intrinsic myocardial dysfunction during development of left ventricular pressure-overload hypertrophy in conscious sheep. Systolic dysfunction precedes diastolic dysfunction. *Circulation* 1993;88:2415–2425.

40. Rajguru SU, Yeargans GS, Seidler NW. Exercise causes oxidative damage to rat skeletal muscle micro-somes while increasing cellular sulfhydrils. *Life Sci* 1994;54:149–157.

41. Venditti P, Piro MC, Artiaco G, Di Meo S. Effect of ex-ercise on tissue anti-oxidant capacity and heart electri-cal properties in male and female rats. *Eur J Appl Physiol* 1996;74:322–329.

42. Sen CK, Atalay M, Hanninen O. Exercise-induced ox-idative stress: glutathione supplementation and defi-ciency. *J Appl Physiol* 1994;77:2177–2187.

43. Atalay M, Seene T, Hänninen O, Sen CK. Skeletal mus-cle and heart antioxidant defences in response to sprint training. *Acta Physiol Scand* 1996;158:129–134.

44. Kumar CT, Reddy VK, Prasad M, Thyagaraju K, Red-danna P. Dietary supplementation of vitamin E pro-tects heart tissue from exercise-induced oxidant stress. *Mol Cell Biochem* 1992;111:109–115.

45. Goldfarb AH, McIntosh MK, Boyer BT. Vitamin E at-tenuates myocardial oxidative stress induced by DHEA in rested and exercised rats. *J Appl Physiol* 1996;80: 486–490.

46. Koyama T, Keatisuwan W, Kinjo M, Saito H. Suppres-

sive effect of coenzyme Q10 on phospholipase A2 activation in cardiac cells after prolonged swimming. *Life Sci* 1992;51:1113–1118.

47. Anversa P, Ricci R, Olivetti G. Effects of exercise on the capillary vasculature of the rat heart. *Circulation* 1987;75:I-12–I-18.

48. Baker BJ, Wilen MM, Boyd CM, Dinh H, Franciosa JA. Relation of right ventricular ejection fraction to exercise capacity in chronic left ventricular failure. *Am J Cardiol* 1984;54:596–599.

49. Kulik TJ, Bass JL, Fuhrman BP, Moller JH, Lock JE. Exercise induced pulmonary vasoconstriction. *Br Heart J* 1983;50:59–64.

50. Epstein SE, Beiser GD, Goldstein RE, et al. Hemodynamic abnormalities in response to mild and intense upright exercise following operative correction of an atrial septal defect or tetralogy of Fallot. *Circulation* 1973;42:1065–1075.

51. Colan SD. Mechanics of left ventricular systolic and diastolic function in physiologic hypertrophy of the athlete heart. *Cardiol Clin* 1992;10:227–240.

52. Colan SD, Sanders SP, Borow KM. Physiologic hypertrophy: effects on left ventricular systolic mechanics in athletes. *J Am Coll Cardiol* 1987;9:776–783.

53. Pelliccia A, Maron BJ, Culasso F, Spataro A, Caselli G. Athlete's heart in women. Echocardiographic characterization of highly trained elite female athletes. *JAMA* 1996;276:211–215.

54. Menapace FJ, Hammer WJ, Ritzer TF, et al. Left ventricular size in competitive weight lifters: an echocardiographic study. *Med Sci Sports Exerc* 1982;14:72–75.

55. Roy A, Doyon M, Dumesnil JG, Jobin J, Landry F. Endurance vs. strength training: comparison of cardiac structures using normal predicted values. *J Appl Physiol* 1988;64:2552–2557.

56. Cohen JL, Segal KR. Left ventricular hypertrophy in athletes: an exercise-echocardiographic study. *Med Sci Sports Exerc* 1985;17:695–700.

57. Douglas PS, O'Toole ML, Hiller WD, Reichek N. Left ventricular structure and function by echocardiography in ultraendurance athletes. *Am J Cardiol* 1986;58:805–809.

58. Crouse SF, Rohack JJ, Jacobsen DJ. Cardiac structure and function in women basketball athletes: seasonal variation and comparisons with nonathletic controls. *Res Q Exerc Sport* 1992;63:393–401.

59. Stratton JR, Levy WC, Cerqueira MD, Schwartz RS, Abrass IB. Cardiovascular responses to exercise: effects of aging and exercise training in healthy men. *Circulation* 1994;89:1648–1655.

60. Douglas PS, O'Toole M. Aging and physical activity determine cardiac structure and function in the older athlete. *J Appl Physiol* 1992;72:1969–1973.

61. Anversa P, Capasso JM. Loss of intermediate-sized coronary arteries and capillary proliferation after left ventricular failure in rats. *Am J Physiol Heart Circ Physiol* 1991;260:H1552–H1560.

62. Cooper G, Kent RL, Mann DL. Load induction of cardiac hypertrophy. *J Mol Cell Cardiol* 1989;21[Suppl 5]:11–30.

63. Grossman W, Jones D, McLaurin LP. Wall stress and patterns of hypertrophy in the human left ventricle. *J Clin Invest* 1975;56:56–64.

64. Sugishita Y, Koseki S, Matsuda M, Yamaguchi T, Ito I. Myocardial mechanics of athletic hearts in comparison with diseased hearts. *Am Heart J* 1983;105:273–280.

65. Elzinga G, Westerhof N. How to quantify pump function of the heart. The value of variables derived from measurements on isolated muscle. *Circ Res* 1979;44:303–308.

66. Weber KT, Janicki JS, Hunter WC, et al. The contractile behavior of the heart and its functional coupling to the circulation. *Prog Cardiovasc Dis* 1982;24:375–400.

67. Ross JJ. Afterload mismatch and preload reserve: a conceptual framework for the analysis of ventricular function. *Prog Cardiovasc Dis* 1976;18:255–264.

68. Braunwald E, Ross JJ. Control of cardiac performance. In: Berne RM, Sperclakis N, Geiger SR, eds. *Handbook of physiology, Section 2: The cardiovascular system,* vol 1. Baltimore: Williams & Wilkins, 1979:533–580.

69. Fagard R, Van den Broeke C, Vanhees L, Staessen J, Amery A. Noninvasive assessment of systolic and diastolic left ventricular function in female runners. *Eur Heart J* 1987;8:1305–1311.

70. Moore RL, Korzick DH. Cellular adaptations of the myocardium to chronic exercise. *Prog Cardiovasc Dis* 1995;37:371–396.

71. Colan SD, Sanders SP, MacPherson D, Borow KM. Left ventricular diastolic function in elite athletes with physiologic cardiac hypertrophy. *J Am Coll Cardiol* 1985;6:545–549.

72. Varani E, Rapezzi C, Binetti G, et al. [Analysis of the diastolic function of the left ventricle by Doppler echocardiography in athletes engaged in competitive sports activities]. *Cardiologia* 1989;34:855–860.

73. Gregoire JM, Vandenbossche JL, Messin R, Englert M. Diastolic function and modifications of left ventricular architecture in ultraendurance athletes. *Acta Clin Belg* 1989;44:388–395.

74. Cuspidi C, Sampieri L, Lonati L, Bocciolone M, Leonetti G. [The characteristics of left ventricular filling in a mild grade of physiological and pathological hypertrophy. A Doppler echocardiographic study]. *G Ital Cardiol* 1990;20:625–630.

75. Finkelhor RS, Hanak LJ, Bahler RC. Left ventricular filling in endurance-trained subjects. *J Am Coll Cardiol* 1986;8:289–293.

76. Pearson AC, Schiff M, Mrosek D, Labovitz AJ, Williams GA. Left ventricular diastolic function in weight lifters. *Am J Cardiol* 1986;58:1254–1259.

77. Missault L, Duprez D, Jordaens L, et al. Cardiac anatomy and diastolic filling in professional road cyclists. *Eur J Appl Physiol* 1993;66:405–408.

78. Yeater R, Reed C, Ullrich I, Morise A, Borsch M. Resistance trained athletes using or not using anabolic steroids compared to runners: effects on cardiorespiratory variables, body composition, and plasma lipids. *Br J Sports Med* 1996;30:11–14.

79. Cohen A, Diebold B, Raffoul H, et al. [Evaluation by Doppler echocardiography of systolic and diastolic functions of the left ventricle of the athlete's heart]. *Arch Mal Coeur* 1989;82 Spec No 2:55–62.

80. Harrison MR, Clifton GD, Pennell AT, DeMaria AN, Cater A. Effect of heart rate on left ventricular diastolic transmitral flow velocity patterns assessed by Doppler echocardiography in normal subjects. *Am J Cardiol* 1991;67:622–627.

81. Panidis IP, Kotler MN, Ren JF, et al. Development and regression of left ventricular hypertrophy. *J Am Coll Cardiol* 1984;3:1309–1320.

82. Kramer PH, Djalaly A, Poehlmann H, Schiller NB. Abnormal diastolic left ventricular posterior wall motion in left ventricular hypertrophy. *Am Heart J* 1983;106:1066–1069.

83. Pearson AC, Pasierski T, Labovitz AJ. Left ventricular hypertrophy: diagnosis, prognosis, and management. *Am Heart J* 1991;121:148–157.

84. Lorell BH, Grossman W. Cardiac hypertrophy: the consequences for diastole. *J Am Coll Cardiol* 1987;9: 1189–1193.

85. Mann DL, Urabe Y, Kent RL, Vinciguerra S, Cooper G. Cellular versus myocardial basis for the contractile dysfunction of hypertrophied myocardium. *Circ Res* 1991;68:402–415.

86. Perloff JK. Development and regression of increased ventricular mass. *Am J Cardiol* 1982;50:605–611.

87. Olivetti G, Ricci R, Anversa P. Hyperplasia of myocyte nuclei in long-term cardiac hypertrophy in rats. *J Clin Invest* 1987;80:1818–1821.

88. Pfeffer MA, Pfeffer JM. Adult myocyte hyperplasia: divided they fail? *J Am Coll Cardiol* 1994;24:150–151.

89. Anversa P, Ricci R, Olivetti G. Quantitative structural analysis of the myocardium during physiologic growth and induced cardiac hypertrophy: a review. *J Am Coll Cardiol* 1986;7:1140–1149.

90. Limas CJ. Biochemical aspects of cardiac hypertrophy. *Fed Proc* 1983;42:2716–2721.

91. Rabinowitz M, Zak R. Mitochondria and cardiac hypertrophy. *Circ Res* 1975;36:367–376.

92. Bishop SP, Melsen LR. Myocardial necrosis, fibrosis, and DNA synthesis in experimental cardiac hypertrophy induced by sudden pressure overload. *Circ Res* 1976;39:238–245.

93. Weber KT, Janicki JS, Pick R, et al. Collagen in the hypertrophied, pressure-overloaded myocardium. *Circulation* 1987;75:I40–I47.

94. Jalil JE, Doering CW, Janicki JS, et al. Fibrillar collagen and myocardial stiffness in the intact hypertrophied rat left ventricle. *Circ Res* 1989;64:1041–1050.

95. Motz W, Strauer BE. Left ventricular function and collagen content after regression of hypertensive hypertrophy. *Hypertension* 1989;13:43–50.

96. Moore GW, Hutchins GM, Bulkley BH, Tseng JS, Ki PF. Constituents of the human ventricular myocardium: connective tissue hyperplasia accompanying muscular hypertrophy. *Am Heart J* 1980;100:610–616.

97. Gaasch WH, Bing OH, Mirsky I. Chamber compliance and myocardial stiffness in left ventricular hypertrophy. *Eur Heart J* 1982;3[Suppl A]:139–145.

98. Harrison DG, Barnes DH, Hiratzka LF, et al. The effect of cardiac hypertrophy on the coronary collateral circulation. *Circulation* 1985;71:1135–1145.

99. Bache RJ. Effects of hypertrophy on the coronary circulation. *Prog Cardiovasc Dis* 1988;30:403–440.

100. Tomanek RJ. Response of the coronary vasculature to myocardial hypertrophy. *J Am Coll Cardiol* 1990;15: 528–533.

101. Hittinger L, Shannon RP, Bishop SP, Gelpi RJ, Vatner SF. Subendomyocardial exhaustion of blood flow reserve and increased fibrosis in conscious dogs with heart failure. *Circ Res* 1989;65:971–980.

102. Goldstein RA, Haynie M. Limited myocardial perfu-

sion reserve in patients with left ventricular hypertrophy. *J Nucl Med* 1990;31:255–258.

103. Marcus ML, Harrison DG, Chilian WM, et al. Alterations in the coronary circulation in hypertrophied ventricles. *Circulation* 1987;75:I19–I25.

104. Borkon AM, Jones M, Bell JH, Pierce JE. Regional myocardial blood flow in left ventricular hypertrophy. An experimental investigation in Newfoundland dogs with congenital subaortic stenosis. *J Thorac Cardiovasc Surg* 1982;84:876–885.

105. Kanatsuka H, Lamping KG, Eastham CL, Dellsperger KC, Marcus ML. Comparison of the effects of increased myocardial oxygen consumption and adenosine on the coronary microvascular resistance. *Circ Res* 1989;65:1296–1305.

106. Izumo S, Nadal-Ginard B, Mahdavi V. Protooncogene induction and reprogramming of cardiac gene expression produced by pressure overload. *Proc Natl Acad Sci U S A* 1988;85:339–343.

107. Nair KG, Cutilletta AF, Zak R, Koide T, Rabinowitz M. Biochemical correlates of cardiac hypertrophy, I: experimental model; changes in heart weight, RNA content, and nuclear RNA polymerase activity. *Circ Res* 1968;23:451–462.

108. Simpson PC. Proto-oncogenes and cardiac hypertrophy. *Annu Rev Physiol* 1989;51:189–202.

109. Morgan HE, Baker KM. Cardiac hypertrophy: mechanical, neural, and endocrine dependence. *Circulation* 1991;83:13–25.

110. Stephens NL, Swynghedauw B. Cardiovascular adaptations to mechanical overload. *Mol Cell Biochem* 1990; 93:1–6.

111. Borow KM, Colan SD, Neumann A. Altered left ventricular mechanics in patients with valvular aortic stenosis and coarctation of the aorta: effects on systolic performance and late outcome. *Circulation* 1985; 72:515–522.

112. Leman RB, Spinale FG, Dorn GW II, et al. Supernormal ejection performance is isolated to the ipsilateral congenitally pressure-overloaded ventricle. *J Am Coll Cardiol* 1989;13:1314–1319.

113. Dorn GW II, Donner R, Assey ME, et al. Alterations in left ventricular geometry, wall stress, and ejection performance after correction of congenital aortic stenosis. *Circulation* 1988;78:1358–1364.

114. Donner R, Carabello BA, Black I, Spann JF. Left ventricular wall stress in compensated aortic stenosis in children. *Am J Cardiol* 1983;51:946–951.

115. Assey ME, Wisenbaugh T, Spann JFJ, Gillette PC, Carabello BA. Unexpected persistence into adulthood of low wall stress in patients with congenital aortic stenosis: is there a fundamental difference in the hypertrophic response to a pressure overload present from birth? *Circulation* 1987;75:973–979.

116. Colan SD, Parness IA, Spevak PJ, Sanders SP. Developmental modulation of myocardial mechanics: age- and growth-related alterations in afterload and contractility. *J Am Coll Cardiol* 1992;19:619–629.

117. Schwitter J, Eberli FR, Ritter M, Turina M, Krayenbuehl HP. Myocardial oxygen consumption in aortic valve disease with and without left ventricular dysfunction. *Br Heart J* 1992;67:161–169.

118. Carroll JD, Carroll EP, Feldman T, et al. Sex-associated differences in left ventricular function in aortic stenosis of the elderly. *Circulation* 1992;86:1099–1107.

119. Carabello BA, Green LH, Grossman W, et al. Hemodynamic determinants of prognosis of aortic valve replacement in critical aortic stenosis and advanced congestive heart failure. *Circulation* 1980;62:42–48.

120. Douglas PS, Reichek N, Hackney K, Ioli A, St. John Sutton M. Contribution of afterload, hypertrophy, and geometry to left ventricular ejection fraction in aortic valve stenosis, pure aortic regurgitation and idiopathic dilated cardiomyopathy. *Am J Cardiol* 1987;59: 1398–1404.

121. Hwang MH, Hammermeister KE, Oprian C, et al. Preoperative identification of patients likely to have left ventricular dysfunction after aortic valve replacement: participants in the Veterans Administration Cooperative Study on Valvular Heart Disease. *Circulation* 1989; 80[Suppl]:I65–I76.

122. Wisenbaugh T, Booth D, DeMaria A, Nissen S, Waters J. Relationship of contractile state to ejection performance in patients with chronic aortic valve disease. *Circulation* 1986;73:47–53.

123. Huber D, Grimm J, Koch R, Krayenbuehl HP. Determinants of ejection performance in aortic stenosis. *Circulation* 1981;64:126–134.

124. Orsinelli DA, Aurigemma GP, Battista S, Krendel S, Gaasch WH. Left ventricular hypertrophy and mortality after aortic valve replacement for aortic stenosis: a high risk subgroup identified by preoperative relative wall thickness. *J Am Coll Cardiol* 1993;22:1679–1683.

125. Chilian WM, Marcus ML. Coronary vascular adaptations to myocardial hypertrophy. *Annu Rev Physiol* 1987;49:477–487.

126. Bache RJ, Alyono D, Sublett E, Dai X-Z. Myocardial blood flow in left ventricular hypertrophy developing in young and adult dogs. *Am J Physiol Heart Circ Physiol* 1993;251:H949–H956.

127. Flanagan MF, Fujii AM, Colan SD, Flanagan RG, Lock JE. Myocardial angiogenesis and coronary perfusion in left ventricular pressure-overload hypertrophy in the young lamb: evidence for inhibition with chronic protamine administration. *Circ Res* 1991;68: 1458–1470.

128. Rakusan K, Flanagan MF, Geva T, Southern J, Van Praagh R. Morphometry of human coronary capillaries during normal growth and the effect of age in left ventricular pressure-overload hypertrophy. *Circulation* 1992;86:38–46.

129. Aoyagi T, Mirsky I, Flanagan MF, et al. Myocardial function in immature and mature sheep with pressure-overload hypertrophy. *Am J Physiol Heart Circ Physiol* 1992;262:H1036–H1048.

130. Fujii AM, Aoyagi T, Flanagan MF, et al. Response of the hypertrophied left ventricle to tachycardia: importance of maturation. *Am J Physiol Heart Circ Physiol* 1993;264:H983–H993.

131. Rakusan K, Wicker P, Abdul-Samad M, Healey B, Turek Z. Failure of swimming exercise to improve capillarization in cardiac hypertrophy of renal hypertensive rats. *Circ Res* 1987;61:641–647.

132. St. John Sutton MG, Plappert TA, Hirshfeld JW, Reichek N. Assessment of left ventricular mechanics in patients with asymptomatic aortic regurgitation: a two-dimensional echocardiographic study. *Circulation* 1984;69:259–268.

133. Gaynor JW, Feneley MP, Gall SA Jr, et al. Measurement of left ventricular volume in normal and volume-overloaded canine hearts. *Am J Physiol Heart Circ Physiol* 1994;266:H329–H340.

134. Vandenbossche J-L, Massie BM, Schiller NB, Karliner JS. Relation of left ventricular shape to volume and mass in patients with minimally symptomatic chronic aortic regurgitation. *Am Heart J* 1988;116:1022–1027.

135. Donaldson RM, Florio R, Rickards AF, et al. Irreversible morphological changes contributing to depressed cardiac function after surgery for chronic aortic regurgitation. *Br Heart J* 1982;48:589–597.

136. Greenberg B, Massie B, Bristow JD, et al. Long-term vasodilator therapy of chronic aortic insufficiency: a randomized double-blinded, placebo-controlled clinical trial. *Circulation* 1988;78:92–103.

137. Scognamiglio R, Fasoli G, Ponchia A, Dalla-Volta S. Long-term nifedipine unloading therapy in asymptomatic patients with chronic severe aortic regurgitation. *J Am Coll Cardiol* 1990;16:424–429.

138. Villari B, Hess OM, Kaufmann P, et al. Effect of aortic valve stenosis (pressure overload) and regurgitation (volume overload) on left ventricular systolic and diastolic function. *Am J Cardiol* 1992;69:927–934.

139. Goldberg B, Fripp RR, Lister G, et al. Effect of physical training on exercise performance of children following surgical repair of congenital heart disease. *Pediatrics* 1981;68:691–699.

140. Bradley LM, Galioto FMJ, Vaccaro P, Hansen DA, Vaccaro J. Effect of intense aerobic training on exercise performance in children after surgical repair of tetralogy of Fallot or complete transposition of the great arteries. *Am J Cardiol* 1985;56:816–818.

141. Rowland TW. Trainability of the cardiorespiratory system during childhood [Review]. *Can J Sport Sci* 1992; 17:259–263.

142. Ruttenberg HD, Adams TD, Orsmond GS, Conlee RK, Fisher AG. Effects of exercise training on aerobic fitness in children after open heart surgery. *Pediatr Cardiol* 1983;4:19–24.

143. Gutgesell HP, Gessner IH, Vetter VL, Yabek SM, Norton JBJ. Recreational and occupational recommendations for young patients with heart disease. A statement for physicians by the Committee on Congenital Cardiac Defects of the Council on Cardiovascular Disease in the Young, American Heart Association. *Circulation* 1986;74:1195A–1198A.

144. Strauzenberg SE. Recommendations for physical activity and sports in children with heart disease. A statement by the Scientific Commission of the International Federation of Sportsmedicine (FIMS) approved by the Executive Committee of the FIMS. *J Sports Med* 1982;22:401–406.

145. Freed MD. Recreational and sports recommendations for the child with heart disease. *Pediatr Clin North Am* 1989;31:1307–1320.

146. Graham TP Jr, Bricker JT, James FW, Strong WB. Task Force 1: Congenital heart disease. *J Am Coll Cardiol* 1994;24:867–873.

147. Burke AP, Farb A, Virmani R. Causes of sudden death in athletes. *Cardiol Clin* 1992;10:303–317.

148. Driscoll DJ. Cardiorespiratory responses to exercise after the Fontan operation. *Circulation* 1990;81: 2016–2017.

149. Maron BJ, Shirani J, Poliac LC, et al. Sudden death in young competitive athletes. Clinical, demographic, and pathological profiles. *JAMA* 1996;276:199–204.

150. Taylor AJ, Rogan KM, Virmani R. Sudden cardiac death associated with isolated congenital coronary artery anomalies. *J Am Coll Cardiol* 1992;20:640–647.

151. Gillette PC, Garson A Jr. Sudden cardiac death in the pediatric population. *Circulation* 1992;85[Suppl]:I64–I69.

152. Siscovick DS, Laporte RE, Newman JM. The disease-specific benefits and risks of physical activity and exercise. *Pub Health Rep* 1985;100:180–188.

153. Friedewald VE Jr, Spence DW. Sudden cardiac death associated with exercise: the risk-benefit issue. *Am J Cardiol* 1990;66:183–188.

154. Viitasalo MT, Kala R, Eisalo A. Ambulatory electrocardiographic recording in endurance athletes. *Br Heart J* 1982;47:213–220.

155. Siscovick DS, Weiss NS, Fletcher RH, Lasky T. The incidence of primary cardiac arrest during vigorous exercise. *N Engl J Med* 1984;311:874–877.

156. Kohl HW, Powell KE, Gordon NF, Blair SN, Paffenbarger RS. Physical activity, physical fitness, and sudden cardiac death. *Epidemiol Rev* 1992;14:37–58.

157. Keane JF, Driscoll DJ, Gersony WM, et al. Second Natural History Study of Congenital Heart Defects: Results of treatment of patients with aortic valvar stenosis. *Circulation* 1993;87[Suppl]:I16–I27.

158. Oakley DG, Oakley CM. Significance of abnormal electrocardiograms in highly trained athletes. *Am J Cardiol* 1982;50:985–989.

159. Hanne-Paparo N, Wendkos MH, Brunner D. T wave abnormalities in the electrocardiograms of top-ranking athletes without demonstrable organic heart disease. *Am Heart J* 1971;81:743–747.

160. Spirito P, Maron BJ, Bonow RO, Epstein SE. Prevalence and significance of an abnormal S-T segment response to exercise in a young athletic population. *Am J Cardiol* 1983;51:1663–1666.

161. Zeppilli P, Pirrami MM, Sassara M, Fenici R. T wave abnormalities in top-ranking athletes: effects of isoproterenol, atropine, and physical exercise. *Am Heart J* 1980;100:213–221.

162. Lewis JF, Maron BJ, Diggs JA, et al. Preparticipation echocardiographic screening for cardiovascular disease in a large, predominantly black population of collegiate athletes. *Am J Cardiol* 1989;64:1029–1033.

163. Epstein SE, Maron BJ. Sudden death and the competitive athlete: perspectives on preparticipation screening studies. *J Am Coll Cardiol* 1986;7:220–230.

164. Maron BJ, Bodison SA, Wesley YE, Tucker E, Green KJ. Results of screening a large group of intercollegiate competitive athletes for cardiovascular disease. *J Am Coll Cardiol* 1987;10:1214–1222.

165. Maron BJ, Poliac LC, Roberts WO. Risk for sudden cardiac death associated with marathon running. *J Am Coll Cardiol* 1996;28:428–431.

166. Kitchiner DJ, Jackson M, Walsh K, Peart I, Arnold R. Incidence and prognosis of congenital aortic valve stenosis in Liverpool (1960–1990). *Br Heart J* 1993; 69:71–79.

167. Otto CM, Pearlman AS, Kraft CD, et al. Physiologic changes with maximal exercise in asymptomatic valvular aortic stenosis assessed by Doppler echocardiography. *J Am Coll Cardiol* 1992;20:1160–1167.

168. Cueto L, Moller JH. Hemodynamics of exercise in children with isolated aortic valvular disease. *Br Heart J* 1973;35:93–98.

169. Cyran SE, James FW, Daniels S, et al. Comparison of

the cardiac output and stroke volume response to upright exercise in children with valvular and subvalvular aortic stenosis. *J Am Coll Cardiol* 1988;11:651–658.

170. Iwasaka T, Nakamura S, Morita Y, et al. Left ventricular function during exercise after aortic valve replacement. *Cardiology* 1993;82:301–308.

171. Movsowitz C, Kussmaul WG, Laskey WK. Left ventricular diastolic response to exercise in valvular aortic stenosis. *Am J Cardiol* 1996;77:275–280.

172. Oldershaw PJ, Dawkins KD, Ward DE, Gibson DG. Diastolic mechanisms of impaired exercise tolerance in aortic valve disease. *Br Heart J* 1983;49:568–573.

173. Martin GR, Soifer SJ, Silverman NH, Dae MW, Stanger P. Effects of activity on ascending aortic velocity in children with valvar aortic stenosis. *Am J Cardiol* 1987;59:1386–1390.

174. Hossack KF, Neilson GH. Exercise testing in congenital aortic stenosis. *Aust N Z J Med* 1979;9:169–173.

175. Alpert BS, Kartodihardjo W, Harp R, Izukawa T, Strong WB. Exercise blood pressure response—a predictor of severity of aortic stenosis in children. *J Pediatrics* 1981;98:763–765.

176. James FW, Schwartz DC, Kaplan S, Spilkin SP. Exercise electrocardiogram, blood pressure, and working capacity in young patients with valvular or discrete subvalvular aortic stenosis. *Am J Cardiol* 1982;50: 769–775.

177. Barton CW, Katz B, Schork MA, Rosenthal A. Value of treadmill exercise test in pre- and postoperative children with valvular aortic stenosis. *Clin Cardiol* 1983; 6:473–477.

178. Cumming GR. Maximal exercise capacity of children with heart defects. *Am J Cardiol* 1978;42:613–619.

179. Goldberg SJ, Mendes F, Hurwitz R. Maximal exercise capability of children as a function of specific cardiac defects. *Am J Cardiol* 1969;23:349–353.

180. Whitmer JT, James FW, Kaplan S, Schwartz DC, Sandker-Knight MJ. Exercise testing in children before and after surgical treatment of aortic stenosis. *Circulation* 1981;63:254–263.

181. Goforth D, James FW, Kaplan S, Donner R, Mays W. Maximal exercise in children with aortic regurgitation: an adjunct to noninvasive assessment of disease severity. *Am Heart J* 1984;108:1306–1311.

182. Boucher CA, Wilson RA, Kanarek DJ, et al. Exercise testing in asymptomatic or minimally symptomatic aortic regurgitation: relationship of left ventricular ejection fraction to left ventricular filling pressure during exercise. *Circulation* 1983;67:1091–1100.

183. Wilson RA, Greenberg BH, Massie BM, et al. Left ventricular response to submaximal and maximal exercise in asymptomatic aortic regurgitation. *Am J Cardiol* 1988;62:606–610.

184. Gerson MC, Engel PJ, Mantil JC, et al. Effects of dynamic and isometric exercise on the radionuclide-determined regurgitant fraction in aortic insufficiency. *J Am Coll Cardiol* 1984;3:98–106.

185. Kawanishi DT, McKay CR, Chandraratna PA, et al. Cardiovascular response to dynamic exercise in patients with chronic symptomatic mild-to-moderate and severe aortic regurgitation. *Circulation* 1986;73:62–72.

186. Spain MG, Smith MD, Kwan OL, DeMaria AN. Effect of isometric exercise on mitral and aortic regurgitation as assessed by color Doppler flow imaging. *Am J Cardiol* 1990;65:78–83.

187. Shen WF, Roubin GS, Hirasawa K, et al. Abnormal left ventricular response to isometric exercise in pure, isolated aortic regurgitation: beneficial effects of nifedipine. *Am J Cardiol* 1984;54:605–609.

188. Shen WF, Roubin GS, Hirasawa K, et al. Noninvasive assessment of acute effects of nifedipine on rest and exercise hemodynamics and cardiac function in patients with aortic regurgitation. *J Am Coll Cardiol* 1984; 4:902–907.

189. Cheitlin MD, Douglas PS, Parmley WW. Task Force 2: Acquired valvular heart disease. *J Am Coll Cardiol* 1994;24:874–880.

190. Lambert EC, Menon VA, Wagner HR, Vlad P. Sudden unexpected death from cardiovascular disease in children. *Am J Cardiol* 1974;34:89–96.

191. Thornback P, Fowler RS. Sudden unexpected death in children with congenital heart disease. *Can Med Assoc J* 1975;113:745–748.

192. Doyle EF, Arumugham P, Lara E, Rutkowski MR, Kiely B. Sudden death in young patients with congenital aortic stenosis. *Pediatrics* 1974;53:481–489.

193. Bastianon V, Del Bolgia F, Boscioni M, et al. Altered cardiac repolarization during exercise in congenital aortic stenosis. *Pediatr Cardiol* 1993;14:23–27.

194. Arnold R, Kitchiner D. Left ventricular outflow obstruction [Review]. *Arch Dis Child* 1995;72:180–183.

195. Kveselis DA, Rocchini AP, Rosenthal A, et al. Hemodynamic determinants of exercise-induced ST-segment depression in children with valvar aortic stenosis. *Am J Cardiol* 1985;55:1133–1139.

196. Driscoll DJ, Wolfe RR, Gersony WM, et al. Cardiorespiratory responses to exercise of patients with aortic stenosis, pulmonary stenosis, and ventricular septal defect. *Circulation* 1993;87[Suppl]:I102–I113.

197. Chandramouli B, Ehmke DA, Lauer RM. Exercise-induced electrocardiographic changes in children with congenital aortic stenosis. *J Pediatr* 1975;87:725–730.

198. von Olshausen K, Schwarz F, Apfelbach J, et al. Determinants of the incidence and severity of ventricular arrhythmias in aortic valve disease. *Am J Cardiol* 1983; 51:1103–1109.

199. Klein RC. Ventricular arrhythmias in aortic valve disease: analysis of 102 patients. *Am J Cardiol* 1984;53: 1079–1083.

200. Schwartz LS, Goldfischer J, Sprague GJ, Schwartz SP. Syncope and sudden death in aortic stenosis. *Am J Cardiol* 1969;23:647–658.

201. Kulbertus HE. Ventricular arrhythmias, syncope and sudden death in aortic stenosis. *Eur Heart J* 1988;9: 51–52.

202. Yano K, Kuriya T, Hashiba K. Simultaneous monitoring of electrocardiogram and arterial blood pressure during exercise-induced syncope in a patient with severe aortic stenosis. *Angiology* 1989;40:143–148.

203. Chen J-S, Wang W, Cornish KG, Zucker IH. Baro- and ventricular reflexes in conscious dogs subjected to chronic tachycardia. *Am J Physiol Heart Circ Physiol* 1992;263:H1084–H1089.

204. Edwards WD, Leaf DS, Edwards JE. Dissecting aortic aneurysm associated with congenital bicuspid aortic valve. *Circulation* 1978;57:1022–1025.

205. Edwards JE. Aneurysms of the thoracic aorta complicating coarctation. *Circulation* 1973;48:195–201.

206. Roberts CS, Roberts WC. Dissection of the aorta associated with congenital malformation of the aortic valve. *J Am Coll Cardiol* 1991;17:712–716.

207. Pachulski RT, Weinberg AL, Chan K-L. Aortic aneurysm in patients with functionally normal or minimally stenotic bicuspid aortic valve. *Am J Cardiol* 1991; 67:781–782.

208. Basso C, Frescura C, Corrado D, et al. Congenital heart disease and sudden death in the young. *Hum Pathol* 1995;26:1065–1072.

209. Milewicz DM, Michael K, Fisher N, et al. Fibrillin–1 (FBN1) mutations in patients with thoracic aortic aneurysms. *Circulation* 1996;94:2708–2711.

210. Shimizu G, Zile MR, Blaustein AS, Gaasch WH. Left ventricular chamber filling and midwall fiber lengthening in patients with left ventricular hypertrophy: overestimation of fiber velocities by conventional midwall measurements. *Circulation* 1985;71:266–272.

211. Shimizu G, Hirota Y, Kita Y, et al. Left ventricular midwall mechanics in systemic arterial hypertension: myocardial function is depressed in pressure-overload hypertrophy. *Circulation* 1991;83:1676–1684.

212. Palmon LC, Reichek N, Yeon SB, et al. Intramural myocardial shortening in hypertensive left ventricular hypertrophy with normal pump function. *Circulation* 1994;89:122–131.

213. Schwartzkopff B, Motz W, Vogt M, Strauer BE. Heart failure on the basis of hypertension. *Circulation* 1993;87[Suppl 4]:IV66–IV72.

214. Clarkson PM, Nicholson MR, Barratt-Boyes BG, Neutze JM, Whitlock RM. Results after repair of coarctation of the aorta beyond infancy: a 10 to 28 year follow-up with particular reference to late systemic hypertension. *Am J Cardiol* 1983;51:1481–1488.

215. Moskowitz WB, Schieken RM, Mosteller M, Bossano R. Altered systolic and diastolic function in children after "successful" repair of coarctation of the aorta. *Am Heart J* 1990;120:103–109.

216. Krogmann ON, Kramer HH, Rammos S, Heusch A, Bourgeois M. Non-invasive evaluation of left ventricular systolic function late after coarctation repair: influence of early vs late surgery. *Eur Heart J* 1993;14: 764–769.

217. Carpenter MA, Dammann JF, Watson DD, et al. Left ventricular hyperkinesia at rest and during exercise in normotensive patients 2 to 27 years after coarctation repair. *J Am Coll Cardiol* 1985;6:879–886.

218. Leandro J, Smallhorn JF, Benson L, et al. Ambulatory blood pressure monitoring and left ventricular mass and function after successful surgical repair of coarctation of the aorta. *J Am Coll Cardiol* 1992;20:197–204.

219. Ong CM, Canter CE, Gutierrez FR, Sekarski DR, Goldring DR. Increased stiffness and persistent narrowing of the aorta after successful repair of coarctation of the aorta: relationship to left ventricular mass and blood pressure at rest and with exercise. *Am Heart J* 1992;123:1594–1600.

220. Gidding SS, Rocchini AP, Moorehead C, Schork MA, Rosenthal A. Increased forearm vascular reactivity in patients with hypertension after repair of coarctation. *Circulation* 1985;71:495–499.

221. Sehested J, Baandrup U, Mikkelsen E. Different reactivity and structure of the prestenotic and poststenotic aorta in human coarctation. Implications for baroreceptor function. *Circulation* 1982;65:1060–1065.

222. Gardiner HM, Celermajer DS, Sorensen KE, et al. Arterial reactivity is significantly impaired in normotensive young adults after successful repair of aortic coarctation in childhood. *Circulation* 1994;89:1745–1750.

223. Markel H, Rocchini AP, Beekman RH, et al. Exercise-induced hypertension after repair of coarctation of the aorta: arm versus leg exercise. *J Am Coll Cardiol* 1986; 8:165–171.

224. Smith RTJ, Sade RM, Riopel DA, et al. Stress testing for comparison of synthetic patch aortoplasty with resection and end to end anastomosis for repair of coarctation in childhood. *J Am Coll Cardiol* 1984;4:765–770.

225. McCrindle BW. Independent predictors of long-term results after balloon pulmonary valvuloplasty. *Circulation* 1994;89:1751–1759.

226. Perrault H, Drblik SP, Montigny M, et al. Comparison of cardiovascular adjustments to exercise in adolescents 8 to 15 years of age after correction of tetralogy of Fallot, ventricular septal defect or atrial septal defect. *Am J Cardiol* 1989;64:213–217.

227. Reybrouck T, Bisschop A, Dumoulin M, Van der Hauwaert LG. Cardiorespiratory exercise capacity after surgical closure of atrial septal defect is influenced by the age at surgery. *Am Heart J* 1991;122:1073–1078.

228. Rosenfeld HM, Van der Velde ME, Sanders SP, et al. Echocardiographic predictors of candidacy for successful transcatheter atrial septal defect closure. *Cathet Cardiovasc Diagn* 1995;34:29–34.

229. Gilljam T, Eriksson BO. Maximal exercise test in long-term follow-up after atrial redirection for complete transposition in a population-based cohort. *Cardiol Young* 1996;6:208–215.

230. Reybrouck T, Gewillig M, Dumoulin M, Van der Hauwaert LG. Cardiorespiratory exercise performance after Senning operation for transposition of the great arteries. *Br Heart J* 1993;70:175–179.

231. Carvalho JS, Shinebourne EA, Busst C, Rigby ML,

Redington AN. Exercise capacity after complete repair of tetralogy of Fallot: deleterious effects of residual pulmonary regurgitation. *Br Heart J* 1992;67:470–473.

232. Paridon SM, Sullivan NM, Schneider J, Pinsky WW. Cardiopulmonary performance at rest and exercise after repair of total anomalous pulmonary venous connection. *Am J Cardiol* 1993;72:1444–1447.

233. Weindling SN, Wernovsky G, Colan SD, et al. Myocardial perfusion, function and exercise tolerance after the arterial switch operation. *J Am Coll Cardiol* 1994;23:424–433.

234. Tanel RE, Wernovsky G, Landzberg MJ, Perry SB, Burke RP. Coronary artery abnormalities detected at cardiac catheterization following the arterial switch operation for transposition of the great arteries. *Am J Cardiol* 1995;76:153–157.

235. Bricker JT. Sudden death and tetralogy of Fallot: risks, markers, and causes. *Circulation* 1995;92:158–159.

236. Gatzoulis MA, Till JA, Somerville J, Redington AN. Mechanoelectrical interaction in tetralogy of Fallot: QRS prolongation relates to right ventricular size and predicts malignant ventricular arrhythmias and sudden death. *Circulation* 1995;92:231–237.

237. Garson A Jr, McNamara DG. Sudden death in a pediatric cardiology population, 1958 to 1983: relation to prior arrhythmias. *J Am Coll Cardiol* 1985;5: 134B–137B.

238. Neuspiel DR, Kuller LH. Sudden and unexpected death in childhood and adolescence. *JAMA* 1985;254: 1321–1325.

239. Steinberger J, Lucas RV Jr, Edwards JE, Titus JL. Causes of sudden unexpected cardiac death in the first two decades of life. *Am J Cardiol* 1996;77:992–995.

The Athlete and Heart Disease:
Diagnosis, Evaluation & Management,
edited by R. A. Williams.
Lippincott Williams & Wilkins, Philadelphia © 1999.

8

Recreational and Competitive Athletics in Older Adults with Cardiovascular Disease

Luther T. Clark, George Nseir, and Roseann M. Chesler

Division of Cardiovascular Medicine, State University of New York Health Science Center, Brooklyn, New York 11203

During recent decades there has been an increasing consciousness of physical fitness among individuals of all ages in the United States. Participation in moderate and strenuous exercises has been increasing, and health clubs and other opportunities for recreational and competitive athletics have proliferated. Furthermore, several groups of national experts have recently emphasized the benefits of regular exercise for cardiovascular fitness and health (1–4), and recommended increased physical activity for all adults. Even so and despite the national emphasis on fitness, physical inactivity remains an important concern, particularly among middle-aged and older adults. Only about one in four adults are active at the level recommended for meaningful health benefits and fewer than 10% of adults exercise vigorously at an intensity sufficient to promote improved cardiovascular fitness (1,3).

The United States is a graying nation and the proportion of older and elderly individuals in the U.S. population is increasing with each census. In the 1990 census, 12.5% of the U.S. population was 65 years of age and older with a disproportionate increase among the group aged 85 years and older. This chapter focuses on recreational and competitive athletics in mature and aging adults, the effects of aging on exercise capacity, the benefits and risks of exercise in

individuals with and without cardiovascular disease, and recommendations for preparticipatory evaluation, prescribing, and monitoring of exercise in this group.

PHYSIOLOGIC CHANGES ASSOCIATED WITH AGING

Aging is associated with progressive changes in cardiovascular, respiratory, musculoskeletal, and central nervous system functions that impact on functional capacity and the types of exercises that individuals can perform. In addition, aging is associated with an increased prevalence of disease and physical inactivity. Some of the changes in functional capacity that are attributed to aging are due to physical inactivity and disease.

Phases of Growth and Aging

As listed in Table 1, growth and aging can be divided into three phases (5). Phase I is the phase of growth and development and includes the toddler/preschool, preadolescence, and adolescence categories. Phase II is the maturity phase and includes the postadolescent and young adult years. Phase III is the aging phase and includes the middle age and elderly categories. The focus of this chapter is primarily on the changes that occur during phase III.

TABLE 1. *Phases of growth and aging*

Category	Years
Phase I: Growth and Development	
Toddler and preschooler	<5
Preadolescent	5–11
Adolescent	12–14
Phase II: Maturity	
Postadolescent	15–19
Young adult	20–30
Phase III: Aging	
Early middle age	30–45
Late middle age	45–65
Young elderly	65–75
Middle elderly	75–85
Very old	>85

Adapted from ref. 6, with permission.

TABLE 2. *Age-related central and physiologic changes that impact on physical work performance and exercise*

Cardiovascular
Decline in $\dot{V}O_{2\ max}$
Decline in max heart rate
Decline in cardiac output
Decreased myocardial muscle mass
Reduction in peripheral blood flow capacity resulting from a decrease in capillary-to-muscle ratio
Pulmonary
Deterioration in static and dynamic lung function
Neurologic
Decline in the number of spinal cord axons, in the nerve conduction velocity with a significant loss in the elastic properties of connective tissue, which affects simple and complex reaction and movement times
Musculoskeletal
Body composition and bone density
Increased body composition and percent fat
Decreased lean body mass
Loss of bone mass
Deterioration of joint structure and decreased collagen
Loss of flexibility
Decrease in muscle mass

Adapted from ref. 10, with permission.

Fitness, Endurance, and Aging

Fitness can be defined in many ways, but usually refers to the ability of an individual to perform moderate to vigorous physical activity without undue fatigue and the capability of maintaining such ability throughout life (6). On the other hand, cardiopulmonary endurance refers to the ability to perform moderate-to-high-intensity work using a large muscle mass for relatively long periods of time. Maximum oxygen consumption ($\dot{V}O_{2\ max}$) is the accepted measure of cardiopulmonary endurance and is a marker of fitness and clinical status. $\dot{V}O_{2\ max}$ is determined by the capacity of the cardiovascular system to deliver oxygen to working muscles and the ability for muscles to use oxygen. It requires functional involvement from the cardiovascular, pulmonary, and musculoskeletal systems and is used as an index by which to evaluate overall maximal cardiovascular functional capacity.

Aerobic Capacity and Maximum Oxygen Consumption

The decline in function that accompanies aging is primarily a consequence of age-related decrements in cardiovascular, pulmonary, and musculoskeletal function. Table 2 and Figure 1 summarize the major physiologic changes that occur with aging that may impact on exercise capacity (5,7–8). There is a linear decline in

the maximum work capacity and the maximal oxygen consumption with aging, at a rate of about 1% per year. Aerobic activity declines about 0.45 mL/O_2/kg/minute per year between the ages of 20 and 65 years in men and 0.3 mL/O_2/kg/minute per year for women. Thus, by age 55 years, the $\dot{V}O_{2\ max}$ in both males and females decreases approximately 30% below values reported for 20- to 30-year-olds.

Figure 2 shows the decline in $\dot{V}O_{2\ max}$ with age for a variety of physical activity groups. The rate of decline in $\dot{V}O_{2\ max}$ with increasing age is nearly twofold faster in sedentary individuals than in athletes (9–11). Physically active individuals and athletes have higher baseline $\dot{V}O_{2\ max}$ values and less decrease with aging (9).

Cardiac Output, Peripheral Vascular Resistance, and Blood Pressure

Maximum attainable heart rate declines with age, as do stroke volume, cardiac output, and the magnitude of increase in arterial pres-

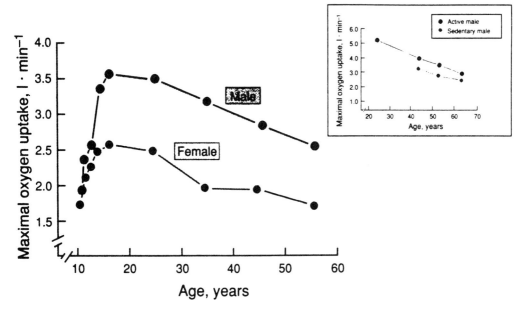

FIG. 1. Rate of decline in $\dot{V}O_2$ as a function of aging. From ref. 7, with permission.

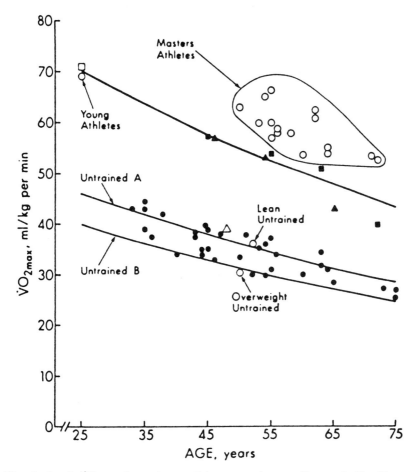

FIG. 2. The decline in $\dot{V}O_{2\ max}$ for various activity groups by age. From ref. 10, with permission.

sure during exercise. Decreased left ventricular compliance, impaired diastolic filling, decreased cardiac contractility, and impaired chronotropic responses to exercise contribute to the reduction in cardiac output. Reductions in vascular smooth muscle compliance caused by calcification and connective tissue infiltration of the aorta and arteries result in increased systolic pressure. The systolic hypertension and impaired diastolic function contribute further to reduced stroke volume, increased myocardial oxygen demand, and limitation of cardiovascular function. There is a modest decline in peripheral oxygen extraction with aging.

Muscular Strength and Flexibility

Muscular strength decreases with aging and correlates with a decrease in muscle mass and force (7). Muscle mass begins to decline at about age 30 years and muscular strength may decrease 30% to 50% with aging. Flexibility also decreases with age and is exacerbated by physical inactivity.

Training and Age-Related Decrease in Exercise Capacity

Exercise training can delay and partially reverse some of the age-associated decline in cardiac functional capacity. Chesler et al. (12) showed that aerobic training prescribed at 75% of maximum heart rate reserve produced increases in $\dot{V}O_{2\ max}$ in women aged 55 to 70 years who were previously sedentary. Hagberg and coworkers (9) showed a 14% increase in $\dot{V}O_{2\ max}$ following a 3-month training program in healthy men aged 67 to 76 years. These same investigators also found that a 6-month program of walking at 40% heart rate reserve resulted in a 12% increase in $\dot{V}O_{2\ max}$ in men and women who had an average age of 63 years. Subjects who continued to walk at higher intensities (85% max heart rate reserve for an additional 6 months) demonstrated another 18% increase. Badentop and coworkers (13) reported similar $\dot{V}O_2$ peak during bicycle ergometry in men and women whether they exercised at 57% or at 70% of max $\dot{V}O_2$ during a 9-week training program. DeVries (14) showed that more than one-third of 60- to 79-year-old men who completed a 6-week walking-jogging program at 41% to 51% of heart rate reserve increased their $\dot{V}O_2$ peak. Thus, low-intensity aerobic training can elicit an increase in $\dot{V}O_{2\ max}$, a finding that is of particular importance for developing exercise programs for the elderly and others who cannot, or who choose not to, engage in vigorous physical activity.

Highly Trained Individuals and Elite Athletes

In cross-sectional and longitudinal studies of the older elite athlete, it has been shown that the decrease in $\dot{V}O_{2\ max}$ with aging can be blunted by approximately one-half (5% per decade versus 10% per decade) with continued hard training. Highly trained older and elderly individuals can maintain stroke volume, peripheral oxygen extraction, and body composition at or near the levels they possessed in their 20s and 30s.

The decline in $\dot{V}O_{2\ max}$ with aging is similar in men and women (15). Drinkwater and colleagues (15) examined aerobic capacity in female subjects aged 10 to 68 years and found that, when women who were categorized as physically fit were compared to those who were unfit, the fit women had superior $\dot{V}O_{2\ max}$, oxygen debt, and postexercise blood lactate. However, there were no differences across age between fit and unfit on maximum heart rate, excess carbon dioxide, and respiratory exchange ratios. The sharpest decline in most variables occurred after age 50 years.

EXERCISE PATTERNS IN OLDER MALES AND FEMALES

Physical Activity Levels

Participation rates in physical exercise have increased substantially during recent years among older (more than 30 years) and elderly (more than 65 years) individuals. It is not uncommon to see individuals of all ages engaging in recreational, low-intensity exercise (e.g., brisk walking, doubles tennis, bicycling) and in vigorous aerobic exercises such as jogging or singles tennis. Even so, overall participation rates remain below national goals. Figure 3 summarizes the physical activity levels among adults in the United States (16). Less than 40% of U.S. adults engage in the recommended amount of physical activity. Approximately 25% of adults are inactive and engage in little or no physical activities. The prevalence of physical inactivity is greater among women than men, among African Americans and Hispanics than among Caucasians, among older than among younger individuals, and among the less affluent rather than more affluent individuals.

Physical inactivity increases with age and by age 75 years, approximately one in three men and one in two women do not engage in physical activity. Among those adults aged 65 years and older who choose to exercise, walking, gardening, and yard work are the most common forms of physical activity. In a report that investigated the physical activity trends among adults within 26 states between 1986 and 1990 (17), leisure time activity was divided into four categories: (a) physical inactivity (no leisure time physical activity), (b) irregularly active (activity performed less than three times per week, less than 20 minutes per session, or both), (c) regularly active, not intensive (more than three times per week, more than 20 minutes per session at less than 60% max capacity, rhythmically contracting, large muscle groups), and (d) regularly active, intensive (more than three times per week, greater than 20 minutes per session, greater than 60% max capacity). According to this report, approximately 6 of 10 adults were physically inactive or irregularly active. Among those who were regularly active, only one of ten were performing exercise at a level known to promote cardiovascular fitness, a finding similar to reports by others (18–21).

Figure 4 summarizes activity status among adults and older individuals classified as physically inactive and regularly active, intensive (17). In general, older men and women showed similar declines in being physically inactive. However, men did not increase significantly in the regularly active, intensive category in the same manner as women. There were no statistically significant changes in the prevalence of several common activities (e.g., walking, cycling, and swimming) for men and women to explain the declines over the 5 years in being physically inactive. It is uncertain whether the choice of competitive or highly vigorous exercise has changed since this study.

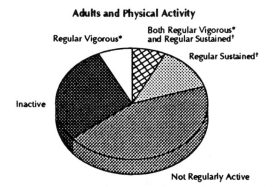

FIG. 3. Summary of the physical activity habits of U.S. adults. *Regular Vigorous–20 minutes 3 times per week of vigorous intensity. †Regular Sustained–30 minutes 5 times per week of any intensity. (Source: CDC, 1992, Behavioral Risk Factor Survey.)

Factors Influencing Choice of Activity among the Elderly

Although it has not been determined what specific factors go into choosing most activities for recreational and competitive athletics among the elderly, those factors that contribute to selection of walking for fitness have been studied (22–23). Women and older adults (older than 50 years) report significantly more walking as physical activity than younger respondents. For the most sedentary subgroups, self-efficacy, family and friend support, and consumption of a heart-healthy diet were associated with the choice of walking for exercise. Thus, interest in walking for exercise appears to be related primarily to

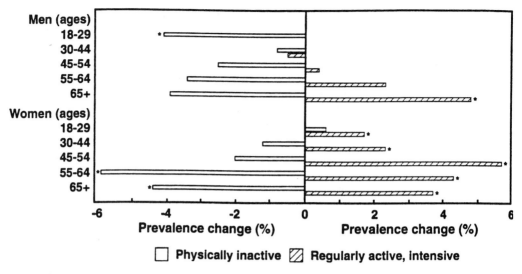

FIG. 4. Summary of the change in two physical activity patterns for men and women by age. From BRFSS 1986–1990. National Center for Chronic Disease Prevention and Health Promotion. Center for Disease Control.

factors other than prevention of cardiovascular disease. Exercise history (participation in physical activity and physical education at younger ages) was negatively associated with minutes of walking. Respondents who were more involved in sports and exposed to physical education classes in childhood were less likely to walk for exercise, but more likely to choose vigorous exercises for fitness. Age was the most powerful demographic variable that correlated with walking for fitness.

Competitive Athletics in Older Individuals

Whereas organized team sports are the primary focus of young athletes, in older athletes (35 years and older), the primary focus is on individual endeavors such as long-distance running—the most common form of vigorous exercise in this group. In patients with known cardiac disease who are enrolled in cardiac rehabilitation programs, regular mild to moderate exercise is the primary objective. However, some cardiac rehabilitation programs (24) go beyond such relatively mild exercises as running in gymnasiums, swimming indoors, and calisthenics at home to more strenuous and competitive outdoor activities. Occasionally, patients who have had

a myocardial infarction can compete in such vigorous competitive sports as marathon running (25). Although marathon running is not a recommended component of the postmyocardial infarction rehabilitative program, with proper training and supervision, some patients who were long distance runners before their infarction may return to this activity if their cardiac status permits.

Patient Perception of Activity Level

Most older individuals overestimate the amount of physical activity they participate in. They often perceive that their level of activity is moderate to high, when in fact it is low (26). In a study by Clarke (27), 71% of persons older than 60 years believed that they were engaged in a sufficient amount of physical activity (performing daily chores and slow walking) and did not see a need for increasing the level of their activity. In addition, those activities which were undertaken were typically gentle walking rather than brisk walking and the vigor was rarely sufficient to be considered vigorous sport or to reach an appropriate activity threshold.

Perceptions of one's physical fitness and exercise activity is important in selection of whether to exercise and what type of exercise to select. Data from participants at one senior citizen's club (ages 63 to 82 years) indicated that participation in physical activities and exercise depended on a number of factors, including adequate time, the presence of other persons, and selection of an enjoyable activity (28). Sustained lower levels of exercise were often more suitable to the situations and functional capabilities of these older adults.

BENEFITS OF EXERCISE IN OLDER ADULTS

Healthy men and women as well as many of those with cardiovascular disease derive benefit from regular physical activity. These benefits include improved exercise capacity, primary and secondary prevention of cardiovascular disease, and lower cardiovascular and overall mortality rate. Recommendations for increased physical activity have been made by the American Heart Association (4), the American College of Sports Medicine (2), the U.S. Department of Health and Human Services (1,16), and others. These groups have recommended that all Americans engage in a program of regular physical activity tailored to their health status and personal lifestyle.

A lifetime of physical activity ameliorates many of the effects of aging. Cardiovascular and overall mortality rates are decreased, and quality of life is improved. In the ongoing study of Harvard College alumni (29), physically active subjects and those who changed from a sedentary to an active life in middle age (and even at advanced age) showed benefit. For those who changed from a sedentary to an active lifestyle, the overall reduction in risk of death was comparable to those who had always been active, no matter how late one started—at least to age 90 years.

Physiologic Benefits

The specific physiologic benefits of regular exercise in older individuals include improvements in physical performance and functional capacity, maximal exercise capacity, maximal oxygen consumption, and cardiac output; a decline in resting heart rate and blood pressure; and increased cardiovascular fitness (30–31). These improvements are due to peripheral and cardiac adaptation, but, in older individuals and in patients with heart or lung disease, peripheral adaptations are especially important. Minute ventilation and vital capacity, muscle strength and flexibility, and bone density also improve. Increased flexibility and muscle strength help maintain mobility and may reduce the incidence of falls and bed sores. The magnitude of the benefits of physical exercise is related to baseline status, and the frequency and intensity of exercise. Recently, it has also been shown that exercise-induced increases in blood flow and shear stress enhance vascular function and structure (32). The increase in endothelial shear stress causes increased nitric oxide and prostacyclin release with augmentation of endothelium-dependent vasodilation and inhibition of multiple processes involved in atherogenesis (32).

Metabolic Benefits

Regular exercise improves lipid profile with an increase in high density lipoprotein, and decreases in total low density lipoprotein, and very low density lipoprotein cholesterol levels (31,33). The increase in high density lipoprotein is strongly associated with changes in body weight and higher levels of exercise. In overweight men and women, regular exercise also enhances the beneficial effects of low saturated fat and low cholesterol diets on blood lipoprotein levels. Exercise training also improves carbohydrate metabolism, glucose tolerance, and insulin sensitivity. In addition, regular physical activity results in lower catecholamine responses to exercise, a salutary effect on fibrinogen levels of healthy older men (34), and reduced risk of osteoporosis and certain neoplastic diseases (35).

Psychological Benefits

The psychological benefits of regular exercise include feeling better, looking better, having more energy, having improved memory and concentration, having improved mood and self-confidence, and having reduced depression and improved overall psychological well-being (4). The nature of the relationship between exercise and mental health is poorly understood. However, improved levels of self-esteem reported in physically active persons may be largely due to improved personal appearance and self-image.

Patients with Cardiovascular Disease

In patients with known coronary heart disease, exercise has similar benefits as in individuals without cardiovascular disease. These include improvements in exercise tolerance, muscle strength, and endurance; decrease in blood pressure; improvement in blood lipid levels; improvement of symptoms; reduction in cigarette smoking; improvement in psychosocial well-being; reduction of stress and mortality rate; and ability to return to work (36). Exercise training also decreases myocardial oxygen demands for a given level of work (as demonstrated by a decrease in the product of heart rate and systolic blood pressure), a particularly beneficial change in patients with coronary artery disease.

RISKS OF EXERCISE

Musculoskeletal

The most common risk in exercising is injury to the muscles and joints. Such injuries are usually due to exercising too hard for too long, particularly if a person has been inactive. In older athletes, factors that contribute to increased risk for musculoskeletal injury include decreasing flexibility with aging, decreased nerve conduction and reaction time, decreased hearing or vision, joint disease, decreased muscle mass, and osteoporosis. The risk of injury increases with increased intensity, frequency, duration, and type of activity. Exercise-related injuries can be reduced by moderating these parameters. Elevations in the intensity and amount of physical activity from moderate to vigorous may increase ben-

efit; however, it is associated not only with a greater risk of injury but also with discontinuation of activity and acute cardiac events.

Cardiovascular Risks of Vigorous Physical Activity

Although the absolute incidence of cardiovascular events and deaths during exercise is low, the cardiovascular risks of exercise remain a major concern for physicians. In addition to the responsibility of evaluating patients before participation in vigorous athletics, physicians face potential legal liability both for failing to detect cardiac abnormalities and for restricting athletic participation (37). Several investigators have evaluated the risks of major cardiovascular complications during recreational activities (e.g., court games, jogging). Individuals who engage in vigorous physical activity have a slight increase in risk of sudden cardiac death during activity. The risk is greatest among sedentary individuals performing sudden, unregulated, strenuous exercises (33,37–44). In a 5-year retrospective investigation (39) conducted on 155 YMCAs and Jewish Community Centers throughout the United States, it was concluded that a small acute risk of cardiovascular complication exists in the general public during recreational activity and that the incidence of cardiovascular complications during exercise training is greater among cardiac patients. Those activities most often associated with fatal and nonfatal cardiovascular complications include racquetball, handball, squash, and jogging, with lower rates associated with swimming, basketball, calisthenics, soccer, and walking. The higher incidence of cardiac events during court games and jogging probably reflect the greater relative participation in these sports. In the study by Siskovick and colleagues (40), among men with habitual low levels of activity, the relative risk of cardiac arrest during exercise, compared with all other times, was 56, whereas among men with habitual high levels of exercise, it was 5.

In younger individuals who die suddenly during athletic activities, hypertrophic cardiomyopathy is the most common cause, whereas, in older adults, coronary artery disease is most frequently implicated (40). Among more than 90 cases of death in joggers and marathon runners that have been reported, coronary artery disease was present in 75%. The most frequently reported diseased artery is the left anterior descending (LAD) coronary artery and the most frequent combination is the LAD and right coronary arteries (41). The incidence of death during jogging is estimated to be one death for every 396,000 hours of jogging or one in 15,000 joggers and one death for every 50,000 marathon runners (43,44).

In studies of death during exercise, the most important variable associated with risk of death was the individual's normal activity pattern. Those who had the highest intensity and frequency of activity were least likely to die at rest and during activity. On the other hand, those who were sedentary with no regular physical activity had the greatest risk of death during physical exertion and at rest. Individuals who exercise on a regular basis have a very, very low risk of sudden death during exercise. In fact, in postmyocardial infarction patients, exercise is an important component of their rehabilitation programs.

GUIDELINES FOR EXERCISE PRESCRIPTION FOR OLDER AND ELDERLY ADULTS

Goals of Exercise Training and Rehabilitation

Many of the functional decrements in exercise capacity observed in older and elderly individuals result from decreased physical activity and physical inactivity (6). In elderly individuals who are healthy, the cardiovascular and musculoskeletal systems respond to exercise training in a manner similar to that of younger individuals. Therefore, the goal of regular exercise is primary prevention with the specific objectives of (a) maintaining or improving fitness and (b) maintaining or improving health. The goals of exercise programs for older and elderly patients with cardiovascular disease are (a) restoration of physical function and health, (b) reduction of risk of cardiovascular morbidity, and (c) reduction of cardiovascular and all-cause mortality.

All adults should participate in regular physical activity at a level appropriate to their abilities, needs, and interests (1–4). The long-term activity goal should be to accumulate at least 30 minutes or more of moderate-intensity physical activity on most, or preferably all, days of the week. Shorter bouts of activity of at least 10 minutes (occupational and nonoccupational) may also provide cardiovascular and other health benefits if performed at a level of moderate intensity (brisk walking, cycling, swimming, home repair, and yard work) with an accumulated duration of at least 30 minutes per day.

Preparticipatory Evaluation

The main purpose of the preparticipatory evaluation is to detect underlying medical problems that may limit one's ability to exercise or that place the individual at increased risk (45). Another potential use of the preparticipatory assessment is to assess fitness so that appropriate exercise counseling may be provided and performance maximized safely. Because the risks of physical activity are very low compared with health benefits, routine medical consultation and pretesting before starting a moderate-intensity physical activity program is not necessary for all adults. However, previously sedentary older adults should be medically evaluated before beginning a vigorous physical activity program. Men older than age 40 years and women older than age 50 years who plan to begin a new program of vigorous activity should have a careful screening to detect cardiovascular or other health problems that may increase risk. In addition, previously sedentary individuals older than 40 years old should also have a baseline exercise stress test before participation in a vigorous exercise program (higher intensity than walking at 50% to 60% maximum heart rate reserve). Asymptomatic individuals younger than 40 years old with no risk factors and no history of coronary artery disease do not require a preparticipatory exercise stress test. When a definite cardiovascular diagnosis is made, the consensus guidelines of the 26th Bethesda Conference (46) should be referred to for specific recommendations for participation in competitive sports.

Frequency, Duration, Intensity

Guidelines for exercise fitness and rehabilitation for adults have been developed and published by the American Heart Association (4), the American College of Sports Medicine (47), the Centers for Disease Control (3), and the American Association for Cardiovascular and Pulmonary Rehabilitation (48). These are summarized in Table 3. The frequency, intensity and duration of activity are interrelated. Higher intensity or longer duration activity should be performed approximately three times weekly, and low intensity or shorter duration activity should be performed more often to achieve cardiovascular benefits. Traditional advice has been for patients to exercise to heart rates between 70% and 85% of maximum. However, training intensities in the 50% to 70% range have been shown to give comparable improvement in functional capacity and endurance, may be safer during unsu-

pervised exercise, and may lead to better adherence to prescribed exercise. A moderate-intensity program of physical activity confers health benefits but activity must be performed regularly to maintain these effects. Moderate-intensity activities are more likely to be continued than high-intensity activity.

Type of Activity

The specific type of activity is best determined by the individual's preferences and what will be sustained. Reduction of cardiovascular risk factors and other health benefits of physical activity do not require a structured or vigorous exercise program because the majority of benefits can be gained from moderate-intensity activities. There should be clear communication of the types of exercise and effective strategies to promote physical activity. The type of exercise program performed by individuals can consist of several types such as the following:

1. Aerobic-type exercise is defined as a constant but not overly strenuous activity in which oxygen delivery to the muscles does not exceed its demand. Aerobic activities include brisk walking, cycling, singles tennis, low- or high-impact aerobics, and swimming. It is generally ac-

TABLE 3. *Exercise training guidelines*

	AHA	ACSM	CDC/ACSM	AACVPR
Aerobic activities				
Frequency (days/week)	≥3	3–5	Daily	3–5
Intensity	50%–60% $\dot{V}O_{2\ max}$ or HR max	55%–90% HR max or 40%–85% $\dot{V}O_{2\ max}$ or HR max reserve	Moderate	50% $\dot{V}O_{2\ max}$
Duration per episode, min	30	15–16	30	30–45
Resistance training				
Activity	Repetitions, 8–10 exercises, major muscle groups	1 set, 8–12 repetitions, 8–10 exercises, major muscle groups	—	1–3 sets, 10/12–15 repetitions, exercises not specified
Frequency	2–3	≥2	Most days preferably all	2–3

ACSM, American College of Sports Medicine Guidelines; AHA, American Heart Association Exercise Standards; CDC/ACSM, Center for Disease Control and American College of Sports Medicine Public Health Statement; AACVPR, American Association for Cardiovascular and Pulmonary Rehabilitation exercise standards.
Adapted from ref. 2, with permission.

cepted, based on the American College of Sports Medicine guidelines, that this be performed 15 to 20 minutes three to four times per week.

2. Low-intensity activities are considered recreational and include such activities as doubles tennis, yoga, dance, and properly prescribed calisthenics.

The chosen program should offer participants a good variety of activities designed for overall body conditioning (cardiovascular and musculoskeletal) and provide fun and enjoyment. Allowing participants to help select the specific exercises improves compliance and adherence to the exercise program.

In designing exercise programs for older and elderly individuals, it is important to give consideration to their special needs. Their musculoskeletal system should be carefully assessed before exercise because disorders such as osteoarthritis affect exercise capacity. Some exercises, such as swimming, yoga, moderate aerobics, and square dancing, are particularly well suited to the physical limitations of the elderly. On the other hand, more strenuous activities, such as jogging or unmodified racquet sports, may require a level of fitness that follows only after years of conditioning and are not appropriate for the first-time exerciser whether older or elderly. Older athletes display a decreased movement pattern, which is seen in stance and in running, walking, jumping, and throwing. Some older pitchers and tennis players cannot get their arms behind their heads or fully extend their elbows, and some aging basketball players cannot maintain a long stride. However, the older tennis player accommodates for these movements by decreasing the range, taking shorter steps, and decreasing the arc of the tennis serve. Also, a softer tennis surface, such as soft clay or synthetic court surface, may be chosen for the elderly tennis player. This not only reduces trauma to bones and joints but also is easier on the feet and reduces risk of injury in case of falls.

In patients older than 65 years, an energy expenditure per week of greater than 500 calories beyond basal requirements should be the goal. A program of rhythmic exercise such as walking, cycling, or swimming, performed three to four times per week for 5 to 30 minutes at intensities of 50% to 60% maximum, is safe and easily maintained. Vigorous sports (e.g., racquetball, marathon running) remain a choice among many older and elderly individuals who have maintained a high level of fitness. These are rarely chosen by individuals who are first-time exercisers.

Thus, despite physical losses, training can help promote increased physical capacity and enhance one's ability to sustain an active lifestyle regardless of age. Older patients require longer warm-up and cool-down periods. Stretching should include muscle groups that are directly related to the exercise to be performed and should be static, as opposed to phasic. Some exercises shorten a muscle, especially when fatigued. Therefore, a period of stretching following the exercise workout serves to lengthen the muscles and prevent postexercise spasm. If joint injury or swelling occurs, exercise should be restricted until ligaments and tendons heal and swelling is reduced.

Improving Adherence with the Exercise Program

Although many older individuals are self-motivated, every effort should be made to gain patient acceptance and adherence with the recommended exercise program. Long-term adherence to exercise programs remains problematic with only approximately 50% of all persons who initiate exercise programs continuing the program for more than 6 months (49). The goals of the program should be clear, realistic, and attainable. In elderly patients, the primary goal of exercise should be to improve their quality of life. Subjects should be educated about the benefits of exercise. Programs should be developed that are enjoyable, promote socialization, and increase interactions with family and peers. Group activities should be recommended over individual activities. Spouses and other family members should be enlisted to help motivate patients to begin and adhere to the program.

Safety measures should be instituted to minimize risk of injury. In elderly patients in particular, emphasis should be placed on low-impact, low- to moderate-intensity exercise with slow progression. The exercise area should be comfortable and well lit, and the temperature should be comfortable. Patients should also be counseled regarding appropriate clothing and footwear.

EXERCISE GUIDELINES FOR PATIENTS WITH CORONARY HEART DISEASE: CARDIAC REHABILITATION

Enrollment of patients into prescribed exercise training and education/counseling for risk factor modification following recovery from uncomplicated myocardial infarction has classically been referred to as *cardiac rehabilitation*. However, the scope of cardiac rehabilitation is broader and can refer to the comprehensive, long-term programs of prescribed exercise and cardiac risk factor modification in patients who have had a myocardial infarction, coronary artery bypass surgery, chronic stable angina, congestive heart failure (CHF), and other forms of cardiovascular disease. Also included are elderly coronary patients, high-risk coronary patients with combinations of myocardial ischemia, arrhythmia, or compensated heart failure, and a variety of other medically complex patients.

The risk of a cardiac event or death during supervised cardiac exercise training programs is very low. However, those who exercise infrequently and have poor functional capacity at baseline may be at somewhat higher risk during exercise training. Cardiac rehabilitation programs have both medical and economic benefits with achievement of optimal outcomes when exercise training is combined with educational messages and feedback about changing lifestyle. Patients who participate in cardiac rehabilitation programs show a lower incidence of rehospitalization and lower charges per hospitalization. A compre-

hensive set of clinical practice guidelines for cardiac rehabilitation was recently published by the U.S. Department of Health and Human Services (36). These should be referred to for guidance in developing rehabilitation programs for specific patients with known coronary heart disease.

Cardiac Rehabilitation

Rehabilitation of cardiac patients includes comprehensive, long-term programs involving prescribed exercise, cardiac risk factor modification, education, and counseling (36). These programs have been traditionally prescribed for patients who have had a myocardial infarction, coronary bypass surgery, or chronic stable angina. The physical activity (exercise) component of cardiac rehabilitation has traditionally been divided into four phases. Phase I is the inpatient program, beginning as soon after the cardiac event or surgery as possible and when the patient is stable. Phase II is the immediate outpatient program. It lasts up to 12 weeks and begins when the patient is discharged from the hospital. This may be hospital-based, community-based, private clinic, or home-based with continuous electrocardiographic (ECG) telemetry monitoring during exercise. Phase III is the intermediate outpatient phase for low-risk patients and can be home- or community-based. This phase is of variable length with intermittent or no ECG monitoring. Phase IV is the maintenance phase; it is generally home- or community-based with no ECG monitoring and limited supervision.

Phase I

Patients qualify for the rehabilitation program only if their hospital course has been uncomplicated and they are free of recurrent angina, significant arrhythmia, and CHF. The optimal amount of exercise depends on the patient's clinical status and symptoms. The exercise stress test provides an objective basis for determining the patient's physical condition as well as a safety monitor for the prescribed activity. Because of the detrimental effects of their cardiac event and bed rest, patients with cardiac disease generally require longer warm-up periods. The focus of phase I is on range-of-motion exercises (upper and lower body) for improved musculoskeletal conditioning, flexibility, and strength. Aerobic conditioning also begins during this phase with self-care and short periods of ambulation several times per day. Multiple short episodes are recommended because patients are usually unable to perform long-duration exercises at this time.

Phase II

Phase II begins following hospital discharge and usually consists of 4 to 12 weeks of hospital or community-based rehabilitation with ECG telemetry monitoring. Aerobic exercise episodes are extended for longer periods and carried out once or twice daily. As the patient's conditioning improves, once-daily exercising 3 to 5 days per week becomes the goal. Emphasis should be placed on aerobic conditioning rather than strength training during the first several weeks of exercise training. The intensity of exercise should be based on the peak heart rate achieved during exercise testing. Low-intensity exercise should be prescribed initially to allow the patient to complete sessions without exercise fatigue. Later, the intensity should be approximately 50% to 85% of maximal oxygen consumption. A target heart rate of 65% of predicted peak heart rate is a common starting point, except after cardiac surgery, because the resting heart rate is usually high. In these cases, 75% of peak heart rate is used initially.

Musculoskeletal conditioning focuses on dynamic, strengthening exercises. This usually involves calisthenics, free weights, and resistance exercise machines. Light dumbbells (1 to 5 pounds) are used during the first 3 to 6 weeks.

Phases III and IV

During phases III and IV, patients progress to fewer monitored exercises and into the long-term maintenance period. Aerobic conditioning is carried out with a single, longer duration episode of continuous exercise. Activities should progress as tolerance is demonstrated, with approximate increases in duration by 5-minute increments per week. Later, intensities can be increased as heart rate response to exercise decreases with conditioning.

The amount of time allotted for musculoskeletal conditioning is increased to allow for total body conditioning. The warm-up for patients with cardiac disease is similar to that for healthy adults with a low level of fitness and elderly individuals. In patients with cardiac disease, a longer cool-down period is recommended in all phases of rehabilitation. Although cardiac events are rare, approximately 40% occur during the recovery period (6,50). Following exercise, a minimum of 15 minutes should be allowed for cool-down and surveillance.

The risk status and rate of progression of exercises vary among patients as do the type and duration of required supervision and monitoring. Low-risk patients can progress more rapidly and those at higher risk should progress more cautiously. Exercise activities and patient status should be assessed every several months. A follow-up treadmill exercise test should be performed approximately 8 weeks after the beginning of exercise training.

Compliance with Cardiac Rehabilitation

As with exercise programs in general, compliance with cardiac rehabilitation is also problematic. Reported dropout rates range from 30% to 85% over 4 years, and medical contraindications to continued participation in exercise programs develop in another 10% to 35% of patients. Adherence to cardiac rehabilitation services may improve patient outcome. Efforts to improve adherence should include clear communication, emotional support, understanding of the patient's values, viewpoints, and preferences, and integration of the program into the patient's lifestyle (36).

Myocardial Infarction and Stable Angina

Each year, there are approximately 1 million survivors of myocardial infarction in the

United States. Another 350,000 individuals are newly diagnosed with stable angina pectoris. The benefits of exercise training following myocardial infarction have been well established (36) and patients with uncomplicated myocardial infarction are ideal candidates for cardiac rehabilitation programs. Exercise training programs significantly reduce overall mortality rate as well as rate of death caused by myocardial infarction. The reported reductions in mortality rate have been highest—approximately 25%—in cardiac rehabilitation programs that have included control of other cardiovascular risk factors. Rehabilitation programs using both moderate and vigorous physical activity have been associated with reductions in fatal cardiac events, although the minimal or optimal level and duration of exercise required to achieve beneficial effects remains uncertain.

Postbypass Surgery and Angioplasty

More than 300,000 patients per year have coronary artery bypass surgery and approximately 360,000 have percutaneous transluminal coronary angioplasty or other transcatheter revascularization procedure. Approximately two-thirds of patients receiving bypass surgery and 45% of those receiving transcatheter revascularizations are 65 years of age or older. Increased physical activity appears to benefit each of these groups. Benefits include reduction in cardiovascular mortality rate, reduction of symptoms, improvement in exercise tolerance and functional capacity, and improvement in psychological well-being and quality of life.

Congestive Heart Failure

There are approximately 400,000 patients with newly diagnosed CHF each year. Patients with CHF appear to show improvement in symptoms, exercise capacity, and functional well-being in response to exercise training, even though left ventricular systolic function appears to be unaffected. In patients with impaired left ventricular function, most adaptations to exercise training appear to be pe-

ripheral and may occur with low-intensity training. In patients with stable heart failure New York Heart Association (NYHA) Class I-III, regular exercise such as walking or cycling should be encouraged (51). Until recently, bed rest was a standard component of therapy for patients with CHF. However, it has come to be recognized that, although there might be some short-term benefits (diuresis), physical inactivity in the long-term is detrimental, and even short periods of bed rest may result in reduced exercise tolerance and aerobic capacity as well as muscular weakness and hypertrophy. Recent studies have shown that patients with CHF can exercise safely, and regular exercise may improve functional status and decrease symptoms (51). Although supervised rehabilitation programs may benefit some patients with heart failure (those who are dyspneic at low work levels, have angina, a recent myocardial infarction, or a recent revascularization), there is insufficient evidence to recommend the routine use of supervised rehabilitation for patients with heart failure.

Morbidity, Mortality, and Safety Issues

The safety of exercise rehabilitation has been well established (36). The rates of myocardial infarction and other cardiovascular complications during exercise training are very low. In randomized trials of approximately 5,000 patients with coronary heart disease (36), there were no increases in cardiovascular complications or serious adverse outcomes with exercise training. Two meta-analyses of 21 randomized, controlled trials of more than 4,000 patients with coronary disease in cardiac rehabilitation programs showed a 25% reduction in mortality rate over 3 years in rehabilitation patients compared with control subjects (36).

EXERCISE IN PATIENTS WITH ACQUIRED VALVULAR HEART DISEASE

The prevalence of acquired valvular heart disease increases with age. Clinically, acquired valvular heart disease is manifest as either valvular stenosis or regurgitation. The diagnosis can usually be made on physical examination alone, and the severity can be estimated from the patient history, physical examination, and noninvasive laboratory studies (ECG, echocardiogram). Considerable information exists regarding the determinants of sudden death and the development of symptoms during exercise in patients with valvular heart disease. However, little is known regarding the influence of exercise on rates of progression and severity of valvular disease or the effects of strenuous exercise on the development and progression of associated ventricular dysfunction (52). Evaluation and guidelines for participation in competitive athletics for patients with acquired valvular heart disease were reviewed in detail by the 26th Bethesda Conference (52). A summary of those recommendations are provided in the following discussion.

Mitral Stenosis

Mitral stenosis is virtually always rheumatic in origin. During exercise, there is an increase in heart rate and cardiac output, which, if sustained for periods of time, can produce marked elevations of left atrial and pulmonary capillary pressures. Patients with severe mitral stenosis are usually symptomatic and do not attempt to participate in vigorous exercise or athletic activities. Patients with mild to moderate mitral stenosis, however, may be asymptomatic, even during vigorous exercise. Based on the recommendations of the 26th Bethesda Conference regarding athletics in patients with acquired heart disease, (a) in the presence of mild mitral stenosis and sinus rhythm, participation in all sports and vigorous exercises is permitted, (b) in the presence of mild mitral stenosis and atrial fibrillation or moderate mitral stenosis (sinus rhythm or atrial fibrillation), only participation in low and moderate static and low and moderate dynamic competitive sports is permitted, and (c) competitive athletics and vigorous exercises should be avoided in patients with severe mitral stenosis.

In addition, those athletes taking anticoagulant therapy should avoid all competitive sports that have a danger of bodily collision.

Mitral Regurgitation

Mitral regurgitation has a number of origins, including mitral valve prolapse, rheumatic heart disease, coronary heart disease, connective tissue disorders (e.g., Marfan syndrome), and dilated cardiomyopathy. Mild degrees of mitral regurgitation are common and frequently found in otherwise normal individuals. Exercise recommendations for patients whose mitral regurgitation is primarily a consequence of ischemic heart disease or ventricular dilatation and dysfunction should be made based on the severity and risks of these conditions. In patients with primarily valvular mitral regurgitation, aerobic exercise is usually associated with little or no change in ejection fraction and regurgitant fraction. However, static exercises are probably deleterious in that they increase arterial pressure with worsening of the regurgitation and elevation of left atrial pressure. Recommendations regarding participation in vigorous exercise for individuals with mitral regurgitation are (a) participation in all competitive athletics permitted if left ventricular size and function are normal and sinus rhythm is present, (b) low and moderate static and low and moderate dynamic athletics permitted when there is sinus rhythm or atrial fibrillation with mild ventricular enlargement and normal ventricular function, and (c) avoidance of vigorous athletics and competitive sports if there is definite ventricular enlargement or any degree of left ventricular dysfunction at rest.

Aortic Stenosis

Aortic stenosis may be rheumatic, congenital, or a result of calcific or degenerative changes. The severity of aortic stenosis can usually be determined by clinical and noninvasive laboratory evaluations. Severe aortic stenosis may produce left ventricular failure, syncope, or angina. The risk of sudden death is greater in symptomatic patients. Although sudden death is rare in patients with mild aortic stenosis, it may occur in completely asymptomatic individuals. Regarding participation in athletics, the guidelines of the 26th Bethesda Conference are that (a) participation in vigorous athletics are permitted in athletes with mild aortic stenosis, (b) low-intensity competitive sports are permitted in athletes with mild aortic stenosis, and (c) competitive athletics should be avoided in patients with severe aortic stenosis or symptomatic patients with moderate aortic stenosis.

Aortic Regurgitation

Aortic regurgitation may be due to a variety of causes, including rheumatic heart disease, congenital bicuspid aortic valve, infective endocarditis, and aortic root diseases. During exercise, there is a decrease in diastolic filling time, increase in heart rate, and decrease in peripheral vascular resistance. These contribute to increased forward flow and a decrease in the aortic regurgitant volume. In patients with severe aortic regurgitation, however, angina pectoris, ventricular arrhythmias, syncope, and sudden death can occur. Regarding participation in competitive athletics, (a) participation in all competitive sports is permitted in patients with mild or moderate aortic regurgitation whose left ventricular size is normal or only mildly increased, (b) participation in low-intensity competitive sports is only permitted in athletes with mild or moderate aortic regurgitation and ventricular arrhythmias at rest or with exertion, and (c) participation in competitive sports and vigorous exercises is not permitted in athletes with severe aortic regurgitation, moderate aortic regurgitation and symptoms, or aortic regurgitation and marked dilation of the proximal ascending aorta.

Postoperative Patients with Prosthetic or Bioprosthetic Cardiac Valves

Although most patients improve following valve replacement and many become asymp-

tomatic, the long-term mortality rate of these patients remains greater than that of the general population. Also, a transvalvular gradient of varying severity is present in most patients. Although hemodynamic variables at rest may be essentially normal following valve replacement, these patients often have an abnormal response to exercise. Before engaging in vigorous exercise, an exercise stress test to at least the level of the planned activity should be conducted. Recommendations for participation in athletics include the following: (a) low and moderate static and low and moderate dynamic competitive athletics are permitted in athletes with a prosthetic or bioprosthetic mitral valve who are not taking anticoagulants and who have normal valvular function and near-normal left ventricular function, (b) low-intensity competitive sports are permitted in athletes with a prosthetic or bioprosthetic aortic valve who are not taking anticoagulant agents, and (c) athletes with a prosthetic or bioprosthetic mitral or aortic valve who are taking anticoagulant agents should not engage in any sport in which there is a danger of bodily collision.

SPECIAL CONSIDERATIONS FOR COEXISTING MEDICAL DISORDERS

Older and elderly patients often have coexisting medical disorders that may affect exercise capacity, including hypertension, peripheral vascular disease, diabetes, and obesity.

Hypertension

Exercise may reduce the risk of development of hypertension, and regular physical exercise usually results in lowered baseline blood pressure. The exercise prescription may need to be modified according to the prescribed antihypertensive medications, and any adjustment of medications requires reassessment of the patient's response to exercise and appropriate modification of the exercise prescription. In patients with known cardiovascular disease who begin exercise training, one of the goals of training is to lower blood pressure.

Peripheral Vascular Disease

Obstructive peripheral arterial disease is common among older and elderly individuals. Careful examination of the peripheral pulses should be a routine component of the preparticipatory examination. Patients with peripheral vascular disease often have atherosclerotic disease elsewhere, particularly in the coronaries. In patients found to have peripheral vascular disease, appropriate medical evaluation and therapy should be carried out. Therapy may include interval exercise training with low-level aerobic exercises, which may improve claudication, if present.

Diabetes

Physical activity is associated with increased insulin sensitivity and glucose clearance, and epidemiologic studies suggest that physical inactivity and obesity may contribute to risk for non–insulin-dependent diabetes. Hemodynamic responses to exercise are frequently abnormal in diabetic patients because of coexistent neuropathy. Heart rate, blood pressure, cardiac output, and peripheral blood flow responses to dynamic and static exercise may be attenuated, and postural hypotension and postexertional orthostatic hypotension are common. Special considerations in diabetic patients include the need for frequent monitoring of blood glucose when initiating an exercise program. Patients should not exercise when they are hypoglycemic or hyperglycemic, and insulin dose may need to be modified depending on exercise level and carbohydrate intake. Insulin should be injected into an area that is not active during exercise (e.g., abdomen), exercise should be done with a partner, and particular attention should be paid to proper footwear. Patients should know the signs and symptoms of hypoglycemia and should discontinue exercise if they occur.

Obesity

Regular exercise improves caloric balance and helps in preventing obesity. Physical activity is associated with improved weight control, even after controlling for dietary factors. There is an inverse relationship between measures of physical activity and indexes of obesity in most U.S. population studies. Studies that have examined the relationship between physical activity and body fat distribution suggest an inverse relationship between physical activity and visceral fat. Physical activity facilitates weight loss and the addition of physical activity to dietary energy restriction can increase and help maintain loss of body weight and body fat mass.

In obese individuals, the benefits of exercise extend beyond weight control. Physical activity in this group lowers the risk of heart disease, stroke, high blood pressure, and diabetes, and it boosts self-control, self-confidence, and well-being. To reach the final goal, exertion must be associated with an appropriate diet and modification of lifestyle. Potential barriers to regular exercise in overweight persons include lack of motivation or confidence, previous negative experience, poor balance, anxiety, discomfort, pain, and injury. These barriers must be taken into consideration when developing the exercise program.

Elderly and Frail Patients

Exercise of low to moderate intensity, when performed on a regular basis by previously sedentary older adults, can result in improved functional status, as well as lowered blood pressure and improved psychological well-being. The aim of physical activity in this group is to maintain functional capacity for independent living, reduce cardiovascular disease, and prevent and manage chronic diseases. The exercise prescription should be individualized, taking into consideration the specific problems related to aging such as vision impairment, balance problems, and limitations in mobility. The usual exercises should consist of short periods and include simple movements related to mobility (standing, balance, walking, getting into and out of vans). This should be followed by exercise and stretching movements to increase range of motion and flexibility in the neck, trunk, arms, hands, legs, and feet. Movements can be alternated between standing and sitting to reduce stress in frail individuals.

Alternatively, water exercises, swimming, or cycling may be more appropriate for those with bone and joint problems. Other considerations include ensuring that there is adequate participant input regarding the types of activities undertaken, that facilities have adequate lighting and ventilation, that there is minimal background noise (because of the greater prevalence of hearing impairment), and that there is a resilient floor surface and well-cushioned mats for floor exercise. A well-trained and empathetic staff that is certified in cardiopulmonary resuscitation and familiar with the major medical disorders associated with the elderly are other key considerations.

SPECIAL CONSIDERATIONS REGARDING EXERCISE AND MEDICATIONS

Older and elderly patients frequently take medications, and the effects of their medications on exercise capacity and safety should be considered when recommending exercise.

Nitrates

Nitrates are frequently used in patients with coronary heart disease. Nitrates relax vascular smooth muscle, with the main effect being on the venous system rather than the arterial system. Nitrates, taken before exercise or on a chronic basis, reduce cardiac workload and improve exercise performance. This is evidenced by an increased tolerance for activity before the onset of angina or ischemic ECG changes.

Nitrates may increase heart rate and decrease blood pressure at rest with similar or no effects during exercise. In patients with angina or CHF, exercise capacity may increase with delayed onset of ischemia. Hemodynamically, nitrates decrease myocardial oxygen consumption. They also increase myocardial oxygen supply by increasing collateral flow or decreasing ventricular diastolic pressure. Nitrates may improve myocardial contractility indirectly by the reduction of impedance to ventricular systolic emptying. Prophylactic use of sublingual nitroglycerin is often effective in preventing angina pectoris before exertion. However, postural hypotension may result from peripheral vasodilation, especially in the postexercise period.

Beta-Blockers

Beta-blockers are used in a variety of cardiovascular conditions, including hypertension and coronary artery disease. Beta-blockers may reduce exercise tolerance and the level of perceived exertion associated with each level of exercise. In patients with ischemic heart disease, beta-blockers may improve exercise capacity. This is achieved by a decrease in both resting and submaximal heart rates and blood pressure, therefore resulting in a decrease in the rate pressure product and myocardial oxygen demand.

Calcium Channel Blockers

Calcium channel blockers exert little impact on exercising adults. They may decrease myocardial oxygen demand and improve myocardial blood supply. The dihydropyridines may increase heart rate and decrease blood pressure at rest and during exercise. In patients with ischemic heart disease, exercise capacity may improve. The nondihydropyridines (verapamil and diltiazem) decrease the heart rate and blood pressure at rest and during exercise. They also may increase exercise capacity in patients with ischemic heart disease. Calcium channel blockers do not limit the ability of an individual to achieve a training effect.

Cardiac Glycosides

Cardiac glycosides (digoxin) are often used in patients with heart failure and systolic dysfunction. They may improve exercise tolerance, because of the increased efficiency of ventricular function and oxygen utilization. Digoxin decreases heart rate in patients with atrial fibrillation; it does not affect the blood pressure at rest or during exertion.

Diuretics

Diuretics are frequently used in patients with cardiovascular disease, particularly hypertension. Diuretics may not be the best choice in the exercising athlete. Dehydration, a side effect of chronic exercise, may be exacerbated by diuretics. Hypokalemia also may be exacerbated during acute vigorous exercise when relatively high levels of catecholamines are released. In patients with CHF, diuretics may help improve exercise capacity.

Vasodilators

Vasodilators may increase the heart rate at rest and during exertion and decrease blood pressure. The angiotensin-converting enzyme inhibitors and the α-adrenergic blockers have a low side-effect profile and are associated with very few side effects in exercising adults. However, patients receiving these medications should be monitored carefully for hypotension after exercise.

Antiarrhythmic Agents

Except for the beta-blockers and calcium channel blockers, antiarrhythmic agents in general do not affect the heart rate, blood pressure, exercise capacity, or exercise training.

SPECIAL CONSIDERATIONS IN WOMEN

Regular physical exercise has similar benefits and training effects in both men and women. Although many studies in recent years have focused on the role of physical activity, exercise training, and physical fitness for primary and secondary prevention of coronary heart disease, most research has been conducted on men. However, there are gender differences that may be important when developing exercise programs for women. Female athletes are usually smaller than men, have less muscle mass, more body fat, and less muscle strength (particularly in the upper extremities). Women are also more predisposed to osteoporosis. Women also live longer than men and are disproportionately represented in the oldest age groups.

In women interested in beginning an exercise program and in female athletes who engage in vigorous competitive sports, the preparticipation evaluation is an important screening tool for the detection of medical conditions and musculoskeletal problems that may lead to increased risk of illness or injury. As in men, the examination should consist of a careful history and physical examination. Body weight and anthropometric measurements should be made and the musculoskeletal evaluation should include an assessment of risk of osteoporosis. In high-risk individuals, a bone density study should be considered. Although the risk of CHD and sudden death are lower for women than men, the preparticipatory evaluation and assessment for CHD should be the same as that done for men. Careful cardiac auscultation should be performed to help differentiate functional from pathologic murmurs. Mitral valve prolapse is more common in women, and the presence of chest pain, shortness of breath, or palpitations may suggest the presence of mitral valve prolapse.

Strength Training

The musculoskeletal benefits of regular exercise may be of particular benefit in women because of their greater predisposition to osteoporosis, lower muscle mass, and decreased strength. Progressive strength training is beneficial in men and women. The difference in muscle strength between trained women and men is due to muscle mass size and not to differences in muscle fiber type or distribution. Improved strength, flexibility, and energy result from strength training. Women can gain great improvements with strength training without gaining noticeable muscle mass. This is probably because of their lower androgen levels.

Osteoporosis

Osteoporosis is four times more likely to develop in women than men because of their thinner, lighter bones, rapid bone loss after menopause, and longer life span. The two areas of concern are amount of peak bone mass attained and the rate of bone loss. The physical activity program should be used to maximize peak bone mass and to serve in conjunction with other treatment modalities such as estrogen replacement therapy. The exercise program may need to be tailored to include activities that are non–weight-bearing and protective and enhancing to bone density. These include exercises that are noncompetitive and moderate, use large muscle mass, and are rhythmic.

The best treatment for premature osteoporosis is prevention and reduction of risk factors. The critical window of opportunity for the establishment of strong and healthy bones is in the adolescent and young adult years. Adequate calcium intake is essential. Regular weight-bearing exercises are important in female athletes of all ages. Regular exercise may also enhance the effects of estrogen replacement therapy in decreasing bone loss following menopause. However, in women with osteoporosis, exercises involving flexion of the spine should be avoided to prevent the risk of vertebral compression fractures.

Weight Loss

The total energy expenditure of the exercise period should be considered when weight loss is a goal of the exercise program. A higher percentage of fat fuel is used with low-intensity exercise. However, the total caloric expenditure is less than higher-intensity programs of the same duration. Low- to moderate-intensity exercise (40% to 60% $\dot{V}O_{2\,max}$) is tolerated more easily by novice exercisers, improving long-range exercise adherence.

A major problem among some female athletes is that of low body fat. The consequence of this, particularly in the athlete, is a negative caloric balance as a result of food restriction and training. This may become a serious problem because, if left uncorrected, it can contribute to a number of problems, including disordered eating, iron-deficiency anemia, premature osteoporosis, and injuries.

Anemia

Women are at greater risk of iron deficiency and resultant anemia than men. Red blood cells, hemoglobin, and hematocrit values are an important consideration for physical activity participation. In general, adult men have approximately 6% more red blood cells and 10% to 15% higher hemoglobin concentrations and hematocrit levels compared with those of women. Women with anemia may have a decreased oxygen-carrying capacity because of the lower concentration of hemoglobin. Women also have lower blood volumes, lower iron stores, decreased dietary iron uptake, increased absorption, and increased loss of iron compared to men.

SUMMARY

Regular exercise is beneficial to adults of all ages and a regular program of physical activity is recommended for all adults. Regular aerobic physical activity improves exercise capacity and plays an important role in the primary and secondary prevention of cardiovascular morbidity and mortality. As one ages, physical inactivity increases and many of the decrements in functional capacity are due to this physical inactivity. These decrements can be delayed or prevented with regular physical activity. The benefits of regular exercise in older and elderly individuals are similar to those in younger persons. These include improvement in exercise tolerance, improvement in psychosocial well-being, reduction in cardiovascular morbidity, and reduction in cardiovascular and total mortality rate. Regular exercise not only improves the number of years of life but also may improve the quality of life during the years that one lives.

REFERENCES

1. NIH Consensus. *JAMA* 1996;276:241–246.
2. American College of Sports Medicine. *ACSM's guidelines for exercise testing and prescription,* 5th ed. Baltimore: Williams & Wilkins, 1995.
3. Pate RP, Prat M, Blair SN, et al. Physical activity and public health: a recommendation from the Centers for Disease Control and Prevention and the American College of Sports Medicine. *JAMA* 1995;273:402-407.

4. Fletcher GF, Balady G, Blair SN, et al. Statement on exercise: benefits and recommendations for physical activity programs for all Americans. A statement for health professionals by the Committee on Exercise and Cardiac Rehabilitation of the Council on Clinical Cardiology, American Heart Association. *Circulation* 1996; 94:857–862.
5. Shephard R. *Physiologic changes over the years: ACSM resource manual,* 3rd ed. Philadelphia: Lea & Febiger, 1993:397.
6. Brechue WF, Pollock ML. Exercise training for coronary artery disease in the elderly. *Clin Geriatr Med* 1996; 12:207–229.
7. McArdle WD, et al. *Exercise physiology energy, nutrition and human performance,* 3rd ed. Philadelphia: Lea & Febiger, 1991:221.
8. Buskirk ER, Hodgson JL. Age and aerobic power: the rate of change in men and women. *Fed Proc* 1987;46: 1824–1829.
9. Hagberg JM. Effect of training on the decline of $VO_{2\,max}$ with aging. *Fed Proc* 1987;46:1830–1833.
10. Heath GW, et al. A physiological comparison of young and older endurance athletes. *J Appl Physiol* 1977;42: 372–376.
11. Rodeheffer RJ, et al. Exercise cardiac output is maintained with advancing age in healthy human subjects: cardiac dilatation and increased stroke volume compensate for a diminished heart rate. *Circulation* 1984;69: 203–213.
12. Chesler R, Stein RA. Personal communication 1990.
13. Badentop DT, et al. Physiological adjustments to higher or lower intensity exercise in elders. *Med Sci Sports Exerc* 1983;15:496–502.
14. DeVries HA. Exercise intensity threshold for improvement of cardiovascular-respiratory function in older men. *Geriatrics* 1971;26:94–101.
15. Drinkwater BL, et al. Aerobic power of females, ages 10–68. *J Gerontol* 1975;30:385–394.
16. *Surgeon General's Report on Physical Activity and Health.* U.S. Department of Health and Human Services Centers for Disease Control and Prevention. Division of Nutrition and Physical Activity, MS K-46, Atlanta, GA 1992.
17. Caspersen CJ, Merrit RK. Physical activity trends among 26 states 1986–1990. *Med Sci Sports Exerc* 1990;27:713–720.
18. Caspersen CJ, et al. Status of the 1990 physical fitness and exercise objectives—evidence from NHIS 1985. *Public Health Rep* 1986;101:587–592.
19. Caspersen CJ, et al. International physical activity patterns: a methodological perspective. In: Dishman RK, ed. *Exercise adherence and public health.* Champaign, IL: Human Kinetics Publishers, 1994:71–108.
20. Stephens T. Secular trends in adult physical activity: exercise boom or bust. *Res Q Exerc Sport* 1987;58:94–105.
21. Stephens T, et al. A descriptive epidemiology of leisure-time physical activity. *Public Health Rep* 1985;100: 147–158.
22. Hovell MF, et al. Identifying correlates of walking for exercise: an epidemiologic prerequisite for physical activity promotion. *Prev Med* 1989;18:856–866.
23. Dishman RK, et al. The determinants of physical activity and exercise. *Public Health Rep* 1984;100: 158–171.
24. Gottheiner V. Long-range strenuous sports training for cardiac reconditioning and rehabilitation. *Am J Cardiol* 1968;22:426–434.
25. Kavanagh T, et al. Marathon running after myocardial infarction. *JAMA* 1974;229:1602–1605.
26. Sidney KH, et al. Activity patterns of elderly men and women. *J Gerontol* 1977;32:25–32.
27. Clarke HH. Circulatory-respiratory endurance improvement. *Phys Fitness Dig* 1974;4:1–16.
28. Melillo KD, et al. Perceptions of physical fitness and exercise activity among older adults. *J Adv Nurs* 1996; 23:542–547.
29. Paffenbarger RS, Kampert JB, Lee IM, Hyde RT, Leung RW, Wing AL. Chronic disease in former college students: LII. Changes in physical activity and other lifeway patterns influencing longevity. *Med Sci Sports Exerc* 1994;26:857–865.
30. Detry JM, Rousseau M, Vandenbroeke G, Kusmin F. Increased arteriovenous oxygen difference after physical training in coronary heart disease. *Circulation* 1971; 44:101–118.
31. Rousseau MF, Brasseur LA, Detry JM. Hemodynamic determinants of maximal oxygen intake in patients with healed myocardial infarction and the influence of physical training. *Circulation* 1973;48:943–951.
32. Niebauer J, Cooke JP. Cardiovascular effects of exercise: role of endothelial shear stress. *J Am Coll Cardiol* 1996;28:1652–1660.
33. Vander L. Cardiovascular complications of recreational physical activity. *Physician Sports Med* 1982;10:89–97.
34. Stratton JR, Chandler WL, Schwartz RS, et al. Effects of physical conditioning on fibrinolytic variables and fibrinogen in young and old healthy adults. *Circulation* 1991;83:1692–1697.
35. Lee IM. Physical activity, fitness, and cancer. In: Bouchard C, Shephard RJ, Stephens T, eds. *Physical activity, fitness, and health: International Proceedings and Consensus Statement.* Champaign, IL: Human Kinetics Publishers, 1994:814–831.
36. Wenger NK, Froelicher ES, et al. *Cardiac rehabilitation. Clinical practice guideline number 17.* U.S. Department of Health and Human Services. AHCPR Publication No. 96-0672. October 1995.
37. Thompson PD. The cardiovascular complications of vigorous physical activity. *Arch Intern Med* 1996;156: 2297–2302.
38. Cantwell JD, et al. Cardiac complications while jogging. *JAMA* 1969;210:130–131.
39. Vander L. Cardiovascular complications of recreational physical activity. *Physician Sports Med* 1982;10:89–97.
40. Siscovick DS, Weiss NS, Fletcher RM, Lasky T. The incidence of primary cardiac arrest during vigorous exercise. *N Engl J Med* 1984;311:874–877.
41. Maron B, Epstein S, Roberts W. Causes of sudden death in competitive athletes. *J Am Coll Cardiol* 1986;7: 204–214.
42. Virmain R, McAllister HA. Coronary heart disease at young age: a report of 187 autopsy patients who died of severe coronary atherosclerosis. *Cardiovasc Rev Rep* 1984;5:799–809.
43. Thompson PD, Fink EJ, Carleton RA, Sturner WQ. Incidence of death during jogging in Rhode Island from 1975 through 1980. *JAMA* 1982;247:2535–2538.
44. Epstein S, Maron B. Sudden death and the competitive athlete. Perspectives on preparticipation screening studies. *J Am Coll Cardiol* 1986;7:220–230.

45. Maron BJ, Thompson PD, Puffer JC, et al. Cardiovascular preparticipatory screening of the competitive athlete. A statement for health professionals from the Sudden Death Committee (clinical cardiology) and Congenital Cardiac Defects Committee (cardiovascular disease in the young), American Heart Association. *Circulation* 1996;94:850–856.

46. Maron BJ, Isner JM, McKenna WJ. 26th Bethesda Conference: Recommendations for determining eligibility for competition in athletes with cardiovascular abnormalities. Task Force 3: Hypertrophic cardiomyopathy, myocarditis and other myopericardial diseases and mitral valve prolapse. *J Am Coll Cardiol* 1994;24: 880–885.

47. American College of Sports Medicine. The recommended quantity and quality of exercise for developing and maintaining cardiorespiratory and muscular fitness in healthy adults. *Med Sci Sports Exerc* 1990; 22:265.

48. American Association for Cardiovascular and Pulmonary Rehabilitation. *Guidelines for cardiac rehabilitation programs,* 2nd ed. Champaign, IL: Human Kinetics Publishers, 1995.

49. Dishman RK. Compliance/adherence in health related exercise. *Health Psychol* 1982;1:237–267.

50. Haskel WL. Cardiovascular complications during exercise training of cardiac patients. *Circulation* 1978;57: 920.

51. Heart failure: Evaluation and care of patients with left ventricular systolic dysfunction. *Clinical Practice Guideline Number 11*; U.S. Department of Health and Human Services, PHS, AHCPR, Rockville, MD, June 1994. [AHCPR Publication No. 94-0612; Norman A. Konstam, M.D. (Co-chair) and Kathleen Dracup, DNSc, RN (Co-Chair)].

52. Cheitlin MD, Douglas PS, Parmley WW. 26th Bethesda Conference: Recommendations for determining eligibility for competition in athletes with cardiovascular abnormalities. Task Force 2: Acquired valvular heart disease. *J Am Coll Cardiol* 1994;24:874–880.

The Athlete and Heart Disease:
Diagnosis, Evaluation & Management,
edited by R. A. Williams.
Lippincott Williams & Wilkins, Philadelphia © 1999.

9

Substance Abuse in Sports: The Impact of Cocaine, Alcohol, Steroids, and Other Drugs on the Heart

Louis L. Cregler

Dean's office, Academic Affairs, City University of New York Medical School, New York,
New York 10031; Department of Medicine, Division of Cardiology, Maimonides Medical Center,
Brooklyn, New York 11219

HISTORICAL PERSPECTIVE

Athletes, coaches and trainers have searched for ways to improve performance for as long as humans have participated in sports. The abuse of drugs has been implicated at every level of competition. Drug use has been reported in high school and noncompetitive individuals. Ancient Greeks in the third century consumed herbs and mushrooms in an attempt to improve athletic performance. Caffeine-based sugar cubes dipped in nitroglycerin were taken before competition by European cyclists in the nineteenth century (1). A mixture of coca leaves and wine called *vin mariani* was also used. In the early 1950s, amphetamine use was suspected in athletes participating in the summer and winter Olympics. By the late 1950s, athletes from the United States and the Soviet Union began experimenting with anabolic steroids. Amphetamines were linked to two deaths during the 1960 summer Olympics in Rome. The International Olympic Committee (IOC) instituted drug use control measures at the 1968 Olympic games. Nineteen athletes were disqualified for drug use during the 1983 Pan American games in Caracas.

Drug abuse among athletes is a recognized problem in sports. The professional athlete's lifestyle, high visibility, high income, frequent travel, and vast amounts of free time have been postulated as risk factors for substance abuse. Athletes use drugs for therapeutic indications, recreational or social reasons, as ergogenic aids, or to mask the presence of other drugs during drug testing (1). Sophisticated pharmacologic methods exist to enhance athletic performance in ways that threaten the meaning and integrity of competition. Nowhere has cocaine, alcohol, anabolic steroids, and other abused substances been given more publicity, and even been glamorized to a certain extent, than by highly visible competitive athletes (2). After falling into obscurity, smokeless tobacco use began to increase with the reduction in cigarette smoking after the Surgeon General's first report in 1964. Consumption of smokeless tobacco was stimulated by media attention using professional athletes promoting it as a safe alternative to cigarettes. Many of these abused agents can have catastrophic effects on the cardiovascular system (3–7).

Drugs that enhance exercise capacity or athletic performance are called *ergogenic,* whereas drugs that impair function are referred to as *ergolytic.* Ergogenic drug use, or doping, is defined by the IOC as the administration of or use of any substance foreign to the body or any physiologic agent taken in abnormal quantities or taken by an abnormal entry into the body with the intent of increasing performance in competition by an athlete (1). Ergogenic drugs include testosterone, anabolic steroids, human growth hormone, amphetamines, and recombinant human erythropoietin (8). Cocaine, the champagne of drugs, is believed to be ergogenic by some athletes. Ergolytic drugs used by athletes include alcohol, cocaine, marijuana, smokeless tobacco, antihypertensives, eye drops, and diuretics. Some antidepressants, antihistamines, and even coffees are considered ergolytic.

The death of a young athlete during competition is rare but such a death can have a devastating impact on peers, coaches, parents, health care providers, and the general public (9–13). Public awareness of sudden death in elite athletes such as Len Bias and Don Rogers owing to substance abuse has increased. During the past decade, sudden death in highly celebrated athletes has magnified both psychological and medicolegal issues (14).

Cocaine-related cardiovascular events escalated during the 1980s as cocaine became purer, cheaper, and easier to obtain. Cocaine abuse is a risk factor for myocardial ischemia or infarction, cardiac arrhythmias, pulmonary edema, ruptured aortic aneurysm, cerebral infarction, infective endocarditis, vascular thrombosis, myocarditis, and dilated cardiomyopathy. All routes and forms of cocaine abuse are potentially cardiotoxic and can be lethal. Fatal cardiac complications occur in first-time users.

Alcohol is the most widely used drug among athletes and has been linked to sports since ancient times. In the 1800s, some marathoners drank alcohol during races. Brandy was still used as a stimulant until 1935. The role of alcohol abuse in the development of heart disease has been reported for more than a century. Adverse consequences of alcohol are hypertension, stroke, coronary events, lipid abnormalities, cardiac rhythm disturbances, and cardiac dysfunction preceding the development of dilated cardiomyopathy.

Anabolic steroids are ergogenic agents used by athletes to enhance performance and increase muscle mass. In 1976, the IOC banned the use of these agents. Anabolic-androgenic steroid abuse receives international media attention when an elite competitive athlete such as Canadian sprinter Ben Johnson tests positive for steroids. Adverse effects of anabolic steroids include fatal and nonfatal myocardial infarction; cardiomyopathy; hepatic, renal, and genital conditions; and lipid abnormalities, as well as vascular thrombotic disease.

Drug testing programs must address short-acting stimulants, beta-blockers, diuretics, anabolic steroids, and drugs affecting the identification of other drugs. Drug testing is performed by three main sporting organizations, the National Collegiate Athletic Association (NCAA), National Football League (NFL), and the United States Olympic Committee (USOC). Drug control and testing for abused substances is an important part of the Olympic games. During the 1996 centennial Olympic games in Atlanta, GA, urine sampling was performed for prohibited substances, including stimulants, narcotics, anabolic steroids, diuretics, peptides, and glycoprotein hormones. Testing was also performed to detect methods of enhancing performance, including blood doping and pharmacologic, chemical, and physical manipulation of the urine (15).

COCAINE AND CARDIOVASCULAR DISEASE

Cardiopulmonary complaints are the most common presenting manifestation of cocaine abuse (16–18) (Fig. 1). Many complaints do not result in hospital admission or require specific treatment. Cardiovascular complaints or events account for 20% of individuals presenting to emergency departments and ambulatory centers for medical attention (3,19,20). The mechanisms responsible for the cardiotoxic effects of cocaine remain unknown (21).

Believing that cocaine was a harmless, nonaddicting, aphrodisiac drug, millions of people tried it and cocaine abuse escalated. In 1985, 30 million Americans used cocaine and 6 million were regular users (22,23). As

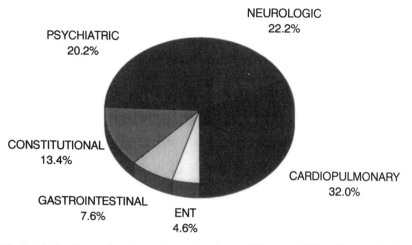

FIG. 1. Medical complications of cocaine abuse. (From ref. 228, with permission.)

medical and social complications (24) of cocaine became evident (Table 1), and with the growing negative image of cocaine, the number of first-time users declined (6,25). The frequency of cocaine use decreased to 4.5 million Americans by 1992, one-third of whom used cocaine at least monthly (26). Seven percent of adults between 18 and 34 years of age admit using cocaine once during the past 12 months (27). The use of cocaine as a stimulant can be traced to 600 A.D. to tombs of South American mummies where the re-

TABLE 1. *Complications associated with cocaine use*

Cardiac	Cerebral atrophy
Chest pain	Cerebral vasculitis
Myocardial infarction	Pulmonary
Arrhythmias	Pneumothorax
Cardiomyopathy	Pneumomediastinum
Myocarditis	Pneumopericardium
Endocrine	Pulmonary edema
Hyperprolactinemia	Exacerbation of asthma
Gastrointestinal	Pulmonary hemorrhage
Intestinal ischemia	Bronchiolitis obliterans
Gastroduodenal perforations	"Crack Lung"
Colitis	Psychiatric
Head and neck	Anxiety
Erosion of dental enamel	Depression
Gingival ulceration	Paranoia
Keratitis	Delirium
Corneal epithelial defects	Psychosis
Chronic rhinitis	Suicide
Perforated nasal septum	Renal
Aspiration of nasal septum	Rhabdomyolysis
Midline granuloma	Obstetric
Altered olfaction	Placental abruption
Optic neuropathy	Lower infant weight
Osteolytic sinusitis	Prematurity
Neurologic	Microcephaly
Headaches	Others
Seizures	Sudden death
Cerebral hemorrhage	Sexual dysfunction
Cerebral infarctions	Hyperpyrexia

Adapted from ref. 24, with permission.

mains of coca leaves were discovered (28–30). For centuries, the natives of Peru and Bolivia chewed coca leaves for their euphoric effects (31). Freud wrote the first major report on the effects of cocaine in 1884 (28).

In the United States, in the early 1900s, many nonprescription medications, cough syrups, tonics, home remedies, and soft drinks contained cocaine. Coca-Cola contained cocaine until it was replaced by caffeine in 1906 (29,32). Mariani's famous cocaine-wine advertisements included testimonials from two popes and several reigning monarchs (33). It was known in 1911 that cocaine use during dental procedures could induce severe myocardial damage, leading to death (34). The Harrison Narcotic Act in 1914 classified cocaine as a narcotic and it became illegal for nonmedicinal purposes. Topical cocaine anesthesia is used today by otolaryngologists in rhinolaryngologic procedures (35,36).

Pharmacology

Cocaine is an alkaloid extracted from the leaves of the Erythroxylon Coca plant grown in South America. This drug belongs to a class of agents known as local anesthetics and each anesthetic contains a benzene ring, an alcohol molecule, and an amino side chain. The differences in potency, euphoric effect, and addictive properties lie in the terminal amino side chain. Euphoric properties of cocaine are due to its action on neurotransmitters in the brain.

Cocaine acts primarily on norepinephrine found in the central and peripheral nervous systems. Cocaine blocks the reuptake of norepinephrine, producing an excess of neurotransmitter in the synapse to stimulate receptors. Higher norepinephrine levels can produce tachycardia, vasoconstriction, an acute elevation in blood pressure, ventricular arrhythmias, and seizures (37) (Fig. 2).

Cocaine hydrochloride is prepared by dissolving the alkaloid in hydrochloric acid to form a water-soluble salt. The molecular weight of this compound is 339.81, and it is 89% cocaine by weight, decomposes on heating, and melts at 195°C. Cocaine alkaloid ("free-base" or "crack") is soluble in alcohol, acetone, ether, and oils, but it is insoluble in water. Crack is easily manufactured in "home" laboratories by combining the hydrochloride

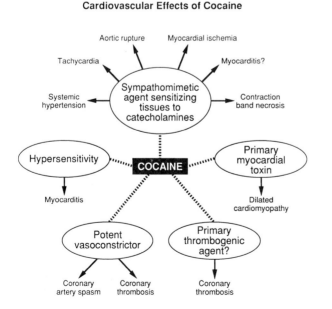

Cardiovascular Effects of Cocaine

FIG. 2. Diagram showing the effects of cocaine on the heart. (From ref. 37, with permission.)

salt with baking soda by the following chemical reaction: Cocaine-HCl + NaHCO$_3$→ Cocaine + NaCl + H$_2$O + CO$_2$ (30). Because cocaine alkaloid melts at 98°C and vaporizes at higher temperatures without decomposing, it can be smoked. The molecular weight of the alkaloid is 303.36 and aqueous solutions of this substance are alkaline. The alkaloid is well absorbed from all mucous membranes and the gastrointestinal tract. Crack became more popular than other illicit drugs abused during the 1980s. The increased demand, availability, and decreased price of cocaine made it profitable to convert cocaine hydrochloride back to the alkaloid (38). The metabolism of cocaine by plasma cholinesterase (pseudocholinesterase), which is genetically determined, may be responsible for cardiotoxic effects (39).

Pathophysiology of Cardiovascular Effects

Myocardial Ischemia and Infarction

After 1982, there were multiple reports of patients with acute myocardial infarction related to cocaine abuse (41–61). Cardiac catheterization was performed in many of these individuals, and approximately half had evidence of atherosclerotic coronary artery disease. The mean age of the patients who experienced cocaine-induced myocardial infarction was 33 years and 25% had no risk factors for coronary artery disease. Two-thirds of the patients were cigarette smokers. The occurrence of an acute myocardial infarction in any young athlete who does not have cardiovascular risk factors should raise suspicion of occult cocaine abuse (3). Two-thirds of the cocaine-induced infarctions are Q-wave infarctions, and the mortality rate is approximately 10% (62). Myocardial infarction has been reported in first-time and chronic cocaine users, with all routes of administration. Occurrence of myocardial infarction is not dependent on cocaine dose. Most patients younger than 40 years of age have no evidence of coronary artery disease (44–46, 51,58). The incidence of myocardial infarction following cocaine use is unknown.

Cocaine can produce myocardial infarction in patients with normal and abnormal coronary arteries (6). Cocaine causes intense vasoconstriction of diseased and normal coronary artery segments, but its effect is markedly enhanced at the site of atherosclerotic narrowing (63). An individual with abnormal coronary artery segments who abuses cocaine is at even higher risk for myocardial infarction. The pathophysiologic features of cocaine-induced myocardial infarction remain unclear but evidence suggests a transient focal coronary event such as a spasm or thrombus (58,64,65). The pathophysiologic mechanisms probably include the triad of (a) an increase in myocardial oxygen demand (increased heart rate and blood pressure) when the supply is fixed, (b) coronary vasospasm, and (c) an increase in thrombotic potential. Coronary artery thrombosis may cause acute myocardial infarction in normal coronary arteries (66). Patients differ pathophysiologically from those with Prinzmetal's angina (62). Coronary spasm has not been induced by ergonovine in patients with normal coronary arteries. Chokshi et al. (67) described a patient in whom the coronary arteries were normal and ergonovine provocative testing was negative after a cocaine-related ischemic event. However, graded doses of intranasal cocaine provoked severe focal spasm of the right coronary artery in the same individual. Nademanee et al. (68) performed ambulatory Holter monitoring and exercise tests in male cocaine abusers admitted for treatment and rehabilitation. Only 3% had ischemic changes induced by exercise testing, but 40% had transient episodes of ST segment elevation by Holter monitor during the first week of cocaine withdrawal.

Cocaine may act independently of the endothelium and adrenergic stimulation to produce calcium-dependent vasoconstriction of vascular smooth muscle (69). Pretreatment with alpha-blockers had no appreciable effect on cocaine-induced contraction, whereas a calcium channel blocker markedly inhibited contractions (63). Calcium channel and α-adrenergic blockade may be useful in the treatment of cocaine-related ischemia (62).

Ruptured Aortic Aneurysm

Ruptured aortic aneurysms have also been reported in cocaine abusers (70,71). Aortic aneurysm rupture was reported in a man who smoked crack and had preexisting hypertension (72). Aortic rupture was probably due to a large increment in systemic arterial pressure secondary to cocaine use. Another patient had chest pain and acute aortic dissection requiring replacement of the aortic valve and a segment of the ascending aorta (73). Acute rupture of an aortic aneurysm represents a potentially fatal complication if it is not recognized and prompt treatment is not instituted.

Pulmonary Edema

Pulmonary edema is a frequent postmortem finding in cocaine-related deaths (74). However, this entity has been reported infrequently before death (75,76). Several patients with pulmonary edema on chest radiograph have been described. In these individuals, pulmonary edema developed after they smoked crack (77, 78). Increased endothelial permeability of the capillaries is the probable cause for the development of pulmonary edema related to cocaine use. It may be similar to heroin toxicity or neurogenic pulmonary edema. In both disorders, increased protein concentration is reported in bronchoalveolar lavage fluid (79,80). The occurrence of pulmonary edema in any young individual who has no cardiopulmonary disease should alert the physician to the possibility of crack abuse (75).

Cardiac Arrhythmias

Experimental studies have demonstrated the arrhythmic potential of cocaine; this property may be due to a primary effect of the drug or be secondary to its effects on catecholamines. Cardiac arrhythmias occur after large and small therapeutic doses of cocaine (81). Arrhythmias may occur during myocarditis (82) or after cocaine-induced myocardial infarction (6). Cocaine intoxication results in hyperpyrexia, leading to seizures and arrhythmias. In some instances, arrhythmias occur after seizures and metabolic acidosis (83,84). Impaired impulse conduction has been noted in the A-V node as well as the His-Purkinje system after cocaine use (85,86). Rhythm disturbances are probably related to the sympathomimetic and local anesthetic properties of cocaine (Fig. 3). Cocaine acts as a local anesthetic by inhibiting sodium influx into cardiac cells, which impairs impulse conduction and creates a substrate for reentrant tachyarrhythmias (21).

Arrhythmias related to cocaine use include ventricular premature beats, sinus bradycardia, sinus tachycardia, ventricular tachycardia/fibrillation, and asystole (49,81,87–89). Geggel (90) described ventricular tachycardia in a neonate born to an addicted mother. Cocaine metabolite was detected in the urine of the baby for several days, and no heart defects were detected by echocardiography.

Few data are available on electrophysiologic evaluation of patients with cocaine-related arrhythmias and sudden death. Isner et al. (51) reported on a college athlete who experienced tachycardia at 300 beats per minute after intranasal cocaine use. An electrophysiologic study identified the presence of two atrioventricular accessory pathways. Both antidromic and orthodromic types of reciprocating tachycardia were induced in response to programmed ventricular pacing. Cocaine has the potential to unmask accessory pathways, resulting in life-threatening cardiac arrhythmias.

Myocarditis and Dilated Cardiomyopathy

Myocarditis is a common autopsy finding in cocaine abusers and may represent microvascular injury (51,52,91). Virmani and colleagues (92) studied 40 autopsy patients with cocaine metabolites in their body fluids and compared the findings with those of patients dying of sudden traumatic injuries without evidence of cocaine use. There was a 20% incidence of myocarditis in patients dying of cocaine overdose.

Cocaine may cause myocarditis and necrosis by several mechanisms. This drug may have a direct effect on lymphocyte activity. Intravenous cocaine can increase natural killer

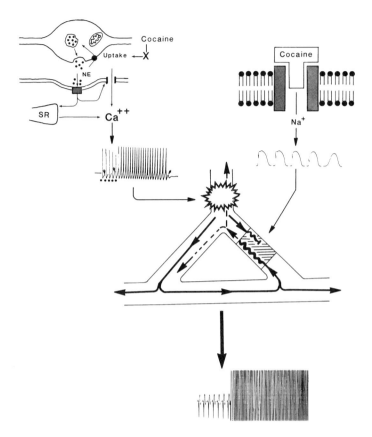

FIG. 3. A schematic representation of a mechanism responsible for cocaine-induced arrhythmia. The upper left-hand portion represents the effects of cocaine on the neural uptake of norepinephrine (NE). Cocaine blocks the neuronal uptake of NE, accentuating the catecholamine effects postsynaptically. By activating α- and β-adrenergic receptors, cytosolic calcium levels increase, triggering oscillatory after-potentials and extrasystoles. Cocaine has local anesthetic properties blocking fast sodium channels, thereby altering impulse conduction. This leads to conduction delays combined with unidirectional impulse blockade, creating a substrate for reentrant circuits and lethal tachyarrhythmias can ensue. (From ref. 21, with permission.)

cell activity in blood that may be cytotoxic to cardiac myocytes (93). The presence of an eosinophilic infiltrate may suggest a hypersensitivity reaction to cocaine (92). Catecholamine administration can induce a focal myocarditis in experimental animals (94). The cause of myocarditis is unknown and an infectious agent has not been excluded.

More and more data are being published on dilated cardiomyopathy in association with cocaine abuse (52,95–101). Weiner (52) described the first two patients with dilated cardiomyopathy associated with chronic cocaine abuse in the absence of coronary artery disease. However, one individual had a long history of heroin and alcohol abuse. Cocaine exerts a profound sympathomimetic effect related to blocked presynaptic reuptake of norepinephrine and dopamine. Chokshi et al. (99) described a 35-year-old woman with acute dilated cardiomyopathy and seizures related to prolonged crack smoking (99). Left ventricular systolic function improved markedly over several weeks. Peng et al. (100) studied seven cocaine abusers whose cardiac evaluation included right ventricular endomyocardial biopsy. Three of the seven patients had biopsy-proven cardiomyopathy.

The pathogenesis of acute cocaine-induced myocardial dysfunction is multifactorial and may be due to destruction of myofibrils, resulting in monocyte necrosis. Chronic cocaine abuse may also lead to interstitial fibrosis and congestive heart failure. Six patients with asymptomatic left ventricular dysfunction resulting from cocaine abuse were described by Bertolet and colleagues (101). Left ventricular dysfunction was unsuspected and unrecognized on routine examination.

Cocaine-related ventricular dysfunction may be consistent with a toxic cardiomyopathy. Tazelaar reported a 93% frequency of contraction-based necrosis in the myocardium of victims of cocaine-related deaths (102). They attributed contraction bands to cocaine-induced catecholamine myocardial injury. It is well established that sympathomimetic amines can be cardiotoxic in individuals with pheochromocytoma. Catecholamine-induced dilated cardiomyopathy is often reversible when the toxic agent is eliminated (103).

Acute depression of myocardial function is yet another cocaine-related complication (104) (Fig. 4). Cocaine abuse should be considered in any young patient with unexplained heart failure and dilated cardiomyopathy (99,101).

Infective Endocarditis

Intravenous cocaine users are at high risk for development of infective endocarditis. Chambers and colleagues (105) reviewed 102 records of cocaine abusers with fever and found a relation with cocaine use and endocarditis. Prolonged cocaine use may cause interstitial or endothelial valvular damage, leading to platelet and fibrin deposition. This is a fertile milieu for bacterial seeding from contaminated needles. The risk for infective endocarditis appears to be greater with cocaine than with heroin or other drugs of abuse (105). Why cocaine abuse leads to endocarditis more often than other injected drugs is not clear. The possibilities include a shorter drug half-life with

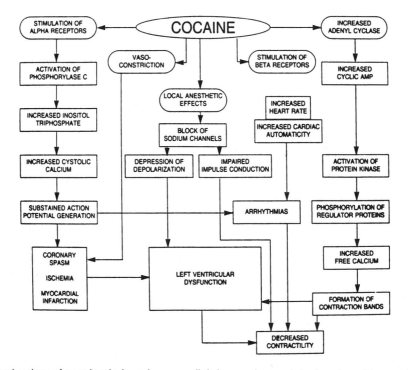

FIG. 4. Mechanism of cocaine-induced myocardial depression and dysfunction. (From ref. 227, with permission.)

more frequent use, differences in bacterial flora, or a direct effect of cocaine itself (105).

Vascular Thrombosis

Deep venous thrombosis of the upper extremity (Paget-Schroetter syndrome) related to cocaine abuse was reported in 12 male individuals (106). Forty-two percent of these patients were intravenous cocaine users without risk factors for deep venous thrombosis of the upper extremity. Another patient exhibited cocaine-related arterial thrombosis associated with protein C and antithrombin III depletion (67). The possibility of a procoagulant effect of cocaine has been raised. Thrombosis caused by cocaine-induced procoagulant effects may provide an explanation for acute infarction in patients with normal coronary arteries (64), cocaine-related stroke, pulmonary hemorrhage, and rhabdomyolysis. Several syndromes associated with cocaine use that may be thrombotic have been described. Renal artery thrombosis has also been described in relation to cocaine abuse (107). Intravenous cocaine abuse associated with superficial thrombophlebitis has also been reported (108).

Cerebrovascular Accidents

Although the incidence of cocaine-related stroke is unknown and is probably low, cocaine is the illicit drug most commonly associated with stroke (109). A growing number of individuals with cocaine-induced stroke have been described (3,110–137). In a 1986 review of five cases of stroke associated with cocaine abuse, Cregler and Mark (19) found that the most likely mechanism was a sudden increase in arterial blood pressure as a result of adrenergic stimulation in an asymptomatic person with a berry aneurysm or arteriovenous malformation. Subarachnoid hemorrhage, intracerebral hemorrhage, and ischemic stroke located in all vascular distributions have been described (138). Severe headache after cocaine use should alert the physician to the possibility of an intracranial hemorrhage (19). Strokes have been described in young patients with normal cerebral vessels (114). Patients with diseased cerebral vessels are at even greater risk for having a stroke (124). Chasnoff (139) described an infant in whom cerebral infarction developed after birth, and the infant's urine was positive for cocaine metabolites. In another case, stroke was described in a neonate following prenatal cocaine exposure (140). The incidence of cocaine-related stroke is unknown but is probably low.

Diagnostic and Therapeutic Considerations

The evaluation of any young athlete with chest pain or an arrhythmia is challenging. Clinical clues that suggest cocaine abuse include tachycardia, dilated pupils, combativeness, altered mental status, or seizures. Chest pain should be presumed to be of ischemic origin until proven otherwise (141). Pleuritic chest pain is common in young cocaine abusers and is of unknown origin (142). The differential diagnoses should include bronchitis, pneumomediastinum pneumothorax, dissecting aneurysm, and myocardial infarction. These individuals should be admitted and monitored while serial CK-MB and other cardiac enzyme levels are obtained (143). Electrocardiograms should be performed on all patients with chest pain or an arrhythmia. The electrocardiograms should be read with "caution" because persistent juvenile ST segment repolarization changes may represent myocardial ischemia (142).

The short half-life of cocaine allows observation and conservative therapy with benzodiazepines in many patients with anxiety, agitation, tremor, or seizure (144). Haloperidol is a useful agent for acute psychosis (145). Patients with unexplained cardiovascular symptoms, including hypertension-related problems, should be asked about cocaine use and, if indicated, drug screening should be done (3, 19,20,146). Self-reports denying the use of cocaine are unreliable (147). The major metabolite of cocaine (benzoylecgonine) is detectable in urine samples by gas chromatography for 3 days or by radioimmunoassay technique for 6 days after intranasal use (148).

Recommendations concerning the treatment of cardiac events that result from cocaine abuse are based on a paucity of clinical data. There are no randomized trials to support the specific use of any class of drugs in acute cocaine-related events. Nitroglycerin has been documented to reverse cocaine-related coronary vasoconstriction (149,150). Phentolamine, an alpha-blocker, and verapamil, a calcium channel blocker, are two other drugs that reverse cocaine-related coronary vasoconstriction (151, 152). Streptokinase and tissue plasminogen activator have been given to a small number of patients with acute infarction who had "normal" coronary arteries on angiography (53,56, 57,59). In one patient, a large intracranial hemorrhage developed after the patient received thrombolytic therapy, and, at autopsy, a ruptured mycotic aneurysm was found (153). Some clinicians advocate the use of thrombolytic therapy (59,142), but others suggest that it is contraindicated in intravenous cocaine abusers (141).

Beta-blockers have been advocated because of their effects on hyperadrenergic states and their antihypertensive and negative chronotropic actions (154,155). Nonselective beta-blockade may result in unopposed α-adrenergic stimulation and may worsen myocardial ischemia (62,156). Labetolol, an alpha-beta blocker, is used as an intravenous bolus or constant infusion to control moderate hypertension associated with cocaine use (157). Severe hypertension may require an intravenous nitroprusside drip. Phentolamine is effective for the treatment of chest pain and elevated blood pressure, but its use should be monitored carefully because it may cause hypotension (156). Beta-blockers are recommended for use in treating supraventricular and ventricular arrhythmias induced by cocaine (142). In an acute myocardial infarction, the use of a short-acting beta-blocker such as esmolol may be helpful (84).

CARDIOVASCULAR EFFECTS OF ALCOHOL

In 1982, the American College of Sports Medicine issued a position statement against the use of alcohol in sports. Alcohol impairs psychomotor skills, reaction time, balance, accuracy, hand-eye coordination, and complex coordination (8). Alcohol decreases strength, speed, power, muscular endurance, and cardiovascular endurance (158). However, it is often consumed to reduce anxiety or tremor before competitive events. Beer is the main alcoholic beverage that athletes drink. The sports literature extols beer as a good fluid and caloric replacement after exercise (159); in fact, it is a poor fluid replacement because of its diuretic effect on the kidneys. A common misconception is that alcoholic beverages are also rich in carbohydrates. A 12-ounce can of beer contains 150 calories and only 50 calories are carbohydrate (159). The only sport that prohibits ethanol is modern pentathlon (which includes shooting events).

Few studies have documented the incidence of alcohol use among university and professional athletes. Toohey and Corder reviewed data on intercollegiate swimmers and found that 91% used alcohol, 25% amphetamines, 70% marijuana, 19% cocaine, and 10% LSD (160). In 1984, the NCAA asked researchers at Michigan State University to study substance abuse habits of collegiate athletes. They surveyed athletes from five men's and five women's sports at all levels of competition. The results indicated that students abuse ergogenic and recreational drugs and that most drug abuse began before college (1) (Table 2).

Alcohol is the oldest social beverage and principal drug of abuse in the United States. Human ancestors have imbibed beer and wine to alter mood and for pleasure since 4,000 B.C. (5,161). Alcoholic beverages include table wines, dessert or cocktail wines, liquors or cordials, beers, and distilled spirits (162). Two-thirds of American adults consume alcohol and at least 10% are heavy drinkers. Moderate drinkers consume one to two drinks per day, one drink being 1¼ ounces of whiskey, 12 ounces of beer, 5 ounces of table wine, or an average cocktail, each of which contains 13 g of alcohol (163). Heavy drinkers are individuals who consume more than five drinks per day. Alcohol abuse has been implicated in the development of heart disease for more than a

TABLE 2. *Substance abuse patterns in college student athletes from 1985 to 1989*

	1985	1989
Number of athletes surveyed	2049	2282
Ergogenic drug use in previous year (%)		
Amphetamines	8	3
Anabolic steroids	4	5
Barbiturates	2	2
Major analgesics	28	34
Weight loss products	n/a	5
Social drug use in previous year (%)		
Alcohol	88	89
Caffeine	68	64
Cocaine/crack	17	5
Psychedelics	4	4
Marijuana	36	28
Smokeless tobacco	20	28

n/a, not assessed. Adapted from ref. 159, with permission.

century (164–166). Adverse consequences of alcohol abuse are hypertension, stroke, coronary events, lipid abnormalities, cardiac rhythm disturbances, systolic dysfunction, and dilated cardiomyopathy (167,168).

Alcohol has predictable dose-dependent consequences on the heart and blood vessels. The relationship between chronic alcohol intake, dilated cardiomyopathy, and atrial arrhythmias is well established. Epidemiologic studies suggest a beneficial effect of moderate alcohol consumption on coronary artery disease and a link between alcohol consumption and hypertension. Hemorrhagic stroke rates are associated with a history of alcohol use. Alcohol has a favorable effect on high density lipoprotein (HDL) level. The use of alcohol may impose a favorable, neutral, or unfavorable risk on genesis of various cardiovascular diseases (167).

ALCOHOL AND BLOOD PRESSURE

Epidemiologic studies demonstrate an association between alcohol use and arterial blood pressure (5). The Los Angeles Heart Study, the Chicago Western Electric Study, the Framingham Heart Study, and the Kaiser-Permanente Multiphasic Health Examination Study reported higher blood pressure and a higher prevalence of hypertension among subjects with a history of heavy alcohol consumption than in those with a history of light or no drinking. In the Kaiser-Permanente study, the association of alcohol consumption and blood pressure for black men and women was not as strong as among whites (169–174).

The hypertensive effect of alcohol is more pronounced in men than in women (175). Among women, those who consume moderate amounts of alcohol have lower blood pressures than those who are abstinent. Blood pressure decreased in women who consumed up to 20 g of alcohol daily, but the average blood pressure is higher in women who consume more than 30 g daily (167).

Moderate alcohol consumption may be the most common cause of secondary hypertension (176,177). Alcohol abuse should be considered in an athlete with new onset hypertension. A blood alcohol and urinary drug screen for cocaine metabolites should be considered in all patients with resistant hypertension. Systolic blood pressure in heavy drinkers is 5 to 10 mm Hg higher than in moderate and nondrinkers (3). The increase is greater in systolic than in diastolic blood pressure. The prevalence of hypertension resulting from chronic alcohol consumption ranges from 5% to 30% in studies. In more than half of alcoholic patients admitted for detoxification, blood pressure exceeds 140/90 mm Hg (4, 5,178) and, in one-third, it is greater than 160/90 mm Hg (179). Blood pressure is highest on admission when most patients still have high blood alcohol levels; blood pressure level usually declines over several days of abstinence. However, persistent elevation in 10% of these patients characterizes them as a subset with essential hypertension. In hypertensive patients, drinking alcohol elevates blood pressure and makes control more difficult. Abstinence or reduced intake may result in a gradual decrease in blood pressure, starting as early as 1 week (4).

Hypertension is transitory in most heavy drinkers but it may not be benign. Clark demonstrated an exaggerated response in blood pressure, heart rate, and catecholamine levels to the cold pressor test in alcoholics with transitory hypertension (179). Some investigators believe that chronic heavy drinking produces abnormal vascular responsiveness. Reducing intake of alcohol can produce modest reductions in blood pressure, with major implications in the goal of reducing the prevalence of hypertension-related morbidity (5).

The precise mechanism by which alcohol produces hypertension is unknown. Some investigators suggest that it is the result of alcohol withdrawal on a subclinical level. Alcohol metabolites acetate and acetaldehyde are vasodilators, but vasoconstriction has been reported in animal data (180,181).

Alcohol-Induced Stroke

Alcohol was first mentioned as a risk factor for stroke in 1725 (182). Since then, epidemiologic studies have shown a link between alcohol consumption and stroke, a relationship found to be independent of hypertension (5, 183,184). In the Honolulu Heart Study, increasing alcohol intake was associated with greater hemorrhagic stroke risk. Moderate and heavy drinkers have a threefold to fourfold risk of development of subarachnoid hemorrhage compared with nondrinkers. Thrombotic stroke risk does not differ between drinkers and nondrinkers. Moderate alcohol consumption is associated with a reduced risk of thrombotic stroke in middle-aged women, but this was not true for men in the Honolulu Heart Study (183). In a study by Gill et al. (185), a marked risk of stroke, including hemorrhagic and thrombotic events, was seen in male heavy drinkers after adjusting for hypertension and smoking.

The highest incidence of stroke occurs in nonalcoholic men who drink more than 300 g of alcohol on weekends (167). Stroke is precipitated during intoxication rather than during withdrawal. Excessive alcohol ingestion may increase the risk of stroke threefold in young athletes (186). Alcoholics suffer stroke at an earlier age than do nondrinkers.

The mechanism of alcohol-induced stroke is complex and unclear. It may include rebound thrombocytosis, activation of the coagulation cascade, hypertension, altered autoregulation of cerebral blood flow, abnormalities of cardiac wall motion, cardiac arrhythmias, and alteration of cerebral metabolism. Older persons with alcohol-induced atrial fibrillation or alcoholic cardiomyopathy are at increased risk for embolic stroke. Unexplained stroke in an athlete without risk factors should trigger a detailed investigation of possible alcohol abuse (5).

Cardiomyopathy

The effects of alcohol on the heart involve the sinus node, atrioventricular node, His-Purkinje system, and atrial and ventricular musculature (167). Congestive heart failure in alcoholics was originally attributed to nutritional and thiamine deficiency (beriberi heart disease) or to cobalt, which enhances foaming in beer. Alcoholic cardiomyopathy has only been considered a separate entity from beriberi heart disease within the past 30 years. It cannot be distinguished clinically or pathologically from dilated cardiomyopathy, and the diagnosis remains one of exclusion. Often a history of alcohol abuse is obtained through repeated questioning of the patient or family (187,188). Unexplained sinus tachycardia may be the only early clue to alcoholism and subclinical cardiomyopathy (5).

Alcoholic cardiomyopathy is a syndrome characterized by dilatation of the chambers, cardiomegaly, and diminished systolic function. Most hearts weigh 600 to 700 g on average. The old adage that alcoholic cardiomyopathy rarely develops in individuals with alcoholic liver disease and vice versa is false (189–191). Alcoholic cardiomegaly is found predominantly in men 30 to 55 years of age with significant histories of alcohol intake. Most have consumed 30% to 50% of their calories as alcohol for 10 to 15 years. The type of alcoholic beverage is not important. The incidence of cardiomyopathy in heavy drinkers may be as high as 30%.

The "holiday heart" syndrome described by Ettinger et al. (192) occurs in chronic alcohol abusers in whom binge drinking leads to paroxysmal arrhythmias. Atrial fibrillation is the most common arrhythmia, but other rhythm disturbances include atrial flutter, junctional tachycardia, paroxysmal atrial tachycardia, premature ventricular contractions, premature atrial contractions, and ventricular tachycardia.

Acute and chronic ingestion of alcohol produces depression of left ventricular systolic function in normal individuals and chronic users of alcohol. The severity of alcohol-induced cardiac dysfunction depends on prior alcohol consumption and underlying heart disease. Gould and colleagues (193) showed that 2 ounces of alcohol impairs cardiac function in patients with heart disease. Asymptomatic alcoholics have abnormalities of systolic time intervals and lower left ventricular ejection fractions than nondrinkers.

Many asymptomatic alcoholics have heart disease that becomes evident on provocation (4). Cregler et al. (194) administered alcohol orally and intravenously to male alcoholics producing left ventricular dysfunction that was manifested by markedly prolonged systolic time intervals. Spodick (195) and Wu (196) and their colleagues also found abnormal systolic time intervals indicative of underlying left ventricular dysfunction in asymptomatic alcoholics. Regan et al. (190) demonstrated an abnormal left ventricular response to angiotensin in chronic alcoholics without cardiac symptoms.

The mechanism of alcohol-induced congestive cardiomegaly is not known. Acetaldehyde, a metabolite of alcohol and a myocardial depressant, can decrease protein synthesis. Several cofactors have been thought to contribute, including hypertension, immunologic disorders, and viral infections (5). The relation of alcohol to cardiovascular disease may be characterized as positive, negative, or neutral depending on quantity, duration, and pattern of consumption, as well as preexisting cardiovascular abnormalities (167).

Alcohol and Coronary Artery Disease

Moderate alcohol consumption has been shown by epidemiologic studies to be associated with a lower risk of coronary atherosclerosis, myocardial infarction, and coronary artery disease. The data regarding the relationship between chronic heavy drinking and coronary artery disease are mixed. Some studies suggest that heavy alcohol consumption increases the risk for fatal and nonfatal myocardial infarctions. This may be related to alcohol-induced hypertension. Heavy drinkers are at increased risk for ischemic heart disease and those with compromised coronary circulation are more likely to suffer sudden death than nondrinkers. Adrenergic activity can produce tachycardia, hypertension, and coronary spasm that can aggravate underlying ischemia.

A Veterans Administration study revealed that angina and myocardial infarction are more likely to develop in heavy drinkers with preexisting coronary heart disease than in those with similar underlying disease who do not consume alcohol (197). Most heavy drinkers also smoke cigarettes, but multivariate analysis showed that heavy drinking influenced the risk of myocardial infarction independent of smoking.

The consumption of one to two alcoholic drinks per day has been shown to reduce the incidence of coronary heart disease (198). This finding is supported by coronary angiographic data that suggest a lower incidence of coronary atherosclerosis in moderate drinkers. The protective mechanism that alcohol exerts against coronary disease is unknown. However, alcohol elevates plasma HDLs and increases fibrinolytic activity that is inversely related to the risk of development of coronary artery disease (199). The effects of alcohol consumption on lipids and lipoprotein depend on the volume consumed, individual susceptibility, age, genetic variables, and dietary factors.

Data from alcoholics suggest that the synthesis of very low density lipoprotein is stimulated and that the level of HDL_2 is increased. Chronic alcoholics may have low or subnormal low density lipoprotein levels. In the general population, moderate consumption of alcohol increases apolipoprotein (apo) AI, AIII, and HDL_3 without affecting other lipoproteins (200,201). Given the complex pathogenesis of coronary artery disease, it is not prudent to recommend alcohol to reduce coronary risk (5).

CARDIOTOXIC EFFECTS
OF STEROIDS

Anabolic steroids are synthetic derivatives of the male sex hormone testosterone. Testosterone was first isolated in 1935 and was used primarily for the treatment of male hypogonadism. Attempts to separate the anabolic form from the androgenic effects have been unsuccessful, and these agents should be referred to as anabolic-androgenic steroids. Sex drive may be affected and some users take human chorionic gonadotrophin to prevent testicular atrophy. Anabolic steroids are ergogenic agents used by athletes to enhance performance and increase muscle mass. Anabolic steroid abuse often receives international media attention when an elite athlete tests positive or suffers an associated adverse event (15,202).

Anabolic steroid usage is a major problem in the United States among children, teen-agers, college students, amateur body builders, and professional athletes of both sexes (160). It is estimated that 1 million Americans have used or are currently using anabolic steroids to promote athletic performance. Adolescents and young adults aged 25 years and younger make up 54% of individuals who use anabolic steroids (203). A recent study examined 12,272 high school students and the relationship between anabolic steroid use, other drugs, sports participation, and school performance. The frequency of anabolic steroid use was significantly associated with the use of cocaine, amphetamines, heroin, tobacco smoking, and alcohol use. The variables that were associated with anabolic steroid use varied by gender and region of the country. These data suggest that anabolic steroid users are more likely to engage in strength training, injection of drugs of abuse, and the use of multiple drugs after controlling for sports participation (204). Human growth hormone may be used for an anabolic effect but data on its effect are limited. Acromegaly is the most common side effect of growth hormone excess. In addition, coronary artery disease and cardiomyopathy have been described.

There are few medical indications for the use of anabolic steroids. Anabolic steroids were first reported to have been used during World War II by German soldiers to increase strength and aggressiveness. In the 1950s, anabolic steroids were administered to male and female Russian competitive athletes. Since that time, many studies have documented the negative physical and psychological side effects of steroids (205–209). Adverse effects of anabolic steroids include cardiac, hepatic, renal, and genital conditions, as well as lipid abnormalities and vascular disease.

Athletes self-administer 10 to 200 times the therapeutic dose prescribed for legitimate medical conditions. The win-at-all-costs mentality in the athletic community emphasizes the personal and high financial stakes involved in the abuse of these agents. Anabolic steroid use was banned by the IOC in 1975. The significant health risks involved in steroid usage prompted the U.S. Congress to discuss the Steroid Trafficking Act of 1990, which considered classifying anabolic steroids as a Schedule-II controlled substance.

Myocardial Infarction

Unfavorable cardiovascular events are linked to anabolic steroid abuse in healthy individuals. These events include nonfatal and fatal myocardial infarctions. The first acute nonfatal myocardial infarction was reported in a 22-year-old weight lifter who received steroids for 6 weeks. Cardiac catheterization revealed normal coronary arteries with apical dyskinesia (210). The first fatal myocardial infarction was reported in a 22-year-old college athlete who had a long history of steroid abuse (211). Additional fatal and nonfatal myocardial infarctions have been reported in male weight lifters and a body builder (212).

Cardiomyopathy

There are reports of cardiomyopathies occurring in body builders using high doses of steroids. The first individual described was a 32-year-old chronic user of high doses of steroids who sustained a right-sided stroke. An echocardiogram and a nuclear cardiac scan were consistent with cardiomyopathy. Ferenchick and colleagues reported on a 37-year-old male body builder who abused multiple agents for years. He was seen with congestive heart failure before he died. An autopsy revealed cardiac hypertrophy, interstitial fibrosis, and an atheroma in his coronary arteries (213).

Other Effects

Two cases were reported from Australia in asymptomatic football players who died suddenly while training (214). The first patient was 18 years old and his autopsy was consistent with hypertrophic cardiomyopathy. The other player, 24 years old, had myocarditis. Normal coronary arteries were present in both individuals and there was no evidence of thrombosis. In each case, a toxicology screen for drugs did not detect evidence of drug use. However, gas chromatographic mass spectrographic analysis of urine detected a metabolite of an anabolic steroid.

Anabolic steroids increase left ventricular mass and responsiveness to catecholamines, therefore increasing the risk of sudden death. Findings of fibrosis and inflammatory changes may be due to a nonspecific myocarditis (214).

Vascular Events

The first report of vascular complications from anabolic steroids was in three patients receiving steroids for hypoplastic anemia. Thrombosis of the superior sagittal sinus developed in each patient (215). Anabolic steroids have been reported to enhance the pressor response to catecholamines in an animal model. Tissue heart preparations have shown that supraventricular and ventricular arrhythmias have varying response to anabolic agents. Alterations of platelet function, fibrinolytic activity, and clotting factors XVII and X have also been reported (216).

Anabolic steroids have been temporally related to myocardial infarction in weight lifters, bilateral pulmonary hemorrhage in a body builder, and cardiomyopathy in a former professional football player (2). There are reports of left ventricular hypertrophy, increased low density lipoprotein, decreased HDL, and sodium and water retention after abuse of steroids.

Contrary to current opinion, acute and chronic steroid usage has a negative impact on exercise performance. The cardiotoxic effect of high-dose administration of one anabolic steroid and stacking of two or more steroids at one time in the sedentary and exercise-trained individuals remains to be determined. The sage clinician considers anabolic steroid abuse in any athlete with an acute vascular event.

MARIJUANA, TOBACCO, AMPHETAMINES AND OTHER DRUGS

Marijuana use is ergolytic; it increases heart rate and decreases cardiac stroke volume and exercise performance. In a study of 161 individuals given marijuana, the group showed a decrease in standing steadiness, simple and complex reaction time, and psychomotor skills. When marijuana is used with alcohol, exercise performance deteriorates more than when either drug is used alone (217). Marijuana is not prohibited by the IOC because of its lack of performance-enhancing activity. However, the argument in favor of testing is that it is an illegal drug in most countries.

Because of the thin line between ergogenic and some therapeutic drug use, agents must be selected carefully in athletes who compete in events in which random drug testing is performed. Stimulants were the first drugs used and studied as ergogenic agents (1). Stimulants are a complex class of drugs because they include the over-the-counter (OTC) preparations widely used for minor ailments. Amphetamines may increase time to exhaustion by masking the physiologic response to fatigue. Despite improved time to exhaustion, lactic acid concentration increases and $\dot{V}O_{2\ max}$ is unchanged (1). Convulsions, coma, and death may occur from using amphetamines. Cardiac complications include stroke, hypertension, angina, and arrhythmias (182). Once amphetamines became prohibited substances, athletes turned to OTC stimulants such as ephedrine and pseudoephedrine. The pharmacologic properties of OTC drugs, in high doses, are very similar to amphetamines. Some antihistamines can make the athlete drowsy. Vicks NyQuil contains an antihistamine and contains 25% alcohol. Diphenhydramine is dangerous for divers and drivers because it produces drowsiness. Anticonvulsants can also impair athletic performance.

Athletes use smokeless tobacco because they believe that nicotine enhances performance. Tobacco may produce psychomotor effects and control appetite that may be helpful to some athletes. Nicotine is a central stimulant that relaxes skeletal muscle, constricts blood vessels, and increases heart rate and blood pressure, making the heart work harder (218). Smokeless tobacco usually takes one or two forms: snuff is placed between the lower lip and gum or chewing tobacco is put in the cheek pouch. Consumption of smokeless tobacco was stimulated by the media, which used professional athletes to promote it as a safe alternative to smoking. The association of athletics with smokeless tobacco remains embodied in the game of baseball (219). The celebrity athlete, as a role model, serves to strengthen the misconception that smokeless tobacco does not impair but rather enhances athletic performance (220). The rate of smokeless tobacco use increased after 1980 from 5% to 16%, with adolescents accounting for the majority of users (221). A survey of college athletes in 1991 revealed that 57% of baseball players, 40% of football players, and 20% of track and field athletes used smokeless tobacco (222).

The predominant active pharmacologic substance in smokeless tobacco is nicotine. Consuming one 34-g (1.2-ounce) container a day is equivalent to smoking 1.5 packs of cigarettes per day. Chewing tobacco or dipping snuff achieves blood nicotine levels equivalent to smoking cigarettes and just as rapidly (219). Nicotine can elevate total cholesterol

and lower HDL. In addition, it alters platelets, resulting in increased coagulability. Other adverse cardiac effects are coronary artery spasm and a reduced threshold for ventricular fibrillation. Reports have described sudden death in athletes using smokeless tobacco following vigorous exercise.

Wrestlers, sprinters, weight lifters, boxers, and jockeys use diuretics shortly before competition in an attempt to dilute the urinary concentration of other prohibited drugs (8). Diuretics can acutely deplete plasma volume and impair performance. These drugs can result in weight loss, deplete potassium, produce premature ventricular contractions, and decrease $\dot{V}O_{2\ max}$. Diuretics may contribute to exertional heat stroke and rhabdomyolysis in distance runners. Skiers and mountain climbers often take acetazolamide in an attempt to avoid mountain sickness. Acetazolamide impairs endurance by producing a mild acidosis that inhibits muscle glycolysis. Another agent, probenecid, blocks renal excretion of anabolic steroids in a fashion similar to how it blocks excretion of penicillins.

Drugs used to treat hypertension include the nonselective beta-blockers that impair exercise performance. Beta-blockers attenuate the exercise-induced increase in blood pressure and heart rate (223). Among elite athletes, beta-blockers can reduce oxygen uptake by as much as 15% (224). They may also curb endurance during submaximal exercise. This is a controversial area because beta-blockers may mask the training effect more than they attenuate it (8).

The use of opiates is prohibited based on their dangers when used as illegal drugs. Opiates are any natural or synthetic drug that has morphine-like properties. Opium is derived from the exudate of the seed capsules of the poppy plant. Heroin is made from morphine by acetylation of the phenolic and alcohol hydroxyl groups (182). Opiates have been used to dull the pain of leg cramps in distance events. Heroin can be smoked, snorted, used orally, sublingually, subcutaneously, rectally, or intravenously. It is usually administered parenterally and has a half-life of 20 minutes. Stroke associated with heroin abuse is ischemic, and intravenous injection is the route of administration. Antiasthma drugs, salbutamol, salmeterol, and terbutaline are widely used in treating asthma, and the IOC prohibition has created some concern in discriminating between medical use and use to enhance performance. The issue has been resolved by allowing the three aforementioned beta-agonists to be taken if their use is declared in advance of the competition and if the drugs are administered only by inhalation. Corticosteroids may also be used by inhalation if declared in advance. Athletes with asthma may also be given theophylline, cromolyn sodium, and anticholinergics without notification. Some sports and countries require athletes with asthma to undergo spirometry before approving the use of beta-agonists. Local anesthetics may be administered only if the IOC has received documentation justifying their use before competition. Topical cocaine use is not allowed. Glucocorticoids may be used by topical, intraarticular, or inhalation routes of administration. The intent to use glucocorticoids must be declared by the physician before competition.

BLOOD DOPING AND PROHIBITED METHODS

Blood doping with native or foreign red blood cells enhances performance by increasing red blood cell mass and delivering more oxygen to muscle (15). The procedure of blood doping involves removing an athlete's red blood cells and giving them back to the person before competition. The increase in red blood cell mass is believed to improve oxygen consumption and benefit endurance. Erythropoietin may be a pharmacologic alternative to blood doping by increasing red blood cell mass. Deaths have been reported in individuals taking erythropoietin. Other complications may include hypertension, congestive heart failure, and stroke. Prohibited methods were created to ban maneuvers such as instilling clean urine in the bladder and stimulating voiding. Prohibited methods were expanded to include drugs that alter testosterone/epitestosterone (T/E) ratio. The T/E ratio is used as an indicator of testosterone use. Epitestosterone lowers the T/E ratio (225).

DRUG TESTING

Drug control and testing have become an important component of athletics and Olympic sports. Most drugs are easy to detect in urine except for the detection of doping with red blood cells. Drug programs must include short- or no-notice testing during training, testing at qualifying competition, and testing during actual competition games. Drug testing is performed for three main sporting organizations (NCAA, NFL, USOC). The USOC was the first sports organization to conduct testing in the United States. It conducts announced testing for all major events. The NFL began testing for illegal drugs and anabolic steroids in the mid-1980s. In 1986, the NCAA instituted a program to test NCAA championship teams, and this policy has been expanded to all sports. The percentage of samples testing positive for stimulants and anabolic steroids annually has stabilized at 0.37% and 1%, respectively. In 1994, diuretics, beta-blockers, and narcotics accounted for 0.17% of positive tests. OTC drugs account for 50% to 60% of all stimulants detected (15).

Prohibited and restricted drugs are listed in three main categories (Table 3). The cate-

TABLE 3. *Classes of substances and methods prohibited by the International Olympic Committee, including substances subject to certain restrictions*

Prohibited classes of substances
  Stimulants
  Narcotics
  Anabolic agents
  Diuretics
  Peptide and glycoprotein hormones and analogues
Prohibited methods
  Blood doping
  Pharmacologic, chemical, and physical manipulation
Classes of drugs subject to restrictions
  Alcohol
  Marijuana
  Local anesthetics
  Corticosteroids
  β-Blockers

Adapted from ref. 15, with permission.

TABLE 4. *Cardiovascular risk factors*

Modifiable	Nonmodifiable
Hypertension	Age
Hyperlipidemia	Sex
Cigarette smoking	Family history
Hyperglycemia	
Left ventricular hypertrophy	
Cocaine use	

Adapted from ref. 228, with permission.

gories include (a) short or immediate-acting stimulants and beta-blockers that affect performance, (b) anabolic steroids that take weeks to obtain training effects and, (c) drugs such as diuretics and probenecid that affect the detection of other drugs (15).

In screening athletes for cardiovascular risk factors and sudden death, all physicians should be alert for cocaine, alcohol, steroids, and other substances of abuse when confronted with unexplained cardiac symptoms (226). These drugs are the newest and often unrecognized risk factors (Table 4) for heart disease in an athlete without traditional cardiovascular risk factors (227,228).

REFERENCES

1. Wagner JC. Enhancement of athletic performance with drugs. An overview. *Sports Med* 1991;12(4):250–265.
2. Welder AA, Melchert RB. Cardiotoxic effects of cocaine and anabolic-androgenic steroids in the athlete. *J Pharmacol Toxicol Methods* 1993;29:61–68.
3. Cregler LL. Cocaine: the newest risk factor for cardiovascular disease. *Clin Cardiol* 1991;14:449–456.
4. Cregler LL, Worner TM, Mark H. Echocardiographic abnormalities in chronic asymptomatic alcoholics. *Clin Cardiol* 1989;12:122–128.
5. Cregler LL. Cardiovascular effects of alcohol. *Primary Cardiol* 1988;14:38–42.
6. Cregler LL, Mark H. Medical complications of cocaine abuse. *N Engl J Med* 1986;315:1495–1500.
7. Worner TM, Cregler LL, Mark H. Cardiac dysfunction in alcoholics. *Mt Sinai J Med (NY)* 1987;4:317–322.
8. Eichner ER. Ergolytic drugs in medicine and sports. *Am J Med* 1993;94:205–209.
9. Maron BJ, Shirani J, Poliac LC, et al. Sudden death in young competitive athletes: clinical, demographic, and pathological profiles. *JAMA* 1996;276:199–204.
10. Del Rosario JD, Strong WB. Sudden cardiac death in young athletes. How to identify patients at risk. *Consultant* 1996:2272–2284.
11. Maron BJ, Epstein SE, Roberts WC. Causes of sudden death in competitive athletes. *J Am Coll Cardiol* 1986; 7:204–214.
12. Bradeen D, Strong WB. Preparticipation screening for

sudden cardiac death in high school and college athletes. *Physician Sports Med* 1988;16:128–140.
13. Strong WB, Steed D. Cardiovascular evaluation of the young athlete. *Pediatr Clin North Am* 1982;29: 1325–1339.
14. Maron BJ. Sudden death in young athletes. Lessons from the Hank Gathers affair. *N Engl J Med* 1993;329: 55–57.
15. Catlin DH, Murray TH. Performance-enhancing drugs, fair competition, and Olympic sport. *JAMA* 1996; 276(3):231–237.
16. Lowenstein DH, Massa SM, Rowbotham MC, Collins SD, McKinney HE, Simon RP. Acute neurologic and psychiatric complications associated with cocaine abuse. *Am J Med* 1987;83(1):841–846.
17. Cregler LL. Acute neurologic and psychiatric complications associated with cocaine abuse [Letter]. *Am J Med* 1988;84(5):978–979.
18. Brody SL, Slovis CM, Wrenn KD. Cocaine-related medical problems. Consecutive series of 233 patients. *Am J Med* 1990;88(5):325–331.
19. Cregler LL, Mark H. Cardiovascular dangers of cocaine abuse [Editorial]. *Am J Cardiol* 1986;57:1185–1186.
20. Cregler LL. The heart and cocaine. *Primary Cardiol* 1989;15(4):23–24.
21. Billman GE. Mechanisms responsible for the cardiotoxic effects of cocaine. *FASEB J* 1990;4: 2469–2475.
22. Abelson HI, Miller JD. A decade of trends in cocaine use in the household population. *Natl Inst Drug Abuse Res Monogr Ser* 1985;61:35–49.
23. Fishburn PM. National survey on drug abuse: main findings 1979. Rockville, MD: National Institute of Drug Abuse, 1980. [DHHS publication no. (ADM) 80–976].
24. Warner WA. Cocaine abuse. *Ann Intern Med* 1993; 119:226–235.
25. Gawin FH, Ellinwood EH Jr. Cocaine and other stimulants. *N Engl J Med* 1988;318(18):1173–1182.
26. 1993 National Household Survey on Drug Abuse. Advance report No 2. Rockville, MD: Substance Abuse and Mental Health Services Administration, Office of Applied Studies, 1994;29.
27. National Institute on Drug Abuse. National Household Survey on Drug Abuse. Population Estimates 1990. Washington, DC: U.S. Department of Health and Human Services, 1991. [NDHHS Publication No. (ADM) 91–1732].
28. Freud S. Ueber Coca. *Centralbl Therap.* 1884;2: 289–314.
29. Idem. On coca. In: Byck R, ed. *Cocaine papers.* New York: Stonehill Publishing Co, 1974:49–73.
30. Siegel RK. Cocaine smoking. *J Psychoactive Drugs* 1982;13:271–343.
31. Ritchie JM, Greene NM. Local anesthetics. In: Gilman AG, Goodman LS, Rall TW, Murad F, eds. *The pharmacological basis of therapeutics,* 7th ed. New York: MacMillan, 1985;309–310.
32. Bouknight LB, Bouknight RR. Cocaine—a particular addictive drug. *Postgrad Med* 1988;83:115–131.
33. Musto D. *The American disease—origins of narcotic control.* New Haven, CT: Yale University, 1973.
34. Price FW, Leaky AB. Grave and prolonged cardiac failure following the use of cocaine in dental surgery. *Lancet* 1911;1:797–799.

35. Fairbanks DN, Fairbanks GR. Cocaine uses and abuses. *Ann Plast Surg* 1983;10:452–457.

36. Lange RA, Cigarroa RG, Yancy CW Jr, et al. Cocaine-induced coronary-artery vasoconstriction. *N Engl J Med* 1989;321(23):1557–1562.

37. Waller BF. Cocaine and the heart. *Indiana Med* 1988; 81(11):956–959.

38. Jekel JF, Allen DF, Podlewski H, Clarke N, Dean-Patterson S, Cartwright P. Epidemic free-base cocaine abuse: case study from the Bahamas. *Lancet* 1986;1: 459–462.

39. Devenyi P. Cocaine complications and pseudocholinesterase. *Ann Intern Med* 1989;110(2):167–168.

40. Coleman DL, Ross TF, Naughton JL. Myocardial ischemia and infarction related to recreational cocaine abuse. *West J Med* 1982;136:444–446.

41. Pasternack PF, Colvin SB, Baumann FG. Cocaine-induced angina pectoris and acute myocardial infarction in patients younger than 40 years. *Am J Cardiol* 1985; 55:847.

42. Cregler LL, Mark H. Relation of acute myocardial infarction to cocaine abuse. *Am J Cardiol* 1985;56:794.

43. Kossowsky WA, Lyon AF. Cocaine and acute myocardial infarction. A probable connection. *Chest* 1984;85: 729–731.

44. Howard RE, Hueter DC, Davis GJ. Acute myocardial infarction following cocaine abuse in a young woman with normal coronary arteries. *JAMA* 1985;254:95–96.

45. Schachne JS, Roberts BH, Thompson PD. Coronary-artery spasm and myocardial infarction associated with cocaine use. *N Engl J Med* 1984;310:1665–1666.

46. Wilkins CE, Matur VS, Ty RC, Hall RJ. Myocardial infarction associated with cocaine abuse. *Tex Heart Inst J* 1985;12:385–387.

47. Cregler LL, Mark H. Myocardial infarction associated with cocaine abuse: a case report. *Tex Heart Inst J* 1986;13:174.

48. Gould L, Gopalaswamy C, Patel C, Betzu R. Cocaine-induced myocardial infarction. *N Y State J Med* 1985; 85:660–661.

49. Weiss RJ. Recurrent myocardial infarction caused by cocaine abuse. *Am Heart J* 1986;111:793.

50. Simpson RW, Edwards WD. Pathogenesis of cocaine-induced ischemic heart disease. *Arch Pathol Lab Med* 1986;110:479–484.

51. Isner JM, Estes NAM III, Thompson PD, et al. Acute cardiac events temporally related to cocaine abuse. *N Engl J Med* 1986;315:1438–1443.

52. Weiner RS, Lockhart JT, Schwart RG. Dilated cardiomyopathy and cocaine abuse. Report of two cases. *Am J Med* 1986;81:699–701.

53. Ring RE, Butman SM. Cocaine and premature myocardial infarction. *Drug Ther* 1986;57:117–125.

54. Cantwell JD, Rose FD. Cocaine and cardiovascular events. *Physician Sports Med* 1986;13(11):77–82.

55. Rollinger IM, Belzberg AS, MacDonald IL. Cocaine-induced myocardial infarction. *CMAJ* 1986;135:45–46.

56. Rod JL, Zucker RP. Acute myocardial infarction shortly after cocaine inhalation. *Am J Cardiol* 1987; 59:161.

57. Wehbie CS, Vidaillet HJ Jr, Navetta FI, Peter RH. Acute myocardial infarction associated with initial cocaine use. *South Med J* 1987;80(7):933–934.

58. Zimmerman FH, Gustafson GM, Kemp HG. Recurrent myocardial infarction associated with cocaine abuse in a young man with normal coronary arteries. Evidence for coronary artery spasm culminating in thrombosis. *J Am Coll Cardiol* 1987;9(4):964–968.

59. Smith HWB, Liberman HA, Brody SL, Battey LL, Donahue BC, Morris DC. Acute myocardial infarction temporally related to cocaine use. *Ann Intern Med* 1987;107:13–18.

60. Mathias DW. Cocaine-associated myocardial ischemia. *Am J Med* 1986;81:675–678.

61. Kossowsky WA, Lyon AF, Chou SY. Acute non-Q wave cocaine-related myocardial infarction. *Chest* 1989;96(3):617–621.

62. Lange RA, Flores ED, Cigarroa RG, Hillis LD. Cocaine-induced myocardial ischemia and infarction. *Cardiology* 1990;7(8)74–79.

63. Flores ED, Lange RA, Cigarroa RG, Hillis LD. Effect of cocaine on coronary artery dimensions in atherosclerotic coronary artery disease: enhanced vasoconstriction at sites of significant stenoses. *J Am Coll Cardiol* 1990;16:74–79.

64. Vincent GM, Anderson JL, Marshall HW. Coronary spasm producing coronary thrombosis and myocardial infarction. *N Engl J Med* 1983;309:220–223.

65. Stenberg RG, Winniford MD, Hillis LD, Dowling GP, Buja LM. Simultaneous acute thrombosis of two major coronary arteries following intravenous cocaine use. *Arch Pathol Lab Med* 1989;113(5):521–524.

66. Fernandez MS, Pichard AD, Marchant E, Lindsay J Jr. Acute myocardial infarction with normal coronary arteries: in vivo demonstration of coronary thrombosis during the acute episode. *Clin Cardiol* 1983;6: 553–559.

67. Chokshi SK, Miller G, Rongione A, Isner JM. Cocaine and cardiovascular diseases. The leading edge. *Cardiology* 1989;76[Suppl 3]:1–6.

68. Nademanee K, Gorelick DA, Josephson MA, Robertson HA, Mody FV, Intarachot V. Transient ischemic episodes among cocaine users: evidence of coronary vasospasm. *Ann Intern Med* 1989;111(11):876–880.

69. Isner JM, Chokski SK. Cocaine and vasospasm [Editorial]. *N Engl J Med* 1989;321(23):1604–1606.

70. Grannis FW Jr, Bryant C, Caffaratti JD, Turner AF. Acute aortic dissection associated with cocaine abuse. *Clin Cardiol* 1988;11(8):572–574.

71. Cregler LL. Acute aortic dissection associated with cocaine abuse [Letter]. *Clin Cardiol* 1988;11(11):806.

72. Barth CW III, Bray M, Roberts WC. Rupture of the ascending aorta during cocaine intoxication. *Am J Cardiol* 1986;57:496.

73. Gadaleta D, Hall MH, Nelson RL. Cocaine-induced acute aortic dissection. *Chest* 1989;96(5):1203–1205.

74. Wetli CV, Wright RK. Death caused by recreational cocaine use. *JAMA* 1979;24:2519–2522.

75. Cucco RA, Yoo OH, Cregler LL, Chang JC. Nonfatal pulmonary edema after "freebase" cocaine smoking. *Am Rev Respir Dis* 1987;136:179–181.

76. Efferens L, Palat D, Meisner J. Nonfatal pulmonary edema following cocaine smoking. *N Y State J Med* 1989;89:415–416.

77. Hoffman CK, Goodman PC. Pulmonary edema in cocaine smokers. *Radiology* 1989;172:463–465.

78. Eurman DW, Potash HI, Eyler WR, Paganussi PJ, Beute GH. Chest pain and dyspnea related to "crack" cocaine smoking. Value of chest radiography. *Radiology* 1989;172:459–462.

79. Frand UI, Shin CS, Williams MH. Methadone-induced pulmonary edema. *Ann Intern Med* 1972;76:975–979.

80. Frand UI, Shim CS, Williams MH. Heroin-induced pulmonary edema: sequential studies of pulmonary function. *Ann Intern Med* 1972;77:29–35.

81. Young D, Glauber JJ. Electrocardiographic changes resulting from acute cocaine intoxication. *Am Heart J* 1947;34:272–279.

82. Vignola PA, Aonuma K, Swaye PS, et al. Lymphocytic myocarditis presenting as unexplained ventricular arrhythmias. Diagnosis with endomyocardial biopsy and response to immunosuppression. *J Am Coll Cardiol* 1984;4(4):812–819.

83. Jonsson S, O'Meara M, Young J. Acute cocaine poisoning. Importance of treating seizures and acidosis. *Am J Med* 1983;75:1061–1064.

84. Gradman AH. Cardiac effects of cocaine. A review. *Yale J Biol Med* 1988;61:137–147.

85. Blumenthal RS, Flaherty JT. Recognizing cardiac crisis in cocaine abusers. *J Crit Illness* 1990;5(3): 225–239.

86. Cregler LL, Swartz MH, Go A, Lee L, Mark H. The effects of cocaine on the electrocardiogram. *Alcohol Clin Exper Res* 1988;12(1):191.

87. Nanji AA, Filipenko JD. Asystole and ventricular fibrillation associated with cocaine intoxication. *Chest* 1984;85:132–133.

88. Benchimol A, Bartall H, Desser KB. Accelerated ventricular rhythm and cocaine abuse. *Ann Intern Med* 1978;88:519–520.

89. Billman GE, Hoskins RS. Cocaine-induced ventricular fibrillation: protection afforded by the calcium antagonist verapamil. *FASEB J* 1988;2(14):2990–2995.

90. Geggel RL, McInerny J, Estes NAM III. Transient neonatal ventricular tachycardia associated with maternal cocaine use. *Am J Cardiol* 1989;63:383–384.

91. Jentzen JM. Cocaine-induced myocarditis [Letter]. *Am Heart J* 1989;117(6):1398–1399.

92. Virmani R, Robinowitz M, Smialek JE, Symth DF. Cardiovascular effects of cocaine. An autopsy study of 40 patients. *Am J Med* 1988;115(5):1068–1076.

93. Dyke CV, Stesis A, Jones R, Chuntharapai A, Seaman W. Cocaine increases natural killer cell activity. *J Clin Invest* 1986;77:1387.

94. Pearce RM. Experimental myocarditis. A study of the histological changes following intravenous injections of adrenalin. *J Exp Med* 1906;8:400.

95. Duell PB. Chronic cocaine abuse and dilated cardiomyopathy [Letter]. *Am J Med* 1987;83:601.

96. Hoffman CK, Goodman PC. Pulmonary edema in cocaine smokers. *Radiology* 1989;172:463–465.

97. Morcos NC, Fairhurst AS, Henry WL. Direct but reversible effects of cocaine on the myocardium [Abstract]. *J Am Coll Cardiol* 1988;11:71A.

98. Hague N, Perreault C, Morgan JP. Effects of cocaine on intracellular Ca++ handling in mammalian myocardium [Abstract]. *Circulation* 1988;78:359.

99. Chokshi SK, Moore R, Pandian NG, Isner JM. Reversible cardiomyopathy associated with cocaine intoxication. *Ann Intern Med* 1989;11(12):1039–1040.

100. Peng SK, French WJ, Pelikan PC. Direct cocaine cardiotoxicity demonstrated by endomyocardial biopsy. *Arch Pathol Lab Med* 1989;113(8):842–845.

101. Bertolet BD, Freund G, Martin CA, Perchalski DL, Williams CM, Pepine CJ. Unrecognized left ventricular dysfunction in an apparently healthy cocaine abuse population. *Clin Cardiol* 1990;13(5):323–328.

102. Tazelaar HD, Karck SB, Stephens BG, Billinghan ME. Cocaine and the heart. *Hum Pathol* 1987;18:195–199.

103. Imperato-McGinley J, Gautier T, Ehlers K, Zullo MA, Goldstein DS, Vaughan ED Jr. Reversibility of catecholamine-induced dilated cardiomyopathy in a child with pheochromocytoma. *N Engl J Med* 1987;316: 793.

104. Birnbach DJ. Cardiovascular disease in the pregnant patient. A new risk factor. *Cardiovasc Risk Factors Int J* 1994;4(1):28–33.

105. Chambers HF, Morris DL, Tauber MG, Modin G. Cocaine use and the risk for endocarditis in intravenous drug users. *Ann Intern Med* 1987;106(6):833–836.

106. Lisse JR, Davis CP, Thurmond-Anderle M. Cocaine abuse and deep venous thrombosis [Letter]. *Ann Intern Med* 1989;110(7):571–572.

107. Wohlman RA. Renal artery thrombosis and embolization associated with intravenous cocaine injection. *South Med J* 1987;80(7):928–930.

108. Stuck RM, Doyle D. Superficial thrombophlebitis following parenteral cocaine abuse. *J Podiatr Med Assoc* 1987;77:351–353.

109. Sloan MA, Kittner SJ, Rigamonti D, Price TR. Occurrence of stroke associated with use/abuse of drugs. *Neurology* 1991;41:1358–1364.

110. Schwartz KA, Cohen JA. Subarachnoid hemorrhage precipitated by cocaine snorting. *Arch Neurol* 1984; 41:705.

111. Brust JC, Richter RW. Stroke associated with cocaine abuse? *N Y State J Med* 1977;77:1473–1475.

112. Lichtenfeld PJ, Rubin DB, Feldman RS. Subarachnoid hemorrhage precipitated by cocaine snorting. *Arch Neurol* 1984;41:223–224.

113. Caplan LR, Hier DB, Banks G. Current concepts of cerebrovascular disease-stroke. Stroke and drug abuse. *Stroke* 1982;13:869–872.

114. Golbe LI, Merkin MD. Cerebral infarction in a user of free-base cocaine ("crack"). *Neurology* 1986;36: 1602–1604.

115. Wojak JC, Flamm ES. Intracranial hemorrhage and cocaine use. *Stroke* 1987;18(4):712–715.

116. Tuchman AJ, Daras M, Zalzal P, Mangiardi J. Intracranial hemorrhage after cocaine abuse. *JAMA* 1987; 257(9):1175.

117. Levine SR, Welch KMA. Cocaine and stroke. *Stroke* 1988;19(6):779–783.

118. Seaman ME. Acute cocaine abuse associated with cerebral infarction. *Ann Emerg Med* 1990;19(1):34–37.

119. Nolte KB, Gelman BB. Intracerebral hemorrhage associated with cocaine abuse. *Arch Pathol Lab Med* 1989;113(7):812–813.

120. Meza I, Estrada CA, Montalvo JA, Hidalgo WN, Andersen J. Cerebral infarction associated with cocaine use. *Henry Ford Hosp Med J* 1989;37(1):50–51.

121. Levine SR, Washington JM, Moen M, Kieran SN, Junger S, Welch KM. Crack-associated stroke [Letter]. *Neurology* 1987;37(6):1092–1093.

122. Klonoff DC, Andrews BT, Obana WG. Stroke associated with cocaine use. *Arch Neurol* 1989;46(9): 989–993.

123. Mangiardi JR, Daras M, Geller ME, Weitzer I, Tuchman AJ. Cocaine-related intracranial hemorrhage. *Acta Neurol Scand* 1988;77(3):177–180.

124. Cregler LL, Mark H. Relation of stroke to cocaine abuse. *N Y State J Med* 1987;87:129–130.

125. Lundberg GD, Garriott JC, Reynolds PC, Cravey RH, Shaw RF. Cocaine-related death. *J Forensic Sci* 1977; 22:402–408.

126. Rogers JN, Henry TE, Jones AM, Froede RC, Byers JM. Cocaine-related deaths in Pima County, Arizona, 1982–1984. *J Forensic Sci* 1986;31:1404–1408.

127. Kaye BR, Fainstat M. Cerebral vasculitis associated with cocaine abuse. *JAMA* 1987;258:2104–2106.

128. Altes-Capella J, Cabezudo-Artero JM, Forteza-Rei J. Complications of cocaine abuse [Letter]. *Ann Intern Med* 1987;107:940.

129. Henderson CE, Torbey M. Rupture of intracranial aneurysm associated with cocaine abuse during pregnancy. *Am J Perinatol* 1988;5:142–143.

130. Chynn KY. Acute subarachnoid hemorrhage. *JAMA* 1975;233:55–56.

131. Tardiff K, Gross E, Wu J, Stajic M, Millman R. Analysis of cocaine-positive fatalities. *J Forensic Sci* 1989; 34:53–63.

132. Jacobs IG, Roszler MH, Kelly JK, Klein MA, Kling GA. Cocaine abuse: neuromuscular complications. *Radiology* 1989;170:223–227.

133. Lehman LB. Intracerebral hemorrhage after intranasal cocaine use. *Hosp Physician* 1987;7:69–70.

134. Mody CK, Miller BL, McIntyre HB, Cobb SK, Goldberg MA. Neurologic complications of cocaine abuse. *Neurology* 1988;38:1189–1193.

135. Mercado A, Johnson G Jr, Calver D, Sokol RJ. Cocaine, pregnancy and postpartum intracerebral hemorrhage. *Obstet Gynecol* 1989;73:467–468.

136. Rowley H, Lowenstein D, Rowbotham M. Thalamo-mesencephalic strokes after cocaine abuse. *Neurology* 1989;39:428–430.

137. Nalls G, Disher A, Daryabagi J, Zant Z, Eisenman J. Subcortical cerebral hemorrhages associated with cocaine abuse. CT and MR findings. *J Comput Assist Tomogr* 1989;13:1–5.

138. Rowbotham MC. Neurologic aspects of cocaine abuse. *West J Med* 1988;149:442–448.

139. Chasnoff IJ, Bussey ME, Savich R, Stack CM. Perinatal cerebral infarction and maternal cocaine use. *J Pediatr* 1986;108:456–459.

140. Spires MC, Gordon EF, Choudhuri M, Maldonado E, Chan R. Intracranial hemorrhage in a neonate following prenatal cocaine exposure. *Pediatr Neurol* 1989; 5(5):324–326.

141. Goldfrank L. Consultations. *Ann Emerg Med* 1987;16: 240.

142. Brody SL. Cocaine. Actions, abuse, and emergencies. *Emery University J Med* 1988;2(4):257–271.

143. Hollander JE, Hoffman RS, Burstein JL, et al. Cocaine-associated myocardial infarction: mortality and complications. *Arch Intern Med* 1995;155:1081–1086.

144. Gay GR. Clinical management of acute and chronic cocaine poisoning. *Ann Emerg Med* 1982;11:562–572.

145. Derlet RW, Albertson TE, Rice P. The effect of haloperidol in cocaine and amphetamine intoxication. *J Emerg Med* 1989;7:633–637.

146. Drug Abuse Warning Network (DAWN). Advance report no. 2. Rockville, MD: Substance Abuse and Mental Health Services Administration. Office of Applied Studies, 1993.

147. McNagny SE, Parker RM. High prevalence of recent cocaine use and the unreliability of patient self-report in an inner-city walk-in clinic. *JAMA* 1992;267: 1106–1108.

148. Hamilton HE, Wallace JE, Shimek EL Jr. Cocaine and benzoylecgonine excretion in humans. *J Forensic Sci* 1977;22:697–707.

149. Brogan WC III, Lange RA, Kim AS, et al. Alleviation of cocaine-induced coronary vasoconstriction by nitroglycerine. *J Am Coll Cardiol* 1991;18:581–586.

150. Hollander JE. The management of cocaine-associated myocardial ischemia. *N Engl J Med* 1995;333: 1267–1272.

151. Negus BH, Willard JE, Hillis LD, et al. Alleviation of cocaine-induced coronary vasoconstriction with intravenous verapamil. *Am J Cardiol* 1994;73:510–513.

152. Hollander JE, Carter WA, Hoffman RS. Use of phentolamine for cocaine-induced myocardial ischemia [Letter]. *N Engl J Med* 1992;327:361.

153. Bush H. Cocaine-associated myocardial infarction. A word of caution about thrombolytic therapy. *Chest* 1988;94:878.

154. Gay GR. Clinical management of acute and chronic cocaine poisoning. *Ann Emerg Med* 1982;11:562–572.

155. Rapport R, Gay GR, Inaba DS. Propranolol: a specific antagonist to cocaine. *Clin Toxicol* 1977;10:265–271.

156. Lange RA, Cigarroa RG, Flores ED, et al. Potentiation of cocaine-induced coronary vasoconstriction by beta-adrenergic blockade. *Ann Intern Med* 1990;112: 897–903.

157. Dusenberry SJ, Hicks MG, Marian PJ. Labetalol treatment of cocaine toxicity. *Ann Emerg Med* 1987;16: 235–236.

158. American College of Sports Medicine. The use of alcohol in sports. *Med Sci Sports Exerc* 1982;14: 481–482.

159. O'Brien CP. Alcohol and sport. Impact of social drinking on recreational and competitive sports performance. *Sports Med* 1993;15(2):71–77.

160. Toohey JV, Corder BW. Intercollegiate sports participation and non-medical drug use. *Bull Narcotics* 1981; 33:23–27.

161. Stimmel B. Psychotropic drug use: defining the problem. In: *Cardiovascular effects of mood-altering drugs.* New York: Raven Press, 1979.

162. Feinman L, Lieber CS. Toxicity of ethanol and other components of alcoholic beverages. *Alcohol Clin Exp Res* 1988;12(1):2–6.

163. Kagan A, Yano K, Rhodes GG, et al. Alcohol and cardiovascular disease: the Hawaiian experience. *Circulation* 1981;64:27–31.

164. Lieber CS, Branchey L, Worner T. A multidisciplinary approach to alcoholism. *Mt Sinai J Med* 1979;46(2): 91–94.

165. Lie JT. Alcoholic cardiomyopathy. *Primary Cardiol* 1983;9(3):179–197.

166. Rahimtoola SH. Digitalis and William Withering, the clinical investigator. *Circulation* 1975;52:969–971.

167. Brown J, King A, Francis CK. Cardiovascular effects of alcohol, cocaine and acquired immune deficiency. In: *Cardiovascular diseases in blacks.* Philadelphia: FA Davis, 1991:341–357.

168. Lange LG, Kinnunen PM. Cardiovascular effects of alcohol. *Adv Alcohol Subs Abuse* 1987;6(3):47–52.

169. Clark VA, Chapman JM, Coulson AH. Effects of various factors on systolic and diastolic blood pressure in

the Los Angeles Heart Study. *J Chronic Dis* 1967;20: 567.

170. Dyer AR, Stamler J, Paul O. Alcohol consumption, cardiovascular risk factors and mortality in two Chicago epidemiologic studies. *Circulation* 1977;56:1067.

171. Kannel WB, Sorlie P. Hypertension in Framingham. In: Paul O, ed. *Epidemiology and control of hypertension.* Stratton: NY, 1974:553.

172. Klatsky AL, Friedman GD, Siegelaub AB, et al. Alcohol consumption and blood pressure. Kaiser-Permanente Multiphasic Health Examination data. *N Engl J Med* 1977;296:1194–1200.

173. Criqui MH, Wallace RB, Mishkel M, et al. Alcohol consumption and blood pressure: the Lipid Research Clinics Prevalence Study. *Hypertension* 1981;3:557.

174. Klatsky AL, Friedman GD, Armstrong MA. The relationship between alcohol beverage use and other traits to blood pressure: a new Kaiser-Permanente Study. *Circulation* 1986;73:628.

175. Harburg E, Ozgoren F, Hawthorne VM, et al. Community norms of alcohol usage and blood pressure: Tecumseh, Michigan. *Am J Public Health* 1980;70: 813–820.

176. Clark LT. Alcohol-induced hypertension. Mechanisms, complications, and clinical implications. *J Natl Med Assoc* 1985;77(5):385–389.

177. Jackson G, Suljaga K, Kaswan M, et al. Alcohol withdrawal and blood pressure. *Mt Sinai J Med* 1986;53(4): 267–270.

178. Saunders JB, Beevers DG, Paton A. Alcohol-induced hypertension. *Lancet* 1981;2:653–656.

179. Clark LT, Friedman HS. Alcohol-induced hypertension. Evidence for vascular hyperreactivity as a mechanism. *Clin Res* 1983;31:688.

180. Altura BT, Pohorecky LA, Altura BM. Demonstration of tolerance to ethanol in non-nervous tissue: effects of vascular smooth muscle. *Alcohol Clin Exp Res* 1980;4: 62–69.

181. Altura BM, Altura BT. Microvascular and vascular smooth muscle actions of ethanol, acetaldehyde and acetate. *Fed Proc* 1982;41:P2447–2451.

182. Kelly MA, Gorelick PB, Mirza D. The role of drugs in the etiology of stroke. *Clin Neuropharmacol* 1992; 15(4):249–275.

183. Kagan A, Popper JS, Rhoads GG. Factors related to stroke incidence in Hawaii Japanese men. The Honolulu Heart Study. *Stroke* 1980;11:14.

184. Donahue RP, Abbott RD, Reed DW, et al. Alcohol and hemorrhagic stroke. *JAMA* 1986;255:2311.

185. Gill GS, Zezulka V, Shipley MJ, et al. Stroke and alcohol consumption. *N Engl J Med* 1986;315:1041–1046.

186. Gorelick PB. Alcohol and stroke. *Stroke* 1987;18(1): 268–271.

187. Burch GE, Walsh JJ. Cardiac insufficiency in chronic alcoholism. *Am J Cardiol* 1960;6:864–874.

188. Brigden W, Robinson J. Alcoholic heart disease. *BMJ* 1964;2:1283–1289.

189. Limas CJ, Guiha NH, Lekagul O, et al. Impaired left ventricular function in alcoholic cirrhosis with ascites. Ineffectiveness of ouabain. *Circulation* 1974;49: 755–760.

190. Regan TJ, Levinson GE, Oldewurtel HA, et al. Ventricular function in noncardiacs with alcoholic fatty liver. The role of ethanol in the production of cardiomyopathy. *J Clin Invest* 1969;48:397–407.

191. Gould L, Shariff M, Zahir M, et al. Cardiac hemodynamics in alcoholic patients with chronic liver disease and presystolic gallop. *J Clin Invest* 1969;48:860–868.

192. Ettinger PO, Wu CF, DeLaCruz C, et al. Arrhythmias and the "holiday heart." Alcohol related cardiac rhythm disorders. *Am Heart J* 1978;95:555–562.

193. Gould L, Gopalaswamy C, Yang D, et al. Effects of oral alcohol on left ventricular ejection fraction, volumes, and segmental wall motion in normals and in patients with recent myocardial infarction. *Clin Cardiol* 1985;8:576–582.

194. Cregler LL, Worner TM, DiPadova C, et al. Alcohol administration unmasks latent left ventricular dysfunction in male alcoholics. *Alcohol Clin Exp Res* 1985; 9(1):87.

195. Spodick DH, Pigott VM, Chirife R. Preclinical cardiac malfunction in chronic alcoholism. *N Engl J Med* 1972; 287:677–780.

196. Wu CF, Sudhaker M, Jaferi G, et al. Preclinical cardiomyopathy in chronic alcoholics. A sex difference. *Am Heart J* 1976;91:281–286.

197. Deutscher S. The effects of heavy drinking on ischemic heart disease. *Primary Cardiol* 1986;12(4): 40–48.

198. Stason WB, Neff RK, Miettinen IS, et al. Alcohol consumption and nonfatal myocardial infarction. *Am J Epidemiol* 1976;104:603–608.

199. Yano K, Rhoads GG, Kagan A. Coffee, alcohol and risk of coronary heart disease among Japanese men living in Hawaii. *N Engl J Med* 1977;297(8):405–409.

200. Taskinen MR, Nikkila EA, Valimaki, et al. Alcohol induced changes in serum lipoproteins and their metabolism. *Am Heart J* 1987;113(2):458–464.

201. Cauley JA, Kuller LH, LaPorte RE, et al. Studies on the association between alcohol and high density lipoprotein cholesterol. Possible benefits and risks. *Adv Alcohol Subs Abuse* 1987;6(3):53–67.

202. Huie MJ. An acute myocardial infarction occurring in an anabolic steroid user. *Med Sci Sports Exerc* 1994; 26(4):408–413.

203. Yesalis CE, Kennedy NJ, Kopstein AN, Barrke MS. Anabolic-androgenic steroid use in the United States. *JAMA* 1993;270:1217–1221.

204. DuRant RH, Escobedo LG, Heath GW. Anabolic-steroid use, strength training, and multiple drug use among adolescents in the United States. *Pediatrics* 1995;2:23–28.

205. Dickerman RD, Schaller F, Prather I, McConathy WJ. Sudden cardiac death in a 20-year old bodybuilder using anabolic steroids. *Cardiology* 1995;86: 172–173.

206. Council on Scientific Affairs. Medical and non-medical uses of anabolic-androgenic steroids. *JAMA* 1990; 264:2923–2927.

207. Overly WL, Dankoff JA, Wang BK, Singh UD. Androgens and hepatocellular carcinoma in an athlete. *Ann Intern Med* 1984;100:158–159.

208. Prat J, Gray GF, Stolley PD. Wilms' tumor in an adult associated with androgen abuse. *JAMA* 1977;237: 2322–2323.

209. Appleby M, Fisher M, Martin M. Myocardial infarction, hyperkalemia and ventricular tachycardia in a young male body-builder. *Int J Cardiol* 1994;44: 171–174.

210. McNutt RA, Ferenchick GS, Kirlin PC, Hamlin NJ.

Acute myocardial infarction in a 22 year old world class weight lifter using anabolic steroids. *Am J Cardiol* 1988;62:164.

211. Ferenchick GS. Are androgenic steroids thrombogenic? [Letter]. *N Engl J Med* 1990;322:476.

212. Bowman SJ, Tanna S, Fernando S, et al. Anabolic steroids and infarction. *BMJ* 1989;299:632.

213. Ferenchick GS, Adelman S. Myocardial infarction associated with anabolic steroid use in a previously healthy 37 year old weight lifter. *Am Heart J* 1992; 124:507–508.

214. Kennedy MC, Lawrence C. Anabolic steroid abuse and cardiac death. *Med J Aust* 1993;158:346–348.

215. Shiozawa Z, Yamada H, Mabuchi C, et al. Superior sagittal sinus thrombosis associated with androgen therapy for hypoplastic anemia. *Ann Neurol* 1982;12: 580–587.

216. Ferenchick GS. Anabolic/androgenic steroid abuse and thrombosis. Is there a connection? *Med Hypothesis* 1991;35:27–31.

217. Bird KD, Boleyn T, Chesher GB, Jackson DM, Starmer GA, Teo RKC. Inter-cannabinoid and cannabinoid-ethanol interactions and their effects on human performance. *Psychopharmacology* 1980;71:181–188.

218. Jones RB. Prohibit smokeless tobacco use in athletic competition. *Physician Sports Med* 1987;15:149–152.

219. Guggenheimer J. Implications of smokeless tobacco use in athletes. *Dental Clin North Am* 1991;35(4): 797–808.

220. Glover ED, Edwards SW, Christen AG, et al. Smokeless tobacco research. An interdisciplinary approach. *Health Values* 1984;8:21.

221. Department of Health and Human Services. The health consequences of using smokeless tobacco. A report of the Advisory Committee to the Surgeon General. [NIH Publication No. 86-2874]. Bethesda, MD: National Institutes of Health, 1986.

222. Glover ED, Edmundson EW, Edwards SW, Schroeder KL. Implications of smokeless tobacco use among athletes. *Physician Sports Med* 1986;14:95–105.

223. Joyner MJ, Freund BJ, Jilka SM, et al. Effects of beta-blockers on exercise capacity of trained and untrained men: a hemodynamic comparison. *J Appl Physiol* 1986;60:1429–1434.

224. Wilmore JH. Exercise testing, training and beta-adrenergic blockade. *Physician Sports Med* 1988;16: 45–52.

225. Dehennin L. Detection of simultaneous self-administration of testosterone and epitestosterone in healthy men. *Clin Chem* 1994;40:106–109.

226. Combs AB, Acosta D. Toxic mechanisms of the heart: a review. *Toxicol Pathol* 1990;18:583–596.

227. Birnbach DJ. Cardiovascular disease in the pregnant patient. A new risk factor. *Cardiovasc Risk Factor Int J* 1994;4(1):28–33.

228. Cregler LL. Cocaine: a risk factor for cardiovascular disease in women. *Cardiovasc Risk Factors Int J* 1994; 4(1):39–44.

The Athlete and Heart Disease:
Diagnosis, Evaluation & Management,
edited by R. A. Williams.
Lippincott Williams & Wilkins, Philadelphia © 1999.

10

Echocardiographic Profiles of Diseases Associated with Sudden Cardiac Death in Young Athletes

Craig R. Asher and Harry M. Lever

Department of Cardiology, The Cleveland Clinic Foundation, Cleveland, Ohio 44195

Echocardiography plays an essential role in the diagnosis of cardiovascular disorders that may predispose young athletes to sudden cardiac death during sports-related activities. With this modality, structural abnormalities involving the myocardium, aorta, and cardiac valves can be detected and followed for progression of disease that may preclude safe participation in sports. Furthermore, a benign adaptive response of the myocardium to strenuous activity (i.e., "athlete's heart," or AH), can be differentiated from the pathologic hypertrophy of hypertrophic cardiomyopathy (HCM). Whether the use of preparticipation echocardiography is feasible and cost effective in identifying young people at risk for fatal cardiac events remains controversial.

This chapter reviews the echocardiographic features of the most common cardiovascular diseases that may lead to nontraumatic sudden death in young athletes (younger than 35 years of age). Unexpected death occurring in middle-aged athletes is generally due to coronary artery disease and is not addressed.

ATHLETE'S HEART

General Principles

The AH syndrome is a composite of physiologic and structural changes that occur in response to repetitive athletic training (1–4). Cardiopulmonary and peripheral circulatory manifestations predominate. Left ventricular (LV) systolic performance is maintained at rest despite rigorous exercise (5–10). A growing body of literature on echocardiographic diagnosis of AH has distinguished changes in LV chamber size, wall thickness and mass (5,11–15). These changes in LV dimensions are particular for age, gender, and race, and are further dependent on the type, intensity, and duration of sporting activity performed (12,16–21). Complementing other clinical information, echocardiography plays a vital part in differentiating these physiologic responses to exercise, from the pathologic forms of hypertrophy, such as HCM.

Echocardiographic Features

Echocardiographically, AH is distinguished by the determination of increased LV mass (5, 11,12,14). LV mass can be calculated by multiplying the volume of LV myocardium times the density of the myocardium. The volume of the LV myocardium is estimated by subtracting chamber volume from total volume (wall thickness plus chamber volume). Methods of LV mass determination are available for clinical application (22,23). The Penn convention formulation is illustrated in Fig. 1 (23). LV mass normal ranges adjusted for body surface area and height are available (24–27). Whereas most studies demonstrate increased LV mass in AH, indexed LV mass based on body size or lean body mass may not differ substantially from matched controls, particularly in weight lifters (5,11,12,14,21,28). In weight lifters, LV mass seemingly augments proportionately with increases in body mass.

The increased LV mass in AH is manifested by hypertrophy with or without cavity dilatation. Generally, eccentric hypertrophy occurs in predominantly endurance athletes (isotonic exercise) as a result of a volume-loading effect on the ventricles, and concentric hypertrophy is seen in strength athletes (isometric exercise) resulting from a pressure-loading effect (2,5,14,20,21,28). Some authors contend that the predominant stimulus to the myocardium in AH is a volume-loading effect and that morphologic changes are greater following endurance compared to

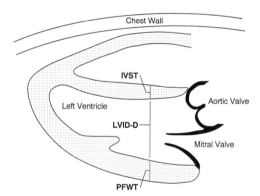

FIG. 1. Schematic of the parasternal long-axis view of the left ventricle. Left ventricular mass can be estimated echocardiographically by the Penn convention measurements. Wall thickness and diameters of the left ventricle are made at the end of diastole (the peak of the R wave on electrocardiogram). Left ventricular mass (grams) is determined by the following equation: 1.04[(LVIDd + IVST + PFWT)³ – (LVIDd)]³ – 13.6. LVIDd, left ventricular internal dimension in end-diastole; IVST, interventricular septal thickness; PFWT, posterior free wall thickness. (Adapted from Lauer MS. Left Ventricular Hypertrophy and Cardiovascular Prognosis *Cleveland Clinic J Med* 1995;62: 169–175, with permission.)

strength training (11,29). Isometric exercise is usually sustainable for only short intervals of time and therefore may be less likely to impart long-lasting effects. Figure 2 illustrates an example of eccentric LV hypertrophy and enlargement seen on the echocardiogram of a professional basketball player.

There are physiologic limitations to the extent in which augmentation of LV cavity dimensions can be considered a consequence of AH (5,12,14,19). With AH, enlargement of the LV cavity size may occur with increases in end-diastolic dimension and volume (10% and 33%, respectively) (5). Increases in LV diastolic cavity size rarely exceed 60 mm; therefore, substantial overlap exists with normal control subjects (5,12). Although, the LV end-systolic dimension may also be increased with AH relative to controls, this occurs to a less significant degree and is not consistent in all studies (5). In comparison, the LV cavity size and volume of patients with HCM is generally normal or reduced in both systole and diastole. Table 1 compares the typical features of AH and HCM.

Similar to LV cavity size, increased LV wall thickness resulting from AH has physiologic limitations. Wall thickness is uncommon to exceed 12 mm (particularly in women) and rarely exceeds 16 mm (5,12,14,17,19). Generally, wall thickening is symmetric in the involvement of the ventricular septum and posterior wall. The ratio of septal to free wall thickness is usually less than 1.3 among individuals with AH (5,12). In contrast, HCM patients most typically have wall thickness greater than 15 mm, with asymmetric involvement of the ventricular septum and posterior wall.

A morphologic "gray zone" characterized by mild increases in LV mass and wall thickness in the range of 13 to 15 mm has been described by Maron and colleagues (5,13). The diagnosis of nonobstructive HCM versus AH may be difficult to distinguish in these individuals. Clinical and echocardiographic data may be required to differentiate primary pathologic hypertrophy from AH. A study of 947 elite Italian athletes revealed that 16

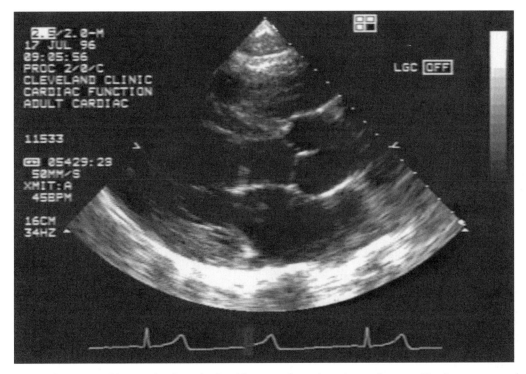

FIG. 2. Parasternal long-axis view obtained by transthoracic echocardiogram. The images are of a young healthy professional basketball player. LVIDd = 6.0 cm; LVIDs = 4.0 cm, IVST = 1.5 cm; PFWT = 1.5 cm. These findings are consistent with athlete's heart as seen in an individual performing a high level of endurance and strength training. LVIDd, left ventricular dimension in end-diastole; LVIDs, left ventricular dimension in end-systole; IVST, interventricular septal thickness; PFWT, posterior free wall thickness.

TABLE 1. *Comparison of typical features of athlete's heart and nonobstructive hypertrophic cardiomyopathy*

	Athlete's Heart	HCM
LV diastolic dimension	nl or ↑	nl
LV wall thickness	nl or ↑	↑
Septal/posterior LV thickness	<1.3	≥1.3
Septal/LV diastolic dimension	<0.48	≥0.48
LV mass	↑	↑
LV mass index	nl or ↑	↑
LV resting function	nl	nl or ↑
RV diastolic dimension	nl or ↑	nl
RV wall thickness	nl	nl or ↑
LA size	nl or ↑	nl or ↑
Diastolic function	nl	nl or ↓

nl, normal; ↑, increased; ↓, decreased; HCM, hypertrophic cardiomyopathy; LV, left ventricle; RV, right ventricle; LA, left atrium.

(1.7%) of those evaluated fell within this morphologic gray zone of increased wall thickness. Notably, among these athletes, the LV end-diastolic cavity size was increased (range 55 to 63 mm, mean 59 mm), marking a distinct difference from HCM (12). Therefore, some investigators have proposed the usefulness of a septal wall thickness to LV end-diastolic or-systolic dimension to distinguish these two entities (a septal wall thickness to LV end-diastolic ratio of greater than 0.48 is considered markedly abnormal) (3,30,31).

Evaluation of mitral inflow and pulmonary vein flow profiles may provide useful information to differentiate normal from pathologic hypertrophy. Diastolic function is normal in AH, often with increased parameters of compliance, in contrast to the usual impaired relaxation pattern seen with HCM (32–38). Therefore, even though a normal mitral inflow profile may not differentiate AH from HCM, an abnormal pattern of impaired relaxation would be unexpected in AH. However, the slightly shortened deceleration time and blunted systolic pulmonary venous flow typical of young people may not be easily distinguishable from a pseudonormal filling pattern more likely to occur in HCM. Future attention to additional indices of diastolic function such as the propagation velocity of color M-mode LV filling and pulmonary vein atrial reversal may provide important clues to characterize these two forms of hypertrophy.

Several other factors suggest the diagnosis of AH and not HCM. Mild degrees of mitral and tricuspid regurgitation were found in most young athletes studied by Douglas and colleagues (39). Cardiac chamber enlargement in AH includes mild increases in right ventricular size and mild left atrial enlargement (5). Right ventricular hypertrophy would be unexpected in AH. Finally, the increased LV cavity dimensions and septal hypertrophy caused by AH typically regresses in the weeks to months following cessation of training (40–43). Therefore, serial echocardiograms with attention to LV mass correlated with the level of training should be sought when AH and HCM cannot be distinguished.

Echocardiographic determination of ultrasonic backscatter has recently been used to contrast pathologic and physiologic hypertrophy (44–46). Myocardial disarray of collagen fibrils found with HCM results in a characteristic pattern of enhanced ultrasound backscatter compared to the minimal reflectance with normal myocardium. The accuracy of this testing is high; however, the costs and additional requirements for instrumentation and expertise limit this technology to research facilities.

HYPERTROPHIC CARDIOMYOPATHY

General Principles

An early description of HCM by Braunwald (47) characterized the important features of severe hypertrophy associated with fiber disarray and LV outflow tract obstruction. Following further observations regarding the morphologic forms of HCM, several of the fundamental genetic and cellular defects have been identified (48,49). Although initially considered a disease of young people, recent studies suggest that HCM may occur more often in the elderly (50–55). Nonetheless, HCM in young patients is often associated with a more malignant disease and higher mortality rate (56). HCM has been reported to be the most common cause of sudden cardiac death in athletes in the United States (57). However, some series have showed a lower incidence than previously demonstrated (58,59).

Echocardiography has helped define the spectrum of diseases that comprise HCM. Before echocardiography, diagnosis of HCM was limited to invasive study in the cardiac catheterization laboratory (47,50). Various disease entities characterized by asymmetry or symmetry and obstruction or nonobstruction, and typical of young and old patients, have come to be recognized (60–63). The mechanisms contributing to obstruction and the importance of provocation have also been detailed by echocardiographic study (64,65). Noninvasive imaging of the heart has allowed for early detection of HCM in populations at highest risk and thus allowed for clinicians to make informed recommendations to patients regarding recreational activities (66).

Echocardiographic Features

The classic features of HCM are diagnosed readily with echocardiography (Table 2). However, the disease is diverse in its structural manifestations (60–62). The hypertrophic segment or segments are generally equal to or greater than 15 mm in thickness. A septal to free wall LV thickness ratio of 1.3 to 1 is typical of HCM, but symmetric forms do occur. Figure 3*A* is an example of asymmetric septal hypertrophy. HCM is more commonly asymmetric in people younger than age 40 years, with the upper septum having the most pronounced hypertrophy. In older individuals, the proximal septum is hypertrophied and a septal bulge may be seen (61). Variations in the location of hypertrophy include an apical form found most commonly in Japan (67,68).

The size, shape, and function of the left and right ventricle are distinct in HCM. The shape of the LV in HCM has specific patterns in young and old individuals. Normally, the LV is ovoid in shape and the right ventricle is a crescent shape. In young patients with HCM, there is frequently reversal of septal curvature causing the LV to be a crescent shape, whereas the right ventricle is ovoid (61). Figure 3*B* is an example of a young patient with HCM. This pattern is not seen in most older adults. LV function in most patients with HCM is normal or hypercontractile, although the segments of the heart with the greatest hypertrophy may be hypocontractile (69,70). A nondilated LV cavity with a small end-systolic volume is expected in HCM. Similarly, the right ventricle is typically normal in size and function but may be involved with the hypertrophic process.

Other less specific, yet frequent, findings in young patients with HCM are notable. The left atrium is frequently enlarged (64). This is likely due to mitral regurgitation (MR) and/or diastolic dysfunction. Mitral annular calcifications occur often in elderly patients with HCM but infrequently in young patients (61). Papillary muscle hypertrophy and displacement occurs in patients with HCM and may contribute to the degree of obstruction and MR (71).

HCM should be designated as nonobstructive or obstructive for all patients identified with the disorder. LV outflow tract obstruction in HCM typically occurs as a results of systolic anterior motion (SAM) of the mitral valve leaflets or chordae and a narrowed LV outflow tract (72). The mechanism of LV outflow tract obstruction is related to the Venturi effect. Accelerated flow in the outflow tract results in a suction effect in which a portion of the mitral apparatus is drawn into this region (64). The profile of LV outflow tract obstruction is illustrated in Color Plate 1 and Fig. 4.

Classification of patients with HCM as nonobstructers requires that a provocative maneuver such as exercise, isoproterenol, or amyl nitrite inhalation is performed. These maneuvers should be used if the LV outflow tract is narrow in combination with significant hypertrophy of the proximal septum or at least one excessively long mitral leaflet (65). Amyl nitrite is easy to administer and, because its effects are transient, it is very safe. Stress echocardiography has also been helpful in documenting outflow tract obstruction in patients who have little or no resting LV outflow tract obstruction (65). The reported high incidence of nonobstructive disease may be the result of not assessing patients for provokable obstruction (73).

LV outflow tract obstruction results in MR in many patients with HCM. When there is

TABLE 2. *"Classic" echocardiagraphic features of hypertrophic cardiomyopathy*

Hypertrophy with LV wall thickness ≥15 mm
Septal/posterior LV wall thickness ratio ≥1.3
Nondilated LV cavity
SAM of the mitral valve*
LVOT gradient >2.5 m/sec with "dagger-shaped" Doppler profile*
Impaired relaxation pattern of mitral inflow

*At rest or with provocation.
LV, left ventricle; SAM, systolic anterior motion; LVOT, left ventricular outflow tract.

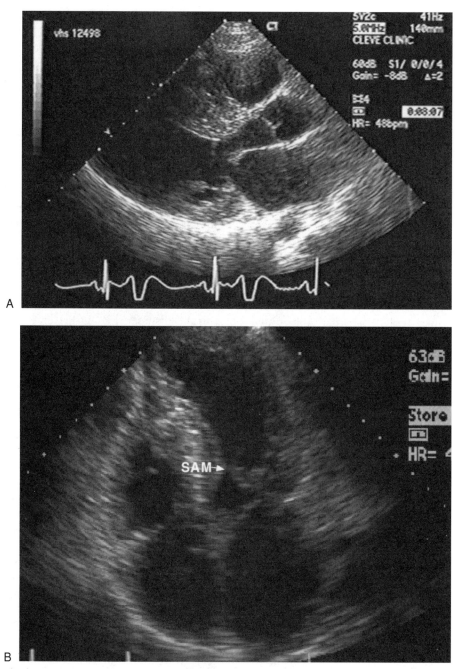

FIG. 3. Transthoracic images of young patients with hypertrophic cardiomyopathy. **A:** Parasternal long-axis view of the left ventricle demonstrating asymmetric hypertrophy. The anterior septum and posterior walls are 2.5 cm and 1 cm in thickness, respectively. **B:** Apical four-chamber view of the left and right ventricle. There is reversal of septal curvature with an ovoid-shaped right ventricle and crescent-shaped left ventricular cavity. Systolic anterior motion (SAM) of the anterior and posterior mitral leaflets are apparent. Mitral regurgitation resulting from the SAM was directed eccentrically posterior and laterally.

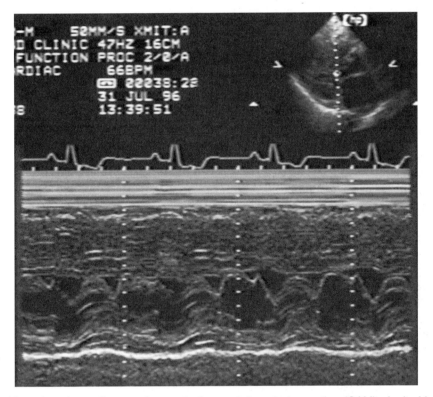

FIG. 4. M-mode echocardiogram demonstrating systolic anterior motion (SAM) of mitral leaflets.

MR, it is caused by the lack of coaptation of the mitral leaflets as a result of their anterior motion. In most patients, both leaflets are involved in the anterior motion, but there can be selective anterior or posterior leaflet SAM. Variability in leaflet length and mobility of the individual leaflets can lead to a mismatch in the coaptation of the leaflets and thus varying degrees of MR (74). The severity of the MR is estimated with the use of color flow Doppler imaging. The MR jet is frequently directed posterolaterally. The LV outflow gradient is calculated using continuous wave Doppler flow imaging, converting the flow velocity (V) obtained in meters/second to mm Hg using the modified Bernoulli equation ($P = 4V^2$) (75). Care must be taken to be sure that the continuous wave Doppler imaging measures the outflow velocity and not the MR profile. Color flow Doppler imaging and the

timing and shape of continuous wave Doppler flow aid in differentiating the outflow tract velocity from the MR velocity (76).

Diastolic function is frequently abnormal in HCM. There is impaired relaxation and increased chamber stiffness. Relaxation abnormalities are usually manifest as prolonged isovolumic relaxation, decreased peak early filling, and a prominent atrial contraction in the mitral inflow velocities (64). Superimposed elevations in left atrial pressure may cause pseudonormal and restrictive filling patterns. Coexistent MR may present a problem in the interpretation of diastolic function. Significant degrees of MR may mask abnormal filling in some patients by elevating the left atrial pressure and pseudonormalizing the mitral inflow pattern. HCM is also associated with decreased compliance; therefore, there is an abnormal increase in LV pressure for a given increase in ventricular volume. This finding is likely reflected on echocardiography by a high amplitude and prolonged duration of the pulmonary vein atrial reversal velocity compared to the mitral *a*-wave duration (77,78). Even though it is clear that there are diastolic filling abnormalities, there has not been a good correlation between the LV filling as measured by Doppler imaging and the LV structure. The reasons for the apparent lack of an association are not clear but are likely attributable to the inability to adjust for the many factors contributing to diastolic function.

Despite the ability to diagnose the different morphologic types of HCM, there are athletes whose echocardiographic findings are in a "gray zone," and it is not clear whether they have HCM (5). In those patients, it may be helpful to have them decondition for a few months and then repeat the echocardiographic study. Borderline hypertrophic patterns may regress. In addition, it may be helpful to study other family members for the presence of HCM. The finding of HCM in a family member would heighten the suspicion that the index case has a mild form of disease. Inability to detect HCM in a family member does not exclude the presence of disease in the patient under evaluation.

ARRHYTHMOGENIC RIGHT VENTRICULAR DYSPLASIA

General Principles

Arrhythmogenic right ventricular dysplasia (ARVD) is a rare, although potentially fatal, condition that may lead to ventricular tachycardia, syncope, and sudden cardiac death in exercising young adults (79–81). Noninvasive recognition of this disorder by echocardiographic examination is possible, but requires a heightened attention and knowledge of specific diagnostic features. The echocardiographic signs of ARVD reflect the pathologic process of adipose and fibrous infiltration of the myocardium, affecting most often the right ventricular outflow tract (anterior infundibulum),

apex, and inferior (diaphragmatic) basal wall, denoted by Marcus, et al. the "triangle of dysplasia" (82,83). Other methods of diagnosis of ARVD include cardiac radionuclear and contrast angiogram, conventional and electron-beam computed tomography, magnetic resonance imaging, and myocardial biopsy (84–88). These studies are more expensive, time-consuming, and invasive than echocardiography.

Echocardiographic Features

Multiple transthoracic echocardiographic findings suggest the diagnosis of ARVD (89–93). The sensitivity of echocardiography for the detection of ARVD is variable and dependent on the clinical history and prevalence of disease in the population being evaluated, the stage of the disorder, the quality of transthoracic images (often optimized with a higher frequency transducer), and the assessment of right ventricular (RV) abnormalities from multiple imaging planes. RV dilatation with hypokinesis occurs in most patients with ARVD; however, a normal echocardiogram does not exclude the diagnosis, and a spectrum of abnormalities may occur (90,91,94–97). In addition, RV enlargement or dysfunction even in selected groups is most often due to cardiac or pulmonary diseases other than ARVD, and thus the specificity of echocardiography for this diagnosis is low in unselected populations (92,93). Although transthoracic echocardiography may only raise the suspicion of ARVD in many cases, other cardiac ischemic, congenital, valvular, and myopathic disorders that cause RV enlargement can be excluded (93). A list of diseases that cause abnormal RV anatomy are listed in Table 3. RV enlargement is often subjectively determined, although specific parameters exist for this diagnosis and comparative dimensions have been described for patients with ARVD (90,98).

RV enlargement and focal or diffuse wall motion abnormalities comprise the most common echocardiographic profile suggesting the diagnosis of ARVD (90,91,93). The inflow tract (parasternal short axis), outflow tract (parasternal long axis), and RV body (apical

TABLE 3. *Cardiac causes of right ventricular enlargement or anomaly*

Atrial septal defect
Partial anomalous venous return
Right ventricular infarction
Tricuspid insufficiency
Pulmonic insufficiency
Ebstein's anomaly
Cardiomyopathy
Pulmonary hypertension
Congenital absence of pericardium
Pulmonary embolism
Right ventricular dysplasia
Uhl's anomaly

four chamber) are the segments most typically enlarged. When dilatation in isolation occurs, the RV outflow tract is the region most frequently involved (90,91). RV function may be reduced or preserved at rest, but characteristically it is dysfunctional with exercise (89,95). Regional or diffuse hypokinesis may range from mild to severe, and akinesis or dyskine-

sis of segments may occur (90). Importantly, follow-up studies of patients with ARVD diagnosed by other modalities have demonstrated the progressive nature of RV enlargement and dysfunction over time (91,99–101). More sophisticated methods of RV chamber size determination such as RV end-diastolic volume and wall motion analysis scores have been used in research laboratories to differentiate ARVD subjects from normal control subjects (89,90).

The pathognomonic findings of ARVD that occur within the triangle of dysplasia are aneurysms (expanding in systole) or bulges (sacculations, outpouchings—expanding in diastole) (83,87,91,93,102). These segments may be single or multiple. Although not a sensitive criteria for the diagnosis of ARVD, focal anomalies are more specific findings, resulting from the infiltration and thinning of myocardium in these regions (Figs. 5 and 6).

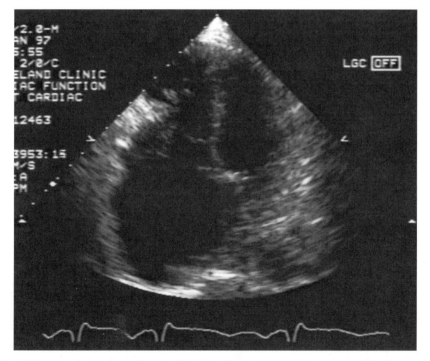

FIG. 5. Apical four-chamber view obtained by transthoracic echocardiogram rotated toward the right ventricle in a patient with arrhythmogenic right ventricular dysplasia and Ebstein's anomaly. The right ventricle is enlarged and there is a right ventricular apical aneurysm, which is pathognomonic of this disease process in the region of the "triangle of dysplasia."

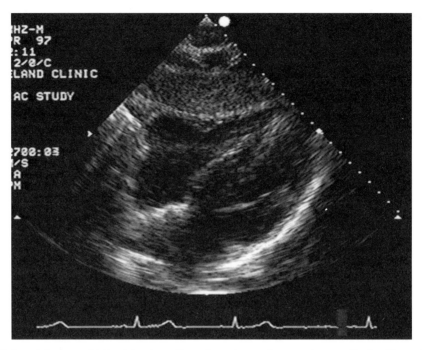

FIG. 6. Subcostal view obtained by transthoracic echocardiogram in a patient with probable arrhythmogenic right ventricular dysplasia. There is a small right ventricular aneurysm at the base of the tricuspid valve. Similar to Fig. 5, this is a region of the "triangle of dysplasia."

Other characteristic findings that aid in the diagnosis of ARVD may be observed. Prominent or irregular trabeculations of the RV wall or moderator band can be identified as coarse and dense echoreflective structures (81,91,97). RV diastolic dysfunction with *e* to *a* reversal of tricuspid inflow despite a normal mitral inflow pattern has been described (103). Premature opening of the pulmonic valve with forward flow in diastole, as seen by M-mode or pulsed Doppler imaging of the pulmonic valve, is a nonspecific finding observed in many patients with ARVD (104). See Table 4 for additional findings suggestive of ARVD.

Although ARVD is most often categorized as a right-sided cardiomyopathy, many pathologic and echocardiographic studies have demonstrated LV abnormalities. Associated LV involvement includes diffuse or focal wall motion dysfunction, which, similar to RV disease, may be progressive in nature (90,101, 105). LV chamber function my be impaired particularly with exercise (89). When LV involvement occurs, segments in continuity with the RV are most often affected.

Despite its limitations, including suboptimal images in some patients, the irregular shape of the right ventricle, and the lack of standard criteria for the diagnosis of ARVD, echocardiography is an effective diagnostic tool. In one study of asymptomatic patients with a suggestive echocardiogram and high clinical suspicion, 90% of patients subsequently received a definitive diagnosis of ARVD by Holter monitor and biopsy (91). Other studies have shown a similar high accuracy of echocardiography in preselected patients (97). However, the value of echocardiographic screening seems less clear because of the low prevalence of ARVD in the population. In a study performed at Duke University Medical Center, RV abnormalities were detected in 18% of nearly 10,000 consecutive echocardiograms performed. From this group, only two were subsequently found to have ARVD (93).

TABLE 4. *Echocardiographic features associated with right ventricular dysplasia*

RV enlargement
RV dysfunction—segmental or diffuse wall motion abnormalities
Localized RV aneurysms (systolic dyskinesis), sacculations or outpouchings (diastolic bulge), involving the "triangle of dysplasia"
Prominent or irregular trabeculations of RV wall or moderator band
RV diastolic dysfunction with normal mitral inflow
Associated LV abnormalities
Premature pulmonic valve opening associated with diastolic forward flow
Abnormal septal motion
Abnormal rotation of the heart

RV, right ventricle; LV, left ventricle.

MARFAN SYNDROME

General Principles

Although Marfan syndrome is characterized by a multisystem involvement including musculoskeletal and ophthalmic abnormalities, it is the cardiovascular manifestations that may render young athletes at risk for life-threatening events (106–108). Cardiovascular involvement as defined by aortic dilatation and mitral valve prolapse occurs in most patients (106,108–112). Abnormalities of the fibrillin component of connective tissue within the aorta and myxomatous degeneration of the cardiac valves constitute the pathologic process active in this disease (113). The natural history of Marfan syndrome includes ascending aortic dilatation and the risk of aortic dissection, rupture, and sudden death (107,108,114). Echocardiography provides a safe, reliable method for screening, diagnosis, and serial measurements for progression of disease.

Echocardiographic features

Transthoracic echocardiography is effective in the evaluation of the aortic valve and proximal ascending aorta, those portions of the aorta most commonly affected by Marfan syndrome (115). Assessment of the aortic valve should focus on the detection of aortic insufficiency and secondary effects of LV enlargement. Evaluation of the aorta must include nonstandard imaging of the left parasternal and right parasternal (ascending aorta) and suprasternal notch (aortic arch)

views. Additional windows for the visualization of the descending aorta (modified apical and subcostal views) can be used, although these segments of the aorta are less typically enlarged in marfanoid patients without dilatation of the proximal aorta.

Measurements of aortic dimensions at the aortic annulus, sinuses of Valsalva, sinotubular junction, and ascending aorta should be recorded in patients undergoing screening for aortic pathologic condition or with known Marfan syndrome. Standardized criteria have been described for the measurement of the aortic root size with M-mode and two-dimensional echocardiography (114,116,117). Adjustments for age (especially in children) and body size should be made (114,118–120). Application of these body size indices for aortic root measurements are important because of the characteristic tall stature of many athletes undergoing preparticipation evaluation.

Aortic root enlargement is the most common cardiac finding of Marfan syndrome, taking the form of an "onion-bulb" malformation with dilatation of the aortic annulus, sinuses of Valsalva, and proximal ascending aorta (110–112). Figure 7 illustrates the characteristic appearance of the proximal aorta in a patient with Marfan syndrome. Effacement of the sinotubular junction may occur with or without aortic dilatation and may be the only sign of aortic pathologic condition. Progression of aortic root dilatation leads to aortic regurgitation and the risk of aortic dissection or rupture. Aortic regurgitation usually occurs when the aortic dimension exceeds 50 mm, and the risk of dissection and rupture

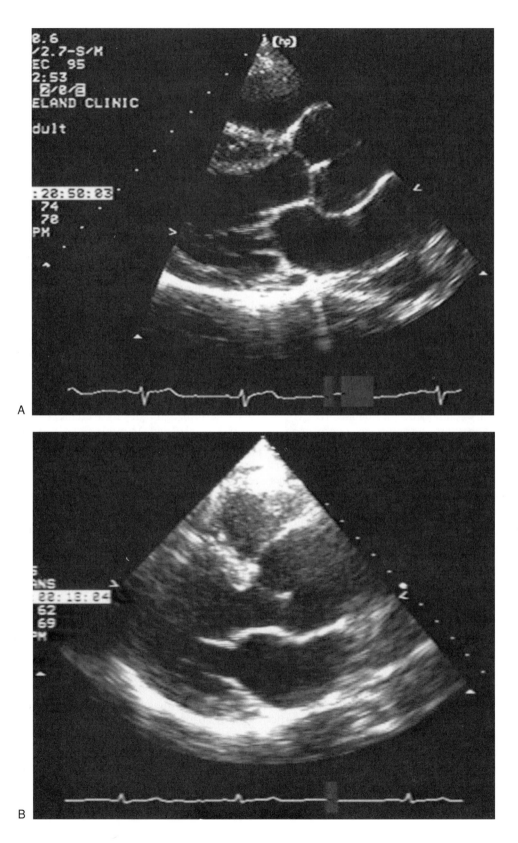

becomes exceedingly large when the aortic dimensions are greater than 60 mm (121, 122). Aortic regurgitation occurring without aortic enlargement should raise the suspicion of unrecognized aortic dissection, and investigations with transesophageal echocardiography or other imaging modalities should be considered.

Substantial variability exists among individuals in the rate of aortic enlargement in patients with Marfan syndrome (123). Aortic dissection can occur with only mild dilatation of the aorta. Clinical and echocardiographic predictors of the rate of aortic dilatation are not well known (124). Therefore, echocardiographic follow-up should be dictated by the size and rate of change of aortic dimensions and generally ranges from every 3 months to 1 year (121). Decisions regarding eligibility or intensity of athletic participation are largely dependent on these measurements, along with integration of clinical criteria.

Because the underlying disorder in Marfan syndrome involves connective tissue destruction, valvular regurgitation is not uncommon. Often this is manifest as prolapse of the mitral, tricuspid, or aortic valve, in order of frequency of occurrence (119). Mitral regurgitation has been observed to occur as a result of mitral valve prolapse with elongation of the chordae and leaflets or as a result of a dilated annulus from LV enlargement and aortic regurgitation (109,114,125,126). Pulmonary artery aneurysms are also associated with Marfan syndrome (111,126,127).

The recognition of aortic dissection in patients with Marfan syndrome is not unlike that seen when caused by other processes. Unrecognized chronic dissections in Marfan patients are not an uncommon finding at the time of prophylactic surgery in many patients (122,128). Although transthoracic echocardiography may be useful in the diagnosis of aortic dissection in some individuals, it is often limited by suboptimal windows and the inability to detect the presence, location, and extent of an intimal flap (127,129–131). Transesophageal echocardiography is highly effective for evaluating these features, and it is additionally advantageous because of the portability and rapidity with which testing can be performed in critically ill patients.

OTHER DISORDERS

Included among the remaining structural congenital or acquired cardiac causes of unsuspected sudden death are coronary artery diseases (Kawasaki disease, hypoplasia, atherosclerosis, anomalous origin or course), annuloaortic ectasia, valvular disease (mitral valve prolapse, aortic stenosis), myocarditis (idiopathic, sarcoidosis), and cardiomyopathies (restrictive and dilated) (57,132). Echocardiography may contribute variably to the detection of these conditions. Clinical suspicion is often required and exclusion of more common disorders may be required for diagnosis.

Often young patients with congenital disorders such as valvular aortic stenosis or dilated cardiomyopathy are seen early in life with symptoms and physical findings that lead to further workup. Therefore, these disorders are usually detected early in life, prohibit individuals from participating in sports, and are not the cause of unexpected sudden cardiac death. Furthermore, these disorders have characteristic echocardiographic features that usually make diagnosis uncomplicated.

FIG. 7. Parasternal long-axis views obtained by transthoracic echocardiogram in two patients with Marfan syndrome. **A:** The aortic sinuses are dilated. The remainder of the proximal aorta is normal in size. This is the classic onion-bulb formation that is typically seen with cystic medial necrosis. There is no effacement of the sinotubular junction. **B:** The aortic annulus, sinuses, and proximal ascending aorta are dilated with a maximal diameter of 4.5 cm. The patient had only mild aortic regurgitation and no evidence of a dissection flap. However, there is effacement of the sinotubular junction, a sign of a more progressive disease process.

Second to pathologic hypertrophy, the leading cause of sudden cardiac death in young athletes in the United States is congenital coronary anomalies (57). Transthoracic echocardiography is not usually used or considered adequate for visualization of coronary arteries. However, one case report and a large prospective screening of a select population has demonstrated a high rate of recognition of the origin of the coronary arteries from the coronary sinuses (133,134). This is achieved with a parasternal short-axis image of the aortic valve. Color Plate 2 illustrates an example of visualization of the origin of the coronary arteries from transthoracic echocardiography. Although not validated by invasive studies, these findings are pertinent to the issue of screening examinations for asymptomatic athletes.

SCREENING ECHOCARDIOGRAPHY

The merits of preparticipation echocardiography for recreational and competitive young athletes remains a topic of continued controversy (17,132,135–141). Echocardiography is likely the most sensitive and specific test available to detect the congenital and acquired abnormalities contributing most commonly to sudden cardiac death in this age group. HCM and most of the remaining causes of sports-related deaths, including Marfan syndrome and valvular disorders, are readily identifiable with echocardiography. Therefore, the dispute over screening echocardiography focuses not on the capability of this modality but rather the cost-effectiveness and feasibility of implementation in millions of young athletes.

The proponents of echocardiography as a universal method of screening advocate the efficacy of a limited examination. These authors contend that history, physical examination, and electrocardiography are not sensitive enough to detect many cardiovascular abnormalities. Two groups have independently reported on limited screening echocardiograms that include two-dimensional parasternal long- and short-axis views (138–140). These views were chosen to exclude primarily HCM, Marfan syndrome, aortic stenosis, and mitral valve prolapse. Further images are obtained if abnormalities are seen. Both investigators claim costs are as low as $15.00 per test, and time required for examination is noted by one author to be only 2 minutes (139). They conclude that these examinations are thus highly sensitive, efficient, and low in costs and can be readily made available by portable echocardiography machines.

Currently, echocardiography is recommended only for patients suspected of having cardiac disease (141). The financial burden of implementation of echocardiographic screening in millions of high school and college athletes is seemingly prohibitive (141). Moreover, there are time constraints related to examining large populations, the need for expert staff to interpret and perform testing, and the difficulty with access to these personnel and equipment. In addition, the unmasking of these new diagnostic dilemmas (such as the "gray zone" between HCM and AH) and of incidental findings such as mitral valve prolapse and small atrial septal defects may add to the burden of subsequent testing and medical care (13,141). This must be counterbalanced with the exceedingly low incidence of asymptomatic congenital heart disease in the population.

CONCLUSION

Sudden unexpected cardiac death in a young athlete is a rare but traumatic event. Potentially life-threatening diseases such as HCM, Marfan syndrome, ARVD, and anomalous coronary arteries may be unrecognized in young people who are active in sports. These diseases, however, can be detected and characterized by clinicians with specific knowledge and attention to their echocardiographic features. Decisions regarding athletic eligibility may therefore be based, in part, on the echocardiographic profiles of these disorders. The application of screening echocardiography in young athletes remains an issue of continued study and debate.

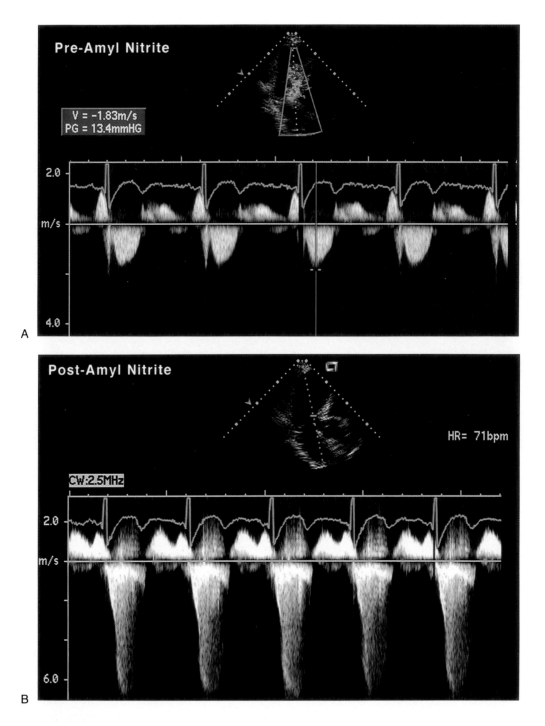

COLOR PLATE 1. Transthoracic echocardiographic continuous wave Doppler flow patterns in a patient with obstructive hypertrophic cardiomyopathy. **A:** Prior to amyl nitrite inhalation the resting gradient is less than 2 m/sec. **B:** Following amyl nitrite, the left ventricular outflow tract gradient is greater than 6 m/sec. with a classic dagger-shaped profile.

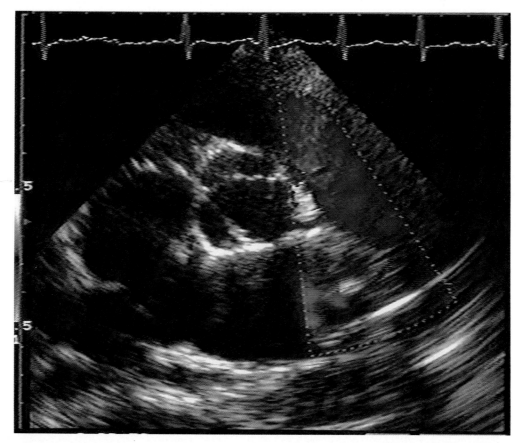

COLOR PLATE 2. Parasternal short axis view at the level of the aortic valve in a healthy adult. The origin of the left main coronary artery can be visualized with color flow Doppler imaging originating from the left coronary sinus.

REFERENCES

1. Cantwell JD. The athlete's heart syndrome. *Int J Cardiol* 1987;17:1–6.
2. Bryan G, Ward A, Rippe JM. Athletic heart syndrome. *Clin Sports Med* 1992;11:259–272.
3. Huston TP, Puffer JC, Rodney WM. The athletic heart syndrome. *N Engl J Med* 1985;313:24–32.
4. Oakley GD. The athletic heart. *Cardiol Clin* 1987;5: 319–329.
5. Maron BJ. Structural features of the athlete heart as defined by echocardiography. *J Am Coll Cardiol* 1986; 7:190–203.
6. Douglas PS, O'Toole ML, Hiller DB, Reichek N. Left ventricular structure and function by echocardiography in ultraendurance athletes. *Am J Cardiol* 1986;58: 805–809.
7. Colan SD, Sanders SP, Borow KM. Physiologic hypertrophy: effects on left ventricular systolic mechanics in athletes. *J Am Coll Cardiol* 1987;9:776–783.
8. Gilbert CA, Nutter DO, Felner JM, Perkins JV, Heymsfield SB, Schlant RC. Echocardiographic study of cardiac dimensions and function in the endurance-trained athlete. *Am J Cardiol* 1977;40:528–533.
9. Nishimura T, Yamada Y, Kawai C. Echocardiographic evaluation of long-term effects of exercise on left ventricular hypertrophy and function in professional bicyclists. *Circulation* 1980;61:832–840.
10. Shapiro LM, Smith RG. Effect of training on left ventricular structure and function: an echocardiographic study. *Br Heart J* 1983;50:534–539.
11. Rost R. The athlete's heart. *Eur Heart J* 1982;3: 193–198.
12. Pelliccia A, Maron BJ, Spataro A, Proschan MA, Spirito P. The upper limit of physiologic cardiac hypertrophy in highly trained athletes. *N Engl J Med* 1991;324: 295–301.
13. Maron BJ, Pelliccia A, Spirito P. Cardiac disease in young trained athletes. Insights into methods for distinguishing athlete's heart from structural heart disease, with particular emphasis on hypertrophic cardiomyopathy. *Circulation* 1995;91:1596–1601.
14. Urhausen A, Kindermann W. Echocardiographic findings in strength- and endurance-trained athletes. *Sports Med* 1992;13:270–284.
15. Shapiro LM. Morphologic consequences of systematic training. *Cardiol Clin* 1992;10:219–226.
16. Pelliccia A, Maron BJ, Culasso F, Spataro A, Caselli G. Athlete's heart in women. Echocardiographic characterization of highly trained elite female athletes. *JAMA* 1996;276:211–215.
17. Lewis JF, Maron BJ, Diggs JA, Spencer JE, Mehrotra PP, Curry CL. Preparticipation echocardiographic screening for cardiovascular disease in a large, predominantly black population of collegiate athletes. *Am J Cardiol* 1989;64:1029–1033.
18. Lewis JF. Considerations for racial differences in the athlete's heart. *Cardiol Clin* 1992;10:329–333.
19. Spirito P, Pelliccia A, Proschan MA, et al. Morphology of the "athlete's heart" assessed by echocardiography in 947 elite athletes representing 27 sports. *Am J Cardiol* 1994;74:802–806.
20. Morganroth J, Maron BJ, Henry WL, Epstein SE. Comparative left ventricular dimensions in trained athletes. *Ann Intern Med* 1975;82:521–524.
21. Fisher AG, Adams TD, Yanowitz FG, Ridges JD, Orsmond G, Nelson AG. Noninvasive evaluation of world class athletes engaged in different modes of training. *Am J Cardiol* 1989;63:337–341.
22. Troy BL, Pombo J, Rackley CE. Measurement of left ventricular wall thickness and mass by echocardiography. *Circulation* 1972;45:602–611.
23. Devereux RB, Reichek N. Echocardiographic determination of left ventricular mass in man. Anatomic validation of the method. *Circulation* 1977;55:613–618.
24. Collins HW, Kronenberg MW, Byrd BF. Reproducibility of left ventricular mass measurements by two-dimensional and M-mode echocardiography. *J Am Coll Cardiol* 1989;14:672–676.
25. Lauer MS, Anderson KM, Larson M, Levy D. A new method for indexing left ventricular mass for differences in body size. *Am J Cardiol* 1994;74:487–491.
26. Daniels SR, Meyer RA, Liang Y, Bove KE. Echocardiographically determined left ventricular mass index in normal children, adolescents and young adults. *J Am Coll Cardiol* 1988;12:703–708.
27. de Simone G, Daniels SR, Devereux RB, et al. Left ventricular mass and body size in normotensive children and adults: assessment of allometric relations and impact of overweight. *J Am Coll Cardiol* 1992;20: 1251–1260.
28. Longhurst JC, Kelly AR, Gonyea WJ, Mitchell JH. Echocardiographic left ventricular masses in distance runners and weight lifters. *J Appl Physiol Respir Environ Exerc* 1980;48:154–162.
29. Roy A, Doyon M, Dumesnil JG, Jobin J, Landry F. Endurance vs. strength training: comparison of cardiac structures using normal predicted values. *J Appl Physiol* 1988;64:2552–2557.
30. Shephard RJ. The athlete's heart: is big beautiful? *Br J Sports Med* 1996;30:5–10.
31. Menapace FJ, Hammer WJ, Ritzer TF, et al. Left ventricular size in competitive weight lifters: an echocardiographic study. *Med Sci Sports Exerc* 1982;14: 72–75.
32. Colan SD, Sanders SP, MacPherson D, Borow K. Left ventricular diastolic function in elite athletes with physiologic cardiac hypertrophy. *J Am Coll Cardiol* 1985;6:545–549.
33. Galanti G, Comeglio M, Vinci M, Cappelli B, Vono MC, Bamoshmoosh M. Echocardiographic Doppler evaluation of left ventricular diastolic function in athletes' hypertrophied hearts. *Angiology* 1993;44: 341–346.
34. Finkelhor RS, Hanak LJ, Bahler RC. Left ventricular filling in endurance-trained subjects. *J Am Coll Cardiol* 1986;8:289–293.
35. Lewis JF, Spirito P, Pelliccia A, Maron BJ. Usefulness of Doppler echocardiographic assessment of diastolic filling in distinguishing "athlete's heart" from hypertrophic cardiomyopathy. *Br Heart J* 1992;68:296–300.
36. Granger CB, Karimeddini MK, Smith VE, Shapiro HR, Katz AM, Riba AL. Rapid ventricular filling in left ventricular hypertrophy: I. Physiologic hypertrophy. *J Am Coll Cardiol* 1985;5:862–868.
37. Pearson AC, Schiff M, Mrosek D, Labovitz AJ, Williams GA. Left ventricular diastolic function in weight lifters. *Am J Cardiol* 1986;58:1254–1259.
38. Nixon JV, Wright AR, Porter TR, Roy V, Arrowood JA. Effects of exercise of left ventricular diastolic perfor-

mance in trained athletes. *Am J Cardiol* 1991;68: 945–949.

39. Douglas PS, Berman GO, O'Toole ML, Hiller WD, Reichek N. Prevalence of multivalvular regurgitation in athletes. *Am J Cardiol* 1989;64:209–212.

40. Maron BJ, Pelliccia A, Spataro A, Granata M. Reduction in left ventricular wall thickness after deconditioning in highly trained Olympic athletes. *Br Heart J* 1993;69:125–128.

41. Martin WH, Coyle EF, Bloomfield SA, Ehsani AA. Effects of physical deconditioning after intense endurance training on left ventricular dimensions and stroke volume. *J Am Coll Cardiol* 1986;7:982–989.

42. Fagard R, Aubert A, Lysens R, Staessen J, Vanhees I, Amery A. Noninvasive assessment of seasonal variations in cardiac structure and function in cyclists. *Circulation* 1983;67:896–901.

43. Ehsani AH, Hagberg JM, Hickson RC. Rapid changes in left ventricular dimensions and mass in response to physiologic conditioning and deconditioning. *Am J Cardiol* 1978;42:52–56.

44. DiBello VD, Lattanzi F, Picano E, et al. Left ventricular performance and ultrasonic myocardial quantitative reflectivity in endurance senior athletes: an echocardiographic study. *Eur Heart J* 1993;14:358–363.

45. Lattanzi F, Spirito P, Picano E, et al. Quantitative assessment of ultrasonic myocardial reflectivity in hypertrophic cardiomyopathy. *J Am Coll Cardiol* 1991; 17:1085–1090.

46. Lattanzi F, Di Bello V, Picano E, et al. Normal ultrasonic myocardial reflectivity in athletes with increased left ventricular mass. A tissue characterization study. *Circulation* 1992;85:1828–1834.

47. Braunwald E, Lambrew CT, Morrow AG, Pierce GE, Rockoff SD, Ross J. Idiopathic hypertrophic subaortic stenosis: a description of the disease based on the analysis of 64 patients. *Circulation* 1964;30[Suppl 4]: 3–119.

48. Clark CE, Henry WL, Epstein SE. Familial prevalence and genetic transmission of idiopathic subaortic stenosis. *N Engl J Med* 1973;289:709–714.

49. Solomon SD, Wolff S, Watkins H, et al. Left ventricular hypertrophy and morphology in familial hypertrophic cardiomyopathy associated with mutations of the beta-myosin heavy chain gene. *J Am Coll Cardiol* 1993;22:498–505.

50. Frank S, Braunwald E. Idiopathic hypertrophic subaortic stenosis: clinical analysis of 126 patients with emphasis on the natural history. *Circulation* 1968;37:759–788.

51. Hardarson T, de la Calzada CS, Curiel R, Goodwin JF. Prognosis and mortality of hypertrophic obstructive cardiomyopathy. *Lancet* 1973;2:1462–1467.

52. Adelman AG, Wigle ED. The clinical course in muscular subaortic stenosis. *Ann Intern Med* 1972;77: 515–525.

53. Krasnow N, Stein RA. Hypertrophic cardiomyopathy in the aged. *Am Heart J* 1978;96:326–336.

54. Fay WP, Taliercio CP, Ilstrup DM, Tajik AJ, Gersh BJ. Natural history of hypertrophic cardiomyopathy in the elderly. *J Am Coll Cardiol* 1990;16:821–826.

55. Whiting RB, Powel WJ, Dinsmore RE, Sanders CA. Idiopathic hypertrophic subaortic stenosis in the elderly. *N Engl J Med* 1971;285:196–200.

56. McKenna W, Deanfield J, Faruqui A, England D, Oakley C, Goodwin J. Prognosis in hypertrophic cardiomyopathy: role of age in clinical electrocardiographic and hemodynamic features. *Am J Cardiol* 1981; 47:532–538.

57. Maron BJ, Epstein SE, Roberts WC. Causes of sudden death in competitive athletes. *J Am Coll Cardiol* 1986; 7:204–214.

58. Waller BF. Exercise-related sudden death in young (age ≤30 years) conditioned subjects. In: *Exercise and the heart*. Philadelphia: FA Davis, 1985:9–73.

59. Phillips M, Bobinowitz M, Higgins JR, Boran KJ, Reed T, Virmani R. Sudden cardiac death in Air Force recruits: a 20 year study. *JAMA* 1986;256:2696–2699.

60. Lewis JF, Maron BJ. Elderly patients with hypertrophic cardiomyopathy: a subset with distinctive left ventricular morphology and progressive clinical course late in life. *J Am Coll Cardiol* 1989;13:36–45.

61. Lever HM, Karam RF, Currie PJ, Healy BP. Hypertrophic cardiomyopathy in the elderly. Distinctions from the young based on cardiac shape. *Circulation* 1989;79:580–589.

62. Maron BJ, Gottdiener JS, Bonow RO, Epstein SE. Hypertrophic cardiomyopathy with unusual locations of left ventricular hypertrophy undetectable by M-mode echocardiography: identification by wide-angle two-dimensional echocardiography. *Circulation* 1981;63: 409–418.

63. Henry WL, Clark CE, Epstein SE. Asymmetric septal hypertrophy: Echocardiographic identification of the pathognomonic anatomic abnormality of IHSS. *Circulation* 1973;47:225–233.

64. Wigle ED, Sasson Z, Henderson MA, et al. Hypertrophic cardiomyopathy: the importance of the site and the extent of hypertrophy. A review. *Prog Cardiovasc Dis* 1985;28:1–83.

65. Marwick TH, Nakatani S, Haluska B, Thomas JD, Lever HM. Provocation of latent left ventricular outflow tract gradients with amyl nitrite and exercise in hypertrophic cardiomyopathy. *Am J Cardiol* 1995;75: 805–809.

66. Maron BJ, Isner JM, McKenna WJ. Task Force 3: Hypertrophic cardiomyopathy, myocarditis and other myopericardial diseases and mitral valve prolapse. *J Am Coll Cardiol* 1994;24:880–883.

67. Louie EK, Maron BJ. Apical hypertrophic cardiomyopathy: clinical and two-dimensional echocardiographic assessment. *Ann Intern Med* 1987;106:663–670.

68. Yamaguchi H, Ishimura T, Nishiyama S, et al. Hypertrophic nonobstructive cardiomyopathy with giant negative T waves (apical hypertrophy): ventriculographic and echocardiographic features in 30 patients. *Am J Cardiol* 1979;44:401–412.

69. Rossen RM, Goodman DJ, Ingham RE, Popp RL. Ventricular systolic septal thickening and excursion in idiopathic hypertrophic subaortic stenosis. *N Engl J Med* 1974;291:1317–1319.

70. Tajik AJ, Guiliani ER. Echocardiographic observations in idiopathic subaortic stenosis. *Mayo Clinic Proceed* 1974;49:89–97.

71. Madu EC, D'Cruz IA. The vital role of papillary muscles in mitral and ventricular function: echocardiographic insights. *Clin Cardiol* 1997;20:93–98.

72. Shah PM, Gramiak R, Kramer DH. Ultrasound localization of left ventricular obstruction in hypertrophic obstructive cardiomyopathy. *Circulation* 1969;40:3–11.

73. Louie EK, Edwards LC. Hypertrophic cardiomyopathy. *Prog Cardiovasc Dis* 1994;36:275–308.
74. Schwammenthal E, Nakatani S, He S, et al. Mechanism of mitral regurgitation in hypertrophic cardiomyopathy: mismatch of posterior to anterior leaflet length and mobility. *Circulation* 1998 (in press).
75. Stewart WJ, Schiavone WA, Salcedo EE, Lever HM, Cosgrove DM, Gill CC. Intraoperative Doppler echocardiography in hypertrophic cardiomyopathy: correlations with the obstructive gradient. *J Am Coll Cardiol* 1987;10:327–335.
76. Nishimura RA, Tajik AJ, Reeder GS, Seward JB. Evaluation of hypertrophic cardiomyopathy by Doppler color flow imaging: initial observations. *Mayo Clinic Proceed* 1986;61:631–639.
77. Rossvoll O, Hatle LK. Pulmonary venous flow velocities recorded by transthoracic Doppler ultrasound: relation to left ventricular diastolic pressures. *J Am Coll Cardiol* 1993:1687–1696.
78. Nishimura RA, Abel MD, Hatke LK, Tajik AJ. Relation of pulmonary vein to mitral flow velocities by transesophageal Doppler echocardiography: effect of different loading conditions. *Circulation* 1990;81:1488–1497.
79. Thiene G, Nava A, Corrado D, Rossi L, Pennelli N. Right ventricular cardiomyopathy and sudden death in young people. *N Engl J Med* 1988;318:129–133.
80. Corrado D, Thiene G, Nava A, Rossi L, Pennelli N. Sudden death in young competitive athletes: clinicopathologic correlations in 22 cases. *Am J Med* 1990;89:588–596.
81. Daliento L, Turrini P, Nava A, et al. Arrhythmogenic right ventricular cardiomyopathy in young versus adult patients: similarities and differences. *J Am Coll Cardiol* 1995;25:655–664.
82. Fontaine G, Fontaliran F, Frank R, Tonet JL, Lascault G, Grosgogeat Y. Right ventricular dysplasia: an overlooked cause of tachyarrhythmias and sudden death. *Cardiologia* 1990;35[Suppl 1]:61–68.
83. Marcus FI, Fontaine GH, Guiraudon G, et al. Right ventricular dysplasia: a report of 24 adult cases. *Circulation* 1982;65:384–398.
84. Hamada S, Takamiya M, Ohe T, Ueda H. Arrhythmogenic right ventricular dysplasia: evaluation with electron-beam CT. *Radiology* 1993;187:723–727.
85. Faitelson L, Marcus F. Unusual forms of ventricular arrhythmias: arrhythmogenic right ventricular dysplasia and repetitive monomorphic ventricular tachycardia. *Cardiovasc Clin* 1992;22:339–348.
86. Ricci C, Longo R, Pagnan L, et al. Magnetic resonance imaging in right ventricular dysplasia. *Am J Cardiol* 1992;70:1589–1595.
87. Robertson JH, Bardy GH, German LD, Gallagher JJ, Kisslo J. Comparison of two-dimensional echocardiographic and angiographic findings in arrhythmogenic right ventricular dysplasia. *Am J Cardiol* 1985;55:1506–1508.
88. Tada H, Shimizu W, Ohe T, et al. Usefulness of electron-beam computed tomography in arrhythmogenic right ventricular dysplasia: relationship to electrophysiological abnormalities and left ventricular involvement. *Circulation* 1996;94:437–444.
89. Manyari DE, Klein GJ, Gulamhusein S, et al. Arrhythmogenic right ventricular dysplasia: a generalized cardiomyopathy? *Circulation* 1983;68:251–257.
90. Blomstrom-Lundqvist C, Beckman-Suurkula M, Wallentin I, Jonsson R, Olsson SB. Ventricular dimensions and wall motion assessed by echocardiography in patients with arrhythmogenic right ventricular dysplasia. *Eur Heart J* 1988;9:1291–1302.
91. Scognamiglio R, Fasoli G, Nava A, Miraglia G, Thiene G, Dalla-Volta S. Contribution of cross-sectional echocardiography to the diagnosis of right ventricular dysplasia at the asymptomatic stage. *Eur Heart J* 1989;10:538–542.
92. Dalal P, Fujisic K, Hupart P, Schwietzer P. Arrhythmogenic right ventricular dysplasia: a review. *Cardiology* 1994;85:361–369.
93. Kisslo J. Two-dimensional echocardiography in arrhythmogenic right ventricular dysplasia. *Eur Heart J* 1989;10:22–26.
94. Kullo IJ, Edwards WD, Seward JB. Right ventricular dysplasia: the Mayo Clinic experience. *Mayo Clinic Proceed* 1995;70:541–548.
95. Manyari DE, Duff HJ, Kostuk WJ, et al. Usefulness of noninvasive studies for diagnosis of right ventricular dysplasia. *Am J Cardiol* 1986;57:1147–1153.
96. Ribeiro PA, Shapiro LM, Foale RA, Crean P, Oakley CM. Echocardiographic features of right ventricular dilated cardiomyopathy and Uhl's anomaly. *Eur Heart J* 1987;8:65–71.
97. Scognamiglio R, Fasoli G, Nava A, Buja G. Two-dimensional echocardiographic features in patients with spontaneous right ventricular tachycardia without apparent heart disease. *J Cardiovasc Ultrasonogr* 1987;6:113–118.
98. Foale R, Nihoyannopoulos P, McKenna W, et al. Echocardiographic measurement of the normal adult right ventricle. *Br Heart J* 1986;56:33–44.
99. Higuchi S, Caglar NM, Shimada R, Yamada A, Takeshita A, Nakamura M. Sixteen-year follow-up of arrhythmogenic right ventricular dysplasia. *Am Heart J* 1984;108:1363–1365.
100. Metzger JT, de Chillou C, Cheriex E, Rodriguez LM, Smeets JL, Wellens HJ. Value of the 12-lead electrocardiogram in arrhythmogenic right ventricular dysplasia, and absence of correlation with echocardiographic findings. *Am J Cardiol* 1993;72:964–967.
101. Pinamonti B, Sinagra G, Salvi A, et al. Left ventricular involvement in right ventricular dysplasia. *Am Heart J* 1992;123:711–724.
102. Baran A, Nanda NC, Falkoff M, Barold SS, Gallagher JJ. Two-dimensional echocardiographic detection of arrhythmogenic right ventricular dysplasia. *Am Heart J* 1982;103:1066–1067.
103. Iliceto S, Izzi M, De Martino G, Rizzon P. Echo Doppler evaluation of right ventricular dysplasia. *Eur Heart J* 1989;10[Suppl D]:29–32.
104. Planinc D, Jeric M, Rudar M. Arrhythmogenic right ventricular dysplasia: mechanocardiographic, echocardiographic and Doppler assessment. *Acta Cardiologica* 1988;XLVIII:289–295.
105. Webb JG, Kerr CR, Huckell VF, Mizgala HF, Ricci DR. Left ventricular abnormalities in arrhythmogenic right ventricular dysplasia. *Am J Cardiol* 1986;58:568–570.
106. Pyeritz RE, McKusick VA. The Marfan syndrome. Diagnosis and management. *N Engl J Med* 1979;300:772–777.
107. Marsalese DL, Moodie DS, Vacante M, et al. Marfan's

syndrome: natural history and long-term follow-up of cardiovascular involvement. *J Am Coll Cardiol* 1989; 14:422–428.

108. Murdoch JL, Walker BA, Halpern BL, Kuzma JW, McKusick VA. Life expectancy and causes of death in the Marfan syndrome. *N Engl J Med* 1972;286:804–808.

109. Pyeritz RE, Wappel MA. Mitral valve dysfunction in the Marfan syndrome. Clinical and echocardiographic study of prevalence and natural history. *Am J Med* 1983;74:797–807.

110. McKusick VA. *Heritable disorders of the connective tissue.* In: Beighton P, ed. St. Louis: Mosby, 1993:68–83.

111. Phornphutkul C, Rosenthal A, Nadas AS. Cardiac manifestations of Marfan syndrome in infancy and childhood. *Circulation* 1973;XLVII:587–596.

112. Hirst AE, Gore I. Marfan's syndrome. A review. *Prog Cardiovasc Dis* 1973;XVI:187–198.

113. Hollister DW, Godfrey M, Sakai LY, Pyeritz RE. Immunohistologic abnormalities of the microfibrillar-fiber system in the Marfan syndrome. *N Engl J Med* 1990;323:152–159.

114. Brown OR, DeMots H, Kloster FE, Roberts A, Menashe VD, Beals RK. Aortic root dilatation and mitral valve prolapse in Marfan's syndrome: an echocardiographic study. *Circulation* 1975;52:651–657.

115. DeMaria AN, Bommer W, Neuman A, Weinert L, Bogren H, Mason DT. Identification and localization of aneurysms of the ascending aorta by cross-sectional echocardiography. *Circulation* 1979;59:755–761.

116. Weyman AE. *Principles and practice of echocardiography.* Philadelphia: Lea & Febiger, 1994:Appendix A.

117. Sahn DJ, DeMaria A, Kisslo J, Weyman A. Recommendations regarding quantitation in M-mode echocardiography: results of a survey of echocardiographic measurements. *Circulation* 1978;58:1072–1083.

118. Roman MJ, Devereux RB, Kramer-Fox R, O'Loughlin J, Spitzer M, Robins J. Two-dimensional echocardiographic aortic root dimensions in normal children and adults. *Am J Cardiol* 1989;64:507–512.

119. Pan CW, Chen CC, Wang SP, Hsu TL, Chiang BN. Echocardiographic study of cardiac abnormalities in families of patients with Marfan's syndrome. *J Am Coll Cardiol* 1985;6:1016–1020.

120. Nidorf SM, Picard MH, Triulzi MO, et al. New perspectives in the assessment of cardiac chamber dimensions during development and adulthood. *J Am Coll Cardiol* 1992;19:983–988.

121. Pyeritz RE. The Marfan syndrome. *Am Fam Physician* 1986;34:83–94.

122. McDonald GR, Schaff HV, Pyeritz RE, McKusick VA, Gott VL. Surgical management of patients with the Marfan syndrome and dilatation of the ascending aorta. *J Thorac Cardiovasc Surg* 1981;81:180–186.

123. Hwa J, Richards JG, Huang H, et al. The natural history of aortic dilatation in Marfan syndrome. *Med J Aust* 1993;158:558–562.

124. Jeremy RW, Huang H, Hwa J, McCarron H, Hughes CF, Richards JG. Relation between age, arterial distensibility, and aortic dilatation in the Marfan syndrome. *Am J Cardiol* 1994;74:369–373.

125. Bowers D. Pathogenesis of primary abnormalities of the mitral valve in Marfan's syndrome. *Br Heart J* 1969;31:679–683.

126. Bowden DH, Favara BE, Donahoe JL. Marfan's syndrome: accelerated course in childhood associated with lesions of mitral valve and pulmonary artery. *Am Heart J* 1965;69:96–99.

127. Mattleman S, Panidis I, Kotler MN, Mintz G, Victor M, Ross J. Dissecting aneurysm in a patient with Marfan's syndrome: recognition of extensive involvement of the aorta by two-dimensional echocardiography. *J Clin Ultrasound* 1984;12:219–221.

128. Svensson LG, Crawford ES, Coselli JS, Safi HJ, Hess KR. Impact of cardiovascular operation on survival in the Marfan patient. *Circulation* 1989;80[Suppl I]:I-233–I-242.

129. Brown OR, Popp RL, Kloster FE. Echocardiographic criteria for aortic root dissection. *Am J Cardiol* 1975; 36:17–20.

130. Iliceto S, Antonelli G, Biasco G, Rizzon P. Two-dimensional echocardiographic evaluation of aneurysms of the descending thoracic aorta. *Circulation* 1982;66:1045–1049.

131. Victor MF, Mintz GS, Kotler MN, Wilson AR, Segal BL. Two-dimensional echocardiographic diagnosis of aortic dissection. *Am J Cardiol* 1981;48:1155–1159.

132. Fahrenbach MC, Thompson PD. The preparticipation sports examination: cardiovascular considerations for screening. *Cardiol Clin* 1992;10:319–328.

133. Maron BJ, Leon MB, Swain JA, Cannon RO, Pelliccia A. Prospective identification by two-dimensional echocardiography of anomalous origin of the left main coronary artery from the right sinus of Valsalva. *Am J Cardiol* 1991;68:140–142.

134. Pelliccia A, Spataro A, Maron BJ. Prospective echocardiographic screening for coronary artery anomalies in 1,360 elite competitive athletes. *Am J Cardiol* 1993;72:978–979.

135. Maron BJ, Bodison SA, Wesley YE, Tucker E, Green KJ. Results of screening a large group of intercollegiate competitive athletes for cardiovascular disease. *J Am Coll Cardiol* 1987;10:1214–1221.

136. Pelliccia A, Maron BJ. Preparticipation cardiovascular evaluation of the competitive athlete: perspectives from the 30-year Italian experience. *Am J Cardiol* 1995;75:827–829.

137. Anderson TM. Echocardiographic screening of the athletic adolescent. *Pediatrician* 1986;13:165–170.

138. Weidenbener EJ, Krauss MD, Waller BF, Taliercio CP. Limited screening echocardiography in athletic exams: economic and administrative aspects. *Indiana Med* 1993;86:514–517.

139. Weidenbener EJ, Krauss MD, Waller BF, Taliercio CP. Incorporation of screening echocardiography in the preparticipation exam. *Clin J Sports Med* 1995;5:86–89.

140. Murry PM, Cantwell JD, Heath DL, Shoop J. The role of limited echocardiography in screening athletes. *Am J Cardiol* 1995;76:849–850.

141. Maron BJ, Thompson PD, Puffer JC, et al. Cardiovascular preparticipation screening of competitive athletes: a statement for health professionals from the Sudden Death Committee (clinical cardiology) and Congenital Cardiac Defects Committee (cardiovascular disease in the young), American Heart Association. *Circulation* 1996;94:850–856.

The Athlete and Heart Disease:
Diagnosis, Evaluation & Management,
edited by R. A. Williams.
Lippincott Williams & Wilkins, Philadelphia © 1999.

11

The Athlete's Electrocardiogram

Gerald F. Fletcher

Department of Medicine, Mayo Medical School, Mayo Clinic, Jacksonville, Florida 32224

The 12-lead electrocardiogram (ECG) continues to be an important diagnostic tool in the cardiovascular evaluation. There are many variations of heart rate, rhythm, conduction, and alteration of both depolarization and repolarization that are considered to be within the range of normal. This discussion expands on these ECG findings in athletes and clarifies such for the observer in the clinical setting.

HEART RATE

Sinus Bradycardia

Sinus bradycardia is the most common rhythm change seen in athletes and should be considered a normal variant rather than an arrhythmia. In one study (1), sinus bradycardia (less than 50 beats/minute) was found in 65% of athletes, and heart rates decreased to less than 40 during sleep. Another study (2) compared 20 trained athletes with untrained control subjects using ambulatory ECG recording. The results showed a significantly lower heart rate ($p<0.01$) in the athletes both during sleep and during other activities. In 20 long-distance runners studied (3), heart rates were 10 beats/minute slower when compared with 50 untrained professional students of similar age, using 24-hour Holter recording during normal activity. Average heart rates during sleep in the runners ranged from 31 to 43 beats/minute (average 36 ± 3) compared to 33 to 55 (average 43 ± 5) in the untrained subjects.

The degree of bradycardia is most profound in athletes engaged in sports requiring the greatest endurance. One study (4) found average heart rates of 56 beats/minute in 74 runners, 57 beats/minute in 53 cyclists, 62 beats/minute in 66 swimmers, and 66 beats/minute in 51 wrestlers. At similar exercise loads, athletes have lower heart rates than untrained subjects, and the exercise heart rate returns to resting levels more rapidly in trained individuals.

Sinus Tachycardia

Sinus tachycardia is a normal rhythm that is most obvious in athletes. However, the rate of the sinus tachycardia is less for a given task in athletes than in nontrained subjects, and in more highly trained athletes, it tends to occur at slower tachycardia rates.

Sinus Arrhythmia

Sinus arrhythmia is frequently present in athletes at rest but usually disappears with exercise (4–7). One group (8) found sinus arrhythmias in 77% of well-conditioned football players. Others found no significant difference in the incidence of sinus arrhythmias in long-distance runners (100%) compared to the normal population (86%) (3).

HEART RHYTHM

Supraventricular Arrhythmias

In one study, 100% of 20 long-distance runners had premature atrial beats on 24-hour continuous ECG recordings, but only one had more than 100 premature atrial beats in 24 hours (3). Another study of 80 healthy runners (9) found ectopic supraventricular complexes in 33 (41%), but again only one athlete had more than 100 supraventricular ectopic beats per 24 hours. Another report revealed tachyarrhythmias in young athletes (10) and found that 10 had supraventricular arrhythmias, all of whom had a documented underlying cause. Five had paroxysmal atrial fibrillation, and five had paroxysmal supraventricular tachycardia. Three had underlying Wolff-Parkinson-White (WPW) syndrome, five mitral valve prolapse, and two a concealed Kent bundle. An unusual case has been reported of an athlete documented to have had a brief run of supraventricular tachycardia in the recovery phase of maximum exercise testing, in which the heart rate reached almost 500 beats/minute (11).

Athletes with supraventricular tachycardias, whether exercise-induced or not, should be evaluated and managed in the same manner as nonathletes. The individual should undergo a complete history and physical examination and other appropriate studies in an effort to discover underlying heart disease. Supraventricular tachycardias generally are not incapacitating in athletic competition, so athletic participation is a function of the ability to control the arrhythmia and the cause of the arrhythmia.

Atrioventricular Junctional Rhythms

There appears to be an increase in atrioventricular (AV) junctional rhythms in athletes. In one study (12), seven of 35 highly trained athletes had AV junctional rhythm during ambulatory recordings. The junctional rhythm was intermittent and occurred when the sinus rate slowed to less than 56 beats per minute. One 31-year-old professional athlete had an AV junctional rhythm at rest but when the sinus rate reached 90 beats/minute, normal conduction resumed. An extensive cardiac evaluation including

electrophysiologic studies failed to detect any underlying cardiac pathology. The rhythm continued in the subject for 8 years without change.

Ventricular Arrhythmias

Ectopic ventricular contractions and ventricular tachycardia have been reported in athletes during exercise and in the immediate postexercise period. In one study during treadmill testing of 60 well-conditioned runners, 27% had ventricular arrhythmias, but only 3% had higher-grade ectopy. In contrast, 60% of the runners had ventricular arrhythmias during a monitored long-distance run: 10% bigeminal, 10% couplets, and 5% multifocal (13). Treadmill testing significantly underestimated the incidence of arrhythmias, in that 57% of the runners who had ventricular arrhythmias while running had none on the treadmill.

In a study of 20 highly trained marathon runners, only one exhibited high-grade arrhythmias (polymorphic ventricular arrhythmias). Six months later, angina pectoris developed in this individual, leading to the conclusion that any high-grade ventricular arrhythmias should be considered abnormal in highly trained athletes (14). Another study of 80 healthy runners found ectopic ventricular couplets in 41 and ectopic supraventricular beats in 33. No relationship was found between the frequency of ventricular ectopy and the amount of weekly running (9). A third study (15) used 24-hour continuous ECG monitoring to compare 20 runners, 20 cyclists, and 40 nonathletic control subjects for the frequency of ventricular ectopy. A slightly higher frequency of premature ventricular beats (70% versus 55%, $p>0.05$) was found in athletes. Complex forms of ectopy also were more common in the athletic groups (25% versus 5%, $p>0.05$). Others, however, reported a frequency of ventricular ectopy of 33.9% in 165 highly trained athletes, but only a 3.6% incidence of complex ventricular arrhythmias.

Ventricular Tachycardia

Among 19 athletes evaluated because of symptomatic tachyarrhythmias, paroxysmal ventricular tachycardia occurred in eight (sustained in five) and ventricular fibrillation occurred in one. All the arrhythmias developed during strenuous exercise (10). Abnormalities of the heart were found in 15 (79%) of the 19 evaluated. Of the nine athletes with ventricular arrhythmias, four had mitral valve prolapse and one had a cardiomyopathy.

Several types of symptomatic ventricular tachycardia have been described in athletes. One can be induced and terminated by programmed ventricular stimulation and probably reflects reentry (16,17). This tachycardia usually occurs in the setting of severe chronic ischemic heart disease and generally arises from the left ventricle or the interventricular septum. Episodes of this variety of tachycardia are usually unrelated to exercise, and treadmill exercise or infusion of isoproterenol rarely provokes the arrhythmia (18).

Another variety of symptomatic ventricular tachycardia is exercise-provoked. Two groups (19,20) first recognized this homogeneous subset of patients. The individuals were young, sometimes athletic, and had minimal heart disease. Their tachycardias originated in the outflow tract of the right ventricle and could not be induced by programmed ventricular stimulation, but could be reproducibly provoked by treadmill exercise or infusion of isoproterenol. Administration of propranolol or verapamil prevented the occurrence of ventricular tachycardia with exercise, whereas class I antiarrhythmic drugs usually were ineffective. It has been suggested that this variety of symptomatic ventricular tachycardia may reflect catecholamine-enhanced automaticity or may be triggered by delayed afterdepolarizations ectopic beats (19,20).

CONDUCTION

Sinus Pauses

Studies have found significantly longer sinus pauses in long-distance runners compared to untrained control subjects both while awake (1.35 to 2.55 seconds) and while asleep (1.6 to 2.8 seconds) (21). One group (22) found that 13 of 35 athletes had sinus pauses greater than 2.0 seconds, whereas only two control subjects exceeded 2.0 seconds. In another series (1), seven of 37 top athletes had sinus pauses greater than 2.6 seconds during 24-hour ECG recording; 51% had pauses of at least 2 seconds (2).

First-Degree Atrioventricular Block

First-degree AV block is a benign conduction problem that is not uncommon in athletes. One study found first-degree block in 37% of athletes, compared to 14% of control subjects (22). Others (2) have found first-degree AV block in three of 20 male athletes aged 14 to 16 years, compared to only one of 20 nonathletic controls.

Second-Degree Atrioventricular Block

Second-degree AV block may be a sign of organic heart disease, but it is not uncommon as a normal variant in the athlete. One marathon runner was reported to have demonstrated AV Wenckebach conduction before, but not after, a 100-yard dash (12). Also, two middle-aged athletes with Wenckebach periods on resting ECG had the disturbance disappear during exercise (23,24). Another study comparing athletes to control subjects found second-degree AV block in eight (23%) of the athletes and two (5.7%) of the control subjects (22). In a study of 20 athletes, second-degree AV block was found in three of the athletes but in only one untrained control (2). Another group applied various forms of sympathetic stimulation to ten male athletes with second-degree Wenckebach block. Of the various forms of stimulation, including exercise, atropine, and isoproterenol infusion, Valsalva, hyperventilation, and position changes, the results were variable with carotid sinus pressure, Valsalva, and hyperventilation. The studies following isoproterenol infusion and exercise with resultant increased sinus rates resulted in normalization of AV conduction in nine of ten individuals (three of whom had mitral valve prolapse) (26).

AV conduction changes in athletes are believed to be related to the intensity and length of training (2). These changes appear to reverse after training is reduced or discontinued. Reversal of ECG changes (including first- and second-degree AV block) has been observed among 95% of 102 Olympic athletes 4 years after they reduced the intensity of training (2). In another single case (27), a 38-year-old marathoner had a high degree of Mobitz type II block, with 2-second pauses and a 6-second pause during sleep, but had a normal coronary angiogram. Five years after decreasing her running to 2 to 5 miles per day, the rhythm had returned to sinus and the AV block disappeared. A report on a 5-year follow-up of 122 intensely active middle-aged cross country skiers concluded that the ECG changes of the athletic heart, including first- and second-degree block, are secondary to intense training and not to underlying coronary artery disease (28).

Complete Atrioventricular Block

Complete AV block is rare in athletes (29,30). In a review of 15,000 ECG tracings at a sports institute (30), only one case of congenital heart block was found. This individual increased his ventricular rate to 155 with treadmill exercise, indicating that ventricular acceleration with exercise was unaffected by the heart block. When the heart block failed to disappear after vigorous (maximum) exercise, it was thought to represent either congenital or organic complete heart block. The same group reviewed previous cases of complete heart block in athletes. In 25% to 50%, there was evidence of an additional cardiac defect. Those individuals with congenital complete heart block but without identified structural cardiac defects usually lead normal lives. If these individuals have no Stokes-Adams attacks and are free of high-grade ectopy at rest and exercise, they can perform strenuous work and participate in sports (30).

Based on these reports, evidence suggests that intensive training of the cardiovascular system may become hazardous to only a few. The symptomatic athlete with a slow heart rate, heart block of any degree, or both deserves further evaluation of his or her cardiovascular system, including an assessment of the intensity of the training program.

DEPOLARIZATION—(QRS CHANGES IN ABSENCE OF HYPERTROPHY PATTERN)

QRS Axis

A summary of several studies (31) reported a QRS frontal plane axis between 0 and +90 degrees in 77.6% of 582 athletes; 74% were between +60 and +90 degrees, and the majority of the remainder were found to have right axis deviation in excess of +90 degrees. A study of 289 professional football players found the mean QRS axis to be +56 degrees, with 5% having right axis deviation. Thus, it appears that vertical and right axis QRS deviations are common findings in highly trained athletes.

Intraventricular Conduction Delays (without Hypertrophy)

Prolongation of intraventricular conduction is commonly seen in athletes, manifesting commonly as incomplete right bundle branch block (BBB). Of 107 Olympic athletes studied, 51.1% had incomplete right BBB (32) and another analysis of ten studies (33) involving 527 athletes showed 84 (16%) with this finding. Of 289 professional football players, 60% had a QRS duration of 0.10 second but only one had complete right BBB (22). Thus, incomplete right BBB is extremely common in highly trained athletes, but complete right and left BBB are rare.

REPOLARIZATION OF THE QRS

Changes in the ECG ST segment, T wave, or both (as manifestations of QRS repolarization) have been reported to occur with increased frequency in both endurance and isometrically trained athletes (22,26,34). The ST segment changes resemble the pattern commonly called early repolarization. Such J point elevation commonly occurs in the anterior and lateral leads (V_3 through V_6); however, these changes may also be seen in the inferior (II, III, aVF) leads. Such changes have been reported in up to 50% of highly trained athletes and in one report were found in the electrocardiogram of 13% of professional football players studied (22). The ST changes of early repolarization can be mistaken for the changes of acute pericarditis or epicardial injury, but the clinical setting and findings are absent.

T wave changes in highly trained athletes are common and variable. The T wave may be tall and peaked, flattened, notched, and slightly or significantly inverted in the precordial leads. The changes may be confused with ischemic changes but are similar to the benign juvenile pattern seen in young adults.

HYPERTROPHY

Ventricular Hypertrophy

ECG evidence of right and left ventricular hypertrophy is commonly observed in well-trained athletes. ECG evidence for ventricular hypertrophy is more common in endurance-trained than in isometrically trained athletes, but as training programs for each group overlap and become less specialized, these differences are becoming less noticeable. Among world class marathon runners in one study (35), 76% were found to have voltage criteria for left ventricular hypertrophy, whereas a summary of several studies involving 952 athletes found 32% to have evidence of left ventricular hypertrophy (range 1% to 76%) (31). Among professional football players, 35% displayed voltage criteria for left ventricular hypertrophy (22).

A summary (31) of five studies of 669 athletes revealed that 19% fulfilled the criteria for right ventricular hypertrophy. Another review of four large studies (36) found criteria for right ventricular hypertrophy to be present in 18% to 69% of athletes, occurring more often in those with dynamic rather than static training. In one study (31), right ventricular hypertrophy was present equally in statically trained athletes and in nonathletic, sedentary control subjects.

Sequential increases in QRS voltage have been shown to occur as training continues. The increase in QRS voltage parallels the intensity and type of training. With cessation of athletic training, the ECG changes of ventricular hypertrophy revert to normal in some instances.

SPECIAL CONCERNS

Preexcitation

Shortening of the PR interval with or without alterations (slurring or delay) in the initial 0.04 second of the QRS are infrequent findings in normal subjects. The most common pattern is the WPW pattern. Whether the incidence of WPW is increased in athletes is debatable. One group has reported a higher incidence in athletes, but fewer episodes of arrhythmias (37). Others who have observed professional athletes estimate the incidence to be close to the 1.5 per 1,000 reported in a large study of the normal population. WPW in the athlete should be approached in a similar manner to WPW in nonathletes. The general approach has been to evaluate completely any symptomatic individual with WPW beyond the routine history and physical examination with tests including Holter recordings, maximal exercise testing, and echocardiography. Electrophysiologic studies should then be considered.

T of the P and T-P Interval

Repolarization of the P wave, or the T of the P, occurs in the terminal part of the QRS complex and early portion of the S-T segment. In certain ECG patterns with tall P waves (often seen best in standard leads II, III, and aVF), there is depression in the late QRS–early S-T segment that may simulate the S-T depression of ischemia. However, this is usually manifest as a depressed upslope rather than the horizontal S-T depression. Such should be considered a normal variant unless there are clinical concerns that suggest otherwise. Another recent observation has regarded the effect of exercise on Q-T dispersion; however, little information on this topic is available.

Holter Recording

Holter long-term ECG recording has been used for many years and has been clinically revealing with regard to cardiac arrhythmias and conduction disturbances seen in athletes, as well as in evaluating the cause of sudden cardiac death (38). This technology is most appropriate for evaluation of athletes because it provides a means to monitor and record the electrical activity of the heart in the dynamic, active state.

Normal Findings in Ambulatory ECG Recording in Athletes

A number of cardiac rhythm alterations have been detected in normal athletes (39). These include sinus bradycardia of 30 to 45 beats per minute, sinus arrhythmia, atrial ectopy, and atrial couplets, as well as ventricular ectopy and ventricular couplets. The heart rate may vary from the 30 to 45 beats per minute at rest to rates of 140 to 160 beats per minute with exercise. However, as athletes become more highly trained, the exercise heart rates are often in the range of 110 to 130 beats per minute. Brief periods of supraventricular rhythm and idioventricular rhythm may also occur. Conduction disturbances also occur in normal athletes (3). First-degree AV block has been described as have AV junctional rhythm and AV Wenckebach conduction.

Several studies have been done in normal runners (3,9,13) (Table 1). In one, the authors (3) obtained 24-hour continuous ECG recordings in 20 young (19- to 28-year old) male long-distance runners (50 miles/week) during activities other than running. All 20 runners had premature atrial complexes, but only one had greater than 100 in 24 hours. Fourteen (70%) had premature ventricular complexes, but only two (10%) had greater than 50 in 24 hours and none had ventricular couplets or tachycardia.

In another study (13), 60 high-level runners (24 to 177 km/week, median 48.5) had ambulatory ECG recordings only during the period of exercise. Sixty percent had ventricular arrhythmias during the recorded run: bigeminy in 10%, couplets in 10%, and multiform premature ventricular contractions in 5%. Forty percent of the group had atrial arrhythmias during the recorded run. Occasional to frequent premature atrial complexes were the most common; however, seven subjects had atrial couplets or paroxysmal atrial tachycardia. This study is limited in scope, however, because of the brief time of Holter recording.

In a larger study (9), 80 healthy runners were studied with continuous Holter ECG recording during both exercise and free activity. In this study, group 1 consisted of 20 runners (0 to <5 miles/week); group 2, 19 runners (≥5 to ≤15 miles/week); group 3, 21 runners (>15 to ≤30 miles/week); and group 4, 20 runners (>30 miles/week). The continuous ECG, both during running and other activity, revealed no significant differences in the occurrence of rhythm and conduction disturbances in the different groups. The most common abnormalities were ventricular ectopic complexes, seen in 40 subjects: less than 50 per minute in 34 and more than 50 per minute in six. The high-grade ventricular ectopic activity—five-beat run of ventricular tachycardia (immediately after exercise) and two instances of ventricular couplets during exercise—were of concern, and subjects were referred for further medical evaluation. However, no data are available on this follow-up.

TABLE 1. *Results of three long-term electrocardiographic studies of apparently healthy runners*

Study and No.of Subjects	Total with ESCs		>100 ESCs/ 24 hr		Atrial Couplets or Tachycardia		Total with EVCs		>50 EVCs/ 24 hr		Paired Ventricular Extrasystoles		Ventric- ular Tachy- cardia		Mobitz 1 AV Block	
	n	%	n	%	n	%	n	%	n	%	n	%	n	%	n	%
Talan et al. 20—FA only	20	100	1	5	2	10	14	70	2	10	0	0	0	0	8	40
Pantano et al. 60—DR only	24	40	—	—	7	12	36	60	—	—	6	10	0	0	0	0
Pilcher et al. 80—DR and FA																
Group I	7	35	0	0	0	0	9	45	0	0	0	0	0	0	0	0
Group II	10	53	0	0	0	0	13	68	1	5	1	5	0	0	0	0
Group III	7	33	1	5	0	0	6	29	1	5	1	5	1	5	0	0
Group IV	9	45	0	0	0	0	13	65	4	20	0	0	0	0	0	0

AV, atrioventricular; DR, during running; ESCs, ectopic supraventricular complexes (predominantly premature atrial); EVCs, ectopic ventricular complexes; FA, during free activity; —, no information.

Indications for Ambulatory ECG Recording

Indications for ambulatory ECG recordings in athletes include but are not limited to the following:

1. History
   a. Syncope and dizziness
   b. Subjective palpitations
   c. Concerns about heart disease in the family
2. Physical examination
   a. Irregular pulse
   b. Certain cardiac murmurs
   c. Evidence of cardiomegaly (with a significant history)

The indications for recording in athletes should be placed in proper perspective. A detailed history should be obtained at the outset with appropriate physical examination emphasizing certain findings, specifically, irregular pulse, heart murmurs, and heart enlargement. A standard 12-lead ECG then may be indicated. If arrhythmias are documented, further analysis may be in order with use of the 24-hour ECG recording. Such may be done during the time of the athletic activity such as running or hurdling. At this time, however, electrode lead systems are not effective in recording the ECG during water sports.

Regardless of the athletic setting, running, gymnastics, or other land sports, the technique of lead application must include proper skin preparation (usually including shaving of hair) and support of the lead system with wrapping of the lead wires and cable securely around the body. In recording of women athletes, the support and stability of the breasts adjacent to the lead system are necessary, usually with tight-fitting undergarments.

Disturbances of heart rate and rhythm are very common and normal in athletes. Such are often related to changes and alterations in parasympathetic and sympathetic tone that develop in athletes as a result of the training effect. Therefore, the proper medical evaluation by health professionals before instigating costly studies should be done as described. This puts the 24-hour ECG recording in the proper perspective in the medical evaluation of athletes.

Telemetry Electrocardiography and Event Recording

Special methods of recording heart rate and rhythm may be effective in detecting ECG changes in athletes. Telemetry or wireless ECG recording may be appropriate in settings in which rate and rhythm can be visually monitored by an ECG technologist: such could be used during game sports such as basketball or soccer. Event recording (with use of a portable personally triggered recording device) may reveal rhythm disturbances in a subject who is symptomatic during the event and can initiate the recording in a clinical setting.

Exercise Testing

An exercise test may be indicated in certain athletes, especially those who have symptoms (of an arrhythmia) during dynamic exercise. Careful observation for the rhythm disturbance and its effect on blood pressure and certain ECG indices can be valuable in determining the potential sequelae of the disturbances if such occurred in real life with various types of activity. In the athlete's performance setting with exercise, certain arrhythmias resolve with increasing sinus rate and others may increase in frequency and severity. These changes (or lack of such changes) may be helpful in the analysis of the impact of rhythm disturbances in the athlete.

SUMMARY

The ECG of the athlete reflects the extremes of normality more than any other test used in a cardiovascular evaluation. This single test is often used in the evaluation of an athlete. In doing so, the ECG wave forms, rate, and rhythm must be evaluated in context of other findings in the history, physical examination, and other tests so as not to designate a cardiac abnormality in a very healthy individual.

REFERENCES

1. Ector H, Bourgois J, Verlinden M, et al. Bradycardia, ventricular pauses, syncope, and sports. *Lancet* 1984;2: 591–594.
2. Kala R, Viitasalo MT. Atrioventricular block, including Mobitz type II-like pattern, during ambulatory ECG recording in young athletes aged 14 to 16 years. *Ann Clin Res* 1982;14:53–56.
3. Talan DA, Bauernfeind RA, Ashley WW, Kanakis C Jr, Rosen KM. Twenty-four hour continuous ECG recordings in long-distance runners. *Chest* 1982;82:19–24.
4. Klemola E. Electrocardiographic observations on 650 Finnish athletes. *Ann Med Intern Fenn* 1951;41:121.
5. Beswick FW, Jordan RC. Cardiological observations at the sixth British Empire and Commonwealth Games. *Br Heart J* 1961;23:113–129.
6. Hantzschel K, Dohrn K. The electrocardiogram before and after a marathon-race. *J Sports Med Phys Fitness* 1966;6:29–32.
7. Hunt BPE. Electrocardiographic study of 20 champion swimmers before and after 100 year sprint swimming competition. *Can Med Assoc J* 1963;88:1251–1253.

8. Balady GJ, Cadigan JB, Ryan TJ. Electrocardiogram of the athlete: an analysis of 289 professional football players. *Am J Cardiol* 1984;53:1339–1343.
9. Pilcher GF, Cook AJ, Johnston BL, Fletcher GF. Twenty-four-hour continuous electrocardiography during exercise and free activity in 80 apparently healthy runners. *Am J Cardiol* 1983;52:859–861.
10. Coelho A, Palileo E, Ashley W, et al. Tachyarrhythmias in young athletes. *J Am Coll Cardiol* 1986;7:237–243.
11. Medved R, Pavisic-Medved V. A rare case of paroxysmal tachycardia during load testing a top-ranking athlete. *J Sports Med Phys Fitness* 1985;25:211–214.
12. Sargin O, Alp C, Tansi C, Karaca L. Electrocardiogram of the month. Wenckebach phenomenon with nodal and ventricular escape in marathon runner. *Chest* 1970;57: 102–105.
13. Pantano JA, Oriel RJ. Prevalence and nature of cardiac arrhythmias in apparently normal well-trained runners. *Am Heart J* 1982;104:762–768.
14. Palatini P, Maraglino G, Sperti G, et al. Prevalence and possible mechanisms of ventricular arrhythmias in athletes. *Am Heart J* 1985;110:560–567.
15. Biffi A, Pelliccia A, Caselli G. Arrhythmias in athletes [Letter]. *Am Heart J* 1986;112:1349–1351.
16. Josephson ME, Horowitz LN, Farshidi A, Kastor JA. Recurrent sustained ventricular tachycardia. 1. Mechanisms. *Circulation* 1978;57:431–440.
17. Josephson ME, Horowitz LN, Farshidi A, Spear JF, Kastor JA, Moore EN. Recurrent sustained ventricular tachycardia. 2. Endocardial mapping. *Circulation* 1978; 57:440–447.
18. Wu D, Kou HC, Hung JS. Exercise-triggered paroxysmal ventricular tachycardia. A repetitive rhythmic activity possibly related to afterdepolarization. *Ann Intern Med* 1981;95:410–414.
19. Palileo EV, Ashley WW, Swiryn S, et al. Exercise provocable right ventricular outflow tract tachycardia. *Am Heart J* 1982;104:185–193.
20. Buxton AE, Waxman HL, Marchlinski FE, Simson MB, Cassidy D, Josephson ME. Right ventricular tachycardia: clinical and electrophysiologic characteristics. *Circulation* 1983;68:917–927.
21. Hiss RG, Lamb LE. Electrocardiographic findings in 122,043 individuals. *Circulation* 1962;25:947–961.
22. Viitasalo MT, Kala R, Eisalo A. Ambulatory electrocardiographic recording in endurance athletes. *Br Heart J* 1982;47:213–220.
23. Grimby G, Saltin B. Physiological analysis of physically well-trained middle-aged and old athletes. *Acta Med Scand* 1966;179:513–526.
24. Grimby G, Saltin S. Daily running causing Wenckebach heart block. *Lancet* 1964;2:729–730.
25. Deleted in proof.
26. Zeppilli P, Fenici R, Sassara M, Pirrami MM, Caselli G. Wenckebach second-degree A-V block in top-ranking athletes: an old problem revisited. *Am Heart J* 1980; 100:281–294.
27. DiNardo-Ekery D, Abedin Z. High degree atrioventricular block in a marathoner with 5-year follow-up. *Am Heart J* 1987;113:834–837.
28. Lie H, Erikssen J. Five-year follow-up of ECG aberrations, latent coronary heart disease and cardiopulmonary fitness in various age groups of Norwegian cross-country skiers. *Acta Med Scand* 1984;216: 377–383.

29. Torkelson L, Jokl E. Complete congenital heart block in an athlete. *J Assoc Phys Ment Rehabil* 1967;21: 54–55.

30. Hanne-Paparo N, Drory Y, Kellermann JJ. Complete heart block and physical performance. *Int J Sports Med* 1983;4:9–13.

31. Ferst JA, Chaitman BR. The electrocardiogram and the athlete. *Sports Med* 1984;1:390–403.

32. Venerando A, Rulli V. Frequency, morphology, and meaning of the electrocardiographic anomalies found in Olympic marathon runners and walkers. *J Sports Med Phys Fitness* 1964;4:135–141.

33. Lichtman J, O'Rourke R, Klein A, Karliner JS. Electrocardiogram of the athlete. Alterations simulating those of organic heart disease. *Arch Intern Med* 1973;132: 763–770.

34. Nishimura T, Kambara H, Chen CH, Yamada Y, Kawai C. Noninvasive assessment of T-wave abnormalities on precordial electrocardiograms in middle-aged professional bicyclists. *J Electrocardiol* 1981;14:357–364.

35. Smith WG, Cullen KJ, Thorburn IO. Electrocardiograms of marathon runners in 1962 Commonwealth Games. *Br Heart J* 1964;26:469–476.

36. Huston TP, Puffer JC, Rodney WM. The athletic heart syndrome. *N Engl J Med* 1985;313:24–32.

37. S'Jongers JJ, Dirix A, Jolie P, Borms J, Segers M. Wolff-Parkinson-White syndrome and sports aptitude. *J Sports Med Phys Fitness* 1976;16:6–16.

38. Fletcher GF. *Dynamic electrocardiographic recording.* Mount Kisco, NY: Futura Publishing, 1979.

39. Fletcher GF. Holter recording in athletes: purposes and applications. In: Waller BF, Harvey WP, eds. *Cardiovascular evaluation of athletes.* Newton, NJ: Laennec Publishing, 1993:87–94.

The Athlete and Heart Disease:
Diagnosis, Evaluation & Management,
edited by R. A. Williams.
Lippincott Williams & Wilkins, Philadelphia © 1999.

12

Noninvasive Testing in Athletes: Signal-Averaged Electrocardiogram and Ambulatory Recordings

Gioia Turitto, Bekir S. Cebeci, Luther T. Clark, and Nabil El-Sherif

Division of Cardiovascular Medicine, State University of New York Health Science Center at Brooklyn, Brooklyn, New York 11203

An analysis of the role of noninvasive testing for stratification of arrhythmic risk in athletes has to take into consideration the fact that the prevalence of cardiovascular disease in a young athletic population is low and sudden cardiac death is rare (1). Given the uncommon occurrence of sports-related sudden death, any screening program is destined to have a relatively low predictive accuracy. An added problem is that the differential diagnosis between nonpathologic cardiac changes associated with training (so-called "athlete's heart") and cardiac disease associated with increased risk for sudden death may be difficult (2). This distinction is important because it can result in decreasing the risk of sudden death by disqualifying athletes with silent organic heart disease from competition and because it avoids unnecessary withdrawal of healthy individuals from sports activity. This chapter discusses the anatomic and electrophysiologic substrate for sudden death in athletes, retrospective studies on athletes surviving cardiac arrest, and the prevalence of abnormal findings on ambulatory and signal-averaged (SA) electrocardiographic (ECG) recordings performed in apparently healthy athletes.

PATHOLOGIC FINDINGS IN ATHLETES WITH SUDDEN CARDIAC DEATH

Autopsy studies have provided valuable insight of the anatomic substrate for fatal arrhythmias by documenting the presence of structural abnormalities in up to 97% of athletes who die suddenly (3–5). On the other hand, the interaction of the fixed anatomic substrate with transient factors that may trigger the terminal arrhythmic event remains unexplored. The demands of competitive sports place the athletes in extreme conditions; they have transient electrolyte abnormalities, significant increase in myocardial oxygen demand predisposing to myocardial ischemia, and heightened activity of the autonomic nervous system. These changes may enhance the risk for life-threatening cardiac arrhythmias in the presence of cardiovascular abnormalities (1). Several reviews of sudden death in athletes have revealed that, in the vast majority of cases, death occurred during or immediately after training or competition (3,6,7).

The distribution of heart diseases found in athletes with sudden death may vary according to their age at the time of death, as well as to the geographic area of data collection. Furthermore, there is some discrepancy between the American and the European, especially Italian, literature regarding the prevalence of different types of organic heart disease in athletes suffering from sudden death (6–8). Based on the Italian experience, arrhythmogenic right ventricular (RV) cardiomyopathy is the most frequently encountered cardiovascular disease in both athletic and sedentary young subjects (younger than 35 years old) dying suddenly. The most recent report by Thiene and colleagues included data on 232 consecutive cases of sudden death occurring in the Veneto region of Italy over a 16-year period (7). Forty-six of the study subjects (20%) were young competitive athletes; in 40 of them, sudden death was attributed to cardiac arrhythmic arrest. Among the 40 athletes with sudden arrhythmic death, RV cardiomyopathy was the most common disease (ten cases, 25%), followed by atherosclerotic coronary artery disease (nine cases), congenital anomalies of the coronary arteries (seven cases), pathology of the conduction system (four cases), mitral valve prolapse (four cases), myocarditis (three cases), hypertrophic cardiomyopathy, dilated cardiomyopathy, and long QT syndrome (one case each). Comparing sports-related events with the remaining cases of sudden death in this population, RV cardiomyopathy ($p = 0.001$) and anomalous origin of a coronary artery ($p < 0.001$) were significantly associated with sudden death in athletes. Studies from the United States are at variance with these data. Hypertrophic cardiomyopathy is identified as the most common cause of sudden death in younger athletes (younger than 35 years old), and atherosclerotic coronary artery disease is identified as the most common cause in older athletes (older than 35 years old) (4). According to Maron et al. (4), hypertrophic cardiomyopathy may account for half of the cases of sudden death in young athletes. In victims of sudden death, hypertrophic cardiomyopathy was significantly more common in athletes than in sedentary individuals (5).

Retrospective questioning of surviving relatives revealed that transient symptoms that could conceivably have been of cardiac origin (lightheadedness, syncope, chest pain) were present in 28% of young athletes studied by Maron et al. (3). On the other hand, 50% of the older athletes with coronary artery disease had experienced prodromal cardiovascular symptoms before sudden death or had a known medical history of coronary artery disease (4). Similarly, the fatal event was preceded by warning symptoms or signs in 39% of the young athletes examined by Thiene's group (7). Athletes with RV cardiomyopathy had a history of warning symptoms (palpitations or syncope) and ECG abnormalities [negative T waves in the precordial leads or ventricular premature complexes (VPCs) with left bundle branch block morphology] more often than athletes who died of coronary artery disease. These findings raise the possibility that, if effective screening for structural heart disease is carried out, a subset of athletes at high risk for sudden death may be identified.

ELECTROPHYSIOLOGIC FINDINGS IN ATHLETES SURVIVING SUDDEN CARDIAC DEATH

Studies on athletes with aborted sudden cardiac death provide the opportunity to test the sensitivity of noninvasive and invasive tests for the detection of an arrhythmogenic substrate. In most of those athletes, the arrhythmic event documented at the time of cardiac arrest was a fast ventricular tachyarrhythmia. The most comprehensive set of data on athletes with aborted sudden death comes from the main referral center for arrhythmologic evaluation of athletes in Italy (9–13). The center studied 1,592 competitive athletes (1,315 male athletes and 277 female athletes) performing all types of sports over a 21-year period (13). All underwent assessment for suspected or documented arrhythmias. Twenty-six of those athletes (23 men, three women, mean age 27 years) were referred after having received cardiopulmonary resuscitation for cardiac arrest. The onset of cardiac arrest was related to physical activity in nearly all cases. Prodromal symptoms were present (and ignored) in 11 of the 26 athletes (42%) (six had palpitations, three syncope, and two presyncope). Cardiac arrest was associated with a ventricular tachyarrhythmia in 23 of the 26 cases (89%) and to asystole in the remaining three. Of the tachyarrhythmic events, six were atrial fibrillation with very fast ventricular conduction through an accessory pathway, leading to ventricular fibrillation (VF), and 17 were ventricular tachycardia (VT) or VF. Two cases of VT/VF were associated with QT prolongation. Structural heart disease was diagnosed in all 15 athletes with primary VT/VF (RV cardiomyopathy in six, dilated cardiomyopathy in three, hypertrophic cardiomyopathy in two, coronary artery disease in two, mitral valve prolapse in one, acute myocarditis in one). The two main conclusions of the study were, first, that sudden death is often heralded by exercise-related symptoms. Thus, a correct evaluation of palpitations, syncope, and presyncope occurring during physical activity is of paramount importance. Second, an anatomic arrhythmogenic substrate is usually identifiable in survivors of sudden death.

FINDINGS IN ATHLETES WITH SUSPECTED OR DOCUMENTED COMPLEX VENTRICULAR ARRHYTHMIAS

The workup of athletes with symptoms likely to be related to arrhythmias, or with documented complex ventricular arrhythmias (frequent VPCs or nonsustained VT), should investigate the possible presence of an arrhythmogenic structural abnormality of the heart and assess the prognostic significance of the arrhythmia. Based on their extensive experience, Furlanello et al. (9) have classified arrhythmias seen in athletes into three categories: benign, paraphysiologic, and pathologic. Benign arrhythmias consist of asymptomatic VPCs or atrial premature complexes that occur in the absence of heart dis-

ease and are similar to those found in an untrained population. Paraphysiologic arrhythmias may result from intensive training (e.g., sinus pauses and Mobitz type 1 second-degree atrioventricular block) and do not require withdrawal from sports activity. Pathologic arrhythmias are characterized by adverse hemodynamic effects on athletic performance or are associated with a potentially arrhythmogenic cardiac substrate. The authors' recommendations are similar to those proposed by the 26th Bethesda Conference on sports eligibility, that is, athletes with organic heart disease or malignant arrhythmias should be excluded from high-level competitive activity (14). There is also agreement on the basic diagnostic workup for athletes with potentially serious arrhythmias, such as frequent VPCs and nonsustained VT, as well as athletes with symptoms possibly related to significant arrhythmias. The first tier of investigative tests should include a 24-hour ambulatory ECG, a stress test, and an echocardiogram (14). The ambulatory ECG should be recorded during the relevant sports activity. There is less consensus on the second tier of investigation, which may include programmed stimulation and coronary angiography.

Little is known of the role of programmed stimulation in evaluating athletes with suspected or documented complex ventricular arrhythmias. A largely unexplored issue is the sensitivity and predictive accuracy of programmed stimulation versus stress testing. For example, in a study by Coelho et al. (15) on 19 athletes with documented arrhythmias, a tachyarrhythmia closely resembling the clinical one was induced by programmed stimulation in 68% of cases and during stress testing in 42% of cases. Furlanello and his group applied a cardiac arrhythmia screening protocol in 110 athletes with documented or suspected arrhythmias (10). The protocol included noninvasive tests [ambulatory ECG, stress test, and signal-averaged ECG (SAECG)] as well as invasive investigations (transesophageal atrial pacing at rest and during exercise, and electrophysiologic study in selected cases). Transient bradyarrhythmias were recorded in six athletes, supraventricular tachyarrhythmias in 21, and ventricular tachyarrhythmias in 67. The latter consisted of frequent or complex VPCs in 46 cases, accelerated idioventricular rhythm in three, nonsustained VT in 17, of whom seven had inducible VT, and sustained VT in one top-level athlete, who had inducible sustained VT. Three athletes (two with spontaneous nonsustained VT and one with syncope but no documented arrhythmia) had inducible VF. An underlying structural heart disease was identified in 33 of 110 study cases (30%). The study demonstrated that the most common arrhythmias documented by noninvasive testing in athletes are ventricular in origin and that programmed stimulation frequently induced VT in those with spontaneous nonsustained VT.

AMBULATORY ECG IN ASYMPTOMATIC ATHLETES

Ambulatory ECG recordings in asymptomatic athletes have shown a low prevalence of complex ventricular arrhythmias (Table 1) (16–21). In most studies, transient bradyarrhythmias were more common than tachyarrhythmias. Bradyarrhythmias were also more frequent in athletes than in age-matched nonathletic control subjects (17,20). In a study including 35 highly trained endurance athletes and an equal number of controls, sinus pauses greater than 2 seconds were recorded in 37% of athletes versus 6% of control subjects. First-degree atrioventricular block occurred in 37% of athletes versus 14% of control subjects, Mobitz type 1 second-degree atrioventricular block in 23% of athletes versus 6% of controls, and Mobitz type 2 in 9% of athletes versus none in the control group (17). Similar results were obtained by Palatini et al. (20) in 40 well-trained healthy endurance athletes and 40 sedentary age-matched control subjects. A first-degree atrioventricular block was present in 28% of athletes versus 5% of control subjects ($p<0.01$), whereas a Mobitz type 1 second-degree atrioventricular block was recorded in 15% of athletes and 3% of control subjects ($p = 0.05$). The presence of bradyarrhythmias in asymptomatic athletes may be considered paraphysiologic in most cases and may be related to the level of training (9). The relevance of bradyarrhythmias to sports eligibility was discussed by Zipes et al. (14) during the Bethesda conference.

Authors comparing the characteristics of ventricular ectopy during 24-hour ambulatory ECG (including at least one exercise period) versus conventional stress ECG found that the

TABLE 1. *Prevalence of arrhythmias during 24-hour ambulatory ECG in asymptomatic athletes with no apparent heart disease*

	20 Long-Distance Runners (16)	35 Endurance Athletes (17)	60 Runners (18)	80 Runners (19)	40 Endurance Athletes (20 Cyclists and 20 Runners) (20)
Sinus pauses > 2 sec	2 (10%)	13 (37%)	—	—	—
Rare APCs	19 (95%)	—	10 (17%)	32 (40%)	24 (60%)
Frequent APCs	1 (5%)	—	6 (10%)	1 (1%)	0
First degree AV block	9 (45%)	13 (37%)	—	—	11 (28%)
Second degree AV block					
Type Mobitz 1	8 (40%)	8 (23%)	—	—	6 (15%)
Type Mobitz 2	0	3 (9%)	—	—	—
AV dissociation	1 (5%)	8 (23%)	—	3 (4%)	—
Rare VPCs	12 (60%)	10 (29%)	15 (25%)	35 (44%)	17 (43%)
Frequent VPCs	2 (10%)*	0*	6 (10%)†	6 (8%)*	1 (3%)*
Ventricular couplets	0	0	6 (10%)	2 (3%)	1 (3%)
Nonsustained VT	0	0	0	1 (1%)	3 (8%)

* > 50/24 hours. † > 30/hour. APCs, atrial premature complexes; AV, atrioventricular; VPCs, ventricular premature complexes; — = not reported; † = defined as > 30/hour or > 1/min; VT, ventricular tachycardia.

latter underestimated the frequency of ventricular ectopy (18). Documentation of organic heart disease in athletes with complex ventricular arrhythmias (frequent VPCs or nonsustained VT) should lead to disqualification from high-intensity competitive sports (14). On the other hand, athletes without structural heart disease and with frequent VPCs may participate in all competitive sports. However, if the frequency of VPCs increases during exercise or stress testing to the extent that they produce symptoms, the athlete may participate only in low-intensity competitive sports. Athletes with VT and without structural heart disease established by noninvasive and invasive tests should not compete for at least 6 months. They may later participate in all competitive sports if they remain asymptomatic and if the VT is not recurrent, or is not inducible by physical activity, stress testing, or programmed ventricular stimulation (14).

More recently, 24-hour ambulatory ECG, as well as stress ECG, have been used to investigate heart rate variability in athletes (22–25). This noninvasive technique can evaluate the autonomic nervous system and measure transient changes in sympathovagal interaction. Traditionally, enhancement of sympathetic activity and vagal withdrawal during physical exercise has been indirectly inferred from the increase in heart rate, systolic blood pressure, and myocardial contractility. This, however, is not adequate for evaluation of sympathovagal interaction. The latter could be more accurately assessed by spectral analysis of heart rate variability (24). The low-frequency (LF, 0.1 Hz) and high-frequency (HF, 0.25 Hz) components of the heart rate spectrum are related, respectively, to the cardiac sympathetic and vagal efferent drives. Spectral analysis of heart rate variability has been investigated in trained athletes, detrained athletes, and young, healthy sedentary subjects (22–24). In one study, 12 competitive swimmers (mean age, 16 years) underwent a treadmill stress test according to a modified Bruce protocol, and spectral analysis was performed during each stage of the protocol and for 15 minutes of recovery (24). As expected,

the gradual decrease in RR interval during exercise was associated with a progressive decrease in the RR variance. Spectral analysis revealed an increase in the LF component and a decrease in the HF component. Fifteen minutes after cessation of exercise, both RR interval and its variance tended to return to control values, although the former variable was still significantly lower compared to preexercise levels. The changes in HF and LF components indicated a prevailing sympathetic modulation of the sinus node in the 15 minutes of recovery following exercise. Thus, a persistent sympathetic activation may significantly outlast the end of a single bout of exercise. To test this hypothesis further, 10 sedentary subjects (mean age, 16 years) were examined 1, 24, and 48 hours after the end of a session of maximal dynamic exercise. The latter consisted of a maximal treadmill stress test, followed by four to six repetitive runs, up to exhaustion. The average exercise time was 30 minutes. This study showed that, 1 hour after exercise, the RR interval was still reduced and the LF component was increased compared to preexercise conditions. After 24 hours, RR values returned to preexercise levels, but the LF component remained significantly elevated, thus indicating an ongoing increased sympathetic activation to the heart. Only 48 hours after exercise did RR variability indices return to baseline (22,24). These findings suggest a more important role for the sympathetic nervous system in the genesis of long-term changes induced by athletic training than was previously considered. Goldsmith et al. (25) used 24-hour ambulatory ECG to investigate parasympathetic activity in eight endurance-trained men and eight age-matched control subjects (25). The authors measured a time-domain variable, the standard deviation of all RR intervals (SDNN), as well as several frequency-domain indices: total power (1.15 × 10^{-5} to 0.40 Hz), LF power (0.04 to 0.15 Hz), and HF power (0.15 to 0.40 Hz). The data were analyzed separately for waking and sleeping hours. All time- and frequency-domain measures of heart rate variability were significantly greater in the trained as compared to the untrained subjects. HF power, a measure of vagal tone, was 4.2 times greater in the trained than in the untrained group over the 24-hour period, whereas LF power was 2.8 times greater in the former than in the latter group. Similar results were obtained when the waking and sleeping hours were analyzed separately. Thus, both parasympathetic and, to a lesser extent, sympathetic activity were substantially higher in trained than in untrained men throughout the 24-hour period. There is evidence that the parasympathetic nervous system may have antiarrhythmic properties in survivors of myocardial infarction (26,27). However, studies are needed to define the pos-sible protective role of enhanced vagal activity against cardiac arrhythmias in athletes.

SIGNAL-AVERAGED ECG IN ATHLETES

The SAECG is a noninvasive technique that can detect the presence of delayed ventricular activation on the body surface, usually referred to as *late potentials* (Fig. 1). The origin of late potentials is believed to be depressed ventricular myocardium with slow and inhomogeneous activation patterns that may provide the anatomic/electrophysiologic substrate for reentrant tachyarrhythmias (28).

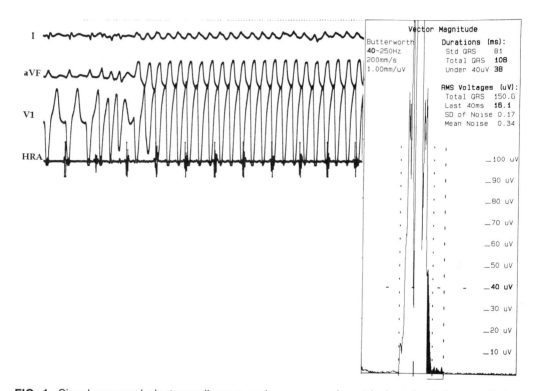

FIG. 1. Signal averaged electrocardiogram and programmed ventricular stimulation results in a 30-year-old basketball player who collapsed during a game. The electrocardiogram recorded at the time of resuscitative efforts showed wide complex tachycardia at a rate of 300/min. A cardiac catheterization showed segmental wall motion abnormalities of the right ventricle, leading to the diagnosis of right ventricular dysplasia. The signal averaged electrocardiogram was abnormal, due to the presence of low-amplitude, low-voltage signals at the end of QRS, consistent with late potentials. Ventricular stimulation with 3 extrastimuli induced sustained monomorphic ventricular tachycardia with a rate of 300/min. This arrhythmia had a left bundle branch block configuration, suggesting its right ventricular origin. Note the atrio-ventricular dissociation during the tachycardia. I, aVF, V1: surface electrocardiographic leads; HRA; intracardiac recording from the high right atrium.

Time-domain analysis of the SAECG derives data from the QRS vector magnitude (the root mean square of three averaged bipolar orthogonal leads, X, Y, and Z). The analysis typically includes the determination of three parameters: (a) the filtered QRS duration, (b) the duration of low-amplitude signals (LAS) of <40 μv, that is, the time that the filtered QRS complex remains below 40 μv; and (c) the root mean square voltage of the terminal 40 msec of the QRS (RMS40). According to the joint Task Force Committee of the European Society of Cardiology, the American Heart Association, and the American College of Cardiology, the definition of an abnormal SAECG has not been fully standardized (29). Using a 40-Hz high-pass filter setting, late potentials may be diagnosed when at least two of the following three criteria are met: (a) QRS duration greater than 114 msec; (b) LAS duration greater than 38 msec; (c) RMS40 voltage less than 20 μv. However, other criteria have been suggested, and the predictive value of the test can vary with the specific criteria that are being applied (30).

Studies of the SAECG in athletes have addressed several issues, including the prevalence of late potentials, the relationship between SAECG parameters and left ventricular mass, and the relationship between an abnormal SAECG and spontaneous or induced ventricular tachyarrhythmias. However, prospective studies on the prognostic value of SAECG to predict sudden death in athletes are lacking.

In healthy sedentary subjects, the prevalence of abnormal SAECG varies from 0% to 26% (29–32). The need to avoid false-positive tests would suggest the use of restrictive criteria for abnormality (e.g., abnormal values of two or three SAECG parameters). On the other hand, an improved specificity would be achieved at the expense of a decreased sensitivity. This may prevent the identification of minor abnormalities that may be related to the presence of a potentially arrhythmogenic substrate in apparently normal athletes (33).

Biffi et al. (34) performed a study to establish the prevalence of late potentials in top-level athletes and to define the relationship between SAECG and athlete's age and body surface values. One hundred top-level male athletes practicing different sports activities were selected. Mean age was 23 ± 2 years and mean body surface area was 2 ± 0.2 m². All underwent a cardiovascular screening to rule out organic heart disease, consisting of clinical evaluation, chest X-ray examination, 12-lead ECG, stress testing, and echocardiogram. If structural heart disease was ruled out, the study subjects had an SAECG. The recordings were analyzed at two filter settings: 25 to 250 and 40 to 250 Hz. Abnormal SAECG was defined as QRS duration greater than 120 msec at 25 Hz and greater than 114 msec at 40 Hz; LAS duration greater than 38 msec for both filters; and RMS40 less than 25 μv at 25 Hz and less than 20 μv at 40 Hz. The prevalence of abnormal SAECG parameters is summarized in Table 2. The table shows that, if the presence of all six SAECG parameters was required to classify a recording as abnormal, the false-positive rate in this

TABLE 2. *Prevalence of abnormal signal-averaged ECG parameters in 100 asymptomatic athletes with no apparent heart disease*

	Filter Setting		
	25–250 Hz	40–250 Hz	25 and 40 Hz
≥ 1 Abnormal parameter	19%	9%	—
≥ 2 Abnormal parameters	11%	6%	—
≥ 3 Abnormal parameters	3%	5%	—
≥ 4 Abnormal parameters	—	—	7%
≥ 5 Abnormal parameters	—	—	4%
6 Abnormal parameters	—	—	2%

Signal-averaged ECG parameters are QRS duration; LAS duration; RMS40 voltage.
Modified from ref. 34, with permission.

healthy athlete population was as low as 2%. By using all three parameters at a single filter setting, the prevalence of an abnormal recording increased to 3% for the 25- to 250-Hz bandpass, and to 5% for the 40- to 250-Hz bandpass. There was no correlation between the type of sports activity and the presence of abnormal SAECG parameters, but there was a weak correlation between these parameters and the athlete's age or body surface area. The highest correlation coefficient was found between QRS duration and body surface area ($r = 0.35$ at 25 Hz, $p<0.0001$; $r = 0.38$ at 40 Hz, $p<0.0001$). However, the presence of abnormal QRS duration was not related to body surface area. The same authors evaluated the correlation between SAECG and left ventricular mass (35). The latter was measured in 153 elite athletes without structural heart disease or cardiac arrhythmias and was indexed to the body surface area. In this population, there was a low prevalence of late potentials (2%) defined as the presence of QRS duration greater than 120 msec, LAS duration greater than 38 msec, and RMS40 less than 25 µv at 25 Hz and less than 20 µv at 40-Hz filter setting. The mean left ventricular mass was 267 ± 64 g (indexed, 133 ± 28 g/m²). There was no significant correlation between left ventricular mass and SAECG. A linear relationship was found only between left ventricular mass and QRS duration, but even extreme ventricular mass (greater than 400 g) was not associated with abnormal QRS duration. Biffi et al. (35) concluded that, given the low prevalence of false-positive results, the SAECG may be a promising test for identifying athletes with potentially arrhythmogenic abnormalities. The same group subsequently studied the prevalence of abnormal SAECG in an athletic population with ventricular arrhythmias, but without apparent heart disease (36). Twenty-five athletes were selected based on the following criteria: normal cardiovascular examination, resting and stress ECG, echocardiogram, radionuclide ventriculography, thallium scintigraphy; and complex ventricular arrhythmias documented by 24-hour ambulatory ECG (defined as greater than

5,000 VPCs and greater than 15 ventricular couplets). Ten athletes consented to programmed ventricular stimulation. The stimulation protocol included the delivery of up to three extrastimuli during three paced cycle lengths (600, 500, and 400 msec) at two RV sites. Criteria for abnormal SAECG were similar to those previously published (34). The documented arrhythmia had a left bundle branch block configuration with inferior frontal plane axis in 20 athletes, a left bundle branch block configuration with superior axis in two, and a right bundle branch block morphology in three. An abnormal SAECG was observed in seven of 25 athletes (28%). There was no significant difference in left ventricular mass between athletes with or without an abnormal recording. Of the ten athletes who underwent programmed stimulation, five had abnormal SAECG. None of the ten athletes had induced sustained VT. Nonsustained VT (six to 25 complexes) was induced in five athletes, of whom four had an abnormal SAECG. In all cases, the morphology of the induced nonsustained VT was similar to the clinical tachycardia. In summary, the study showed a high prevalence of SAECG abnormalities in a population of athletes with apparently normal heart who had significant ventricular arrhythmias. The prevalence of abnormal SAECG was significantly higher than in athletes without documented arrhythmias (28% versus 2%, respectively) (34). Although an abnormal SAECG did not correlate with left ventricular hypertrophy, it was seen more frequently in athletes with nonsustained VT induced by programmed stimulation. The prognostic significance of these findings is, at present, unknown. It is possible that overt heart disease may progress to develop in athletes with complex ventricular arrhythmias and an abnormal SAECG.

The correlation between the SAECG and programmed ventricular stimulation was also investigated by Bettini et al. (33). The study included 78 athletes (69 men, nine women; mean age, 22 years) with ventricular arrhythmias. Twenty-two had sustained VT/VF and 56 had frequent VPCs. In this group, 29

(13%) had no apparent heart disease, 37 (47%) had RV cardiomyopathy, and 12 had other types of heart disease. All 78 athletes underwent SAECG, and 56 had programmed stimulation. The SAECG was analyzed at different filter settings (25, 40, 60, and 80 Hz). For each filter setting, the recording was considered abnormal when at least two of three parameters (QRS duration, LAS duration, and RMS40) were abnormal. By applying these criteria, an abnormal SAECG was recorded in 39% of athletes with arrhythmias. An abnormal recording was more frequent in athletes with heart disease (53%) than in those with no apparent heart disease (14%). It was also more common in athletes with spontaneous sustained VT/VF (73%) than in those with complex ventricular arrhythmias (25%). The sensitivity, specificity, and predictive accuracy of SAECG for spontaneous sustained VT/VF was, respectively, 73%, 86%, and 82%. The sensitivity, specificity, and predictive accuracy of the test for the presence of an underlying arrhythmogenic cardiomyopathy was, respectively, 53%, 86%, and 65%. This high predictive accuracy was probably related to the fact that the vast majority of athletes with organic heart disease had RV cardiomyopathy, a disease which is known to have a high prevalence of late potentials. In the same group, programmed stimulation was performed at two RV sites, with delivery of up to three extrastimuli at three paced cycle lengths (600, 500, and 420 msec) and burst pacing up to a rate of 260 per minute. Sustained VT/VF was induced in 17 cases (30%), including 11 cases with spontaneous sustained VT/VF. Nonsustained VT of at least five complexes was induced in 26 cases (46%), including 18 cases with spontaneous sustained VT/VF. The authors concluded that, given its high predictive accuracy for the presence of cardiomyopathy (65%) and spontaneous sustained ventricular tachyarrhythmias (82%), the SAECG may be viewed as a useful addition to imaging techniques to unmask a clinical or potential arrhythmogenic substrate in athletes (33).

SIGNAL-AVERAGED ECG AS A SCREENING TEST FOR ARRHYTHMOGENIC HEART DISEASES

Published studies on the role of SAECG as a screening test for arrhythmogenic heart disease have some limitations: (a) the study population is usually heterogeneous, including both symptomatic and asymptomatic patients, as well as patients with or without ventricular tachyarrhythmias, (b) the accuracy of the test may be significantly different in mild versus severe forms of the heart disease under investigation, and (c) criteria for recording and analyzing the SAECG are not standardized. The diagnostic yield of the SAECG for the most common types of heart disease found in athletes is discussed in the following paragraphs.

Right Ventricular Cardiomyopathy

Right ventricular cardiomyopathy is a disorder of the RV myocardium that leads to progressive myocardial atrophy with fibrofatty replacement. The electrical instability associated with the disease is explained by disruption of the electrical wavefront as it travels through the diseased RV myocardium. Because the left ventricle is usually spared, cardiac performance is usually normal, thus allowing the patient to endure strenuous physical activities (6). The propensity of patients with RV cardiomyopathy to suffer from arrhythmic death during exercise is most likely linked to the transient hemodynamic and neurohumoral factors associated with exercise. Exercise can result in acute disproportionate increase in RV afterload and dimension. Damage to the subepicardial sympathetic nerve endings may account for a functional or structural sympathetic denervation, resulting in hypersensitivity to catecholamines and enhanced arrhythmogenesis during sympathetic stimulation (7). In approximately 30% of patients with RV cardiomyopathy, a delayed RV activation is evident on the 12-lead ECG as a delayed deflection, which is best seen in the right precordial leads and known as ε wave (37). The sensitivity of the time-domain SAECG is high in RV cardiomyopathy, and the presence of late potentials has been listed as a minor diagnostic criterion for the diagnosis of this disease (38). The prevalence of late potentials varies from 14% to 83% (mean, 62%) (37,39–43). This wide range is probably related to the anatomic extent of the disease, with a lower proportion of abnormal recordings in localized forms and a higher proportion in more advanced stages of RV cardiomyopathy. In a study that may be of some relevance to the athletic population, the characteristics of RV cardiomyopathy were compared in two age categories: a younger group (mean age, 15 ± 5 years) versus an older group (mean age, 38 ± 14 years) (41). Syncope and ventricular arrhythmias on a 24-hour ambulatory ECG were more frequent in the younger group. Time-domain SAECG showed late potentials in 60% of young patients and in 69% of older subjects.

The screening ability of the SAECG for RV cardiomyopathy was tested in family members of patients with known disease (42,43). In an Italian study, 75 members of 11 families, who were classified as either healthy or as having various degrees of RV cardiomyopathy based on echocardiographic criteria, underwent SAECG and 24-hour ambulatory ECG (42). An abnormal SAECG was obtained in 43 of the 75 study subjects: 39 had RV cardiomyopathy and four had normal findings. The SAECG was abnormal in all 16 patients with widespread disease (100%), in 23 of 31 patients with localized disease (74%), and in four of 28 subjects with no evidence of disease (14%) ($p = 0.001$). The overall sensitivity and specificity of the SAECG was, respectively, 83% and 86%. In a French study, conventional ECGs and SAECGs were recorded in 13 patients with RV cardiomyopathy and spontaneous or induced sustained VT and were compared to those from 101 asymptomatic family members (43). The prevalence of ECG abnormalities and late potentials in patients was, respectively, 69% and 62%, whereas in family members it was, respectively, 34% and 16%. These findings strongly suggest that the SAECG may be useful in identifying subjects with asymptomatic RV cardiomyopathy.

Hypertrophic Cardiomyopathy

The arrhythmogenic substrate in hypertrophic cardiomyopathy is represented by a combination of myocardial fiber disarray and postnecrotic ischemic fibrosis (7). The mechanisms by which hypertrophic cardiomyopathy may lead to sudden death may be multiple: (a) slow and inhomogeneous cardiac activation may predispose to reentrant ventricular tachyarrhythmias, (b) transient myocardial ischemia may have a proarrhythmic effect, or (c) acute hemodynamic changes associated with a reduction in left ventricular volume (in the absence of arrhythmias) may precipitate syncope and sudden death. Cripps et al. (44) studied 64 patients with hypertrophic cardiomyopathy and 50 age- and gender-matched control subjects. An abnormal SAECG was more common in patients than in controls (20% versus 4%, $p<0.001$). There was no association between abnormal SAECG and family history of premature sudden death, history of syncope/ presyncope, maximal left ventricular wall thickness, systolic anterior motion of the mitral valve, or maximal rate of oxygen uptake on exercise. A more recent report from the same group included 121 patients with hypertrophic cardiomyopathy and 44 age-matched normal individuals (45). Time-domain SAECG was abnormal in six patients (5%) at 25-Hz filter setting and in ten patients (8%) at 40-Hz filter setting. None of the nine patients with cardiac arrest (of whom eight were 30 years of age or younger) had an abnormal recording. The low prevalence of abnormal SAECG in known patients with hypertrophic cardiomyopathy may limit its usefulness as a screening test for this disease.

Coronary Artery Disease

Congenital or acquired coronary artery disease may precipitate acute myocardial ischemia and fatal ventricular tachyarrhythmias. In patients with congenital coronary anomalies, the acute takeoff angle of the artery may result in narrowing of the coronary ostium. The increased stroke volume associated with physical activity can cause dilatation of the ascending aorta, which, in turn, may lead to an even greater acute takeoff angle of the artery with the coronary ostium assuming a slitlike configuration. This would result in diminished coronary blood flow and myocardial ischemia. It is also possible that dilatation of the aorta and the pulmonary trunk during exercise squeezes the coronary artery with anomalous origin as it passes between these two great vessels.

There is no evidence to support a role of the SAECG as a screening test for silent coronary artery disease. It is unlikely that repetitive episodes of transient myocardial ischemia may create sufficient conduction slowing in localized myocardial zones to generate late potentials (46). On the other hand, acute ischemic syndromes are not associated with transient SAECG abnormalities (47–49). Several studies have documented that myocardial ischemia, occurring spontaneously or during pharmacologic or stress testing, did not induce late potentials on the SAECG. This finding was independent of the presence or absence of abnormal SAECG parameters at baseline, the mechanism of induced ischemia (pharmacologic versus stress testing), the type of ischemia (transmural versus nontransmural), and the presence of complex ventricular arrhythmias during ischemia.

Primary Electrical Disease

Primary electrical disease refers to ventricular tachyarrhythmias occurring in the absence of documented organic heart disease (50–55). The exclusion of unrecognized RV cardiomyopathy is important, especially in patients with right-sided VT (left bundle branch block configuration). The fact that body surface QRST integral mapping and cine magnetic resonance imaging may reveal concealed abnormalities in these patients raises the possibility that some "idiopathic" right-sided VTs may be related to early RV cardiomyopathy (50,51). It is possible that the

SAECG may have a role in identifying patients with concealed focal structural abnormalities of the RV. Another primary electrical disease that may incorporate at least some cases of RV cardiomyopathy is the syndrome characterized by a variable degree of right bundle branch block, persistent ST segment elevation, and sudden cardiac death (52–54). A small number of patients with this syndrome have been reported to show late potentials on the SAECG (52,54).

The value of the SAECG in patients with idiopathic VT has been investigated by Mehta et al. (56) who performed right and left ventricular endomyocardial biopsies in 38 patients with VT (nonsustained in 23 and sustained in 15) and no evidence of structural heart disease. All patients had programmed ventricular stimulation and SAECG. Late potentials were found in 18% of patients, whereas abnormal biopsy results were obtained in 40% of cases and were more common in patients with sustained rather than nonsustained VT (60% versus 26%, $p<0.05$). An increase in fibrous tissue was the most frequent pathologic abnormality. Late potentials were significantly associated with abnormal biopsy findings ($p<0.01$). Programmed stimulation induced the clinical VT in 50% of patients. The presence of late potentials had a moderate sensitivity for abnormal biopsy findings and inducible VT (63% and 37%, respectively), but a high specificity for these variables (84% and 100%, respectively). In another study, Leclercq and Coumel enrolled 132 patients with idiopathic VT (39). Further testing revealed underlying heart disease in 26 of the patients, including 13 with RV cardiomyopathy. Late potentials were present in 81% of the patients with heart disease and only in 4% of those with normal hearts, yielding a sensitivity of 86% and a specificity of 96% for detecting clinically silent arrhythmogenic heart disease.

CONCLUSION

Definition of the anatomic and electrophysiologic substrates of sports-related sudden death is the first step in the attempt to design programs for primary prevention of this event. General screening of athletes at large by conducting a thorough history and physical examination and by performing a 12-lead ECG and an echocardiogram would probably identify most of the athletes with obvious cardiovascular disease and increased risk for sudden death. However, given the low incidence of sudden cardiac death in competitive athletes, a routine screening of this type may be impractical. Diagnostic investigation should instead focus on individuals with relevant symptoms (palpitations, chest pain, syncope/presyncope) or ECG abnormalities, keeping in mind that, in more than half of the cases, sudden death is unheralded. Optimal noninvasive cardiovascular evaluation should include an echocardiogram, a 24-hour ambulatory ECG, a stress ECG, and an SAECG. Programmed ventricular stimulation may be considered for athletes with abnormal findings, but the predictive accuracy of this technique for future arrhythmic events is presently unknown. In conclusion, an effective risk stratification strategy for sudden death in the athlete population remains to be defined.

REFERENCES

1. Maron BJ, Mitchell JH. Revised eligibility recommendations for competitive athletes with cardiovascular abnormalities. *J Am Coll Cardiol* 1994;24:848.
2. Maron BJ, Pelliccia A, Spirito P. Cardiac disease in young trained athletes. Insights into methods for distinguishing athlete's heart from structural heart disease, with particular emphasis on hypertrophic cardiomyopathy. *Circulation* 1995;91:1596.
3. Maron BJ, Roberts WC, McAllister HA, Rosing DR, Epstein SE. Sudden death in young athletes. *Circulation* 1980;62:218.
4. Maron BJ, Epstein SE, Roberts WC. Causes of sudden death in competitive athletes. *J Am Coll Cardiol* 1986;7: 204.
5. Burke AP, Farb A, Virmani R. Causes of sudden death in athletes. *Cardiol Clin* 1992;10:303.
6. Corrado D, Thiene G, Nava A, Rossi L, Pennelli N. Sudden death in young competitive athletes: clinico-pathologic correlations in 22 cases. *Am J Med* 1990;89:588.
7. Corrado D, Basso C, Thiene G. Pathologic findings in victims of sports-related sudden cardiac death. *New Trends Arrhyth* 1995;11:30.
8. Thiene G, Nava A, Corrado D, Rossi L, Pennelli N. Right ventricular cardiomyopathy and sudden death in young people. *N Engl J Med* 1988;318:129.
9. Furlanello F, Bertoldi A, Bettini R, Dallago M, Vergara G. Life-threatening tachyarrhythmias in athletes. *PACE* 1992;15:1403.
10. Bertoldi A, Furlanello F, Fernando F, et al. Cardioarrhythmologic evaluation of symptoms and arrhythmic manifestations in 110 top level consecutive professional athletes. *New Trends Arrhyth* 1993;9:259.
11. Bettini R, Gramegna L, Visona L, Bertoldi A, Dallago M, Furlanello F. Progress in the assessment of athletes with hyperkinetic ventricular arrhythmias. *New Trends Arrhyth* 1993;9:271.
12. Furlanello F, Bertoldi A, Dallago M, et al. Aborted sudden death in competitive athletes. In: Santini M, ed. *Progress in clinical pacing: 1994.* Armonk, NY: Futura Media Services, 1994:733.
13. Bertoldi A, Furlanello F, Fernando F, et al. Young competitive athletes resuscitated from cardiac arrest on field: what have we learned and what can be done? *New Trends Arrhyth* 1995;11:20.
14. Zipes DP, Garson A Jr. Revised eligibility recommendations for competitive athletes with cardiovascular abnormalities. Task Force 6: Arrhythmias. *J Am Coll Cardiol* 1994;24:892.
15. Coelho A, Palileo E, Ashley W, et al. Tachyarrhythmias in young athletes. *J Am Coll Cardiol* 1986;7:237.
16. Talan DA, Bauernfeind RA, Ashley WW, Kanakis C Jr, Rosen KM. Twenty-four hour continuous ECG recordings in long-distance runners. *Chest* 1982;82:19.
17. Viitasalo MT, Kala R, Eisalo A. Ambulatory electrocardiographic recording in endurance athletes. *Br Heart J* 1982;47:213.
18. Pantano JA, Oriel RJ. Prevalence and nature of cardiac arrhythmias in apparently normal well-trained runners. *Am Heart J* 1982;104:762.
19. Pilcher GF, Cook J, Johnston BL, Fletcher GF. Twenty-four-hour continuous electrocardiography during exercise and free activity in 80 apparently healthy runners. *Am J Cardiol* 1983;52:859.
20. Palatini P, Maraglino G, Sperti G, et al. Prevalence and possible mechanisms of ventricular arrhythmias in athletes. *Am Heart J* 1985;110:560.
21. Zehender M, Meinertz T, Keul J, Just H. ECG variants and cardiac arrhythmias in athletes: clinical relevance and prognostic importance. *Am Heart J* 1990;119:1378.
22. Furlan R, Piazza S, Dell Orto S, et al. Early and late effects of exercise and athletic training on neural mechanisms controlling heart rate. *Cardiovasc Res* 1993;27: 482.
23. Rimoldi O, Furlan R, Pagani MR. Analysis of neural mechanisms accompanying different intensities of dynamic exercise. *Chest* 1992;101:226S.
24. Furlan R, Piazza S, Dell Orto S, et al. Heart rate variability in athletes. In: Santini M, ed. *Progress in clinical pacing: 1994.* Armonk, NY: Futura Media Services, 1994:697.
25. Goldsmith RL, Bigger JT Jr, Steinman RC, Fleiss JL. Comparison of 24-hour parasympathetic activity in endurance-trained and untrained young men. *J Am Coll Cardiol* 1992;20:552.
26. La Rovere MT, Specchia G, Mortara A, Schwartz PJ. Baroreflex sensitivity, clinical correlates, and cardiovascular mortality among patients with a first myocardial infarction. *Circulation* 1988;81:939.
27. Bigger JT Jr, Fleiss JL, Steinman RC, Rolnitzky LM, Kleiger RE, Rottman JN. Frequency domain measures

of heart period variability and mortality after myocardial infarction. *Circulation* 1992;85:164.

28. El-Sherif N, Gough WB, Restivo M. Electrophysiologic correlates of ventricular late potentials. In: El-Sherif N, Turitto G, eds. *High-resolution electrocardiography*. Mount Kisco, NY: Futura Publishing, 1992:279.

29. Breithardt G, Cain ME, El-Sherif N, et al. Standards for analysis of ventricular late potentials using high-resolution or signal-averaged electrocardiography: a statement by a Task Force Committee of the European Society of Cardiology, the American Heart Association, and the American College of Cardiology. *J Am Coll Cardiol* 1991;17:999.

30. Caref EB, Turitto G, Ibrahim BB, Henkin R, El-Sherif N. Role of bandpass filters in optimizing the value of the signal-averaged electrocardiogram as a predictor of the results of programmed stimulation. *Am J Cardiol* 1989;64:16.

31. Raineri AA, Marcello T, Rotolo A. Quantitative analysis of ventricular late potentials in healthy subjects. *Am J Cardiol* 1990;66:1359.

32. Turitto G, Mansoor S, Rao S, Caref EB, El-Sherif N. A comparative analysis of commercial software for signal-averaged electrocardiography. *Ann Noninv Electrocardiol* 1996;1:147.

33. Bettini R, Bonato P, Furlanello F. Prevalence of late potentials in normal and arrhythmic athletes. In: Santini M, ed. *Progress in clinical pacing: 1994*. Armonk, NY: Futura Media Services, 1994:707.

34. Biffi A, Verdile L, Ansalone G, Fernando F, Caselli G, Santini M. Prevalenza di potenziali tardivi ventricolari in una popolazione di atleti di elevato livello agonistico. *Int J Sports Cardiol* 1995;4:101.

35. Biffi A, Verdile L, Fernando F, et al. Influence of left ventricular mass on signal-averaged electrocardiogram in top-level athletes. *New Trends Arrhyth* 1995;11:385.

36. Biffi A, Ansalone G, Verdile L, et al. Ventricular arrhythmias and the athlete's heart. Role of signal-averaged electrocardiography. *Eur Heart J* 1996;17:557.

37. Kinoshita O, Fontaine G, Rosas F, et al. Time- and frequency-domain analyses of the signal-averaged ECG in patients with arrhythmogenic right ventricular dysplasia. *Circulation* 1995;91:715.

38. McKenna WJ, Thiene G, Nava A, et al. on behalf of the Task Force of the Working Group Myocardial and Pericardial Disease of the European Society of Cardiology and of the Scientific Council on Cardiomyopathies of the International Society and Federation of Cardiology, supported by the Schoepfer Association. Diagnosis of arrhythmogenic right ventricular dysplasia/cardiomyopathy. *Br Heart J* 1994;71:215.

39. Leclercq JF, Coumel P. Late potentials in arrhythmogenic right ventricular dysplasia. Prevalence, diagnostic and prognostic values. *Eur Heart J* 1993;14[Suppl E]: 80.

40. Berder V, Vauthier M, Mabo P, et al. Characteristics and outcome in arrhythmogenic right ventricular dysplasia. *Am J Cardiol* 1995;75:411.

41. Daliento L, Turrini P, Nava A, et al. Arrhythmogenic right ventricular cardiomyopathy in young versus adult patients: similarities and differences. *J Am Coll Cardiol* 1995;25:655.

42. Oselladore L, Nava A, Buja G, et al. Signal-averaged

electrocardiography in familial form of arrhythmogenic right ventricular cardiomyopathy. *Am J Cardiol* 1995; 75:1038.

43. Hermida J-S, Minassian A, Jarry G, et al. Familial incidence of late ventricular potentials and electrocardiographic abnormalities in arrhythmogenic right ventricular dysplasia. *Am J Cardiol* 1997;79:1375.

44. Cripps TR, Counihan PJ, Frenneaux MP, Ward DE, Camm AJ, McKenna WJ. Signal-averaged electrocardiography in hypertrophic cardiomyopathy. *J Am Coll Cardiol* 1990;15:956.

45. Kulakowski P, Counihan PJ, Camm AJ, McKenna WJ. The value of time and frequency domain, and spectral temporal mapping analysis of the signal-averaged electrocardiogram in identification of patients with hypertrophic cardiomyopathy at increased risk of sudden death. *Eur Heart J* 1993;14:941.

46. Solomon AJ, Tracy CM. The signal-averaged electrocardiogram in predicting coronary artery disease. *Am Heart J* 1991;122:1334.

47. Caref EB, Goldberg N, Mendelson L, et al. Effects of exercise on the signal-averaged electrocardiogram in coronary artery disease. *Am J Cardiol* 1990;66:54.

48. Turitto G, Zanchi E, Risa AL, et al. Lack of correlation between transient myocardial ischemia and late potentials on the signal-averaged electrocardiogram. *Am J Cardiol* 1990;65:290.

49. Turitto G, Caref EB, Zanchi E, Menghini F, Kelen G, El-Sherif N. Spontaneous myocardial ischemia and the signal-averaged electrocardiogram. *Am J Cardiol* 1991; 67:676.

50. Peeters HAP, SippensGroenewegen A, Schoonderwoerd BA, et al. Body-surface QRST integral mapping. Arrhythmogenic right ventricular dysplasia versus idiopathic right ventricular tachycardia. *Circulation* 1997; 95:2668.

51. Carlson MD, White RD, Trohman RG, et al. Right ventricular outflow tract tachycardia: detection of previously unrecognized anatomic abnormalities using cine magnetic resonance imaging. *J Am Coll Cardiol* 1994; 24:720.

52. Martini B, Nava A, Thiene G, et al. Ventricular fibrillation without apparent heart disease: description of six cases. *Am Heart J* 1989;118:1203.

53. Brugada P, Brugada J. Right bundle branch block, persistent ST segment elevation and sudden cardiac death: a distinct clinical and electrocardiographic syndrome. *J Am Coll Cardiol* 1992;20:1391.

54. Corrado D, Nava A, Buja G, et al. Familial cardiomyopathy underlies syndrome of right bundle branch block, ST segment elevation and sudden death. *J Am Coll Cardiol* 1996;27:443.

55. Leenhardt A, Glaser E, Burguera M, Nurnberg M, Maison-Blanche P, Coumel P. Short-coupled variant of torsade de pointes. A new electrocardiographic entity in the spectrum of idiopathic ventricular tachyarrhythmias. *Circulation* 1994;89:206.

56. Mehta D, McKenna WJ, Ward DE, Davies MJ, Camm AJ. Significance of signal-averaged electrocardiography in relation to endomyocardial biopsy and ventricular stimulation studies in patients with ventricular tachycardia without clinically apparent heart disease. *J Am Coll Cardiol* 1989;14:372.

The Athlete and Heart Disease:
Diagnosis, Evaluation & Management,
edited by R. A. Williams.
Lippincott Williams & Wilkins, Philadelphia © 1999.

13

Cardiac Arrhythmias and Electrophysiologic Observations in the Athlete

Mark Steven Link, Paul J. Wang, and N. A. Mark Estes III

New England Medical Center, Tufts University School of Medicine,
Boston, Massachusetts 02111

The evaluation and management of individuals with the symptoms of or a diagnosis of cardiac arrhythmias represents a challenge for the physician. In the athlete, this issue is made even more complex by the psychological, social, physical, and potential economic ramifications of treating young patients in their prime. Supraventricular arrhythmias (other than atrial fibrillation and atrial flutter) are more common in the young patient compared to the older patient. Ventricular arrhythmias in the younger patient are less common than ventricular arrhythmias in the older patient, and they are less commonly associated with coronary artery disease (CAD). However, these ventricular arrhythmias may be associated with a high risk of sudden death, especially when they are found in patients with structural heart disease, as has been demonstrated in several well-known athletes (1,2). Even though sudden cardiac deaths in well-known athletes have occurred, this problem is uncommon. With estimates of up to 25 million competitive athletes, only 10 to 30 sudden deaths are documented per year in athletes younger than age 30 years (3–6). This chapter discusses the evaluation and treatment of cardiac arrhythmias and of symptoms consistent with cardiac arrhythmias in athletes. Also discussed are the problems of evaluating asymptomatic athletes with a diagnosis of structural heart disease that may increase their risk of sudden death. Recommendations for participating in competitive athletics are based on the 26th Bethesda Conference on Recommendations for Determining Eligibility for Competition in Athletes with Cardiovascular Abnormalities (7).

SYMPTOMS

The importance of the history in the evaluation of the athlete with symptoms of cardiac arrhythmias cannot be overstated (8,9). Athletes may have palpitations, lightheadedness, syncope, or even sudden cardiac death. These symptoms can be associated with exertion or can occur at rest. Symptoms that occur with exertion are generally more likely to be serious or life-threatening than those that occur at rest (10,11). However, recent reports of exercise-induced neurocardiogenic syncope have tempered the clinical dictum that exercise-induced syncope is a malignant arrhythmia until proven otherwise (12–15). The symptoms of palpitations and lightheadedness are less commonly associated with life-threatening arrhythmias than are symptoms of syncope. The duration and frequency of symptoms are also important. Symptoms that are frequent and long-lived are somewhat less likely to be life-threatening compared to those that are minutes in duration and infrequent. Whether to proceed with further noninvasive or invasive evaluation of the athlete with symptoms is largely dependent on the history of the patient and the medical history of the family. In an athlete with symptoms consistent with ventricular arrhythmias (sudden onset, injury associated with syncope, exertionally related symptoms), a full evaluation is usually necessary. In an athlete with symptoms suggestive of less serious conditions such as dehydration or neurally mediated syncope (premonitory symptoms, gradual onset of syncope, frequent symptoms, nonexertional symptoms, orthostatic symptoms), little or no further evaluation may be needed. Because many of the structural heart diseases associated with sudden death are genetic in origin, athletes with a family medical history of early sudden death require a thorough workup almost regardless of their symptoms.

STRUCTURAL HEART DISEASE

In addition to the symptoms and family medical history, the determination of structural heart disease is essential in assessing the clinical significance of spontaneous or induced arrhythmias. Nonsustained ventricular arrhythmias in the absence of structural heart disease generally have no prognostic significance. As in the nonathlete, patients with no organic heart disease or only mitral valve prolapse are at a low risk of sudden death. By contrast, the presence of structural heart disease is associated with an increased risk of sudden death. In most North American series on sudden death, hypertrophic cardiomyopathy (HCM) is the most common underlying heart disease in the young athlete (16). After HCM, which accounts for up to 50% of the sudden death patients in North America, anomalous coronary arteries and CAD are the next most common (3). In the athlete older than 30 years old, CAD is the underlying disease in up to 80% of patients (17). However, the experience in Italy is that arrhythmogenic right ventricular dysplasia (ARVD) is the most common underlying organic heart disease (11). The reasons for this difference in the prevalence of ARVD and HCM in North

America and Europe are not entirely clear. In general, it appears that those young patients with HCM, ARVD, and anomalous origin of the coronary arteries are at the highest risk of life-threatening arrhythmias. Ventricular arrhythmias in the setting of congenital heart disease such as Ebstein's anomaly, tetralogy of Fallot, and other stenotic or regurgitant valvular heart diseases also indicate a higher risk of life-threatening arrhythmic events in the athlete (18). Idiopathic dilated cardiomyopathy and acute myocarditis are also rare causes of sudden death. As the athlete ages, CAD becomes more common and accounts for a higher prevalence of heart disease.

ELECTROCARDIOGRAM AND HOLTER MONITORING

It is well recognized that abnormal electrocardiograms (ECGs) are common in athletes. The spectrum of abnormality includes sinus bradycardia, first- and second-degree heart block, early repolarization, left ventricular hypertrophy, and T-wave inversion (19,20). In the ECGs of 289 professional football players, sinus bradycardia was seen in 77%, first-degree atrioventricular (AV) block was seen in 9%, voltage criteria for left ventricular hypertrophy was seen in 35%, and ischemic ST-T wave changes were seen in 13% (21). However, there are certain ECG abnormalities that are associated with heart disease and an increased risk of life-threatening arrhythmias. These abnormalities include the pseudoinfarct pattern seen in HCM (septal q waves) and Wolff-Parkinson-White (WPW) syndrome (inferior q waves) (Fig. 1) (22,23). ARVD patients typically have precordial T-wave inversion (Fig. 2). In addition, these ARVD patients occasionally possess right ventricular conduction delays with a characteristic late depolarization of the right ventricle known as the epsilon wave or even complete right bundle branch blocks (24). Long QT syndrome (LQTS) patients are recognized almost solely by ECG criteria (Fig. 3) (25).

In addition to abnormal ECGs, Holter monitors on athletes demonstrate atrial premature

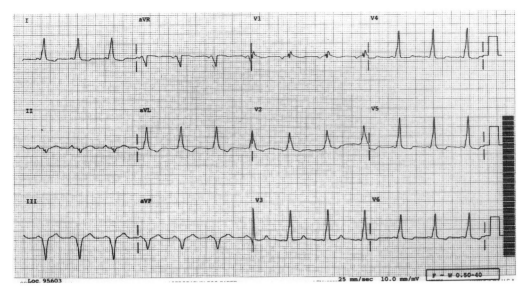

FIG. 1. Surface electrocardiogram of a 40-year-old man with Wolff-Parkinson-White (WPW) syndrome. Note the short PR interval, negative delta waves inferiorly and positive delta waves anteriolaterally. The inferior q waves are typical of a posterior-septal bypass tract and can be misdiagnosed as an inferior wall myocardial infarction. This patient had known WPW syndrome since age 12 years; at age 40 years, he was seen with presyncope, atrial fibrillation, and a ventricular response of up to 300 beats/minute.

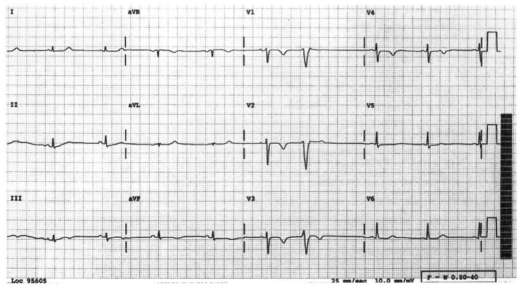

FIG. 2. Surface electrocardiogram of a 35-year-old woman with arrhythmogenic right ventricular dysplasia. Note the inverted T waves anteriorly and a ventricular premature beat with a left bundle morphologic appearance in leads V_1 through V_3. This patient had syncope while jogging. At electrophysiologic evaluation, she was found to have a left bundle morphology ventricular tachycardia. An echocardiogram demonstrated a dilated right ventricle consistent with arrhythmogenic right ventricular dysplasia.

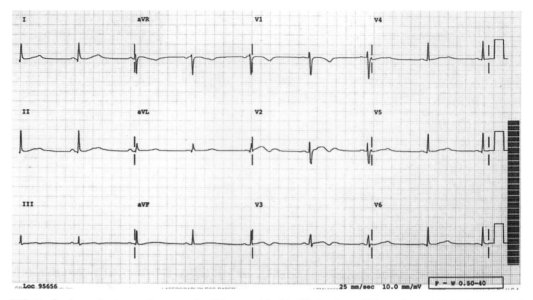

FIG. 3. Surface electrocardiogram of a 17-year-old girl with the long QT syndrome. Note the marked prolongation of the Q-T interval, the prominent U wave, and the unusual appearance of the T and U waves. This patient had recurrent syncope precipitated by bradycardia. With a permanent pacemaker and beta-blocking agents, she has been free of syncope.

contractions, severe sinus bradycardias, first-, second-, and even occasional third-degree heart block, short runs of supraventricular tachycardia, ventricular premature contractions, and short runs of ventricular tachycardia (VT) (19). The bradyarrhythmias and heart block are due to high vagal tone and are reversible with exercise or atropine. Thus, in the absence of symptoms, Holter monitoring is not routinely indicated. Loop monitors in which an ECG recording is initiated by pressing a button on a monitor may be especially useful in those athletes with occasional symptoms.

ELECTROPHYSIOLOGIC OBSERVATIONS

With invasive electrophysiologic testing (EPS), further characterization of the arrhythmia and opportunities for treatment can be made. The principles of EPS are similar in the athlete and the nonathlete. Catheters are placed in the femoral vein and advanced to the right atrium, AV junction, and the right ventricle. A comprehensive EPS evaluation includes evaluation of the sinus node, AV node, His-Purkinje system, assessment for atrioventricular bypass tracts (WPW) and dual AV nodal pathways, and attempts to induce atrial and ventricular arrhythmias. This evaluation is performed in an antiarrhythmic drug-free state. The sensitivity, specificity, and predictive value of EPS are dependent on the clinical presentation, type of abnormality found at EPS, and the underlying organic heart disease.

The evaluation of the sinus node consists of the sinus node recovery time (SNRT). To assess SNRT (and therefore sinus node dysfunction) the high right atrium is paced for 30 to 60 seconds at multiple heart rates. Pacing is then abruptly discontinued. The time from the last paced atrial beat to the first native sinus beat is the sinus node recovery time. SNRT over 1.5 seconds is considered abnormal. However, the sensitivity of the SNRT is poor. Markedly prolonged SNRT is associated with syncope, especially in the patient with sick sinus syndrome. However, the SNRT is affected by vagal influence, and, in the young patient, the significance of a mildly prolonged SNRT is unclear. Specificity in the athlete may also be poor because of the influence of vagal tone. Values of normality and abnormality of the SNRT for athletes are not established.

The evaluation of the AV node includes assessment of conduction, Wenckebach cycle length (heart rate), and assessment for the presence of dual AV nodal pathways that may serve as the anatomic substrate for AV nodal reentrant tachycardia (AVNRT). Wenckebach cycle length is obtained by pacing the atria at faster and faster rates until Wenckebach conduction is seen. Wenckebach cycle lengths are influenced by vagal tone. Vagal tone at rest is often increased in the athlete, and thus the Wenckebach heart rate is often low. However, as exercise is increased, vagal tone is withdrawn. Maximal heart rates with exercise are not affected by the increased vagal tone at rest. Thus, in the athlete, the Wenckebach heart rate is of little predictive value for maximal heart rate with exercise. Testing for dual AV nodal pathways includes decremental atrial stimulation while assessing atrial-His and His-ventricular depolarization. The presence of dual AV nodal pathways is signified by a "jump" in the atrial-His conduction time. This jump signifies conduction block in the fast pathway and conduction over the slow pathway, thus, the presence of dual AV nodal pathways. Dual AV nodal pathways are seen in up to 20% of patients with no clinical AVNRT. Patients with clinical AVNRT are usually inducible during decremental atrial stimulation.

Atrial stimulation can also induce other atrial tachycardias including paroxysmal atrial tachycardia, multifocal atrial tachycardia, atrial fibrillation, atrial flutter, and inappropriate sinus tachycardia. However, the sensitivity and specificity of these tachycardias are low, and often EPS is of little value in the diagnosis or treatment of these tachyarrhythmias.

An EPS also assesses for the presence of atrioventricular accessory pathways. These pathways serve as the anatomic substrate for WPW. Accessory pathways can be manifest on the surface ECG (WPW) or concealed (these pathways only conduct in a retrograde fashion and thus are not seen on the surface ECG). An adenosine infusion can screen for the presence of an antegrade accessory pathway by blocking the AV nodal conduction and thereby making an antegrade bypass tract more manifest. Because accessory pathways are myocardial muscle tissue, fewer than 5% of accessory pathways are affected by adenosine. Rapid atrial pacing frequently unmasks borderline cases of WPW. Accessory pathways conduct more rapidly than the AVN and do not exhibit decremental properties (a property in which the more rapidly the AVN is stimulated, the slower an impulse is conducted). Therefore, as the AVN conduction time lengthens, the accessory pathway becomes more manifest on the surface ECG. The presence of concealed accessory pathways can be assessed by ventricular pacing and the observation of retrograde atrial activation. If accessory pathways are found, it is important to assess for sudden death risk and risk for sustained atrioventricular reentrant tachycardia (AVRT). The risk of sudden death is related to the velocity of impulse conduction antegrade through the accessory pathway. If the conduction is very rapid and the patient has spontaneous atrial fibrillation, the risk of ventricular fibrillation is high (26,27). Refractory times of 250 ms or less (heart rates of 240 or greater) are thought to put the patient at an increased risk of sudden death (28,29).

Ventricular stimulation is performed in an effort to diagnose ventricular arrhythmias and to prognosticate the risk of future arrhythmias, including sudden death. The interpretation of ventricular stimulation is influenced by presenting clinical syndrome, spontaneous arrhythmias, and underlying organic heart disease. The method of ventricular stimulation varies from laboratory to laboratory, but as a rule consists of one to three extrastimuli given in the right ventricular apex or outflow tract at shorter and shorter cycle lengths until refractoriness is observed. These extrastimuli are given in sinus rhythm and after a paced drive train.

Many factors relate to sensitivity, specificity, and predictive value of ventricular stimulation. The first and probably most important determinant of sensitivity is the presence of structural heart disease. Ventricular stimulation is of highest sensitivity in patients with CAD. In CAD patients with spontaneous sustained VT, ventricular stimulation provokes VT in up to 95% of patients (30,31). Furthermore, inducible ventricular arrhythmias after a myocardial infarction predicts new onset of ventricular arrhythmias and sudden death in long-term follow-up (32). Of highest specificity is the induction of sustained monomorphic VT. The induction of VT is rarely seen except in patients who have previously had VT or whose risk of VT in follow-up is quite high (31). However, the significance of inducible nonsustained VT and ventricular fibrillation is less well established. Many authorities claim that the induction of ventricular fibrillation is only significant in patients with a cardiac arrest (33).

Sensitivities and specificities are much lower in patients with HCM, idiopathic dilated cardiomyopathy (IDCM), ARVD, and congenital heart disease than in patients with CAD (34). In the largest series of EPS in HCM patients, 230 patients underwent an EPS evaluation. In these patients, who were not selected based on the occurrence of a clinical arrhythmia, sustained ventricular arrhythmias were induced in 36%. Polymorphic VT was much more common (3:1) than monomorphic VT (35). Of the patients with resuscitated sudden death, a ventricular arrhythmia was induced in 66%. Inducibility in patients with asymptomatic HCM was 30%. Inducible ventricular arrhythmias predicted a higher incidence of cardiac arrest in follow-up, especially in those patients with symptoms of impaired consciousness. However, three of the 17 patients (all three had syncope or resuscitated sudden death) with a subsequent cardiac arrest did not have inducible ventricular arrhythmias (35). It appears that EPS in HCM is most useful in patients with syncope or cardiac arrest. However, even if these patients are noninducible, the risk of sudden death remains high, especially in those with previous syncope or resuscitated sudden death. The use of EPS for screening

asymptomatic HCM patients appears to be quite limited.

In patients with IDCM presenting with spontaneous ventricular arrhythmias, such arrhythmias can be induced in 60% to 70% (36–38). In patients without previous clinical arrhythmias, ventricular arrhythmias can be induced in 10% to 40% (39,40). However, the predictive value of inducible arrhythmias is poor. In most series, patients without inducible arrhythmias have the same risk of subsequent sudden death as those who are inducible (36,38,40). In a review of 377 patients with IDCM undergoing EPS, noninducibility did not confer a high negative predictive value. These noninducible patients have an incidence of sudden death nearly equal (approximately 70%) to that of patients with an induced arrhythmia (34). As in HCM, EPS in IDCM has a poor predictive value and cannot be relied upon to predict future events.

In patients with ARVD who are detected with a ventricular arrhythmia, an arrhythmia can be induced in 70% to 80% (41,42). In these patients with a ventricular arrhythmia, inducibility at EPS increases the risk of subsequent sudden death (43). Yet the use of EPS in ARVD patients who are asymptomatic is unclear. There is even less data on the use of EPS in patients with congenital heart disease. Whereas the occurrence of ventricular arrhythmias and sudden death in patients with repaired tetralogy of Fallot ranges from 1% to 7%, the use of EPS in this situation and other congenital heart disease is unclear (44). In patients with LQTS, programmed electrical stimulation is of limited value and is rarely used (45). Catecholamine infusions and exercise testing have been used to evaluate those patients with suspected LQTS. In patients with LQTS, catecholamine infusions and exercise paradoxically increase the QTc interval (25). In patients with no structural heart disease (idiopathic VT), the sensitivity (46) and specificity (31,47) of EPS are generally high.

Because many athletes with cardiac symptoms have a diagnosis other than CAD, one can see the dilemma of ventricular stimulation with these patients. Whereas EPS in CAD is a useful tool to evaluate symptoms, prognosticate future events, and to guide treatment, the use of EPS in patients with a cardiac diagnosis other than CAD is much less clear. In most of these other conditions, the lower sensitivity and often poor specificity must be taken into account when assessing the results of EPS. However, despite the lower sensitivity and specificity, EPS should be considered in athletes with symptoms that suggest ventricular arrhythmias. EPS should also be considered if these symptoms occur in an athlete with structural heart disease or a family history of early sudden death.

RISK FACTORS FOR SUDDEN CARDIAC DEATH IN SPECIFIC CARDIAC CONDITIONS

Coronary Artery Disease

A number of factors that increase risk of sudden death have been defined for patients with CAD (48). These include more than 10 premature ventricular contractions per hour, nonsustained and sustained VT, inducible VT, low left ventricular ejection fraction, abnormal signal-averaged ECG, and decreased heart rate variability.

Hypertrophic Cardiomyopathy

Risk factors for sudden cardiac death in HCM include family history of sudden death (49), resuscitated sudden death (35,49), and inducible ventricular arrhythmias (35,49). Spontaneous nonsustained VT as a risk factor for sudden death is controversial and may not be an independent risk factor (50,51).

Arrhythmogenic Right Ventricular Dysplasia

In ARVD, risk factors for spontaneous tachyarrhythmias include inducible VT at EPS, drug failure during serial testing, irregular antiarrhythmic drug intake, previous cardiac arrest, and presence of late potentials on signal-averaged electrocardiograms (43). Many patients with ARVD meet one of these criteria.

Risk factors for sudden cardiac death, including syncope (24) and markedly depressed right ventricular function (41), have been described. Furthermore, ARVD is a progressive disease and the patient's risk of sudden cardiac death may increase with time (41,52,53).

Idiopathic Dilated Cardiomyopathy

Although some studies have shown an increased risk of sudden death in IDCM in patients with nonsustained VT and inducible arrhythmias, the most significant risk of sudden death is the degree of LV dysfunction (54). Another factor portending an increased risk of sudden death is the presence of syncope (55).

Long QT Syndrome

Patients with the LQTS are at increased risk of sudden death if there is a family history of sudden death, if they personally have had syncope or resuscitated sudden cardiac death, or if bradycardia is present (25,56).

Anomalous Coronary Arteries

There are no clear risk factors for sudden death in anomalous coronary arteries. Most of the deaths occurring with anomalous coronary arteries occur with exertion.

Normal Hearts

In the individual with a normal heart, the only arrhythmia that is an ominous predictor is clinical sustained VT or ventricular fibrillation (57). Nonsustained VT and frequent premature ventricular contractions, even if exercise induced, do not increase the risk of sudden death (58,59).

TREATMENT OF SUPRAVENTRICULAR TACHYARRHYTHMIAS IN ATHLETES

Although most atrial arrhythmias are not life-threatening, there are occasional occurrences of sudden death due to these tachyarrhythmias. These sudden deaths can occur with WPW, but are also reported in AVNRT and in patients with HCM (60,61). Treatment of supraventricular arrhythmias can be accomplished with beta-blocking agents, calcium channel blocking agents, digoxin, antiarrhythmic agents, and ablative procedures (Table 1). Beta-blockers can be effective in many patients; however, they are banned in some competitive sports and many young patients have intolerable side effects. Calcium channel blocking agents and digoxin are not as effective as beta-blockers in many supraventricular arrhythmias. Antiarrhythmic agents are effective in many supraventricular tachyarrhythmias, but concern about proarrhythmias and long-term use limit their use in this young patient cohort. The two most common supraventricular arrhythmias (AVNRT and WPW) are usually readily cured with radiofrequency ablation (RFA). This procedure can be accomplished with low morbidity, and, in the young athlete, radiofrequency ablation should often be considered as initial treatment. The

Bethesda Conference recommends 6 months of a symptom-free period before a return to competitive athletics in those patients with supraventricular tachyarrhythmias and syncope, near syncope, or significant palpitations (62). However, athletes who undergo RFA can return to competitive athletics in 3 months if they have no recurrence of arrhythmias (62).

Atrioventricular Nodal Reentrant Tachycardia

The treatment of AVNRT has undergone a revolution with the initiation and widespread use of RFA. Whereas medications and cardiac surgery were the only treatment prior to 1990, RFA now has become the opportunity to cure the patient and avoid surgery and pharmacologic treatment. Many authorities consider RFA of AVNRT to be a first line treatment, even before a trial of pharmacologic agents (63,64). With current techniques, RFA can cure patients with AVNRT greater than 95% of the

TABLE 1. *Supraventricular arrhythmias**

Condition	Symptoms	ECG	Diagnosis	Treatment Options	Competitive Athletics
AVNRT	Palpitations LH Syncope	NL	Monitor EPS	BB Digoxin Ca ch ant RFA	After 3 to 6 months of a symptom-free period
WPW	Asymptomatic	Short PR delta waves	ECG EPS	No therapy RFA if high risk	In order to compete athletes should undergo an EPS to stratify risk of SCD.
WPW	Palpitations LH Syncope	Short PR delta waves	ECG EPS	Antiarrhythmics RFA	After 3 to 6 months of a symptom-free period
Atrial fibrillation	Palpitations	Often NL	Monitor	Rate control Anticoagulation Antiarrhythmics	If warfarin is used for anticoagulation, sports with bodily contact should be prohibited.
Atrial flutter	Palpitations	Often NL	Monitor	Rate control Anticoagulation Antiarrhythmics RFA	If warfarin used for anticoagulation, sports with bodily contact should be prohibited.
APCs	Palpitations	Often WNL	Monitor	Reassurance BB if disabling symptoms	No restrictions

*Recommendations for participating in competitive athletics are based on the 26th Bethesda Conference on Recommendations for Determining Eligibility for Competition in Athletes with Cardiovascular Abnormalities.

ECG, electrocardiogram; AVNRT, atrioventricular reentrant tachycardia; LH, lightheadedness; NL, normal; EPS, electrophysiologic study; BB, beta-blockers; Ca ch ant, calcium channel antagonists; RFA, radiofrequency ablation; WPW, Wolff-Parkinson-White syndrome; SCD, sudden cardiac death; APC, atrial premature complex.

time, eliminating the need and risk of drugs. The procedure is of relatively low risk. The most common serious complication is complete heart block requiring a permanent pacemaker. This complication is seen in less than 1% of patients (64). In the athlete with a cultural fear of medicines and with the problems with prohibited drugs (including beta-blockers) and the frequent recurrences of this tachyarrhythmia, RFA should be offered as an early option.

Wolff-Parkinson-White/Concealed Accessory Pathways

As with AVNRT, RFA should be considered as the initial treatment of patients with *symptomatic* WPW (63,64). Symptoms of WPW include palpitations, presyncope, syncope, and even resuscitated sudden cardiac death. Whereas pharmacologic treatment can be ef-

fective, the lifelong risk of antiarrhythmic drugs and chance of arrhythmia breakthrough outweigh the short-term risk of RFA. In the patient at risk for sudden death (rapidly conducting accessory pathways), pharmacologic therapy should not be relied upon, especially in the athlete (Fig. 4). Pharmacologic treatment may still have a role in patients with accesory pathways very near their AVN (increased risk of permanent pacemaker) and in patients unwilling to undergo RFA. Pharmacologic therapy surely has a role in the short-term management of the symptomatic patient with WPW.

Controversy exists with patients who have a manifest accessory pathway on their surface ECG but are without symptoms. It appears that the risk of sudden death in these completely asymptomatic patients is low (28,65). Sudden death is an uncommon first manifestation of this syndrome (27). Electrophysiologic testing in selected patients has been proposed to eval-

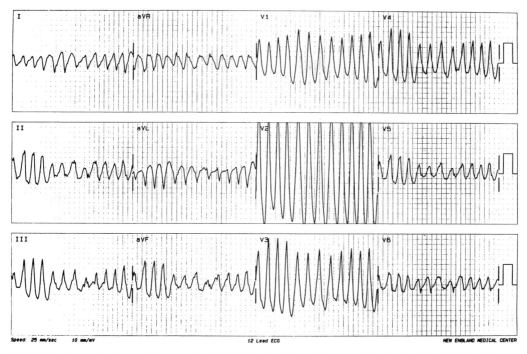

FIG. 4. Surface electrocardiogram of atrial fibrillation in a 29-year-old patient with Wolff-Parkinson-White syndrome and multiple bypass tracts. Note the slight changes in morphology of the QRS complex depending on which accessory pathway contributes most to the depolarization of the ventricle. In atrial fibrillation, ventricular depolarization is up to 270 beats/minute. This patient presented with recurrent presyncope and palpitations and underwent a radiofrequency ablation of several accessory pathways.

uate the risk of sudden death in asymptomatic patients with WPW. If the accessory pathway is able to conduct atrial impulses to the ventricle at greater than 240 bpm, then the patient is at higher risk of sudden death. Approximately 20% of asymptomatic patients have these rapidly conducting accessory pathways, and it is in these individuals that ablation would be advised. If the accessory pathway conducts impulses at rates lower than 240 bpm, it is thought that the risk of sudden death in follow-up is extremely low (28,29). Because of the low risk of sudden death in asymptomatic patients, most authorities recommend electrophysiologic evaluation only in those patients with high-risk occupations (e.g., airline pilots, bus drivers). Many, if not most, authorities include athletes in those high-risk occupations because, with increased adrenergic stimulation, it is feared that accessory pathways may conduct even more rapidly (27,66,67).

Atrial Fibrillation/Atrial Flutter

Atrial fibrillation and atrial flutter are the most common arrhythmias seen in the general population, although they are unusual in younger patients. Treatment of these arrhythmias is more difficult in the athlete because of the frequent need for anticoagulation. Options for treatment include rate control alone (predominantly in those with lone atrial fibrillation), rate control with anticoagulation, antiarrhythmic agents to prevent atrial fibrillation recurrences, or RFA. In patients without structural heart disease or other risk factors for stroke (hypertension, previous thromboembolism), aspirin alone may be adequate (68). In the athlete, especially with Paroxysmal Atrial Fibrillation (PAF), this would likely be the most reasonable choice. Coumadinization in patients with structural heart disease or risk factors for stroke, lowers the risk of stroke. However, coumadinization increases the risk of bleeding and is contraindicated in competitive sports that have a risk of bodily contact or trauma (62). There is concern that all antiarrhythmic agents other than amiodarone increase sudden death risk (68). Therefore, an-

tiarrhythmic therapy is not an attractive alternative in young athletes. Ablative techniques for atrial fibrillation and atrial flutter are rapidly evolving, and cure rates for atrial flutter are as high as 90% (69). In the athlete with atrial flutter, early ablation may be preferable to anticoagulation and antiarrhythmic agents. However, in those athletes with atrial fibrillation, curative catheter techniques are not yet sufficiently advanced to be of clinical utility.

Paroxysmal Atrial Tachycardia, Inappropriate Sinus Tachycardia

With these more unusual arrhythmias, pharmacologic therapy with beta-blocking agents or calcium channel blockers is the initial therapy. These tachycardias do not increase the risk of sudden death or of embolic events. Antiarrhythmic agents can also be effective, but the risk of proarrhythmia with these agents is of concern for treatment of such relatively benign conditions. The experience of RFA for these tachyarrhythmias is limited and generally should be considered only after standard therapy has failed (64).

TREATMENT OF VENTRICULAR ARRHYTHMIAS IN THE ATHLETE

The alternatives and options for the treatment of ventricular arrhythmias (Tables 2 and 3), are not as appealing as for the supraventricular arrhythmias mainly because very few ventricular tachyarrhythmias are curable and the lifetime risk of sudden cardiac death remains high. Perhaps the only real cures are seen in those patients with no underlying heart disease and idiopathic VT or right ventricular outflow tract VT (64). In these patients without structural heart disease, cure rates with RFA approach 90% with a low incidence of complications (70,71). Thus, in the athlete with no structural heart disease and VT, RFA is an ideal treatment. On the other hand, in patients with underlying organic heart disease, cure of the underlying disease and thus of their predisposition to ventricular arrhythmias is unlikely. RFA in ventricular arrhythmias in the presence of heart disease is investigational and cannot be

TABLE 2. *Diagnosis and management of ventricular arrhythmias in athletes**

Condition	Symptoms	ECG	Diagnosis	Treatment Options	Competitive Athletics
VPCs	Palpitations	NL	Monitor	Reassurance BB	No restrictions
NSVT	Palpitations	Often NL	Monitor	Assess for SHD If no SHD, reassure. If SHD, further evaluation is needed	No restrictions if no SHD If SHD present, see table
VT/VF	Palpitations Syncope Sudden death	Can be NL or reflective of underlying disease	Monitor	RFA if no SHD ICD or AAD if SHD present	No restrictions if no SHD and cure by RFA Restricted to low-intensity sports for all others

*Recommendations for competitive athletics are based on the 26th Bethesda Conference.
ECG, electrocardiogram; VPC, ventricular premature contractions; NL, normal, SHD, structural heart disease; BB, beta-blockers; NSVT, nonsustained ventricular tachycardia; VT, ventricular tachycardia; VF, ventricular fibrillation; RFA, radiofrequency ablation; ICD, implantable cardioverter defibrillator; AAD, antiarrhythmic drugs.

TABLE 3. *Ventricular arrhythmias in different forms of structural heart disease*

Condition	Symptom	ECG	VT morph	Treatment Options	Competition Athletics
Idiopathic LV-VT	Palpitations LH, syncope	Nl	RB, left axis	RFA	No restrictions 3 months after RFA
Idiopathic RVOT VT	Palpitations LH, syncope	Nl	LB, inf axis	RFA	No restrictions 3 months after RFA
HCM	Palpitations Syncope SCD	Q's-ant		BB AAD Myomectomy ICD	Only low intensity
ARVD	Palpitations Syncope SCD	T-inv ant RBBB Epsilon wave	LB, inf axis	Sot or amio ICD RFA	Only low intensity
CAD	Palpitations Syncope SCD	Infarcts Ischemic ST	RB or LB	AAD ICD Surgery	Only low intensity
IDCM	Palpitations Syncope SCD	Often LBBB	RB or LB	Amio ICD	Only low intensity
LQTS	Palpitations Syncope SCD	Long QTc	Torsades	BB PPM ICD	Only low intensity
Anomalous CAD	SCD	NL	VF	CABG	No restrictions after CABG

ECG, electrocardiogram; VT, ventricular tachycardia; LV, left ventricle; LH, lightheadedness; Nl, normal; RB, right bundle; RFA, radiofrequency ablation; RVOT, right ventricle outflow tract VT; LB, left bound; HCM, hypertrophic cardiomyopathy; SCD, sudden cardiac death; BB, beta-blockers; AAD, antiarrhythmic drugs; ICD, implantable cardioverter defibrillator; ARVD, arrhythmogenic right ventricular dysplasia; RBBB, right bundle branch block; LBBB, left bundle branch block; sot, sotalol; amio, amiodarone; PPM, permanent pacemaker, CABG, coronary artery bypass surgery.

relied upon to protect against sudden death (70). According to the Bethesda Conference, only low-intensity competitive athletics is permitted in athletes with structural heart disease and sustained ventricular arrhythmias, without regard to the method of treatment (62).

Hypertrophic Cardiomyopathy

In the patient with HCM, several strategies have been developed and include surgery, beta-blockers, antiarrhythmic agents, permanent pacemakers, and implantable cardioverter defibrillators (ICDs) (22). Although surgery decreases the risk of sudden cardiac death, it does not eliminate it. The same can be said of beta-blockers, amiodarone, and pacemakers. Indeed, implantation of the ICD is the surest way to prevent sudden cardiac death in the patient with HCM. In athletes with HCM who survive sudden death, an ICD should be offered. In others thought to be at high risk

based on family medical history of sudden death or with inducible ventricular arrhythmias, an ICD may be appropriate. In patients with a lower risk of sudden death, an ICD is an option, but it is not universally agreed upon. In most individuals with HCM, competitive athletics should be prohibited and beta-blockers should be prescribed (72).

Arrhythmogenic Right Ventricular Dysplasia

In the patient with ARVD, there are limited options for treatment. Because ARVD is a likely progressive disease, treatments effective at one point may become ineffective later in time (41,52). RFA is rarely curative (53,73,74). Sotalol is thought to be particularly effective in these patients (75). Current opinions of the optimal treatment of these patients vary, but in those of sufficiently high risk for sudden death, an ICD should be considered (Figs. 5 and 6)

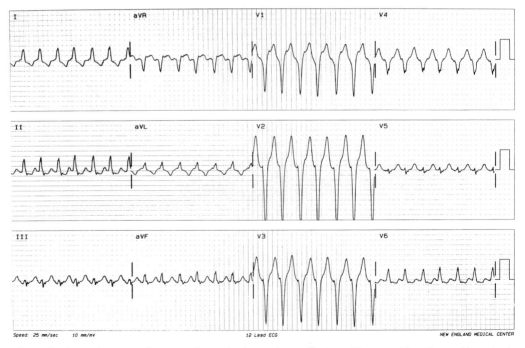

FIG. 5. Surface electrocardiogram of ventricular tachycardia in a 33-year-old patient with arrhythmogenic right ventricular dysplasia. Note the left bundle morphology and inferior axis of the ventricular tachycardia. This patient presented with a cardiac arrest during skiing at age 25 years. She was initially given antiarrhythmic agents, but because of recurrent events she underwent implantation of an implantable cardioverter defibrillator.

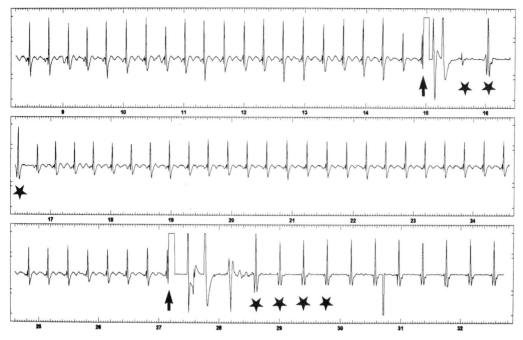

FIG. 6. Continuous intracardiac tracings from an implantable cardioverter in a 36-year-old patient with arrhythmogenic right ventricular dysplasia. **Top panel:** A ventricular tachycardia of 180 beats/minute is seen. In the last few seconds of the top panel, a cardioversion by the implantable cardioverter defibrillator (ICD) is seen (*arrow*). The patient has three beats of a sinus rhythm (*stars*) followed by reinitiation of his ventricular tachycardia (**middle panel**). **Lower panel:** Successful cardioversion of the ventricular tachycardia is seen.

(24,76). Moderate- and high-level competitive athletics are contraindicated in view of the frequent provocation of arrhythmias with exercise (62).

Idiopathic Dilated Cardiomyopathy

In the patient with IDCM, the optimal treatment is not yet clear, but several principles are generally agreed upon. Class 1 antiarrhythmic agents are rarely effective and are possibly toxic; thus, they should be avoided. Beta-blockers are probably quite effective in this patient group and should be prescribed to all patients who can tolerate them. Angiotensin-converting enzyme inhibitors lower the risk of all-cause mortality and sudden death and should also be prescribed to all patients. Amiodarone may have the highest efficacy of all antiarrhythmic agents for life-threatening ventricular arrhythmias in this condition (77). However, the optimal place of amiodarone and ICD therapy is yet

to be determined (78). In patients with IDCM and a prior spontaneous sustained ventricular arrhythmia, competitive athletics of moderate or high intensity should be avoided (62).

Long QT Syndrome

Certainly, most patients with the LQTS should be placed on beta-blockers (Fig. 7). Whether permanent pacemakers should be first-line therapy is controversial, but it is generally agreed that bradycardia or recurrent symptoms with beta-blocker therapy are indications for permanent pacemaking. More controversial treatments include ganglionectomy and ICD therapy (79).

Coronary Artery Disease

In the patient with CAD and ventricular arrhythmias (Fig. 8), EPS is more predictive of

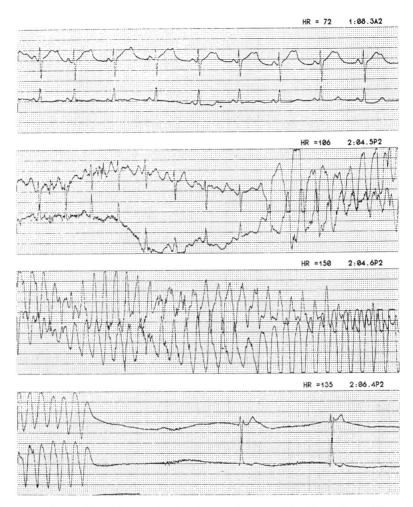

FIG. 7. Electrocardiographic Holter monitoring from a 17-year-old with the long QT syndrome. **Top panel:** Marked prolongation of the T wave is seen. After the peak of the T wave, a U wave is seen. **Second panel:** Torsades de pointes begins. This torsades continued for a full 2 minutes at 300 beats/minute and terminated spontaneously **(bottom panel)**. This patient presented with multiple syncopal episodes at the age of 15 years. She was initially diagnosed with a seizure disorder, but with this Holter monitor and electrocardiograms, the diagnosis of the long QT syndrome was made. This patient was initially given a β-adrenergic blocking agent. After recurrent presyncope and palpitations, the patient underwent a sympathetic ganglionectomy and implantation of a permanent pacemaker.

response to antiarrhythmic therapy. However, even those patients made noninducible by an antiarrhythmic agent have a yearly sudden death incidence of 5% to 10% (48). Class I agents currently have little role in the management of arrhythmias in these patients. Amiodarone is more effective than these conventional agents in the prevention of sudden death. Currently, ICDs may offer the best protection against sudden death. However, whether ICDs or amiodarone prolong life is being tested in three major randomized trials, the results of which are pending (80). In athletes with CAD and ventricular arrhythmias, only low-intensity competitive athletics are permitted (62).

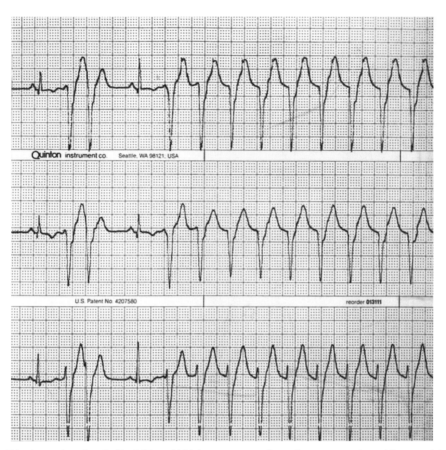

FIG. 8. Rhythm strips (leads II, aVF, and V$_5$) from an exercise tolerance test in a 49-year-old patient with coronary artery disease. Ventricular tachycardia occurred in the recovery period. This patient presented with recurrent symptomatic nonsustained ventricular tachycardia during cardiac rehabilitation. During evaluation with an exercise tolerance test, sustained ventricular tachycardia was seen. At electrophysiologic evaluation, this patient was inducible to ventricular tachycardia and received an implantable cardioverter defibrillator.

BRADYARRHYTHMIAS

Sinus bradyarrhythmias are almost universal in the athlete and should be considered normal (Table 4). Multiple studies have shown heart rates as low as 25 bpm during sleep. First-degree and Mobitz I second-degree block are frequently seen. Mobitz II heart block and third-degree heart block are reported, but are much rarer (19,81). Increased vagal tone is thought to be the basis for most of these bradyarrhythmias. Although resting bradycardia is often extreme, maximal

sinus rates are preserved. Permanent pacemakers should rarely be needed in those patients with first-degree or Mobitz I heart block. According to the Bethesda Conference guidelines, athletes with first-degree or Mobitz I heart block that does not worsen with exercise do not need treatment or restriction of competitive athletics. However, athletes with Mobitz II or complete heart block should have competitive athletics prohibited until permanent pacing is accomplished (Fig. 9). Athletes with permanent pacemakers should not participate in competitive athletics with a danger

TABLE 4. *Algorithm for bradyarrhythmias**

Condition	Symptoms	Diagnosis	Treatment Options	Competitive Athletics
1st degree HB	None	ECG	None	No restrictions
Wenckebach	None	Monitor, ECG	None	No restrictions
Wenckebach	LH, syncope	Monitor, ECG	PPM	No bodily collision if PPM present
Mobitz II or CHB	None	Monitor, ECG	PPM	No bodily collision
Mobitz II or CHB	LH, syncope	Monitor, ECG	PPM	No bodily collision

*Note should be made of the recommendation for prophylactic pacemaker insertion for those patients with Mobitz II heart block or higher. Note should also be made of the recommendations for avoiding sports with bodily contact after a pacemaker is inserted (Based on the 26th Bethesda Conference).

HB, heart block; ECG, electrocardiogram; LH, lightheadedness; PPM, permanent pacemaker; CHB, complete heart block.

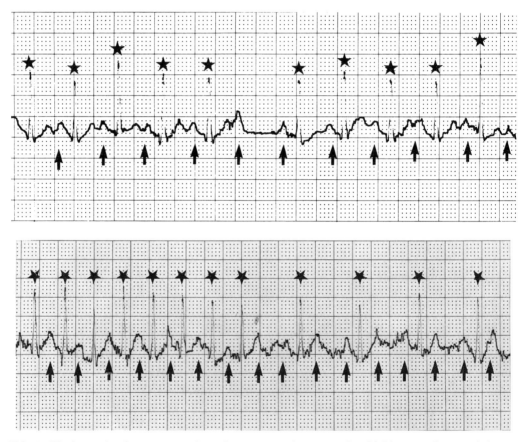

FIG. 9. Rhythm strips from an exercise tolerance test demonstrating Mobitz type II second degree heart block in a 19-year-old defensive end. The P waves are marked by arrows and the QRS complexes are marked by stars. Early in the test (**top panel**), a single nonconducted sinus beat is seen. **Bottom panel:** An abrupt change from 1:1 AV conduction to 2:1 AV conduction is seen. This fit young man complained of dyspnea on exertion.

of bodily collision (62). Although case reports of asystole following exercise have been reported (82), these cases are too rare to have an impact on general therapy.

SYNCOPE

Syncope is seen in up to 20% of the general population. The incidence increases with age. Syncope in the athlete is not as common as in the general population and must be fully evaluated. A prior history of syncope is frequently found in the young patient who experiences sudden death (83). Benign conditions such as hyperventilation and dehydration rarely cause syncope in the athlete and should be considered a diagnosis of exclusion. Neurocardiogenic syncope is the most common cause of syncope seen in the young and therefore it is the most probable cause of syncope in the young athlete. Syncope that occurs at peak exercise should be considered pathologic until proven otherwise (11,83,84). Patients with HCM, ARVD, anomalous coronary arteries, and CAD frequently have syncope at maximal exertion. This syncope can be hemodynamically caused in HCM, but it is often of arrhythmic origin. ARVD and CAD exercise-induced syncope is most frequently arrhythmic in origin. Therefore in the athlete with syncope, the evaluation for organic heart disease is of paramount importance. If there is organic heart disease or a family medical history of sudden death, then more testing, often including EPS, is necessary.

Neurocardiogenic syncope is almost certainly the most common cause of syncope in the young patient, and the diagnosis is usually readily apparent from the history. Most cases of neurocardiogenic syncope occur after prolonged standing, fright, or anxiety. A prodrome of a sensation of warmth, sweating, and lightheadedness is frequent. Acute drop attacks are unusual. The loss of consciousness is short-lived and unlikely to be associated with injury, loss of bowel or bladder continence, or postevent confusion. Recently, cases of exercise-induced neurocardiogenic syncope have been reported (12–15). In these se-

ries, syncope occurs during exercise or within 1 minute of stopping exercise. Most of these patients had abnormal tilt tests. The long-term prognosis with medical treatment in these patients was generally excellent and many of these patients returned to athletics. (See Chapter 14 for further details on head-upright tilt testing.)

CONCLUSION

The athlete with arrhythmias or symptoms of arrhythmias shares many characteristics with the nonathlete. Foremost of these similarities are the similar physiology and pathophysiology of syncope, presyncope, and cardiac arrhythmias. However, there are important differences between athletes and nonathletes. Many of the athletes are young. There is a lower incidence of coronary disease and a higher incidence of various other cardiomyopathies. It is in these patients with nonischemic cardiomyopathies that electrophysiologic testing is not as predictive as in the patient with coronary disease. Therefore, one is often unsure of the true origin of symptoms and the risk of sudden death in subsequent follow-up. The treatment of arrhythmias for the athlete offers some unique challenges; often an attempt is made to avoid pharmacologic therapy and to maximize the athlete's ability to play. RFA should be offered to those athletes with conditions in which a cure is possible. In those in whom a cure is unlikely or in whom the diagnosis remains in doubt, a difficult decision awaits the athlete, the coaches, and the physicians. Whether to allow play depends on several factors, including the relative certainty of diagnosis, the hazards of play, and the consequences if the presumptive diagnosis is wrong (85).

REFERENCES

1. Kassirer JP. Diagnosis in the public domain. *N Engl J Med* 1993;329:50–51.
2. Maron BJ. Sudden death in young athletes: lessons from the Hank Gathers affair. *N Engl J Med* 1993;329:55–57.
3. McCaffrey FM, Braden DS, Strong WB. Sudden cardiac death in young athletes. *Am J Dis Child* 1991;145: 177–183.

4. Driscoll DJ, Edwards WD. Sudden unexpected death in children and adolescents. *J Am Coll Cardiol* 1985;5: 118B–121B.

5. Epstein SE, Maron BJ. Sudden death and the competitive athlete: perspectives on preparticipation screening studies. *J Am Coll Cardiol* 1986;7:220–230.

6. Rich BSE. Sudden death screening. *Med Clin North Am* 1994;78:267–288.

7. 26th Bethesda Conference: Recommendations for determining eligibility for competition in athletes with cardiovascular abnormalities. *J Am Coll Cardiol* 1994; 24:845–899.

8. Kapoor WN. Evaluation and outcome of patients with syncope. *Medicine* 1990;69:160–175.

9. Calkins H, Shyr Y, Frumin H, Schork A, Morady F. The value of the clinical history in the differentiation of syncope due to ventricular tachycardia, atrioventricular block, and neurocardiogenic syncope. *Am J Med* 1995; 98:365–373.

10. McGovern BA, Liberthson R. Arrhythmias induced by exercise in athletes and others. *S Afr Med J* 1996;86: C78–C82.

11. Corrado D, Thiene G, Nava A, Rossi L, Pennelli N. Sudden death in young competitive athletes: clinicopathologic correlations in 22 cases. *Am J Med* 1990;89: 588–596.

12. Sneddon JF, Scalia G, Ward DE, McKenna WJ, Camm AJ, Frenneaux MP. Exercise induced vasodepressor syncope. *Br Heart J* 1994;71:554–557.

13. Sakaguchi S, Shultz JJ, Remole SC, Adler SW, Lurie KG, Benditt DG. Syncope associated with exercise, a manifestation of neurally mediated syncope. *Am J Cardiol* 1995;75:476–481.

14. Calkins H, Siefert M, Morady F. Clinical presentation and long-term follow-up of athletes with exercise-induced vasodepressor syncope. *Am Heart J* 1995;129: 1159–1164.

15. Kosinski D, Grubb BP, Kip K, Hahn H. Exercise-induced neurocardiogenic syncope. *Am Heart J* 1996; 132:451–452.

16. Maron BJ, Shirani J, Poliac LC, Mathenge R, Roberts WC, Mueller FO. Sudden death in young competitive athletes: clinical, demographic, and pathologic profiles. *JAMA* 1996;276:199–204.

17. Maron BJ, Epstein SE, Roberts WC. Causes of sudden death in competitive athletes. *J Am Coll Cardiol* 1986;7: 204–214.

18. Graham TP Jr, Bricker JT, James FW, Strong WB. Task Force 1: congenital heart disease. *J Am Coll Cardiol* 1994;24:867–873.

19. Zehender M, Meinertz T, Keul J, Just H. ECG variants and cardiac arrhythmias in athletes: clinical relevance and prognostic importance. *Am Heart J* 1990;119: 1378–1391.

20. Oakley CM. The electrocardiogram in the highly trained athlete. *Cardiol Clin* 1992;10:295–302.

21. Balady GJ, Cadigan JB, Ryan TJ. Electrocardiogram of the athlete: an analysis of 289 professional football players. *Am J Cardiol* 1984;53:1339–1343.

22. Wigle ED, Rakowski H, Kimball BP, Williams WG. Hypertrophic cardiomyopathy: clinical spectrum and treatment. *Circulation* 1995;92:1680–1692.

23. Wang K, Asinger R, Hodges M. Electrocardiograms of Wolff-Parkinson-White syndrome simulating other conditions. *Am Heart J* 1996;132:152–155.

24. Marcus FI, Fontaine G. Arrhythmogenic right ventricular dysplasia/cardiomyopathy: a review. *PACE* 1995;18: 1298–1314.

25. Jackman WM, Friday KJ, Anderson JL, Aliot EM, Clark M, Lazzara R. The long QT syndromes: a critical review, new clinical observations and a unifying hypothesis. *Progr Cardiovasc Dis* 1988;31:115–172.

26. Klein GJ, Bashore TM, Sellers TD, Pritchett EL, Smith WM, Gallagher JJ. Ventricular fibrillation in the Wolff-Parkinson-White Syndrome. *N Engl J Med* 1979;301: 1080–1085.

27. Zardini M, Yee R, Thakur RK, Klein GJ. Risk of sudden arrhythmic death in the Wolff-Parkinson-White syndrome: current perspectives. *PACE* 1994;17:966–975.

28. Leitch JW, Klein GJ, Yee R, Murdock C. Prognostic value of electrophysiologic testing in asymptomatic patients with Wolff-Parkinson-White pattern. *Circulation* 1990;82:1718–1723.

29. Sharma AD, Yee R, Guiraudon G, Klein GJ. Sensitivity and specificity of invasive and nonivasive testing for risk of sudden death in Wolff-Parkinson-White syndrome. *J Am Coll Cardiol* 1987;10:373–381.

30. Brugada P, Green M, Abdollah H, Wellens HJJ. Significance of ventricular arrhythmias initiated by programmed ventricular stimulation: the importance of the type of ventricular arrhythmia induced and the number of premature stimuli required. *Circulation* 1984;69: 87–92.

31. Bigger JT, Reiffel JA, Livelli FD, Wang PJ. Sensitivity, specificity, and reproducibility of programmed ventricular stimulation. *Circulation* 1986;73[Suppl II]:73–78.

32. Richards D, Byth K, Ross D, Uther J. What is the best predictor of spontaneous ventricular tachycardia and sudden death after myocardial infarction? *Circulation* 1991;83:756–763.

33. Prystowsky EN. Electrophysiologic-electropharmacologic testing in patients with ventricular arrhythmias. *PACE* 1988;11:225–251.

34. Anderson KP, Mason JW. Clinical value of cardiac electrophysiological studies. In: Zipes DP, Jalife J, eds. *Cardiac electrophysiology.* Philadelphia: WB Saunders, 1995:1133–1150.

35. Fananapazir L, Chang AC, Epstein SE, McAreavey D. Prognostic determinants in hypertrophic cardiomyopathy. *Circulation* 1992;86:730–740.

36. Milner PG, DiMarco JP, Lerman BB. Electrophysiological evaluation of sustained ventricular tachyarrhythmias in idiopathic dilated cardiomyopathy. *PACE* 1988; 11:562–568.

37. Liem LB, Swerdlow CD. Value of electropharmocologic testing in idiopathic dilated cardiomyopathy and sustained ventricular tachyarrythmias. *Am J Cardiol* 1988; 62:611–616.

38. Poll DS, Marchlinski FE, Buxton AE, Josephson ME. Usefulness of programmed stimulation in idiopathic dilated cardiomyopathy. *Am J Cardiol* 1986;58:992–997.

39. Das SK, Morady F, DiCarlo L, et al. Prognostic usefulness of programmed ventricular stimulation in idiopathic dilated cardiomyopathy without symptomatic ventricular arrhythmias. *Am J Cardiol* 1986;58: 998–1000.

40. Turitto G, Ahuja RK, Caref EB, El-Sherif N. Risk stratification for arrhythmic events in patients with nonischemic dilated cardiomyopathy and nonsustained ventricular tachycardia: role of programmed ventricular

stimulation and the signal averaged electrocardiogram. *J Am Coll Cardiol* 1994;24:1523–1528.

41. Peters S, Reil GH. Risk factors of cardiac arrest in arrhythmogenic right ventricular dysplasia. *Eur Heart J* 1995;16:77–80.

42. Wichter T, Martinez-Rubio A, Kottkamp H, et al. Reproducibility of programmed ventricular stimulation in arrhythmogenic right ventricular dysplasia/cardiomyopathy [abst]. *Circulation* 1996;94[Suppl 1]:1–626.

43. Wichter T, Haverkamp W, Martinez-Rubio A, Borggrefe M. Long-term prognosis and risk-stratification of arrhythmogenic right ventricular dysplasia/cardiomyopathy [abstr]. *Circulation* 1995;92:1–97.

44. Perry JC, Garson A. Arrhythmias following surgery for congenital heart disease. In: Zipes DP, Jalife J, eds. *Cardiac electrophysiology*. Philadelphia: WB Saunders, 1995:838–848.

45. Bhandari AK, Shapiro W, Morady F, Shen E, Mason J, Scheinman MM. Electrophysiologic testing in patients with the long QT syndrome. *Circulation* 1985;71:63–71.

46. Brodsky MA, Orlav MV, Winters RJ, Allen BJ. Determinants of inducible ventricular tachycardia in patients with clinical ventricular tachyarrhythmia and no apparent structural heart disease. *Am Heart J* 1993;126:1113–1120.

47. Livelli FD, Bigger JT Jr, Reiffel JA, et al. Response to programmed ventricular stimulation: sensitivity, specificity and relation to heart disease. *Am J Cardiol* 1982;50:452–458.

48. Link MS, Homoud M, Foote CB, Wang PJ, Estes NA III. Antiarrhythmic drug therapy of ventricular arrhythmias: current perspectives. *J Cardiovasc Electrophysiol* 1996;7:653–670.

49. Maron BJ, Fananapazir L. Sudden cardiac death in hypertrophic cardiomyopathy. *Circulation* 1992;85[Suppl I]:57–63.

50. Spirito P, Rapezzi C, Autore C, et al. Prognosis of asymptomatic patients with hypertrophic cardiomyopathy and nonsustained ventricular tachycardia. *Circulation* 1994;90:2743–2747.

51. McKenna WJ, Sadoul N, Slade AKB, Saumarez RC. The prognostic significance of nonsustained ventricular tachycardia in hypertrophic cardiomyopathy. *Circulation* 1994;90:3115–3117.

52. Corrado D, Basso C, Camerini F, et al. Is arrhythmogenic right ventricular dysplasia/cardiomyopathy a progressive heart muscle disease? A multicenter clinicopathologic study. *Circulation* 1995;92:1–470.

53. Shoda M, Kasanuki H, Ohnishi S, Umemura J. Recurrence of new ventricular tachycardia after successful catheter ablation in patients with arrhythmogenic right ventricular dysplasia. *Circulation* 1992;86:1–580.

54. Borggrefe M, Block M, Breithardt G. Identification and management of the high risk patient with dilated cardiomyopathy. *Br Heart J* 1994;72[Suppl]:S42–S45.

55. Middlekauff HR, Stevenson WG, Stevenson LW, Saxon LA. Syncope in advanced heart failure: high risk of sudden death regardless of origin of syncope. *J Am Coll Cardiol* 1993;21:110–116.

56. Moss AJ. Prolonged QT-interval syndromes. *JAMA* 1986;256:2985–2987.

57. Kinder C, Tamburro P, Kopp D, Kall J, Olshansky B, Wilber D. The clinical significance of nonsustained ventricular tachycardia: current perspectives. *PACE* 1994;17:637–664.

58. Kennedy HL, Whitlock JA, Sprague MK, Kennedy LJ, Buchingham TA, Goldberg RJ. Long-term follow-up of asymptomatic healthy subjects with frequent and complex ventricular ectopy. *N Engl J Med* 1985;312:193–197.

59. Busby MJ, Shefrin EA, Fleg JL. Prevalence and long-term significance of exercise-induced frequent or repetitive ventricular ectopic beats in apparently healthy volunteers. *J Am Coll Cardiol* 1989;14:1659–1665.

60. Wang Y, Scheinman MM, Chien WW, Cohen TJ, Lesh MD, Griffin JC. Patients with supraventricular tachycardia presenting with aborted sudden death: incidence, mechanism and long-term follow-up. *J Am Coll Cardiol* 1991;18:1711–1719.

61. Madariaga A, Carmona JR, Mateas FR, Lezaun R, De Los Arcos E. Supraventricular arrhythmia as the cause of sudden death in hypertrophic cardiomyopathy. *Eur Heart J* 1994;15:134–137.

62. Zipes DP, Garson A. Task Force 6: arrhythmias. *J Am Coll Cardiol* 1994;24:892–899.

63. Naccarelli GV, Shih H, Jalal S. Catheter ablation for the treatment of paroxysmal supraventricular tachycardia. *J Cardiovasc Electrophysiol* 1995;6:951–961.

64. Manolis AS, Wang PJ, Estes NA III. Radiofrequency catheter ablation for cardiac tachyarrhythmias. *Ann Intern Med* 1994;121:452–461.

65. Munger TM, Packer DL, Hammill SC, et al. A population study of the natural history of Wolff-Parkinson-White syndrome in Olmsted County, Minnesota, 1953–1989. *Circulation* 1993;87:866–873.

66. Steinbeck G. Should radiofrequency current ablation be performed in asymptomatic patients with the Wolff-Parkinson-White syndrome. *PACE* 1993;16:649–652.

67. German LD, Gallagher JJ, Broughton A, Guarnieri T, Trantham JL. Effects of exercise and isoproterenol during atrial fibrillation in patients with Wolff-Parkinson-White syndrome. *Am J Cardiol* 1983;51:1203–1206.

68. Katcher MS, Foote CB, Homoud M, Wang PJ, Estes NA III. Strategies for managing atrial fibrillation. *Cleve Clin J Med* 1996;63:282–294.

69. Fischer B, Haissaguerre M, Garrigues S, et al. Radiofrequency catheter ablation of common atrial flutter in 80 patients. *J Am Coll Cardiol* 1995;25:1365–1372.

70. Klein LS, Miles WM. Ablative therapy for ventricular arrhythmias. *Progr Cardiovasc Dis* 1995;37:225–242.

71. Calkins H, Kalbfleisch SJ, El-Atassi R, Langberg JJ, Fred M. Relation between efficacy of radiofrequency catheter ablation and site of origin of idiopathic ventricular tachycardia. *Am J Cardiol* 1993;71:827–833.

72. Maron BJ, Isner JM, McKenna WJ. Task Force 3: hypertrophic cardiomyopathy, myocarditis and other myopericardial diseases and mitral valve prolapse. *J Am Coll Cardiol* 1994;24:880–885.

73. Asso A, Farre J, Zayas R, Negrete A, Cabrera JA, Romero J. Radiofrequency catheter ablation of ventricular tachycardia in patients with arrhythmogenic right ventricular dysplasia [abst]. *J Am Coll Cardiol* 1995;25:315A.

74. Leclercq JF, Chouty F, Cauchemez B, Leenhardt A, Coumel P, Slama R. Results of electrical fulguration in arrhythmogenic right ventricular disease. *Am J Cardiol* 1988;62:220–224.

75. Witcher T, Borggrefe M, Haverkamp W, Chen X, Breithardt G. Efficacy of antiarrhythmic drugs in patients with arrhythmogenic right ventricular disease. *Circulation* 1992;86:29–37.

76. Link MS, Wang PJ, Haugh CJ, et al. Arrhythmogenic right ventricular dysplasia: clinical results with implantable cardioverter defibrillators. *J Inter Cardiovasc Elect* 1997;1:41–48.

77. Dec GW, Fuster V. Idiopathic dilated cardiomyopathy. *N Engl J Med* 1994;331:1564–1575.

78. Borggrefe M, Chen X, Martinez-Rubio A, et al. The role of implantable cardioverter defibrillators in dilated cardiomyopthy. *Am Heart J* 1994;127:1145–1150.

79. Tan HL, Hou CJY, Lauer MR, Sung RJ. Electrophysiologic mechanisms of the long QT interval syndromes and torsade de pointes. *Ann Intern Med* 1995;122:701–714.

80. Estes NA III. Clinical strategies for use of the implantable cardioverter defibrillator: the impact of current trials. *PACE* 1996;19:1011–1015.

81. Cooper JP, Fraser AG, Penny WJ. Reversibility and benign recurrence of complete heart block in athletes. *Int J Cardiol* 1992;35:118–120.

82. Fleg JL, Asante AVK. Asystole following treadmill exercise in a man without organic heart disease. *Arch Intern Med* 1983;143:1821–1822.

83. Kramer MR, Drori Y, Lev B. Sudden death in young soldiers: high incidence of syncope prior to death. *Chest* 1988;93:345–347.

84. Williams CC, Bernhardt DT. Syncope in athletes. *Sports Med* 1995;19:223–234.

85. Maron BJ, Brown RW, McGrew CA, Mitten MJ, Caplan AL, Hutter AM. Ethical, legal and practical considerations affecting medical decision-making in competitive athletes. *J Am Coll Cardiol* 1994;24:854–860.

The Athlete and Heart Disease:
Diagnosis, Evaluation & Management,
edited by R. A. Williams.
Lippincott Williams & Wilkins, Philadelphia © 1999.

14

Head-Upright Tilt Testing and Syncope in Athletes

Marc Ovadia

*Division of Pediatric Cardiology, Cornell University College of Medicine/North Shore University,
North Shore University Hospital, Manhasset, New York 11030*

[It is] as true today as when Celsus made the remark, "The dominant view of the nature of disease controls its treatment."

—Sir William Osler, Oxford Medicine (1919)

There is a background incidence of syncope in the normal population (neurocardiogenic, or "vasovagal" mechanism syncope) that also is present in athletes. Most syncope in athletes is a manifestation of such common syncope mechanisms. Their workup is the subject of this chapter.

The physiology of the athlete is, however, different from that of their more sedentary counterparts. In the performance athlete, sinus bradycardia and asymptomatic hypotension are frequent occurrences. There are important electrocardiographic (ECG) changes in the performance athlete as well as certain echocardiographic findings, such as dilation or hypertrophy of the ventricles.

The cardiac changes that characterize the heart of the athlete imitate heart disease. Hypertrophy of the interventricular septum, ST and QT changes in the presence or absence of sinus bradycardia, and isolated bradycardia—features normally present in the performance athlete—may conceal the diagnosis of vasovagal syncope by raising suspicion of organic cardiac disease in the individual, rather than a more benign version of syncope.

The workup of syncope in the athlete is made much more difficult because of the presence of these factors. This chapter discusses in some detail the normal ECG and cardiovascular changes of the athlete in order to facilitate the distinction of normal from abnormal, and to aid proper differential diagnosis of syncope.

CLINICAL EVALUATION

History

The history of the athlete with syncope needs to focus on several factors. The setting of the syncope is important, particularly whether syncope occurred on a hot day when the athlete was dehydrated, whether the athlete was standing when syncope occurred, and whether syncope occurred immediately after exertion (i.e., during cool-down) or at a moment of physical injury. The presence of any of these factors points to neurocardiogenic (vasovagal) syncope as the diagnosis. If, contrariwise, syncope occurred at peak exertion or if syncope occurred in the sitting or recumbent posture, then neurocardiogenic (vasovagal) syncope is less likely and heart disease is more likely.

The characteristics of the syncope (or near-syncope or presyncope) are most important to establish. If the athlete remembers feeling lightheaded before loss of consciousness and describes feeling warm or nauseated (possibly with a headache), then neurocardiogenic syncope is likely (1). On the other hand, if the athlete experienced angina or palpitations or if the athlete has no memory of the period immediately preceding the event, then the common form of neurocardiogenic syncope is less likely. There are exceptions to such rules. For example, neurocardiogenic syncope does occur in athletes who also have heart disease or surgically repaired heart disease, and asystolic (pure cardioinhibitory) syncope occurs without premonitory signs even though it is neurocardiogenic (vagal) in origin (2).

Additional important characteristics of the syncope are whether it was brief, whether it resolved as soon as the athlete was laid down, and whether it was associated with flaccidity and not with rigidity, with patterned motor movements or with frank convulsion. If syncope had the benign characteristics noted then, again, neurocardiogenic syncope is more likely. There are exceptions. Asystolic (pure cardioinhibitory) syncope commonly has motor signs, despite its neurocardiogenic origin, and, in patients with a lowered seizure threshold, generalized tonic-clonic (or other type) convulsions may be triggered secondarily.

The presence of headache and visual changes is useful information to elicit. In neurocardiogenic syncope (as in most syncope associated with severe hypotension), the athlete describes a graying (or yellowing) or a narrowing-in of the visual field from outside-to-inside, with occasional black scotomata. By contrast, the migraine sufferer (*migraineur*) may describe bright scotomata and scintillating zig-zag lines (*teichopsia*) and there may be an associated headache. Neurocardiogenic syncope and migraine can occur in the same patient. Migraine typically does not lead to syncope but only to presyncope as part of the migraine itself. History of prior migraine or other headache may be an important historical factor—more so if the chief presenting symptom is presyncope with unusual subjective sensations than if the presenting symptom is syncope.

Retrograde amnesia occurs not uncommonly in all syncope, including vasovagal syncope in the normal individual (Ovadia M, Bacon-Pajonas K. Unpublished observations). Not infrequently, therefore, the subject

may recall no premonition; he or she may only remember looking up from the ground and being unable to understand how he or she got there. When athletes collapse, witnesses typically are present, a circumstance that is fortunate for the clinician. The witness establishes whether the athlete faltered and appeared confused before losing consciousness, even though the athlete may not recall this phase of the experience.

An observer who is present just prior to syncope in another person can converse with the individual, but the individual would seem somewhat confused. For example, the individual would be able to count down from 100, but he or she might not remember what number was said at the time he or she passed out, if the task is remembered at all once the individual recovers. Athletes endure extremes such as blood pressure to 46mm Hg systolic without immediate loss of consciousness. But retrograde amnesia for these periods (once the patient recovers from syncope) is very common.

Witnesses are useful also for establishing whether the event was syncope or near-syncope. Subjective impressions are mistaken with unexpected frequency, particularly in younger patients and in cases of brief but severe hypotension.

Prior history of syncope should be elicited, as should details about prior events. History of prior syncope or presyncope after long periods of standing upright, or syncope after fright, surprise, or pain, all point to a neurocardiogenic (vasovagal) origin of the event.

History of heart disease is useful but often misleading, in that even people with heart disease or repaired heart disease can have vasovagal syncope. The presence of a diagnosis of heart disease may only guarantee that this particular athlete is referred for specialized evaluation. From the point of view of the cardiologic or neurologic clinician in the syncope clinic, this falsely elevates the frequency of a prior history of heart disease as compared with an unbiased population of people with syncope. This reduces the significance and specificity (from the point of view of mechanism) of this historical finding.

Medication use (including β-adrenergic inhalers for asthma) or caffeine withdrawal may be relevant as well, in that these may predispose to neurocardiogenic syncope. Habits regarding salt intake, particularly the avoidance of salt, must be elicited. Family history of syncope, seizures, or sudden death should be elicited.

Physical Examination

The physical examination is important but usually unrevealing.

Height and habitus should be evaluated thoughtfully because of the possibility of Marfan syndrome or another genetic disease in the athlete with syncope. Blood pressure and heart rate in the lying, sitting, and standing positions should be determined repeatedly.

Typically, the cardiac examination reveals no right ventricular or left ventricular heave. S_3 and S_4 are frequent findings in normal younger athletes (as they are in all adolescents). Auscultation over the carotids for the ejection murmur of bicuspid aortic valve and click should be sought. Repeated precordial auscultation after Valsalva and after standing from squatting are vital for hearing the murmur of hypertrophic cardiomyopathy (idiopathic hypertrophic subaortic stenosis, or IHSS); often the combination of standing from squatting and simultaneous Valsalva is useful for bringing out this ejection murmur when either maneuver alone was not sufficient.

At least one lower extremity pulse should be palpated carefully, simultaneously with each upper extremity, and with one carotid pulse. Extremity examination should look for clubbing or hypertrophic osteopathy, although it is unheard of for a performance athlete to have longstanding primary pulmonary hypertension that has escaped detection.

Hyperventilation with the patient standing is useful in younger patients to elicit *Absence*, thereby curtailing an otherwise lengthy and inconvenient workup in the rare individual with an undiagnosed case of this particular form of idiopathic epilepsy.

Bedside Tests and Laboratory Examination

The ECG should be studied with great attention to certain common athletic variants. These variant findings are detailed in the next section. The clinician should be familiar with the possible ECG manifestations of hypertrophic cardiomyopathy and right ventricular dysplasia (3,4,4a–4e).

Echocardiography is discussed in Chapter 10. Left ventricular dilation and septal hypertrophy are common in athletes (5,6).

Holter examination and event recorder monitoring are useful. Ambulatory blood pressure monitoring is useful rarely, particularly in the teen-aged athlete with documented mild hypertension or chronic orthostatic hypotension.

The single most useful test in the athlete with syncope is the head-upright tilt test. First discussed, however, are the common ECG variants of the athlete and why they occur, because these ECG findings can mislead the clinician and lead to overinterpretation of ECG, Holter, and tilt test results. Also discussed are mechanisms of neurocardiogenic and other tilt-induced syncope.

Electrocardiographic Variants in the Athlete (Athletic Heart Syndrome)

From the practical point of view of a practicing cardiologist, to be an athlete means not to have a normal ECG. This section describes the ECG variations that characterize the heart of the athlete (7,8). Generally, these findings go under the heading of the athletic heart syndrome, but they are too commonly observed to warrant conferring that diagnosis whenever any one of these findings is documented. [That diagnosis is reserved for the patient with echocardiographic hypertrophy that is presumed to regress on detraining (9,10).]

The physiologic changes that underlie the changes reflected in the ECG are often important in the causation of syncope in the athlete. However, it is common for some striking athletic ECG variants to be irrelevant to syncope causation. These athletic ECG variants must be familiar to the clinician so that the findings are not overinterpreted when incidentally discovered in the syncopal patient.

The ECG variations that characterize athletes are of two types: those that may be attributed directly to enhanced parasympathetic tone—increased vagal tone or hypervagotonia (11,12)—and those that are not so related (Table 1).

A broad variety of ECG changes can be attributed to enhanced vagal tone, some of which (such as slow ventricular tachycardia) may not seem to be a normal variant, or vagally mediated, at first blush.

Sinus bradycardia is probably the most common ECG finding in the performance athlete. Found in 75% to 85% of highly trained athletes (13,14), it is characterized by its disappearance on exertion and the absence of symptoms. The sinus bradycardia appears to be due to hypervagotonia (15,16) or to a lower intrinsic heart rate in combination with hypervagotonia. It is found in both endurance- and resistance-trained athletes (17, 18). Because it is a reflection of hypervagotonia in the athlete, it does not indicate the presence of sick sinus syndrome.

Often, sinus bradycardia occurs in the setting of exaggerated respiratory sinus arrhythmia (a common vagal finding even in normal individuals) (19). Whether the increased parasympathetic tone reflected in the lower heart rate is due solely to the reported baroreceptor hypersensitivity attributed to the athlete (20) or whether all parasympathetic reflexes are similarly affected (and baroreceptor hypersensitivity is only secondarily involved) is unknown.

Sinus pauses are an additional manifestation of hypervagotonia in the athlete. The sinus pause indicates both the presence of vagal sinus node suppression and the absence of any atrial, atrioventricular (AV) nodal (junctional), or ventricular autonomous escape mechanism (21).

Intimately connected with sinus bradycardia and sinus pauses are five additional findings: wandering atrial pacemaker, junctional bradycardia, atrial extrasystoles, ventricular extrasystoles, and accelerated idioventricular rhythm ("slow ventricular tachycardia"). All of these, occurring in the setting of vagal suppression of sinus mechanism, are normal escape rhythms. Thus, the presence of any one of these findings is a manifestation of the same hypervagotonia that underlies the sinus bradycardia. In the athlete, these findings do not signify heart disease, sick sinus syndrome, or any of the variants of this syndrome.

Wandering atrial pacemaker is the circumstance in which the predominant rhythm varies in the course of minutes, days, or weeks. Because the rhythm that governs the heart is simply that automatic rhythm whose "escape cycle length" is shortest—that is, it comes from the site characterized by the shortest time till spontaneous depolarization—the effect of increased parasympathetic tone is felt particularly in the innervated cardiac atrial sites that have the shortest intrinsic escape cycle length and

---

TABLE 1. *ECG changes*

Increased vagal tone*
  Effect on automatic tissues
    Sinus bradycardia
    Sinus pauses
    Wandering atrial pacemaker
    Junctional bradycardia
    Accelerated idioventricular rhythm[†]
      (also termed *slow ventricular tachycardia*)
    Atrial extrasystoles (escape)
    Ventricular extrasystoles (escape)
  Effect on conduction
    Prolonged PR interval (1st-degree AV block)
    Wenckebach phenomenon
    Wenckebach (Mobitz I) AV block
    Infra-His block[†]
Nonvagal
    Ventricular premature complexes
    Atrial premature complexes
    Increased QRS amplitude
    Prolonged QT interval
    Prominent U waves
    Abnormalities of intraventricular conduction
    ST segment elevation
    T wave abnormalities

---

  *Hypervagotonia
  [†]Rare

that are most sensitive to parasympathetic stimulation. These sites ordinarily serve as pacemaker for the heart. With increased parasympathetic tone, these sites are one by one silenced: first the sinus node, then the site characterized by the next shortest cycle length, and then the next. Some individuals have more possible distinct pacemaker sites than others, and these individuals show wandering atrial pacemaker when, as athletes, they manifest increased vagal tone. A series of regular sites, with slower and slower intrinsic rates, is seen on the Holter monitor. Thus, from the practical point of view, wandering atrial pacemaker describes the switch from some predominant P-wave morphologic characteristic to another (rarely to a third). From P-wave characteristics alone it may be difficult to ascertain which morphologic characteristic is sinus—the characteristics may appear quite similar. However, a characteristic of wandering atrial pacemaker is that all of the nonsinus morphologic characteristics occur at rates slightly below that of sinus rhythm. The so-called coronary sinus rhythm P-wave pattern is just one of these automatic escape rhythms in the athlete with wandering atrial pacemaker.

Junctional bradycardia is the presence of an AV nodal (junctional) escape rhythm at the time of sinus bradycardia. There is no P wave, but, with electrophysiologic testing, a P wave is found simultaneous with (and therefore buried in) the QRS complex. A complementary relationship between junctional bradycardia and sinus pauses may exist. In patients with particularly slow or absent junctional escape rhythms, sinus pauses are seen. In other patients, the escape rhythm may be junctional—an ECG manifestation of sinus node slowing resulting from hypervagotonia.

Atrial extrasystoles occurring as an escape phenomenon are characterized by escape cycle length longer than sinus and occurrence at a time of sinus bradycardia or other evidence of hypervagotonia.

Ventricular extrasystoles also occur as an escape phenomenon and are similarly characterized by cycle length (measured from the preceding QRS) longer than the sinus cycle length. They are seen at times of vagal sinus slowing.

Accelerated idioventricular rhythm ("slow ventricular tachycardia") (Fig. 1) is a not uncommon manifestation of hypervagotonia in the athlete (22,23). In individuals in whom the junctional pacemakers appear to be vagally innervated (or, contrariwise, in whom the infra-Hisian pacemakers are characterized by particularly short escape cycle lengths, resulting from either increased sympathetic tone or inborn variation), there appears this additional rhythm—ventricular tachycardia. This is typically a monomorphic slow ventricular tachycardia with imperfect cycle length reproducibility, suggestive of an automatic mechanism. It has no clinical significance beyond that of the bradycardia that led to it.

The kinship of these rhythms is due to their reflection of the spontaneous depolarization of a cascade of tissues more and more resistant to parasympathetic slowing. In the absence of such an escape rhythm, sinus asystole and syncope, or convulsive syncope, results.

The aforementioned manifestations of hypervagotonia all reflect vagal suppression of the sinus node and vagal effects on spontaneous depolarization of automatic tissues. The

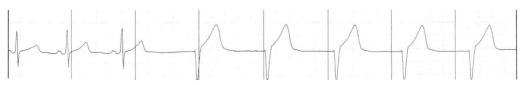

FIG. 1. Accelerated idioventricular rhythm in a juvenile athlete. (Time marker 1 sec.)

next several rhythms to be discussed reflect vagal effects on conduction through tissues.

Prolonged PR interval (first-degree AV block) is the most common manifestation of a vagal effect on the AV node. This reflects increased conduction time between atrium and ventricle. It may not imply the presence of any actual abnormality of AV conduction in the normal athlete. In some individuals, however, the underlying cause is not direct smooth slowing of conduction as a result of heightened parasympathetic tone, but rather the use of a different anatomic route for AV conduction, a so-called "slow pathway," resulting from complete block (conduction failure) in the normal AV node conduction pathway (the "fast" pathway) owing to the heightened tone. The slow pathway in the athlete may not have the same relationship with the fast pathway that it does in other individuals; therefore, the presence of the pathways may not be signaled by the presence of precisely two distinct PR intervals differing by 50 ms in conduction time for similar (differing by $\leq$ 10 ms) atrial cycle lengths—the typical definition used in clinical invasive electrophysiologic testing for the presence of fast and slow pathways in the AV node. A continuous monotonic increase in PR is typical for the athlete undergoing invasive electrophysiologic testing (with standard programmed atrial stimulation protocol), with a PR variation frequently in excess of 150 ms, far exceeding that seen in nonathletes or in patients with supraventricular tachycardia caused by AV nodal reentry (the usual indication for invasive testing). In athletes, the findings may also be variable depending on the patient's degree of alertness. The prolonged PR in these athlete's ECGs remains constant over the course of the ECG but shortens with exercise and with standing.

Infrequently, the prolonged PR is variable in length, without any "dropped" ventricular beats. The PR prolongs progressively (by decreasing increments) over several beats, and then suddenly returns to normal, with preserved AV conduction throughout. This is termed the *Wenckebach phenomenon* (24) (Fig. 2).

More familiar is the Wenckebach type of second-degree AV block. This is a form of true second-degree block. The PR prolongs progressively from beat to beat (again, by decreasing increments) until with one P there is failure to conduct the impulse through the AV node to the ventricle. On the very next beat, the PR returns to normal. This behavior repeats itself a few beats later. When blocked beats occur frequently in normal sinus rhythm (e.g., 3:2 or 2:1 A:V ratio), it is not possible to document all of the aforementioned features. Indeed, the only manifestation of the Wenckebach character of the block may be a slightly shortened PR intermittently noted after the blocked ("dropped" QRS) beat. Another feature of Wenckebach second-degree AV block is that it often occurs at times of sinus bradycardia (reflecting independent vagal suppression of sinus and AV nodes simultaneously). A synonym for Wenckebach type of second-degree AV block is Mobitz type I second-degree AV block.

This phenomenon occurs quite commonly in athletes. In the setting of sinus bradycardia, rather than a sinus beat, occasionally a junctional escape beat terminating the dropped beat interval is seen. This rhythm is of no hemodynamic consequence. It is important to recognize because it can coexist with syncope in the athlete, where *it is of no significance* (except as a sign that the patient is an athlete) and where it should not be interpreted as causative or be suggestive of the intermittent presence of a higher degree of AV block causative of the syncope.

The accepted nomenclature distinguishes Wenckebach type of second-degree AV block, reflecting block at the AV node (due in this case simply to hypervagotonia), from block in the His or infra-His conduction system. It is frequently seen written that the other type of AV block (Mobitz type II second-degree AV block) implies infra-His conduction system disease and risk of life-threatening bradycardia. (Mobitz type II second-degree AV block describes that block in which there is no PR prolongation leading up to block.)

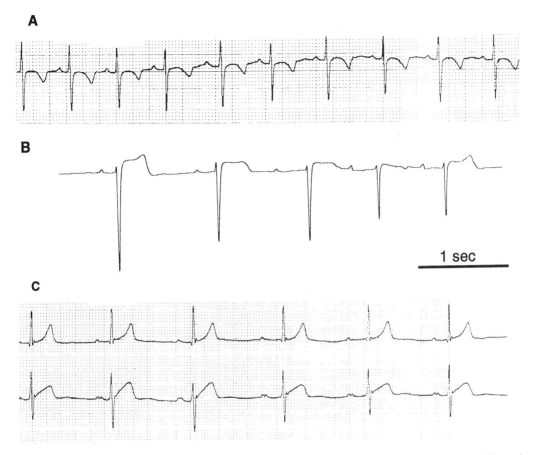

FIG. 2. Wenckebach phenomenon in athletes with syncope. Note PR interval prolongation followed by PR shortening, with no occurrence of AV block. **Panel A:** Basketball player who also herds animals and competes in rodeo. **Panel B:** 14 year old basketball player. **Panel C:** Multiple-sport athlete.

In all likelihood, the implication of apparent Mobitz II block actually depends on the population in which it is seen. [For an interesting discussion of Bayesian probability applied in a different context, see Shaw et al. (25).] In the athlete with a structurally normal heart, the apparent presence of Mobitz II AV block probably represents a false-positive result and an inaccurate diagnosis—usually this is just an unusual variant of block occurring within the AV node. The occasional shortening of the PR after the blocked beat, or the coincidence of this type of block with sinus bradycardia, should point to the correct diagnosis. I have not observed Mobitz type II second-degree AV block in the athlete that in fact correlated with infra-His disease of the conduction system.

Regarding apparent infra-His block, particularly in athletes studied by invasive electrophysiologic testing (Fig. 3), it is well known that AV nodal refractory periods increase with increasing frequency of stimulation. Because of the extremely low sinus rates in the athlete, it is possible during invasive electrophysiologic testing to perform programmed electrical stimulation with unusually slow drive rates, that is, low frequency of stimulation. In this highly artificial setting, the AV node may not manifest block with earlier and earlier

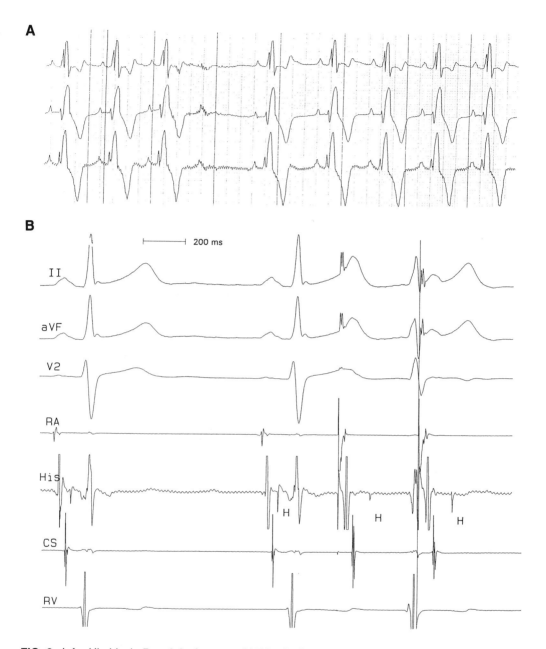

FIG. 3. Infra-His block. **Panel A:** Apparent Möbitz II 2° AV block in an athlete (hockey player). The blocked P wave may not be sinus in origin. The right bundle branch block is due to repaired Tetralogy of Fallot. This man's syncope was proven to be of vagal etiology not related to the finding depicted here. **Panel B:** His buncle electrogram in juvenile athlete documenting infra-His block brought out by programmed electrical stimulation. Note His ventricular interval prolongation (second H), followed by occurrence of infra-His block (third H not followed by any QRS). The significance of this is uncertain.

single atrial extrastimuli. Rather the site of block may move to the infra-His region. This is solely an artifact, brought on by the possibility of programmed extrastimulation at extremely low drive rates in the athlete. The infra-His block encountered in invasive electrophysiologic testing of athletes [or with spontaneous atrial premature complexes (APCs)] is a test finding that does not correlate with anything real.

Higher grades of AV block, for example, advanced second-degree AV block (in which many sinus P waves occur for a single conducted beat) or third-degree AV block (complete heart block), are only rarely observed solely as vagal phenomena. The hypervagotonia of athletes is only rarely severe enough to provoke this, although the hypervagotonia of esophageal or intraabdominal visceral injury may bring on these findings. These findings are seen during provoked vasovagal syncope in the context of tilt-table testing, and thus probably occur in spontaneous syncope as well.

As with any occurrence of protracted asystole, brief atrial flutter or fibrillation may also occur. In the absence of a history of palpitations, this finding may imply a prognosis not much different from the finding of asystole, provided the fibrillation reverts quickly.

As regards long periods of ventricular asystole caused by hypervagotonia, an interesting dichotomy is observed anecdotally that distinguishes younger from older patients. Younger patients tend to have vagal AV block, even advanced second-degree AV block, whereas older patients tend to have sinus arrest. Whether this implies developmental change in vagal effects on the AV node versus the sinus node is unknown.

An important fact relative to hypervagotonia is that rapid parasympathetic withdrawal normally occurs upon standing. Thus, the manifestations of hypervagotonia in the athlete's ECG are more likely to be observed when the athlete is lying on the examination or procedure table or while sleeping during a Holter recording, and they are less likely to occur during real exercise. Such findings are reduced upon sitting or standing. The clinician must recognize this and downplay the significance of recumbent ECG findings that often have little to do with the athlete's status playing (26).

The rhythm and ECG changes so far described are direct consequences of heightened parasympathetic (vagal) tone. The following discussion completes the survey of common variants in athletes with those that are not directly due to hypervagotonia.

In addition to manifestations of hypervagotonia, there are other findings in the ECG of the athlete. These include increased QRS amplitudes (correlating poorly with the presence or absence of hypertrophy or dilation) (27), long QT intervals (28,29) and prominent U waves, and numerous mild abnormalities of intraventricular conduction including incomplete right bundle branch block, myriad ST segment elevations and mild changes (so-called *repolarization changes*), and abnormalities of the T wave.

APCs and ventricular premature complexes (VPCs) are also seen frequently in athletes (30). These must be distinguished from atrial or ventricular escape beats (31). The cycle length preceding the escape beat exceeds that of the underlying rhythm, whereas the cycle length preceding the APC or VPC is shorter than that of the underlying rhythm.

The chief importance of the ECG variants in the athlete is that they should not be overinterpreted as causes of syncope when for the athlete they are merely normal variants. While the hypervagotonia that these ECG changes reflect may be important in syncope, the changes themselves typically are not.

MECHANISMS OF VASOVAGAL (NEUROCARDIOGENIC) SYNCOPE

This section discusses the mechanisms only of the most common upright syncopal syndromes occurring in athletes (which happen to be the same as those for nonathletes), starting with general comments on upright syncope.

The problem of maintaining blood pressure in a normal range when standing erect is addressed by many physiologic systems of the human body. Although the human is akin to other animals in many respects, the ability to respond to upright posture with increased heart rate (the baroreceptor response) and increased vascular return plus somewhat increased peripheral resistance (contraction of lower extremity musculature, gentle Valsalva) is not universal in animals. With respect to some aspects of the latter mechanisms, this may be in part a learned response.

The mechanism of the baroreceptor response is that reduced blood pressure is sensed arterially, and a particular reflex mechanism (whereby higher blood pressure leads directly to tonic vagal inhibition of heart rate) is inhibited whenever blood pressure is reduced. This leads to increased heart rate and maintained blood pressure.

This reflex in this circumstance constitutes a closed-loop system. Numerous diverse factors modulate the system (32). Conceptually, one part of this closed-loop mechanism is the open-loop gain, the amount of effect that a particular experimentally controlled stimulus elicits. Modulation of open-loop gain is the chief mechanism whereby the entire system is modulated, whether in health, in disease, or as a pharmacologic or toxicologic response. (The closed-loop system is not designed to detect posture, vascular tone, or heart rate, although these are relevant parameters. Rather, it is designed to detect changes only in the blood pressure.) In addition to this closed-loop system (the baroreceptor reflex), there are other closed-and open-loop control systems (neural including serotonergic and endogenous opioid pathways, humoral including endocrine, eicosanoid, nitric oxide [NO] and others) and laws of physics (e.g., in diving) that affect the blood pressure and the subject's response to it. All of these systems are always in play.

In this discussion, the forms of syncope are grouped mechanistically as vasovagal, where "vaso" refers to a vasodilatation that appears to be present, and "vagal" refers to the association with slow heart rate. In some instances of the clinical syncope referred to as vasovagal, however, the aforementioned features are not part of the causation of syncope but are mere epiphenomena.

Patterns of Vasovagal Syncope

Vasovagal, or neurocardiogenic, syncope occurs in three basic forms: (a) *vasodepressor type*—wherein the blood pressure decreases in the upright posture, leading to syncope, typically during a period of sinus tachycardia; (b) *mixed type* (i.e., mixed vasodepressor/cardioinhibitory type)—wherein blood pressure decreases and the heart rate decreases in the upright posture prior to syncope: these two changes together cause syncope; and (c) *pure cardioinhibitory syncope*—wherein heart rate suddenly decreases or goes to zero. This may occur in response to prolonged upright posture or some other vagal stimulus (Table 2; Fig. 4). Rarely, it occurs at a time of sitting or even recumbent posture.

The nosologic validity of the tripartite distinction of vagal syncope is supported by the well-studied disorder named the *hypersensitive carotid sinus syndrome* (where these entities were defined) whose causation is more clearly vagal than that of many upright syncopal syndromes.

Postulated Mechanisms

The mechanism of the vasodepressor form of vasovagal (neurocardiogenic) upright syn-

TABLE 2. *Patterns of syncope*

Causative
Vagal mechanisms
  Vasodepressor
  Mixed vasodepressor/cardioinhibitory
  Cardioinhibitory
  (Usual afferent is cardiac mechanoreceptor,
    rare afferent is esophageal or arterial
    baroreceptor, and extremely rare afferent
    is cardiac chemoreceptor*)
Orthostatic hypotension
Delayed orthostatic hypotension
Contributing to manifestations
Vagal mechanisms
  (Typical afferent is arterial baroreceptor, rare
    afferent is mechanoreceptor)

*In which case the reflex is referred to as the Bezold-Jarisch reflex.

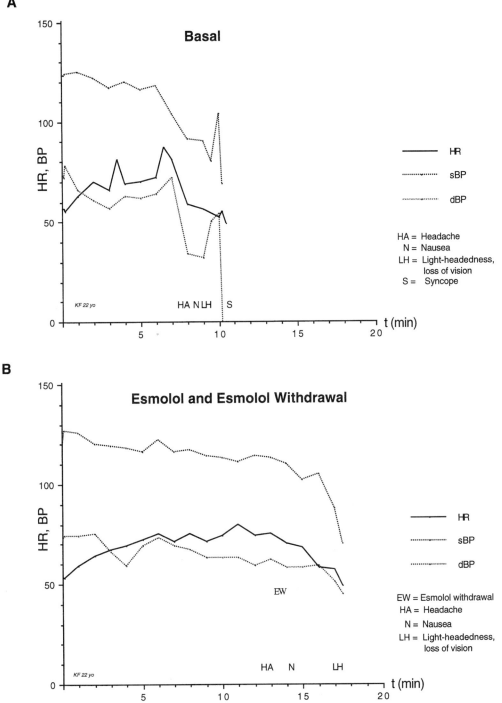

FIG. 4. Head-up tilt responses in mixed syncope in a competitive triathlon athlete with exercise syncope. Tilt occurs at t=0. **A:** Response to basal tilt. Sinus bradycardia with an attenuated heart rate response; by 7 minutes, a lowering of the diastolic blood pressure is noted, reflecting venous pooling, and systolic blood pressure diminishes subsequently (syncope). **B:** Response to esmolol/esmolol-withdrawal testing. The athlete is tilted during esmolol infusion for 15 minutes. When the esmolol infusion is discontinued, blood pressure diminishes, leading to light-headedness and loss of vision (presyncope). (Reproduced with permission. Ovadia M et al. *Circulation* 1995;92:1854. © 1995 The American Heart Association.)

cope is believed to be as follows. Prolonged standing leads to venous pooling in the lower extremities. Incipient hypotension is countered by increased adrenaline and noradrenaline release, and to a lesser extent by baroreceptor mechanisms (reduction of the tonic parasympathetic inhibition of heart rate). The heart rate then increases in response to one or both of these mechanisms, and wall stress is increased in the cardiac chambers. This triggers the activation of mechanoreceptors in the walls of the heart and cardiac vessels, leading to afferent impulses of a cardiodepressor reflex that is well known in animals and humans.[1]

The efferent of this (mechanoreceptor-afferent) cardiodepressor reflex includes sympathetic inhibition via corticospinal pathways and parasympathetic (vagal) cardiac inhibition, which causes reduction of heart rate to greater or lesser degree. The heart rate slowing occurs via the muscarinic-receptor gated K^+ channel ($i_{K,Ach}$, GIRK), a $G_{\beta\delta}$-sensitive 35 pS inwardly rectifying K^+ channel of special importance in specialized atrial tissue. This channel mediates vagal slowing of sinus node impulses.

In the case of vasodepressor syncope, it is believed that this entire mechanoreceptor reflex is active, but that the direct effect on heart rate is relatively mild.

There are, however, alternative explanations for certain cases of vasodepressor phenomena that do not postulate a vagal mechanism and that may be more accurate for particular patients. A research group at my institution and a research group of Fouad-Tarazi at the Cleveland Clinic (33,34) have remarked about the existence of a group of patients with upright syncope who appear to have a pattern of response quite similar to what would be expected in primary autonomic failure or insufficiency, with the sole difference being that, in these patients, hypotension occurs a few minutes after

assuming the upright posture, whereas in the patient with primary autonomic failure or autonomic insufficiency, the hypotension typically occurs immediately. This pattern of response is termed *delayed orthostatic hypotension* or *xx11 syncope* (based on a numbering scheme relevant to our protocol of tilt testing, in which vasovagal syncope is termed *x101*), and Fouad-Tarazi's group was independently led to call it *persistent orthostatic hypotension.* This physiologic characteristic may be identical to that of the patient group described in Mayo Clinic and other publications as postural tachycardia syndrome (POTS). It is our view that, in these patients, the sympathetic mechanisms for maintenance of blood pressure in the upright posture are present, but they quickly become overwhelmed. Adding to this course of events are the normal vasodilatation of exercise (present in normal subjects and in athletes, although not in established hypertensive individuals), the frequency with which athletes become dehydrated (35), and the well-documented mild orthostatic intolerance that can occur in elite athletes (36,37). In our experience, these patients may be differentiated from true vasovagal vasodepressor syncope by the fact that the use of β-adrenergic blocking agents leads to worsening of symptoms, whereas in true vasovagal (neurocardiogenic) vasodepressor syncope, the use of beta-blockers alleviates symptoms.

The historical attribution of vagal mechanisms to all syncope with vasodepressor features is based on the observation that, after syncope has occurred (when typically the patient is supine), the heart rate slows markedly, reflecting presence of a vagal mechanism, at least at that moment. This observation is not inconsistent with the concepts put forth by myself and my colleagues and by Fouad-Tarazi. Syncope may occur after progressive hypotension based on the inadequacy of autonomic (sympathetic) mechanisms to maintain blood pressure, with no vagal mechanism active at the time of syncope. The hypotension that has been present in the period leading up to the syncope will have caused heightening of baroreceptor reflex sensitivity (at all levels of neural integration) during the period of hy-

---

[1]Although often termed the Bezold-Jarisch reflex after Jarisch and von Bezold, such terminology is incorrect. Those authors described a similar reflex whose afferent is chemoreceptor and not mechanoreceptor. That phenyldiguanide sensitive reflex is properly termed the Bezold-Jarisch reflex, and may be present in inferior wall ischemia and during coronary injections of iodinated dye material. The presently discussed reflex has a different afferent.

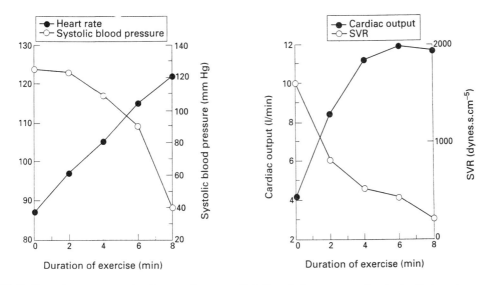

FIG. 5. Exercise syncope due to exercise vasodilatation during an exercise test with invasive monitoring. Decrease of vascular resistance is documented with exercise, with no heart rate slowing in relation to the occurrence of presyncope/syncope at a systolic pressure of 39 mm Hg. This observation may call into question certain hypotheses of causation. (Reproduced with permission. Sneddon JF et al. *Br Heart J* 1994;71:555. © 1994 The BMJ Publishing Group.)

potension. (The presence of a pronounced tachycardia that is unaffected by β-adrenergic blocking drugs supports this assertion.) When suddenly the patient loses consciousness and slumps to the ground, the baroreceptors experience a sudden (relative) hypertension. They then discharge, leading to a vagal discharge that inhibits sinus node impulse formation and slows the heart. Thus, in this conceptual framework, some "vasodepressor" syncope is not due to a vagal mechanism. The postsyncopal cardiac slowing is due to a vagal mechanism, but a mechanism whose afferent is the baroreceptor of the carotid sinus, not the mechanoreceptor of the heart. Furthermore, the vagal contribution is postsyncopal and therefore noncausal.

These comments are important for three reasons. First, the vasodepressor form of so-called vasovagal or neurocardiogenic syncope is the most common form of syncope observed, both in normal individuals and in athletes. Thus, the assertion that within this subgroup there may be a group whose causation is markedly differ-

ent [i.e., the overwhelming of autonomic (sympathetic) reflexes, rather than the presence of a vagal plus sympathoinhibitory neural effect] is potentially important for therapy. That such a group exists among performance athletes has been neatly documented by Sneddon et al. (38) (Fig. 5) who have reported on athletes (particularly Case 1 in their article) in whom the (normal) vasodilatation associated with exercise leads to so great a decrease in peripheral vascular resistance that it outstrips the ability of the heart to compensate via increased contractility and increased heart rate mechanisms. Therefore, hypotension and syncope occur as a specific effect of the overwhelming of autonomic (sympathetic) mechanisms, with no vagal admixture in the chain of causation.

The second important comment coming from the observation that syncope with vasodepressor phenomenology may or may not be of a vagal mechanism is that, in the athlete, hypervagotonia is common; indeed hypervagotonia is the rule in the performance athlete (see Electrocardiographic Variants in the Athlete). It is easy but erroneous to draw the inference from the occurrence of vasodepressor-appearing syncope, in such a setting of hypervagotonia, that the mechanism of the syncope was vagal. The bradycardia may be due to the athlete's hypervagotonia, which may be incidental to— and even in some cases independent of—the mechanism of syncope. The implication of these remarks is that much of what appears to be vasovagal vasodepressor syncope may in fact be due simply to the overwhelming of sympathetic reflexes, even in an athlete. Unrelated manifestations of hypervagotonia are due to the individual's athlete status and are not related to the causation of this syncope.

A third significant remark is a caution to those who perform tilt testing for the elucidation of mechanism in patients or athletes with recurrent syncope. Head-up tilt testing is a procedure used in an effort to observe spontaneous syncope, to elucidate its mechanism, and to guide further workup and therapy. Because of the logistical inconvenience of prolonged periods of head-up tilt, many laboratories shorten the period of basal tilt (tilt with no provocative pharmacologic agents) and subsequently perform additional tilts with pharmacologic agents of various classes to bring on syncope more quickly in susceptible individuals. Agents of several pharmacologic types are used in provocative tilt protocols, but chiefly drugs of three types are used: β-adrenergic agonists, such as isoproterenol; specific vasodilators, such as nitroglycerin; and withdrawal of β-adrenergic blocking drugs, such as esmolol (an ultra–short-acting beta-blocker). [In tilt testing using drugs of the first two classes, the provocative intervention is direct. In tilt testing using drugs of the third class (beta-blockers), the actual provocative intervention may not be the beta-blocker but rather the pharmacologic withdrawal of the drug because of its short (4 to 7 minutes) half-life (39).]

Of these classes of pharmacologic provocative head-up tilt protocols, isoproterenol is the most common. Isoproterenol has consistently been shown to shorten the time till syncope in head-upright tilt testing and to increase the frequency of syncope—hence the utility of pharmacologic provocation with isoproterenol. Its desired mechanism of action is to increase contractility (because of its nonspecific action on β_1-adrenoceptors on the myocardium) and thereby to provoke vagal syncope by mechanoreceptor stimulation. However, isoproterenol also has other adrenergic effects: it provokes a prominent tachycardia and it is a vasodilator as well.

The problem with interpreting isoproterenol-induced upright syncope is that the apparent vasodepressor response may not be real for two reasons. First, cardiac slowing may be blunted or abolished as a result of the positive chronotropic effect of isoproterenol. (This has been partly corrected for by such researchers as R. Sheldon by redefining mixed vasodepressor cardioinhibitory syncope in such fashion as to account for the positively chronotropic effect of isoproterenol.) Second, isoproterenol may cause the false-positive appearance of apparent vasodepressor syncope in normal individuals. In one study by Kapoor (49), isoproterenol was seen to cause syncope in between 45% and 65% of normal individuals when subjected to a standard tilt test protocol with isoproterenol provocation. Whether this is due to vasodilatation or to inordinate pharmacologic β_1-adrenergic stimulation, the results make clear the inherent problem with isoproterenol-induced syncope. There is a question when confronted with a vasodepressor response under isoproterenol provocation whether the response represents vasovagal (neurocardiogenic) syncope. Sometimes there is a question whether it correlates with clinical syncope at all.

Thus, it is clear that, in the causation of phenomenologic vasodepressor syncope, not only vasovagal mechanisms but also overwhelming of autonomic (sympathetic) mechanisms and diverse isoproterenol false-positive mechanisms must be considered. In ostensibly healthy nonathletes, additional mechanisms to be considered include autonomic failure, autonomic insufficiency (intrinsic or pharmacologic), variants of sick sinus syndrome, and other rarer physiologic entities. In women, occult pregnancy may present as syncope.

In athletes, one additional mechanism that should be considered is hypertension-induced hypotension. Although only rarely documented convincingly, the mechanism appears to consist of a period of hypertension that triggers a vagal reflex via a baroreceptor afferent. Following quickly on the heels of the hypertension is a period of modest or profound hypotension. This is vagal but not mechanoreceptor in causation. This has been seen in early (labile) hypertensive patients (40) as well as during isoproterenol infusion, and it has been observed to occur spontaneously and fortuitously during tilt testing (perhaps resulting from "white-coat hypertension" in borderline hypertensive patients) or exercise testing. Two of the cases of Snedden, Camm and McKenna (38) may reflect such an etiologic situation. It is expected that this may be particularly important in athletes, because severe degrees of hypertension normally accompany certain athletic activities: blood pressures in the 200 to 600 mm Hg range have been recorded (41). This may also be relevant in diving and after exposure to prescribed or illicit drugs with hypertensive effects via vasoactive mechanisms.

The mechanism of mixed vasodepressor-cardioinhibitory responses is more definitely vagal *a priori,* in that bradycardia precedes and likely contributes to the causation of the syncope. The presumed mechanism is identical to that already described for vasodepressor vasovagal syncope: venous pooling in the upright posture, perhaps augmented by vasodilatation or hypohydration, leading to a hyperadrenergic state. This in turn leads to activation of the cardiac mechanoreceptors, with consequent reflex action of vagal slowing of the heart as well as sympathoinhibition. The clinical syndrome is one of mild or severe bradycardia and disproportionate hypotension. An alternative (but equivalent) way of viewing the findings is hypotension without appropriate tachycardic response—indeed with paradoxical slowing of the heart rate.

This form of syncope may be more common in athletes, perhaps because of their intrinsic hypervagal state (whether or not this contributes to actual causation of the particular syncope), perhaps because of their ability to tolerate periods of hypotension, thereby postponing their syncope until a phase of bradycardia supervenes.

The third and most interesting canonical form of neurocardiogenic syncope is pure cardioinhibitory syncope (2,42). In this form of syncope, the efferent response (which occurs with any of several afferents) is vagal inhibition of the heart beat, leading to sudden profound sinus slowing or asystole. The wide variety of possible afferents is an interesting aspect of these syndromes. In addition to prolonged upright posture, this response may be elicited by brief upright posture after vigorous exercise, by emotional trauma (even as part of blood-injury phobia), and by esophageal stimulation in some patients, and perhaps by trigeminal stimulation in others (a human counterpart of the diving reflex of lower animals). Both Gillette (43) and the groups of Almquist (44), as well as Benditt (47,47a), have reported competent swimmers who have been fished up from the bottom of a pool unconscious after near-drowning, in whom subsequent evaluation documented sudden asystole in response to head-up tilt testing. In my experience, the syndrome most often presents with convulsions and syncope, rather than just syncope. Rarely, there may be a history of so-called breath holding as a toddler. There is frequently a family history of fainting and of other forms of presumed vagal syncope. It is a defensible (although somewhat extreme) point of view to assert that only these rare pure asystoles are rightly called vagal or vasovagal, in that all the other syncopes may have admixture of nonvagal mechanisms.

THE PRACTICE OF HEAD-UPRIGHT TILT TESTING IN THE EVALUATION OF SYNCOPE

Syncope in the athlete should be viewed with more concern than in the nonathlete. The workup is accordingly more rigorous. There are no accepted international standards for ECG, Holter, echocardiogram, head-up tilt testing, catheterization, coronary angiocardiography, and invasive electrophysiologic testing in this setting. My colleagues and I recommend tilt test for three unexplained syncopes in a nonathlete with otherwise negative findings (ECG, Holter, echocardiogram), but in the athlete, we recommend a tilt test for even one unexplained syncope.

In any sizable syncope practice, eventually one patient dies suddenly. With careful workup, this patient will die having already received a diagnosis of hypertrophic cardiomyopathy, probable hypertrophic cardiomyopathy, pulmonary hypertension, primary or secondary myocardial disease, ischemic heart disease minimally symptomatic (or asymptomatic) Wolf-Parkinson-White Syndrome or nonsustained ventricular tachycardia. And, such a patient will not be an individual carrying the diagnosis "structurally normal heart, benign vagal syncope."

The tilt test is a useful stepping-stone on the way to discontinuing workup in a patient with variant syncope in which structural heart disease, ischemia, arrhythmia, and idiopathic epilepsy appear unlikely, and in which vagal (neurocardiogenic) syncope or delayed orthostatic hypotension seem probable.

Background to Head-Upright Tilt Testing

An early report of tilt testing to provoke vagal syncope was made by Stephen E. Epstein in 1968 (45). Even though tilt table evaluation has been in continuous use in trauma surgery and emergency department medicine to assess volume status in possibly hypovolemic patients, it became important in the evaluation of unexplained syncope only after the widespread use of electrophysiologic testing in syncope workup created a group of undiagnosed patients with syncope and negative findings on programmed electrical stimulation.

Reports by Fitzpatrick and Sutton (46) in Great Britain and by Benditt et al. (47) in the United States initiated the widespread trend to use tilt testing as part of the diagnostic workup of syncope. From the time of the earliest reports of tilt testing, pharmacologic provocation protocols were used (isopro-

terenol) (48). Also, early clinical practice used invasive electrophysiologic testing as part of the same workup that included tilt testing; thus, in Benditt's work, tilt testing is performed as an adjunct to electrophysiologic testing at the same sitting. Benditt's protocol also includes isoproterenol provocation. Certain clinics persist in the practice of recommending cardiac catheterization and invasive electrophysiologic testing as part of the workup of all unexplained syncope, even when the historical features point clearly to a vagal etiology and when the patient is not an athlete. British clinics were the first to dispense with invasive electrophysiologic testing as a routine in patients with unexplained syncope and low pretest probability of arrhythmia or conduction system disease.

Kapoor and Brant (49) and our group (50) have championed the approach of dispensing with isoproterenol provocation and placing more confidence in the results of a prolonged basal tilt. We have also instituted a practice of performing tilt testing as an earlier part of the workup, even in patients with structural heart disease or known arrhythmia (i.e., before diagnostic cardiac catheterization and electrophysiologic testing) if the patient's history suggests vagal syncope or one of the orthostatic hypotension variants (e.g., delayed orthostatic hypotension). In our practice, this approach has been assisted by the introduction of a provocation protocol that could be used safely even in patients with significant occult heart disease—a circumstance in which isoproterenol could not be used as a provocative pharmacologic measure. We introduced and validated the esmolol and esmolol-withdrawal tilt protocols (Table 3), wherein tilt is performed during the withdrawal of an ultra–short-acting beta-blocker (Fig. 6), leading to stimulation of syncope apparently by unmasking the native catecholamines (although the possible added stress of the period of tilt under beta-blockade may contribute as well to the provocative efficacy).

In our clinic, invasive electrophysiologic testing is then reserved for patients in whom the syncope is not explained, or is clinically

TABLE 3. *Esmolol/Esmolol Withdrawal Protocol*

1. **Rest**
2. **Basal tilt**
   60-Degree head upright tilt for 49 minutes or until syncope (*t*).
3. **Rest**
   Esmolol bolus 500 µg/kg IV, and maintenance infusion, 50–300 µg/kg/min IV (may continue to increase during esmolol phase of tilt).
4. **Esmolol tilt**
   60-degree head upright tilt, during which esmolol will be discontinued. Continue esmolol for 15 minutes (if basal negative), or *t* + 5 minutes (if basal positive).
5. **Esmolol withdrawal tilt**
   Stop esmolol and continue tilt 29 minutes, or until syncope supervenes.
6. **Rest**
   Continue if no syncope thus far, and no contraindications to isoproterenol. Isoproterenol drip,* 0.05 µg/kg/min, increase HR ≥ 120% baseline, <150/min
7. **Isoproterenol tilt**
   60-Degree head upright tilt. Continue tilt 15 minutes or until syncope. *Positive tilt test,* hypotension or bradycardia leading to syncope[†] that resolves with recumbency; *transient positive,* severe clinical depression of blood pressure *or* reduction in heart rate without syncope, or brief syncope *that resolves without recumbency.*

*Optional. Reserved for research purposes.
[†]*Or* intolerable presyncope and symptoms identical to clinical symptoms.

only inadequately explained, by tilt test results. In athletes, we have a lower threshold for proceeding to invasive electrophysiologic testing even if tilt results are positive. This is partly based on referring physician preference, partly on the imperfect positive predictive value of the tilt test, and partly, perhaps, on medicolegal concerns.

In patients (athletes or nonathletes) with syncope during exercise or at peak exertion, the tilt test should be only part of the workup. Invasive electrophysiologic testing with coronary angiocardiography or stress testing with radionuclide perfusion imaging should complete the workup.

Alternatives to Head-Upright Tilt Testing

Tilt testing is not the only provocative protocol for eliciting syncope in patients with history of upright syncope. Gillette uses instead a protocol of prolonged standing, in which active tone in the lower extremity musculature is maintained.

Another approach used by some authors is active standing after treadmill testing: this should be regarded as merely a variant of tilt testing in which a provocative maneuver precedes an active standing protocol. Vasodilatation and catecholamines induced by the exercise are the provocative maneuver, in analogy to isoproterenol or nitroglycerin use as pharmacologic provocations as an adjunct to ordinary tilt testing. A third and highly meritorious approach is lower body negative pressure. Lower body negative pressure involves the use of reduced ambient pressure about the lower extremities to induce truncal and central circulatory hypovolemia. Based on the observation in the early modern era of artificial ventilation, when negative pressure ventilators were used, that normovolemic patients may become hypotensive and even syncopal after prolonged negative pressure ventilation, this technique is in fact a highly effective method of inducing hypotension and syncope. However its chief application to date has been in normal subjects to study the physiology of responses to hypovolemia, and no extensive clinical study in syncopal patients has been reported (51). Some interesting work with lower body negative pressure in exercise physiology has appeared (52,53).

Protocols of Head Upright Tilt Testing

The first tilt (the basal tilt) is performed on a tilt table with footplate support, noninvasive blood pressure monitoring, ECG monitoring, and an intravenous line and R_2 external pads to permit pacing or cardioversion.[2]

The angle of tilt is usually 60 degrees, although some laboratories use 80 degrees to increase incidence of syncope and to hasten its appearance. Tilt at 60 degrees with knee or mid-thigh restraint is completely passive tilt.

---

[2]Death as a complication of tilt testing has occurred in other laboratories in the setting of spontaneous or induced ventricular tachycardia or fibrillation.

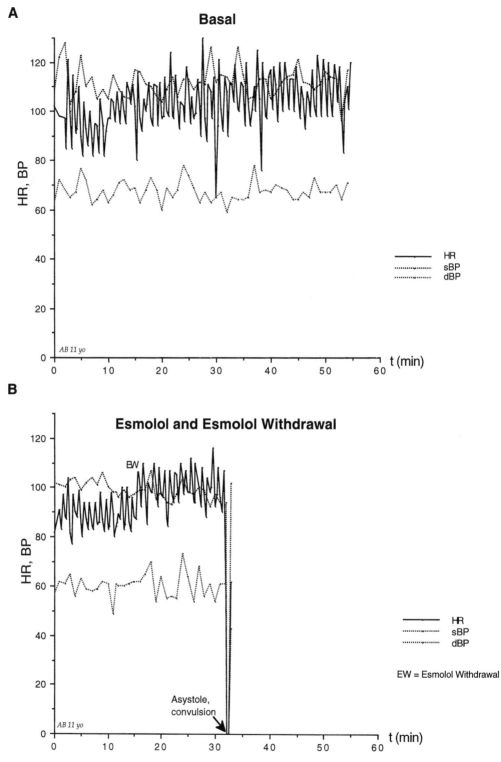

FIG. 6. Head-up tilt test responses in asystolic (pure cardioinhibitory) syncope with history of convulsions showing utility of esmolol-withdrawal as a provocative maneuver. **A:** Basal HUT is negative, though sinus arrhythmia is observed. **B:** Provocative testing with esmolol/esmolol-withdrawal elicits asystolic response after esmolol withdrawal. The presumed mechanism of provocation is that withdrawal of the ultra-short acting β-blocker esmolol unmasks endogenous catecholamines, which trigger syncope. Esmolol-withdrawal as provocative maneuver is superior to isoproterenol.

However, tilt to 80 degrees (even with knee restraint) introduces a component of active muscle contraction and coordination (i.e., it is no longer simply passive tilt). This introduces a perhaps undesirable additional variable.

The duration of the tilt is widely variable in U.S. and Canadian laboratories. In our laboratory, the initial tilt test is for 49 minutes, imitating protocols validated by British workers. If marked sinus arrhythmia with bradycardia or sinus pauses appears only in the last 2 minutes of tilt, then the tilt test is continued for 5 to 10 minutes beyond this.

Other workers use 30 minutes rather than 49. There are also many research workers who use a subsequent multistep isoproterenol tilt protocol and who shorten the initial tilt to a mere 10 minutes. We do not believe that the available data support the validity of such a practice. In our published data (50), the median time to syncope on the initial (basal) tilt is 26 minutes. Therefore, truncating the basal tilt at 10 minutes necessitates an unwarranted reliance on provocative measures to bring on syncope for more than half of patients.

Pharmacologic provocation tilts are used subsequently to the basal tilt. In most laboratories, the provocative tilt is performed only if the basal tilt is negative. In our practice, the mainstay of pharmacologic provocation is esmolol with esmolol-withdrawal during tilt; this is performed irrespective of the results of the baseline tilt. Thus, in our laboratory, a complete data set of tilt responses (baseline, beta-blocker, beta-blocker withdrawal provocation) is obtained for each patient (see Table 3). As discussed earlier, the rationale for the use of beta-blocker withdrawal is that endogenous catecholamines at physiologic levels (rather than exogenous catecholamines at pharmacologic levels) are thereby used to provoke syncope. The avoidance of isoproterenol may increase the sensitivity of the tilt protocol for the true vagal syncopes, those with spontaneously manifest asystolic features, that is, mixed vasodepressor/cardioinhibitory and pure cardioinhibitory syncope (see Fig. 6).

Other laboratories persist in the use of isoproterenol, often using protocols similar to that of Benditt. The rationale for this approach is that, from the logistical standpoint, isoproterenol increases the incidence of syncope and shortens the time to syncope. This should shorten the test. In the extensive experience of myself and my colleagues, however, we believe that it does so only at the expense of masking asystolic syncope (because isoproterenol is a potent positively chronotropic drug) and thus converting true mixed syncope or pure cardioinhibitory syncope into apparent vasodepressor syncope, the most suspect class of finding.

Furthermore, this practice renders the tilt test inaccessible to patients with suspected or known heart disease or tachyarrhythmia, because such patients either should not receive isoproterenol or may be permitted to receive it only after negative invasive electrophysiologic and coronary arteriographic findings, effectively excluding them from a patient pool to which tilt testing can be offered. Thus the routine and widespread use of isoproterenol biases the published reports away from patients with mild or suspected heart disease and falsely increases the proportion of patients with structurally normal hearts, making comparisons particularly difficult for the average patient.

This is a particular problem for performance athletes who have Holter and echocardiographic abnormalities that mimic serious organic heart diseases. For example, an athlete may have evidence of left ventricular hypertrophy and therefore carry the diagnosis of "possible" hypertrophic cardiomyopathy, excluding him from the standard full protocol for tilt testing in those laboratories. The isoproterenol practice introduces an unsatisfactory dichotomy in diagnostic approach: two separate approaches are used in the workup of patients who have the same clinical disease, leading to disparities and hence errors in diagnosis.

Lastly and most compellingly (and this is the reason for which we eschew isoproterenol use outside the research setting), isoproterenol causes false-positive syncope in normal patients without history of syncope (49).

In so doing, an isoproterenol positive result (particularly in an athlete) may well be a false-positive result. This may lead to a mistaken diagnosis, and workup will be terminated prematurely.

Another commonly used provocative pharmacologic maneuver, seen in European and British reports, is the use of nitroglycerin. A highly effective provocative maneuver, nitroglycerin use leads inevitably to interpretational uncertainty, because a hypovolemic patient with apparent vasodepressor syncope subsequent to nitroglycerin administration may have had a normal direct drug effect rather than a triggered vasovagal (neurocardiogenic) event.

Additional procedures performed during or with tilt have included invasive electrophysiologic testing, microneurography, and invasive arterial blood pressure monitoring. Results from these complicated protocols are subject to hard-to-unravel interpretational problems, in that intravascular instrumentation and the associated analgesics—or the fearful anticipation of the same—may alter responses to tilt testing.

Heart rate variability determinations (which require no additional instrumentation or even consent form signatures) have often been used in association with tilt, and for many years were included in our own protocol. The results have only rarely been useful (54,55); this should not be considered a valid part of a standard procedure.

HEAD-UP TILT TESTING IN THE ATHLETE

Tilt test responses of athletes with history of syncope are presented in two series and numerous single cases (either as case reports or as illustrative examples in larger series).

Grubb et al. (56) reported 24 trained athletes with episodes of syncope stated to have occurred during exertion. The patients ranged in age from 14 to 26 years, and they participated in a variety of sports, including running in nine, basketball in four, swimming in three, and various other exercises in the rest.

Because resting heart rates were not reported, there is no objective gauge of the level of training. There was no significant heart disease in the group, although four subjects carried the echocardiographic diagnosis of mitral valve prolapse.

Each patient had experienced at least two episodes of syncope, and the average number of syncopes per patient was 3.0 ± 1.1. In only one was there observed an apparent convulsion at the time of syncope. The patients were studied using a common head-upright tilt testing protocol. There was a 30-minute baseline tilt to 80 degrees.

Subsequently each patient underwent a multistep isoproterenol pharmacologic provocation tilt protocol. Initially, 1 μg/minute of isoproterenol was given, and the patient was subjected to 30 minutes of tilt. If the result of this tilt test was negative, the patient then was returned to the supine position and received 2 μg/minute of the drug, and the patient underwent a repeated 30 minutes of tilt. If this test, in turn, failed to provoke hypotension or bradycardia and their sequelae, then the patient received 3 μg/minute of the drug, and the test was repeated once again.

Using this protocol, Grubb elicited syncope in ten subjects during the baseline tilt (mean time to syncope 18 ± 10 minutes), in three during the first isoproterenol tilt, in four during the second isoproterenol infusion tilt, and in two during the third isoproterenol infusion tilt. Five subjects did not experience hypotension or syncope. Vasodepressor versus mixed versus pure cardioinhibitory responses were not reported, but in light of the frequent need for isoproterenol to induce syncope, it is probable that distinctions based on these data would not be conclusive in any case. It is reported that during the induced syncope in the patient with history of convulsion, similar convulsive movements were observed.

On the basis of these data, vasovagal (neurocardiogenic) syncope was diagnosed in the patients with the induced syncope. Various approaches were used to treat the patients chronically: six received fludrocortisone, three (transdermal) scopolamine, five beta-blockers, two *both* fludrocortisone and beta-blocker therapy, one disopyramide, and two no therapy. Incidentally, repeat tilt testing was used in an attempt to guide therapy.

During a remarkably long follow-up period of 23 ± 7 months, no recurrence of syncope was reported in the patients who received treatment. Only one patient was lost to follow-up. Both patients who received no therapy experienced additional episodes of syncope. Of the five patients in whom tilt testing failed to induce syncope (and who were therefore offered no therapy), two had recurrences of syncope. In this study, only 41% of the patients experienced syncope with the basal tilt.

In the second relevant report, Calkins et al. (57) reported 17 athletes aged 14 to 60 years at the time of symptom onset (mean age 28 ± 17 years) who underwent head-up tilt testing as part of evaluation for syncope that occurred in relation to exercise. Nine were competitive athletes, whereas eight were described as recreational athletes. They participated in the following activities: running in seven, swimming in two, basketball in one, and a variety of other sports in the remainder. One patient had mitral valve prolapse; all other patients had normal noninvasive and (in five patients) invasive evaluation.

Ninety-four percent experienced lightheadedness as a prodrome to syncope. One patient reported incontinence with no observed abnormal motor movements to suggest convulsion.

A 15-minute 70-degree head-up tilt was performed as the initial tilt, followed by repeat tilt during infusion of isoproterenol at increasing dose rates up to 4 μg/minute.

In six of the 17 patients, syncope was induced by baseline tilt alone. All of the other 11 patients experienced syncope after pharmacologic provocation with isoproterenol. Even though junctional rhythm, sinus bradycardia, and asystole were mentioned to have occurred in 14 patients, it was not stated whether these findings preceded, coincided with, or followed the expression of syncope and the return to recumbency. Subclassification of the responses is therefore impossible.

Critical review of these two excellent studies identifies few weaknesses in the studies themselves, but large gaps in existing knowledge. First, it is clear that, in the absence of the study of large and homogeneous groups of athletes engaged in a particular sport and matched with respect to degree of training, it is difficult to assess the specificity of the tilt test findings. It is well known, for example, that performance athletes may have reduced orthostatic tolerance. Therefore, they may be at increased risk for false-positive syncope on head upright tilt testing, particularly with isoproterenol pharmacologic provocation protocols. Secondly, the absence of a gauge of degree of training renders it difficult to extrapolate these results to true performance athletes, particularly because profound hypervagotonia is not specifically commented upon in the aforementioned published reports. Such hypervagotonia is a marked and fairly constant feature of the physiology of athletes trained past a certain point. Third, natural history remains obscure.

Finally, the absence of data on mixed vasodepressor and cardioinhibitory syncope and on pure cardioinhibitory syncope is frustrating. This may be due in part to the fact that these types of syncope occur less frequently than those with vasodepressor findings. Based on the case material presented in the published series, it might erroneously be concluded that pure cardioinhibitory syncope does not occur with significant frequency in the athlete with syncope. However, the use of isoproterenol pharmacologic provocation protocols may have diminished the frequency of such findings in the reported series, and the relative rarity of it may explain its absence in those series.

Other reports of experience with syncope in athletes managed with tilt testing include those of Rechavia (58), Ovadia et al. (59), and Milstein et al (47a). Rechavia reported a case of a basketball player, Ovadia an international competition triathlete (60) with recurrent syncope, and Almquist et al. a swimmer recovered after drowning.

To get some sense of the manner in which mixed syncope and pure cardioinhibitory syncope may present in the athlete, it is necessary to turn to the literature presentations of single cases. Milstein reports a swimmer with asystolic syncope at tilt testing who was presented with drowning (sudden cardiac death) on diving into a pool. Oslizlok and Gillette (43) present a similar case of a swimmer in the pediatric age group. Both of these patients may be regarded as having a variant either of mixed vasodepressor and cardioinhibitory syncope or of pure cardioinhibitory syncope.

Buja et al. (61) have reported symptomatic asystole in response to semiupright hyperventilation in athletes. Although syncope and convulsions were thus induced, the absence of clinical history either of syncope or of convulsions suggests that these findings were nothing more than extreme manifestations of the familiar hypervagotonia of the athlete, and they should not be overinterpreted. In our experience, we have made similar observations, suggesting to us that the Valsalva-like expiratory phase of the forced ventilatory cycle may be the physiologic setting for these asystoles.

Little work has been reported on the significance of exact syncope timing in relation to exercise (i.e., syncope whose symptoms occur during exercise versus syncope whose symptoms occur after exercise). That syncope whose symptoms occur during exercise may be vagal is suggested by the report of Sakaguchi et al. (62). In that study, 12 nonathletes with exercise syncope were studied by head-up tilt testing. Eight of ten had vasodepressor findings on basal tilt, and one had vasodepressor findings with isoproterenol (3 μg/minute). One had negative findings.

Our experience is different, however. Syncope during exercise occurs most likely as a consequence of organic heart disease. We have seen occult hypertrophic cardiomyopathy, occult critical pulmonary obstruction, and occult pulmonary and right ventricular hypertension present as exercise syncope. It is likely that the differences in type of referral practice—our patients have more severe syndromes and higher pretest probability of heart disease—may explain the differences between our experience and that of Sakaguchi.

TREATMENT

The treatment of syncope in the athlete has been based on the treatment of neurocardiogenic (vasovagal) syncope in other populations (Table 4). That therapy is largely empirical. Beta-blockers and disopyramide have been typical drugs used, based on the dominant view of the pathophysiology of the syncope. Other drugs including scopolamine and urecholine have been popular as well. Many drugs have been tested. The group of drugs generally thought to be useful is small compared with the number of drugs still being used.

As discussed previously, there is a group of athletes with tilt positive syncope in whom the repeat tilt test during beta-blockade shows worsening of the manifestations, akin to the expected findings in orthostatic hypotension. In these patients, the premise that syncope is simply vasovagal in causation is suspect. For a group of patients as this, therapy with increased salt, fludrocortisone, or α-agonists may be expected to be reasonable, based on the presumed pathophysiologic condition, and this has led to the introduction of a large additional group of drugs and approaches (63), which are generally far more useful in practice than all other classes of agents, particularly for the athlete.

This section discusses the available approaches based on a reasonable step-by-step approach useful to the clinician, with comments about the range of applicability of each treatment in its place (see Table 4).

The mainstay of therapy is to teach the patient to be aware of situations (settings or premonitory symptoms) in which syncope may occur, so that he or she will have heightened vigilance. Then when the patient becomes aware of any symptoms that may lead to syncope, he or she will sit or lie down immediately to avoid syncope. The clinician should not be discouraged from making such a recommendation in athletes.

A minimal list of situations for the athlete to be aware of includes prolonged standing, standing after suddenly stopping intense exer-

TABLE 4. *Treatment*

Behavioral	Dosage		Comments	
	Initial	Subsequent		
Dietary				
Increased salt	Dietary	1 g NaCl po b.i.d.	Superior	*Avoid in hypertension.*
Beta-Blocker				
with ISA				
Pindolol (Visken™)	5 mg po b.i.d.	10 mg po b.i.d.	Best	*May worsen symptoms.*
Acebutolol (Sectral™)	200 mg po b.i.d.			*May worsen symptoms*
without ISA				
Propranolol (Inderal LA™)	60 to 80 mg po qD			*May worsen symptoms. Avoid in asystolic convulsive syncope. May worsen bradycardia. Typically poorly tolerated in athletes.*
Mineralocorticoid				
Fludrocortisone (Florinef™)	0.05 mg po qD	0.1 mg po qD	Superior	*Avoid in hypertension. Anticipate need for Cortrosyn™ stimulation test to exclude adrenal insufficiency.*
Constrictor				
Arterioconstrictors				
Midodrine (Proamatine™)	2.5 mg po b.i.d.	5 mg 7.5 mg po b.i.d. 7.5 mg po t.i.d.	Superior	*Avoid in preexisting hypertension.*
Pseudoephedrine (Sudafed™)	75 mg po b.i.d.	90 mg po t.i.d.		*Anticipate tachyphylaxis.*
Venoconstrictors				
Ergot derivatives and ergot				*See text and relevant references.*
Other				
Compression stockings		Superior		

cise, dehydration, and times when there is a gastrointestinal or esophageal problem (e.g., gastroenteritis). The athlete is advised to sit or lie down immediately. Frequent vigorous coughing (termed *cough CPR*) may be useful if it will take the athlete more than a moment to find a place to sit or lie down, especially if the athlete's time-to-syncope is known to be extremely short.

Another basic element of therapy is to increase salt intake. This appears to increase the latency till syncope, thus giving the patient a longer and more adequate time to respond to early hypotensive symptoms. (This is not applicable to patients with documented or suspected hypertension.)

There are various ways to take increased salt. We recommend patients have some salt with each meal and have a couple of heavily salted snacks during the day. Even though there are other ways to give salt (e.g., NaCl tablets, typical dose 1–2 g twice daily), this is usually unnecessary, because it is easy to take in 7 g of salt daily by dietary liberalization alone. Salted pretzels (Bachmann's pretzels have almost 1.5 g of salt in a small package), pickles, and other salty snacks can be suggested. Twenty-four-hour urine collection for salt can be performed on an average day to confirm adequate intake once high-salt dietary habits have been instituted, with the objective of taking at least 7 g daily for the adolescent or young adult athlete. Literature reports of targets between 2 and 9 g of NaCl daily have been recorded as part of the efficacious therapy of orthostatic hypotension.

Based on historical practice, beta-blockers are typically considered as the first pharmacologic treatment. However, the utility of beta-blockers is questionable in athletes, both from the point of view of poor patient acceptance and the frequency with which they, in fact, make the situation worse, whether subjectively or confirmed by tilt testing. For straightforward vasodepressor vagal syncope, however, they are often useful.

The first beta-blocker we try for outpatient therapy in an athlete is pindolol (Visken™), a nonselective beta-blocker with intrinsic sympathomimetic activity. Because of the latter action, it is well tolerated, even in athletes, and even in individuals with resting bradycardia. The starting dose is 5 mg twice daily, which may be doubled. (Before going to a much higher dose, we have the patient on salt and on fludrocortisone or an α-agonist.)

An alternative approach, anecdotally less effective, is acebutolol (Sectral™), a cardioselective beta-blocker. Similarly to pindolol, it has intrinsic sympathomimetic activity.

For the nonathletic patient or the athlete in an off-season, standard recommendation may include the beta-blockers propranolol (long-acting preparation Inderal LA™, 60 or 80 mg once daily) or atenolol (Tenormin™, 25 mg once or twice daily). These agents (particularly the latter) are typically ill-tolerated by the true performance athlete and make resting bradycardia worse. To the patient with pure cardioinhibitory response on tilt testing, we do not offer these drugs. (All beta-blockers also may increase the risk of hyperthermia in athletes by impairing mechanisms of heat dissipation.)

A second drug that should be considered is fludrocortisone (Florinef™). This is a mineralocorticoid with considerable glucocorticoid potency (64). Often it is so effective that it is difficult to wean the patient off it, and this circumstance may raise the question of occult adrenal insufficiency. Therefore, as a rigid rule, Cortrosyn™ (ACTH) stimulation testing should be performed before using this in a patient (0.25 mg intramuscularly, with cortisol measured at time 0, 15, and 30 minutes by the same laboratory—more complicated versions of this test also exist).

The goal of fludrocortisone therapy is to increase plasma volume through the sodium-retaining action of that drug. Even in the absence of any change in blood pressure in the asymptomatic period, this leads to attenuated symptoms and longer time from start of hypotensive symptoms to syncope (i.e., longer latency). Undesirable but infrequent side effects include headaches, subjective "bloatedness," lower extremity edema, anomalous weight increase, abnormalities of menses, and hypertension (65). The latter side effect we have seen only when the drug is combined with other medications at high dose.

Fludrocortisone is given at a dose of 0.05 mg daily, increased to 0.1 mg daily, and in some patients the dose may be increased as high as 0.15 mg twice daily. At least 20 mEq daily of KCl can be given concomitantly—the possible side effect of hypokalemia is avoided by administering KCl when fludrocortisone is used at higher doses (66).

The group of patients in whom fludrocortisone is the mainstay of pharmacotherapy is precisely the group of athletes with apparent vasodepressor tilt test responses, but in whom response is worsened after beta-blocker (typically performed as part of the initial tilt workup). This is the group that may be regarded as having delayed orthostatic hypotension, and other of the many therapies familiar in orthostatic hypotension will be useful as well. The fludrocortisone is also effective in true vasovagal syncope because it increases the latency (time-to-syncope) by elevating the blood pressure during this phase.

Alpha-agonists have an important place in therapy for the same reason. Among such drugs, pseudoephedrine (Sudafed™) has enjoyed the longest popularity because of its wide availability, and etilefrine, another similar drug, has been shown to be effective in a controlled trial. The pseudoephedrine dose in an adolescent may reach 75 to 90 mg three times daily. It may be added on to other therapy, including therapy with fludrocortisone, without ill effect.

The alpha-agonist favored in our clinic is the newer agent midodrine (Proamatine™) (67). Unlike pseudoephedrine, midodrine is a pure alpha-agonist, rather than a mixed alpha- and beta-agonist.

Midodrine is surprisingly effective even after many other drugs have failed (68). Its side effects include piloerection (patients complain of "goosebumps") and supine hypertension. Because of the latter, midodrine should be used at the minimal dose at which it is effective. It may be started at 2.5 mg two or three times daily, but in difficult cases, 7.5 mg twice daily may be a reasonable point of departure as well. Therapy should be followed with ambulatory blood pressure monitoring and lying, sitting, and standing blood pressure determination in the physician's office. A maximal dose of 7.5 mg three times daily or 10 mg twice daily is appropriate for the average young adult or adolescent. Midodrine tachyphylaxis is frequently encountered irrespective of dose. In our clinic, we attempt to manage this with a "drug holiday" or period of midodrine abstinence during which pseudoephedrine or fludrocortisone is given.

The typical patient with vasodepressor or mixed responses on tilt testing should respond to one or to a combination of the aforementioned medications. Frequently, several regimens must be tried before finding an effective combination and dose; therefore, patients should be told in advance that they may need to try several medicines or combination regimens for as long as 2 to 3 months each, so that the patient is not disappointed if the first one or two efforts do not work.

A next step is compression stockings. These may be specified in different lengths and degrees of compression. We choose medium compression and have no preference as to length. These may be expensive, and the patient should be made aware that they may or may not help, and often they are not tolerated. Typically, fludrocortisone must be reduced or discontinued (going to alternate day treatment before discontinuation) because of its associated hypertension when compression hose are used.

DDD (AV universal) pacemakers, although considered on the basis of a multicenter study in vagal syncope soon to be published, cannot be recommended at this time to patients other than those with pure cardioinhibitory syncope. Sheldon's study presented at the 1997 North American Society of Pacing and Electrophysiology (NASPE) meetings (without corresponding published abstract, R. Sheldon, 1998 personal communication) demonstrated in a large cohort of patients with predominantly vasodepressor (but rare mixed) syncope that permanent DDD pacemaker implantation (using the Medtronic Thera DR*i*™ unit) the efficacy of pacing with a variant of DDI hysteresis ("rate drop"). Because long-term data are lacking, it would be inappropriate to recommend this for vasodepressor syncope at this time.

The following discussion identifies other drugs used or recommended and includes relevant comments.

Disopyramide is frequently used, because of its anticholinergic effects, but in randomized double-blind study, it has been shown to be inferior to placebo. Given the results of the Cardiac Arrhythmia Suppression Trial (CAST) study (in certain populations, sudden death attended the use of any type I antiarrhythmic agent, presumably owing to bradycardia-dependent or adrenergic-dependent ventricular tachycardia brought out by the type I drug—an effect termed "proarrhythmia") and the facts that (a) disopyramide is a potent type I antiarrhythmic drug and (b) bradycardia is frequent in this population, and because occult heart disease may also be present, it is our practice to avoid this drug and to discontinue its use whenever an equally effective drug could be found. We have always been able to find such a replacement drug or regimen.

Scopolamine by transdermal patches is an intervention based on the assumption that overactive vagal outpouring is the cause of vagal syncope. Still recommended by some clinicians, most workers have found this to be poorly tolerated and rarely effective. Urecholine (Probanthine) has been used by some workers with similar intent, with anecdotal reports of efficacy.

Fluoxetine (Prozac) and similar drugs have been reported to be efficacious in excellent studies by Blair Grubb (68a) that involved repeat head-upright tilt testing as a measure of efficacy. In our own experience, these may be effective in an occasional patient with vasodepressor or mixed vasodepressor and cardioinhibitory syncope, but concerns about proarrhythmia may apply. We have observed atrial proarrhythmia with the use of such drugs.

Indomethacin (Indocin™) has been reported to be efficacious in orthostatic hypotension, but it has not been specifically studied in upright syncope in athletes.

Dihydroergotamine mesylate (DHE 45™) is available in the United States, but superior formulations may be available overseas, and ergot preparations have a definite place in the management of delayed orthostatic hypotension, orthostatic hypotension, and variant vasodepressor-tilt positive neurocardiogenic syncope (69,70). A venoconstrictor, caution should be used because of the risk of supine and ambulatory hypertension at the initiation of therapy. This is the only drug proven equal in efficacy to midodrine, the pure alpha-agonist in managing orthostatic hypotension.

Ritalin™ (methylphenidate) is frequently considered, but its use (although sometimes unexpectedly effective) cannot be generally endorsed at this time.

Table 4 summarizes the chief medications and doses in therapy of neurocardiogenic syncope and delayed orthostatic hypotension.

Cardioinhibitory Syncope: The Role of Pacing

It has long been known that vagally mediated syndromes other than neurocardiogenic syncope, such as the hypersensitive carotid sinus syndrome, may respond to dual-chamber pacing. The hypersensitive carotid sinus syndrome represents an analog of mixed vasodepressor and cardioinhibitory syncope and of pure cardioinhibitory syncope: upright posture is a necessary condition for syncope, and the blood pressure and heart rate findings follow the same patterns as those of neurocar-

diogenic syncope. This is the first vagal condition proven treatable (or curable) with dual-chamber pacing (71,72,72a,72b).

Prior to the work of Sheldon mentioned above, syncope in neurocardiogenic syncope (without convulsions) was believed not to respond to pacing, although some discrepancies persisted in the American versus British and continental medical literatures regarding (a) the ability of pacing to abolish spontaneous syncope versus syncope that occurs during provocative testing and (b) the ability of pacing to reduce syncope in some cases of mixed syncope (cardioinhibitory and vasodepressor features).

However, no such negative results were ever reported for symptoms whose manifestation appeared to be due to primary asystole. In Sra's benchmark article (72c) on the failure of vasodepressor vagal hypotension and syncope to respond to pacing, no patient had convulsive syncope and no patient had a primary cardioinhibitory response to orthostatic stress; in the individuals who had mixed syncope, the cardioinhibitory component appeared later and was mild.

Convulsive syncope (i.e., in which a convulsion is related to asystole) may respond to pacing (72d–f). Whereas convulsions occur in several vagal syndromes spanning the time line from infancy to adulthood, the best studied convulsive syndromes are those occurring in cardioinhibitory syncope (either pure cardioinhibitory syncope or mixed syncope with severe and early cardioinhibitory component). In my experience and that of several others, these convulsive syndromes appear to respond to pacing. In more than 25 patients with syncope and convulsive symptoms, it has been observed that, in cardioinhibitory syncope, permanent dual-chamber pacing abolishes convulsions (2). Because typically these patients are seen with generalized motor convulsions (the clinical features are those of a new onset seizure disorder), these syndromes are not likely to be confused with vasodepressor neurocardiogenic syncope; rather, they are mistaken for idiopathic epilepsy of recent onset. The convulsion typically occurs at the time of reperfusion when the heart starts beating again after a period of asystole (73); thus, the definition of convulsive syncope must be taken to assume a very particular temporal association between asystole and the convulsion. Successful pacemaker therapy of convulsive (asystolic) syncope may not alleviate all syncopal and presyncopal symptoms. Indeed, in some patients, new presyncope may arise concomitant with successful therapy of the seizures, which will have disappeared with the institution of permanent pacing. Pacing is highly effective in abolishing the convulsions (at the expense of replacing those convulsions with presyncope or asymptomatic hypotension). Presumably, vasodepressor responses are still present. That some of these children have been diagnosed only after aborted sudden cardiac death is a further argument for pacing, although it is not specifically known whether pacing confers increased longevity in the majority of patients with these rare syndromes.

The use of pacing for neurocardiogenic syncope remains profoundly limited by the absence of a posture sensor that would permit pacing to be initiated by the assumption of upright posture. The objective of developing a posture sensor is highly relevant and has been approached by several groups in clinical and theoretical published articles (73). (Because increase of heart rate upon assumption of the upright posture in the normal patient is mediated by parasympathetic withdrawal via the arterial baroreceptor reflex, the development of a posture sensor in rate adaptive pacing is the equivalent of restoration of an autonomic reflex in some patients, and is the equivalent of the modulation of this reflex for others by manipulation of open-loop gain.)

In the absence of a posture sensor, clinical practice involves DDD pacer with (a) special variants of DDI hysteresis as described earlier, (b) regular hysteresis, or (c) high lower rate limit settings at all times. [The reported use of pre-ejection interval (PEI) as posture sensor has been proven to be based on invalid theoretical assumptions (73).]

Special Situations

Syncope in the Athlete with Migraine

The migraine patient with vagal syncope represents a special case, and with careful choice of therapy, both problems can be considerably alleviated. Long-acting propranolol preparations (e.g., Inderal LA™ 80 mg daily) are an appropriate initial measure in combination with increased salt. Caffeine-containing preparations and dihydroergotamine are appropriate secondary measures. All forms of vagal syncope can also complicate migraine acutely as a result of pain or esophageal irritation (74). Because this includes asystolic convulsive syncope (75), attempt should be made to document the rhythm during a syncopal attack, to avoid administering beta-blockers. In cases of asystole, it is particularly important to use a long basal tilt and esmolol-withdrawal provocation rather than to rely on isoproterenol provocation in this group of patients.

Syncope in the Athlete with Hypertension

A frequent problem in teen-aged and young athletes is incipient essential hypertension (76–80). When this is documented or suspected on the basis of family history, a beta-blocker is appropriate initial therapy. Salt and Florinef should be avoided. Although for other hypertensive patients angiotensin-converting enzyme inhibitors or diuretics may be an appropriate first-line or first-step choice, in this group of patients, beta-blockers with or without intrinsic sympathomimetic activity appear more appropriate.

Syncope in the Diver and Recreational Swimmer: Underwater Syncope and Syncope During Water Sports

A fascinating group of syndromes has been well documented in the diver and recreational swimmer (81). In the diver, anoxic syncope, decompression syncope, and various postemersion syncopes (including so-called *sincope degli ultimi metri*—syncope of the final yards) are well described and have disparate origins.

In the recreational swimmer, trigeminal stimulation also can lead to asystolic convulsive syncope, which is a rare but well documented cause of sudden death after diving into a pool. Patients with the more common forms of neurocardiogenic syncope or delayed orthostatic hypotension frequently become hypotensive after emersion.

Syncope in relation to water sports thus represents a fascinating differential diagnosis, particularly important because of the immediate risk of drowning. Patients with the same clinical syndrome may be subjected to vastly different approaches to workup and recommendations. To present a clinical approach to such syncope, a discussion of relevant physiology is indispensable, followed by enumeration of classes of syncope that become manifest in relation to water sports.

Entry into the water is accompanied by a shift of blood volume to the cranial vault, the lungs, and certain of the intraabdominal viscera. Diving is accompanied by further shift in the same direction, but of greater magnitude.

In diving, compression of intraalveolar gas results in elevated Pa_{O_2} and an initial sense of well-being. Assuming there is no availability of compressed gas, the Pa_{CO_2} increases progressively as the Pa_{O_2} decreases, depending somewhat on the degree of physical exertion and the ambient temperature, but occurring whether or not the swimmer is at depth. Normally, the Pa_{CO_2} reaches a certain point, different for different individuals, at which diaphragmatic contraction starts to occur (the Pa_{CO_2} breakpoint). At first this can be suppressed voluntarily, but eventually this and related mechanisms become overpowering, and the subject must try to resurface and breathe. Had this CO_2 effect not been preeminent, then the subject would, a bit later, have reached a point when Pa_{O_2} was so depressed (the Pa_{O_2} breakpoint) as to cause a stimulus to breathe less potent than the Pa_{CO_2} stimulus, followed by clouding of consciousness and anoxic syncope.

Elite athlete swimmers differ in two ways from the ordinary individual and even from the ordinary athlete. First, they can voluntarily suppress respiration, thus postponing the Pa_{CO_2} breakpoint and reducing the interval between the Pa_{CO_2} and the Pa_{O_2} breakpoints—indeed, sometimes even inverting it. (Similarly to other athletes, their slower heart rates and efficient metabolisms also may postpone the Pa_{O_2} decrease during apnea; this is not specific to swimmers.)

Second, as a learned—and sometimes *lethal*—behavior, these athletes hyperventilate before immersion. This postpones the Pa_{CO_2} breakpoint and prolongs considerably the period they may stay immersed. What is innocent in a Malibu or Jones Beach surfer may be life-threatening to a diver, because after such preventive hyperventilation, the Pa_{CO_2} breakpoint may be avoided altogether because the Pa_{O_2} breakpoint arrives first, and the elite swimmer then experiences anoxic syncope while underwater.

Another potential mechanism of syncope underwater related to hyperventilation is frank convulsion in the individual with a chronic seizure disorder, related to hyperventilation, respiratory alkalosis, and hypocalcemia.

Additional relevant mechanisms include the inverse blood shift experienced by the diver on coming to the surface, coupled with the reduction in alveolar Pa_{O_2} owing to decompression of the intraalveolar gas. These two mechanisms probably underlie the fascinating syndrome of the syncopal rendez-vous (*le rendez-vous syncopal*) as described in the French literature, and of *la sincope degli ultimi metri*—syncope of the last few yards—of Italian authors.

When the swimmer or diver emerges from the water, there is further inverse blood shift to the extremities and viscera. This is the equivalent of orthostatic stress with provocation and frequently precipitates syncope resulting from orthostatic hypotension or delayed orthostatic hypotension, or less frequently (and perhaps only as a concomitant to orthostatic hypotension or delayed orthostatic hypotension) vagal mechanisms. An additional mechanism of disturbance of consciousness is decompression sickness. Occurring only when compressed gas was used in a dive, this is due to gaseous N_2 microemboli in nervous tissues.

It must always be remembered in dealing with ostensibly vagal syncope in the bradycardic recumbent athlete during the recovery phase from syncope that the vagal bradycardia may be the result and not the cause of the syncope, indeed, that no vagal mechanism may be in evidence. This is true because the loss of consciousness in orthostatic hypotension or delayed orthostatic hypotension may be due solely to intravascular volume contraction exceeding the autonomic compensation (i.e., autonomic or sympathetic failure without sympathetic withdrawal); independently an intact—in the elite athlete, a hyperactive—baroreceptor reflex causes bradycardia after the athlete collapses to the ground. This is a vagal sequela of a nonvagal syncope, as discussed earlier. It is particularly difficult in swimmers to determine the sequence of events (heart rate decrease first versus blood pressure decrease first) in spontaneous syncope.

Even though a so-called diving reflex in mammals has frequently drawn attention, it is not clear that this does exist in humans, although a well-known vagal reflex depends on a trigeminal afferent (and is used in children to terminate episodes of supraventricular tachycardia). Perhaps this trigeminally afferented reflex is implicated in some cases of swimming pool divers losing consciousness in the pool. Alternatively, the Valsalva or acute hypertension may trigger bradycardia (baroreceptor-mediated), or the syncope may be anoxic as previously stated above.

Important history to be obtained includes whether syncope occurred in the water or outside, and if outside, then in what posture. If syncope occurred in the water, then it must be ascertained whether it was likely to have been anoxic syncope and whether hyperventilation may have contributed indirectly or directly. If compressed gas had been used and evaluation is performed soon after the occurrence, then history to suggest decompression sickness must be elicited; referral to a hyperbaric specialist is essential.

If the pattern of syncope fits no syndrome perfectly and occurred soon after emergence from the water, then head-up tilt testing is useful, although often inconclusive. The pattern of syncope on tilt testing is more often that of orthostatic hypotension or delayed orthostatic hypotension than of true vagal syncope, and often therefore worsens with beta-blockade, but may improve with alpha$_1$-agonist therapy [e.g., midodrine (Proamatine™) or the nonselective adrenergic agonist pseudoephedrine (Sudafed™)]. For mixed syncope, as for asystolic (pure cardioinhibitory) syncope, DDD pacemakers should be considered early.

Except for the most straightforward cases with out-of-water syncope, referral to a highly specialized clinic is essential because of the risk of drowning.

REFERENCES

1. Thilenius OG, Ryd KJ, Husayni J. Variations in expression and treatment of transient neurocardiogenic instability. *Am J Cardiol* 1992;69:1193–1195.
2. Ovadia M, Bacon-Pajonas K, Thoele DM, Gear K, Marcus FI. Convulsive syncope of the young: a vagal syndrome with features distinct from mixed vasodepressor/cardioinhibitory syncope and from breath-holding. *J Am Coll Cardiol* 1996;27:396–397A.
3. Batlouni M, Gimenes VM, Ghorayeb N. Ondas T negativas gigantes associadas a hipertrofia isolada dos musculos papilares do ventriculo esquerdo, em atletas. Relato de dois casos. *Arq Bras Cardiol* 1988;50:183–187.
4. Williams RA. Sudden cardiac death in blacks, including black athletes. *Cardiovasc Clin* 1991;21:297–320.
4a. Fontaine G, Guedon-Moreau L, Frank R, Lascault G, Fontaliran F, Tonet J, Himbert C, Grosgogeat Y. La dysplasie ventriculaire droite. *Ann Cardiol Angéiol* (Paris) 1993;42:399–405.
4b. Fontaine G, Umemura J, DiDonna P, Tsezana R, Cannat JJ, Frank R. La durée des complexes QRS dans la dysplasie ventriculaire droite arythmogène. Un nouveau marqueur diagnostique non invasif. *Ann Cardiol Angéiol* (Paris) 1993;42:399–405.
4c. Furlanello F, Bettini R, Bertoldi A, Vergara G, Visona L, Durante GB, Inama G, Frisanco L, Antolini R, Zanuttini D. Arrythmia patterns in athletes with arrhythmogenic right ventricular dysplasia. *Eur Heart J* 1989;10 Suppl D:16–9.
4d. Maron BJ, Pelliccia A, Spirito P. Cardiac disease in young trained athletes. Insights into methods for distinguishing athlete's heart from structural heart disease, with particular emphasis on hypertrophic cardiomyopathy. *Circulation* 1995;91:1596–1601.
4e. Occhetta E, Aina F, Sansa M, Prando MD, Magnani A, Negro R, Rossi P. Anomalie della ripolarizzazione ventricolare e aritmie nell'atleta. Caso clinico di osservazione prolungata. *G Ital Cardiol* 1986;16:439–444.
5. Bryan G, Ward A, Rippe JM. Athletic heart syndrome. *Clin Sports Med* 1992;11:259–272.
6. Zanfardino V, De Simone R, Verza M, et al. Studio elettrocardiografico, vettorcardiografico ed ecocardiografico

del grado di ipertrofia ventricolare sinistra in atleti di fondo e mezzofondo. *Cardiologia* 1988;33:945–948.

7. Beckner GL, Winsor T. Cardiovascular adaptation to prolonged physical effort. *Circulation* 1954;9:835.

8. Mammarella G, D'Urso A, Fraioli AM, Barbieri GE, Rizzo R, Bellisario G. Diversa incidenza delle alterazioni del ritmo cardiaco negli atleti e nei giovani non allenati. *Minerva Cardioangiol* 1987;35:407–410.

9. Macchi G. Effetti a lungo termine sul cuore dell'attivita sportiva agonistica in ex atleti professionisti. *G Ital Cardiol* 1987;17:505–550.

10. Vollmer-Larsen A, Vollmer-Larsen B, Kelbaek H, Godtfredsen J. The veteran athlete: an echocardiographic comparison of veteran cyclists, former cyclists and non-athletic subjects. *Acta Physiol Scand* 1989;135:393–398.

11. Zeppilli P. Cuore d'atleta ed invecchiamento cardiaco. *G Ital Cardiol* 1987;17:511–513.

12. Zeppilli P, Manno V. Vagotonia fisiologica e non fisiologica nell'atleta. *G Ital Cardiol* 1987;17:865–873.

13. Roeske WR, O'Rourke RA, Klein A, Leopold G, Karlimer KS. Noninvasive evaluation of ventricular hypertrophy in professional athletes. *Circulation* 1976; 53:286–292.

14. Casadei B. Effects of athletic training on neural control of heart rate. *Cardiovasc Res* 1993;27:1383–1384.

15. Ekblom B, Kilbom ASA, Soltysiak J. Physical training, bradycardia and autonomic nervous system. *Scand J Clin Lab Invest* 1973;32:251–256.

16. Furlan R, Piazza S, Dell'Orto S, Gentile E, Cerutti S, Pagani M, Malliani A. Early and late effects of exercise and athletic training on neural mechanisms controlling heart rate. *Cardiovasc Res* 1993;27:482–488.

17. Underwood RH, Schwade JL. Noninvasive analysis of cardiac function in elite distance runners—echocardiography, vectorcardiography and cardiac intervals. *Ann N Y Acad Sci* 1977;301:297–309.

18. Ikaheimo MJ, Palatsi IJ, Takkunen JT. Noninvasive evaluation of the athletic heart: sprinters versus endurance runners. *Am J Cardiol* 1979;44:24–30.

19. Reiling MJ, Seals DR. Respiratory sinus arrhythmia and carotid baroreflex control of heart rate in endurance athletes and untrained controls. *Clin Physiol* 1988;8: 511–519.

20. Barney JA, Ebert TJ, Groban L, et al. Carotid baroreflex responsiveness in high-fit and sedentary young men. *J Appl Physiol* 1988;65:2190–2194.

21. Ogawa S, Tabata H, Ohishi S, et al. Prognostic significance of long ventricular pauses in athletes. *Jpn Circ J* 1991;55:761–766.

22. Adbulatif M, Fahkry M, Naguib M, Gyamfi YA, Saeed I. Multiple electrocardiographic anomalies during anaesthesia in an athlete. *Can J Anaesth* 1987;34:284–287.

23. Crowley JS, Hollway JD. Cases from the aerospace medicine residents' teaching file. *Aviat Space Environ Med* 1988;59:183–185.

24. Kinoshita S, Konishi G. Atrioventricular Wenckebach periodicity in athletes: influence of increased vagal tone on the occurrence of atypical periods. *J Electrocardiol* 1987;20:272–279.

25. Shaw LJ, Eagle KA, Gersh BJ, Miller DD. Meta-analysis of intravenous dipyridamole-thallium-201 imaging (1985 to 1994) and dobutamine echocardiography (1991 to 1994) for risk stratification before vascular surgery. *J Am Coll Cardiol* 1996;27:787–798.

26. Karvonen J, Vuorimaa T. Heart rate and exercise intensity during sports activities. Practical application. *Sports Med* 1988;5:303–311.

27. Bjornstad H, Storstein L, Meen HD, Hals O. Electrocardiographic findings of left, right and septal hypertrophy in athletic students and sedentary controls. *Cardiology* 1993;82:56–65.

28. Bjornstad H, Storstein L, Meen HD, Hals O. Electrocardiographic findings in athletic students and sedentary controls. *Cardiology* 1991;79:290–305.

29. Palatini P, Maraglino G, Mos L, et al. Effect of endurance training on Q-T interval and cardiac electrical stability in boys aged 10 to 14. Ventricular arrhythmias in trained boys. *Cardiology* 1987;74:400–407.

30. Visser FC, Mihciokur M, van Dijk CN, den Engelsman J, Roos JP. Arrhythmias in athletes: comparison of stress test, 24 h Holter and Holter monitoring during the game in squash players. *Eur Heart J* 1987;8[Suppl D]:29–32.

31. Palatini P, Scanavacca G, Bongiovi S, et al. Prognostic significance of ventricular extrasystoles in healthy professional athletes: results of a 5-year follow-up. *Cardiology* 1993:82(4):286–293.

32. Sagawa K. Baroreflex control of systemic arterial pressure and vascular bed. In: Shepherd JT, Abboud F, eds. *Handbook of physiology,* section 2: The cardiovascular system, vol III. Bethesda, MD: American Physiological Society, 1983:453–496.

33. Patel C, Wattar AR, Jaeger F, Goren H, Fouad-Tarazi F. Does the systemic hemodynamic profile predict the severity of orthostatic intolerance. *Pacing Clin Electrophysiol* 1997;20:1077.

34. Wattar AR, Patel C, Jaeger F, Fouad-Tarazi F. Gender differences in tilt-induced neurocardiogenic syncope. *Pacing Clin Electrophysiol* 1997;20:1161.

35. Sawka MN, Greenleaf JE. Current concepts concerning thirst, dehydration, and fluid replacement. *Med Sci Sports Exerc* 1992;24:643–644.

36. Giannattasio C, Seravalle G, Bolla GB, et al. Cardiopulmonary receptor reflexes in normotensive athletes with cardiac hypertrophy. *Circulation* 1990;82:1222–1229.

37. Moore GE, Holbein ME, Knochel JP. Exercise-associated collapse in cyclists is unrelated to endotoxemia. *Med Sci Sports Exerc* 1995;27:1238–1242.

38. Sneddon JF, Scalia G, Ward DE, McKenna WJ, Camm AJ, Frenneaux MP. Exercise induced vasodepressor syncope. *Br Heart J* 1994;71:554–557.

39. West DB, Trippel DL, Gillette PC, Garner SS. Pharmacokinetics of esmolol in children. *Clin Pharmacol Ther* 1991;49:618–623.

40. Palombo C, Montereggi A, Genovesi-Ebert A, et al. The Intraarterial blood pressure monitoring in the evaluation of patients with dizziness and/or fainting. *Clin Exper Theory Pract* 1985;A7:423–438.

41. Palatini P. Blood pressure behaviour during physical activity. *Sports Med* 1988;5:353–374.

42. Kreutz JM, Mazuzan JE. Sudden asystole in a marathon runner: the athletic heart syndrome and its anesthetic implications. *Anesthesiology* 1990;73:1266–1268.

43. Oslizlok P, Allen M, Griffin M, Gillette P. Clinical features and management of young patients with cardioinhibitory response during orthostatic testing. *Am J Cardiol* 1992;69:1363–1365.

44. Almquist A, Goldenberg IF, Milstein S, et al. Provocation of bradycardia and hypotension by isoproterenol and upright posture in patients with unexplained syncope. *N Engl J Med* 1989;320:356–351.

45. Epstein SE, Stampfer MD, Beiser GD. Role of the capacitance and resistance vessels in vasovagal syncope. *Circulation* 1968;37:524–533.

46. Fitzpatrick A, Sutton R. Tilting towards a diagnosis in recurrent unexpalained syncope. *Lancet* 1989;1: 658–660.

47. Benditt DG, Remole S, Bailin S, Dunnigan A, Asso A, Milstein S. Tilt table testing for evaluation of neurally-mediated (cardioneurogenic) syncope: rationale and proposed protocols. *Pacing Clin Electrophysiol* 1991; 14:1528–1537.

47a. Milstein S, Buetikoffer J, Lesser J, Goldenberg IF, Benditt DG, Gornick C, Reyes WJ. Cardiac asystole: a manifestation of neurally mediated hypotension-bradycardia. *J Am Coll Cardiol* 1989;14:1626–1632.

48. Waxman MB, Yao L, Cameron DA, Wald RW, Roseman J. Isoproterenol induction of vasodepressor-type reaction in vasodepressor-prone persons. *Am J Cardiol* 1989;63:58–65.

49. Kapoor WN, Brant N. Evaluation of syncope by upright tilt testing with isoproterenol. *Ann Intern Med* 1992; 116:358–363.

50. Ovadia M, Thoele D. Esmolol tilt testing with esmolol withdrawal for the evaluation of syncope in the young. *Circulation* 1994;89:228–235.

51. Hilton F, Giordano J, Fortney S. Vasodepressor syncope induced by lower body negative pressure: possible relevance to +Gz-stress training—a case report. *Aviat Space Environ Med* 1989;60:61–63.

52. Convertino VA. Endurance exercise training: conditions of enhanced hemodynamic responses and tolerance to LBNP. *Med Sci Sports Exerc* 1993;25:705–712.

53. Fortney S, Tankersley C, Lightfoot JT, et al. Cardiovascular responses to lower body negative pressure in trained and untrained older men. *J Appl Physiol* 1992; 73:2693–2700.

54. Costa O, Freitas J, Puig J, et al. Analise espectral da variabilidade da frequencia cardiaca em atletas. *Rev Port Cardiol* 1991;10:23–28.

55. Shin K, Minamitani H, Onishi S, Yamazaki H, Lee M. The power spectral analysis of heart rate variability in athletes during dynamic exercise—part II. *Clin Cardiol* 1995;18:664–668.

56. Grubb BP, Temesy-Armos PN, Samoil D, Wolfe DA, Hahn H, Elliott L. Tilt table testing in the evaluation and management of athletes with recurrent exercise-induced syncope. *Med Sci Sports Exerc* 1993;25:24–28.

57. Calkins H, Seifert M, Morady F. Clinical presentation and long-term follow-up of athletes with exercise-induced vasodepressor syncope. *Am Heart J* 1995;129: 1159–1164.

58. Rechavia E, Strasberg B, Agmon J. Head-up tilt table evaluation in a trained athlete with recurrent vaso-vagal syncope. *Chest* 1989;95:689–691.

59. Ovadia M, Gear K, Thoele D, Marcus FI. Accelerometer systolic time intervals as fast-response sensors of upright posture in the young. *Circulation* 1995;92: 1849–1859.

60. Douglas PS. Cardiac considerations in the triathlete. *Med Sci Sports Exerc* 1989;21[Suppl 5]:S214–S218.

61. Buja G, Folino AF, Bittante M, et al. Asystole with syncope secondary to hyperventilation in three young athletes. *Pacing Clin Electrophysiol* 1989;12:406–412.

62. Sakaguchi S, Shultz JJ, Remole SC, Adler SW, Lurie KG, Benditt DG. Syncope associated with exercise, a manifestation of neurally mediated syncope. *Am J Cardiol* 1995;75:476–481.

63. Cunha EV. Management of orthostatic hypotension in the elderly. *Geriatrics* 1987;42:61–68.

64. Seihara H. 9α-Fluorohydrocortisone as a mineralocorticoid. *Nippon Rinsho* 1994;52:583–586.

65. Whitworth JA, Butkus A, Coghlan JP, et al. 9-Alpha-fluorocortisol-induced hypertension: a review. *J Hypertension* 1986;4:133–139.

66. Salim MA, DiSessa TG. Serum electrolytes in children with neurocardiogenic syncope treated with fludrocortisone and salt. *Am J Cardiol* 1996;78:228–229.

67. McTavish D, Goa KL. Midodrine. A review of its pharmacological properties and therapeutic use in orthostatic hypotension and secondary hypotensive disorders. *Drugs* 1989;38:757–777.

68. Ward C, Kenny RA. Observations on midodrine in a case of vasodepressor neurogenic syncope. *Clin Autonomic Res* 1995;5:257–260.

68a. Grubb BP, Wolfe DA, Samoil D, Temesy-Armos P, Hahn H, Elliott L. Usefulness of fluoxetine hydrochloride for prevention of resistant upright tilt induced syncope. *Pacing Clin Electrophysiol* 1993;16:458.

69. Jennings G, Esler M, Holmes R. Treatment of orthostatic hypotension with dihydroergotamine. *BMJ* 1979;2: 307.

70. Fouad FM, Taruzi RC, Bravo EL. Dihydroergotamine in idiopathic orthostatic hypotension. *Clin Pharmacol Ther* 1981;30:782–789.

71. Fitzpatrick A, Theodorakis G, Ahmed R, Williams T, Sutton R. Dual chamber pacing aborts vasovagal syncope induced by head-up 60° tilt. *Pacing Clin Electrophysiol* 1991;14:13–19.

72. Koyama, S, Matsubara T, Aizawa Y, et al. A case of vasovagal syncope with culsions. The effects of midodrine hydrochloride. *Jpn Circ J* 1992;56:950–9541.

72a. Brignole M, Menozzi C, Lolli G, Oddone D, Gianfranchi L, Bertulla A. Pacing for carotid sinus syndrome and sick sinus syndrome. *Pacing Clin Electrophysiol* 1990;13:2071–2075.

72b. Deschamps D, Richard A, Citron B, Chaperon A, Binon JP, Ponsonaille J. Hypersensibilité sino-carotidienne. Evolution à moyen terme et à longue terme des patients traités par stimulation ventriculaire. *Arch Mal Coeur* 1990;83:63–67.

72c. Sra JS, Jazayeri MR, Avitall B, Dhala A, Deshpande S, Blanck Z, Akhtar M. Comparison of cardiac pacing with drug therapy in the treatment of neurocardiogenic (vasovagal) syncope with bradycardia or asystole. *N Engl J Med* 1993;328:1085–1090.

72d. Fitzpatrick A, Theodorakis G, Ahmed R, Williams T, Sutton R. Dual chamber pacing aborts vasovagal syncope induced by head-up 60° tilt. *Pacing Clin Electrophysiol* 1991;14:13–19.

72e. Arnold LW, Gamble W, O'Connor B, Saul JP, Walsh E. Pacemaker treatment for toddlers and children with severe neurocardiogenic syncope and cardiac asystole. *Pacing Clin Electrophysiol* 1992;15:507.

72f. Benditt DG, Remole S, Asso A, Hansen R, Lurie K. Cardiac Pacing for carotid sinus syndrome and vasovagal syncope. Ch. 2 in Barold SS, Mugica J, eds. New Perspectives in Cardiac Pacing v.3. Mt. Kisco, NY:Futura;1993:15–28.

73. Ovadia M, Gear K. Thoele D, and Marcus FI. Accelerometer systolic time intervals as fast-response sen-

sors of upright posture in the young. *Circulation* 1995; 92:1849–1859.

74. Steiner TJ, Smith FR, Clifford Rose F. Vasomotor reactivity in migraine. In: Clifford Rose F, Zilkua KS eds. Progress in migraine research. Tonbridge Wells: Pitman;1981:33–40.

75. Lewis NP, Fraser AG, Taylor A. Syncope Line 13 while vomiting during [a] migraine attack. *Lancet* 1988;2: 400–401.

76. Franz IW. Belastungsblutdruck bei Hochdruckkranken und Sport. *Forttschr Med* 1998;106:107–110.

77. Franc IW. Hypertonie und Sport, *Dtsch Med Wochenschr* 1987;112:1557–1559.

78. Palatini P. Blood pressure behaviour during physical activity. *Sports Med* 1988;5:353–374.

79. Tanji JL. Tracking of elevated blood pressure values in adolescent athletes at 1-year follow-up. *Am J Dis Child* 1991;145:665–667.

80. Tanji JL. Exercise and the hypertensive athlete. *Clin Sports Med* 1992;11:291–302.

81. Gancia GP, Lin YC. Applied physiology of diving. *Sports Med* 1988;5:41–56,181.

The Athlete and Heart Disease:
Diagnosis, Evaluation & Management,
edited by R. A. Williams.
Published by Lippincott Williams & Wilkins, 1999.

15

The Pathology of Sudden Cardiac Death in Athletes[1]

Renu Virmani, Allen P. Burke, and Andrew Farb

Department of Cardiovascular Pathology, Armed Forces Institute of Pathology, Washington, DC 20306

Cardiovascular disease is the largest killer of adults in the Western world. In this century, remarkable inroads have been made into the understanding of heart disease, leading to a reduction in death rates from cardiac causes. Although the incidence of sudden cardiac death (1), and all coronary artery disease deaths (2), in the United States has shown a decrease in recent decades, it is estimated that 300,000 to 400,000 sudden deaths occur annually as a result of heart disease (3). Clearly, sudden cardiac death remains a health problem of huge proportions.

The exact incidence of sudden death during exercise is unknown, but is very low (4,5). However, the sudden death of a prominent young athlete in the prime of life is a devastating event and is a result of cardiac disease in more than 80% of cases (6). Epidemiologic studies have shown that physical conditioning is beneficial and decreases the incidence of acute coronary events (7,8). Exercise increases the risk of sudden death during or immediately after exertion by a factor of approximately tenfold in sedentary individuals who exercise erratically (5,9,10), but this increase in risk is far less in conditioned athletes. Therefore, a better understanding is needed of the underlying diseases that may predispose athletes to sudden death and of the effects of exercise on the heart.

ADAPTATION OF THE CARDIOVASCULAR SYSTEM TO EXERCISE AND THE ATHLETE'S HEART

There are two forms of exercise—isotonic (dynamic) and isometric (static). Isotonic exercise requires a change in muscle length with little increase in tension or resistance, whereas isometric exercise requires little change in muscle length against an increase in resistance. Examples of isotonic exercise are running, swimming, and bicycling, and examples of isometric exercise are weight lifting, hand grip exercises, and pushing and pulling against a resistance. In isotonic exercise, peripheral resistance declines, resulting in an increase in the heart rate, cardiac output, and venous return to the heart. The mean arterial pressure increases, with an elevated systolic blood pressure and little change in diastolic pressure. In isometric exercise, there is an increase in resistance to blood flow through muscle undergoing static contraction, and this results in an increase in peripheral resistance. Intramuscular pressure increases during contraction while the muscle length is the same, resulting in decreased or no muscle blood flow. Static exercise results in an increase in systolic and diastolic pressure and an increase in mean systolic pressure.

[1]The opinions or assertions contained herein are the private views of the authors and are not to be construed as official or as reflecting the views of the Department of the Army or Navy or the Department of Defense.

Cardiac adaptation to chronic exercise has been recognized for decades. As originally described, the clinical manifestations of "athlete's heart" include sinus bradycardia at rest, a soft systolic murmur, audible third and fourth heart sound, and cardiomegaly by chest radiograph (11). With the emergence of M-mode echocardiography in the 1970s, a large number of studies were published studying cardiac changes in athletes. Within the limits of the technology, it was demonstrated that cardiac dimensions in a group of athletes exceeded those of matched control subjects, although there was an overlap without a bimodal distribution (12). More recent two-dimensional echocardiographic studies have consistently demonstrated increased cardiac mass in professional athletes who train both isometrically and isotonically (12–15). In addition, these studies have demonstrated a difference in cardiac changes in endurance athletes (isometrically trained) compared to weight lifters (isotonically trained athletes).

In athletes who regularly undergo isotonic training, such as swimming and running, two-dimensional echocardiography shows increased left atrial and left ventricular dimensions (13). The increase in end-diastolic dimension persists with adjustment for body surface area and weight. There is also an increase in left ventricular wall thickness of approximately 14% over controls (12). The degree of increase in wall thickness is mild and confined to the septum and posterior wall in end-diastole, as shown in studies on professional cyclists (16).

There are no well-documented autopsy studies that document morphologic abnormalities, such as increased cavity size and increased left ventricular wall thickness, in trained athletes who die of noncardiac causes. We have reviewed the cardiac findings in 13 exercise-related deaths in which no cardiac or noncardiac cause of death could be established (unpublished observations, see Table 3). The mean heart weight was 386 ± 78 g, which was not significantly different from those dying a traumatic death. It is conceivable that they had not engaged in exercise for a long enough period to demonstrate any changes in heart weight or in cardiac dimensions. We also excluded from this group athletes dying of idiopathic left ventricular hypertrophy, a condition which may or may not be related to chronic conditioning (see subsequent discussion).

Echocardiographic studies demonstrate that athletes engaged in chronic isometric exercise have increased left ventricular wall thickness and normal end-diastolic volumes. These same studies show that athletes engaged in isotonic exercise have comparatively mild or no increased wall thickness and increased end-diastolic volumes (12,13). In contrast to endurance athletes, weight lifters demonstrate by echocardiography increased wall thickness during diastole and systole (14). Therefore, the effect on the heart is that of pressure overload, resulting in an increase in left ventricular mass, which results primarily from an increase in left ventricular wall thickness.

The significance and possible pathologic consequences of adaptive cardiac hypertrophy in athletes have been debated (12,17–19). Athletes in the peak of conditioning have an estimated 45% increase in left ventricular mass (12). Because left ventricular hypertrophy is known to predispose to ventricular arrhythmias, it is possible that exercise-related cardiac adaptation is harmful. However, although sinus bradycardia and transient atrioventricular (AV) block are more common in athletes than control subjects, supraventricular, AV nodal, and ventricular ectopic beats are not more frequent in athletes without structural heart disease (20). The current view is that cardiac hypertrophy, especially in isotonically trained athletes, is considered a benign adaptive process (12,16).

The cardiac hypertrophy present in trained athletes is generally concentric. In up to 12% of athletes, however, there is asymmetric hypertrophy, which may be confused with hypertrophic cardiomyopathy (21). The degree of asymmetry in athletes is generally mild, usually within the range of 13 to 15 mm, allowing a distinction from hypertrophic cardiomyopathy (12).

TABLE 1. Causes of sudden cardiac death in exercising individuals (published series including all sports)

Author	Year	n	Age, years	Sports					Causes of Death											
				BG	PT	Run	Swim	OTH	CAD	HCM	LVH	RVC	CAA	SST	MYO	VD	CS	AO	UNK	OTH
Buddington	1974	109[a]	22 (9–39)	30	31	28	6	14	43	5	18	0	7	9	4	0	0	0	0	0
Opie	1975	19[a]	40 (17–58)	11	0	0	0	10	19	0	0	0	0	0	0	0	0	0	0	0
Maron	1980	29	19 (13–30)	21	1	4	1	2	3	14	5	0	4	0	0	0	0	2	1	0
Tsung	1982	4	17 (14–18)	4	0	0	0	0	0	1	0	0	2	0	0	0	0	0	1	0
Kennedy	1984	11	10–49	9	0	2	0	0	7	2	0	0	1	0	0	0	0	1	1	0
Virmani	1985	32	28 (14–60)	13	6	8	2	3	8	2	4	0	3;2[c]	3	4	3	0	0	2	0
Northcote	1986	60[a]	46 (22–66)	60	0	0	0	0	51	1	0	0	0	0	0	4	0	0	2	0
Virmani	1986	13	30 (8–47)	13	9	6	1	4	14	2	2	0	2;1[c]	1	0	2	0	0	6	1[e]
Thiene	1988	10	22 (13–30)	4	1	1	1	3	0	0	0	10	0	0	0	0	0	0	0	0
Niimura	1989	62	<15	0	18	29	7	8	0	8	2[b]	0	0	0	5	0	24[d]	0	23	0
Corrado	1990	22[a]	23 (11–35)	15	1	1	3	2	4	0	0	6	2	0	0	0	3	1	0	2[c]
Burke	1991	25	24 (14–34)	19	3	0	3	2	4	8	2	1	4	0	1	1	0	0	4	1[g]
Maron	1996	134	17 (12–40)	108	0	17	3	6	3	48	14;4[b]	4	25;6[c]	1	5;4[j]	8	0	6	3	3[h]
Total	1974–1996	550[j]		307 (56%)	70 (13%)	96 (17%)	27 (5%)	52 (9%)	156 (30%)	91 (18%)	51 (10%)	21 (4%)	58 (11%)	14 (3%)	25 (5%)	17 (3%)	27 (5%)	10 (2%)	43 (8%)	7 (1%)

[a]Excluding noncardiac deaths: 86 (Buddington), 21 (Opie), 58 (Northcote), 18 (Corrado).

[b]Dilated cardiomyopathy.

[c]Tunnel left anterior descending coronary artery.

[d]5 long QT, 8 ventricular tachycardia, 3 sick sinus syndrome, 4 atrioventricular block, 4 atrial fibrillation.

[e]Myxoma.

[f]Mitral valve prolapse.

[g]Kawasaki disease.

[h]Congenital heart disease (2), not specified (1).

[i]Idiopathic ventricular scars, possibly healed myocarditis.

[j]520=total of cardiac deaths.

BG, Ballgames; PT, physical training; OTH, other; CAD, coronary atherosclerotic disease; HCM, hypertrophic cardiomyopathy; LVH, idiopathic left ventricular hypertrophy; RVC, right ventricular cardiomyopathy; CAA, coronary artery anomalies; SST, sickle cell trait; MYO, myocarditis; VD, valvular disease; CS, conduction disturbances; AO, aortic dissection/rupture; UNK, unknown.

Modified from ref. 33, with permission.

TABLE 2. *Causes of death in published series of joggers and marathon runners*

Author	Year	n	Age, years	Sex	CAD	HCM	RVC	UNK	Other	No. Marathon Runners
Opie	1975	19	—	19M	19*	0	0	0	0	0
Noakes	1979	1	42	M	0	1	0	0	—	1
Noakes	1979	5	27–44 (37 ± 6)	5M	3	0	0	1	1 RVC	5
Thompson	1979	18	—	17M:1F	13	0	0	3	Myocarditis, heat stroke	1
Waller	1980	5	44–53 (46 ± 6)	5M	5	0	0	0	—	1
Morales	1980	2	54,34	2M	0	0	0	0	2 tunnel LAD	2
Virmani	1982	30	18–57 (37 ± 9)	30M	22	0	0	7	1 FMV	0
Thompson	1982	7	28–74	7M	6	0	0	0	1 GI hemorrhage	3
Jackson	1983	9	35–56	9M	8	0	0	0	1	0
Noakes	1984	3	31–45	3M	3	3	0	0	0	2
Virmani	1985	11	19–59	11M	10	1	1	0	0	1
Corrado	1990	1	26	M	0	0	1	0	0	0
Burke	1991	9	14–40 (30)	8M:1F	5	0	0	2	1 LVH, 1 myocarditis	0
Total	1975–1991	120	14–74	118M:2F	94 (78%)	4 (3%)	1 (1%)	13 (11%)	21 (19%)	15 (13%)

*In 12 of these cases, coronary artery disease was assumed but not proved.

CAD, coronary atherosclerotic disease; HCM, hypertrophic cardiomyopathy; RVC, right ventricular cardiomyopathy; LAD, left anterior descending coronary artery; GI, gastrointestinal; LVH, left ventricular hypertrophy; FMV, floppy mitral valve; M, male; F, female; UNK, unknown.

Modified from ref 33, with permission.

TABLE 3. *Causes of sudden death with exercise collected from the state of Maryland from 1989–1996*

Group	Age, years	Age range	Sex M:F	Race W:B:O	Type of Exercise			Cause of Death						
					Basketball	Jogging/running	Other	Ht Wt (g)	LVH	HCM	RVC	CAD	UNK	Other
≤35 years (n=48)	22 ± 6	10–32	43:5	21:24:3	25	6	17	470 ± 126	7	5	4	4	13	15
>35 years (n=14)	46 ± 9	36–65	14:0	8:6:0	5	5	4	473 ± 358	1	0	0	7	0	6
All cases (n=62)	28 ± 13	10–65	57:5	29:30:3	30 (48%)	11 (18%)	21 (34%)	473 ± 111	8 (13%)	5 (8%)	4 (6%)	11 (18%)	13 (21%)	21 (34%)

M, male; F, female; W, white; B, black; O, other; Ht wt, heart weight; g, grams; LVH, left ventricular hypertrophy; HCM, hypertrophic cardiomyopathy; RVC, right ventricular cardiomyopathy; CAD, coronary artery disease; UNK, unknown.

CAUSES OF SPORTS-RELATED SUDDEN CARDIAC DEATH

For the most part, the causes of sudden death in athletes are no different from causes of sudden death in sedentary individuals. However, there are a handful of entities that cause life-threatening arrhythmias more frequently during exercise than at rest, including hypertrophic cardiomyopathy, right ventricular cardiomyopathy, and coronary artery anomalies. These conditions, as well as coronary atherosclerosis (the most common exercise-related cause of sudden death in individuals older than 35 years of age), are emphasized in this chapter.

The causes of sudden death in athletes younger than age 35 years are usually cardiomyopathies or congenital coronary anomalies, whereas in older athletes the cause of sudden death is usually severe atherosclerotic coronary disease (22). There are two overlapping categories of sports-related sudden cardiac death, which generally reflect this age division. The first category includes competitive professional or semiprofessional athletes dying suddenly of cardiac causes. In 90% of such cases, deaths occur during sport activity or immediately thereafter (6), and in 10% the deaths occur during rest. Most of these deaths (at least in the United States) occur in athletes who participate in team sports, such as basketball and football, and who are younger than 30 years of age (6). The causes of death in this group are diverse and are often cardiomyopathies or coronary artery anomalies that are previously undiagnosed. The second category of sports-related sudden death occurs in individuals who die suddenly while jogging or running (or immediately after running) and who are usually, but not necessarily, trained athletes. These people are usually older than 35 years of age and often die of coronary atherosclerosis; they are more likely to have had a clinical diagnosis of heart disease.

Table 1 tabulates series of sudden cardiac deaths in young individuals, most of whom were participating in team sports at the time of death (6,23–34). There is a wide geographic spectrum in these series, and some participants are selected by age (30) or condition (29), introducing a bias in the types of diagnoses. However, the relatively high incidence of cardiomyopathy and coronary artery anomalies is evident. Table 2 presents series of sudden cardiac deaths occurring exclusively during running or jogging, and demonstrates the great preponderance of coronary artery disease. Table 3 presents unpublished data from the Office of the Chief Medical Examiner in Maryland, including all exercise-related sudden deaths without knowledge of the physical conditioning of the individual. In this table, the marked differences in causes of death between people younger and older than 35 years is obvious.

PUBLISHED SERIES OF SUDDEN DEATH IN COMPETITIVE ATHLETES

The largest series of sudden death in competitive athletes is that of Maron et al. (6). The most common diagnosis in this series of more than 100 athletes from the United States is hypertrophic cardiomyopathy, diagnosed at autopsy in 36% of cases. A review of the literature demonstrates that, among cases of exercise-related sudden deaths in a wider range of individuals in several countries, hypertrophic cardiomyopathy was diagnosed in 18% of cases, the largest single group with the exception of persons with coronary atherosclerosis (see Table 1). In this compilation of series, other forms of cardiomyopathy included idiopathic left ventricular hypertrophy (9%), right ventricular cardiomyopathy (4%), and dilated cardiomyopathy (1%) (6,23–31,35).

Anomalous coronary arteries is the cause of death in 10% to 20% of competitive athletes (6,22,35) and is a frequent cause of death only in athletes younger than 30 years of age. After hypertrophic cardiomyopathy, coronary atherosclerosis is the second most frequent cause of sudden death in the collective series from 1974 to 1996, representing 28% of cases (see Table 1). In those series of predominantly coronary artery deaths (25,28), the mean age was 40 years or older, indicating that age is a major determinant of the cause of death even in exercising individuals.

Other causes of death in those engaged in exercise include myocarditis (5%), conduction system abnormalities (5%), valvular disease (3%), aortic dissections (2%), tunnel coronary arteries (2%), and repaired congenital anomalies of the heart (less than 1%). The diagnosis of conduction abnormalities, especially long QT syndrome, is dependent on premortem electrocardiographic data, because autopsy findings are nonspecific. Tunneled coronary artery (usually of the left anterior descending), also termed myocardial bridges, is a type of coronary artery anomaly that is present in up to 30% of the normal population, but which may be implicated as a cause of exercise-related sudden death if it is especially severe (36).

PUBLISHED REPORTS OF SUDDEN DEATH IN JOGGERS AND MARATHON RUNNERS

In the 14 series or case reports published involving 122 individuals dying during or soon after jogging, the age range was from 14 to 74 years (see Table 1), with the mean age greater in those engaged in athletic activities versus sporting activities (see Tables 1 and 2). Probably because of a bias in establishing coronary artery disease in marathon runners, a relatively high percentage of these athletes (12%) had completed at least one marathon. As in most cases of exercise-related sudden death, most of the deaths occurred in men, comprising 95% of cases. The cause of death was overwhelmingly secondary to severe underlying coronary atherosclerosis (78%).

Epidemiologic evidence strongly suggests that regular physical activity is beneficial in increasing cardiovascular functional capacity, reducing risk factors for coronary artery disease, and preventing cardiovascular disease (37). Nevertheless, it has been firmly established that the risk of sudden death is highest during vigorous exercise (especially in men and women who are not conditioned athletes) and in individuals with underlying heart disease (38). It has been recommended that anyone who plans to exercise vigorously should

have a physical examination within 2 years of commencing. Individuals younger than 40 years of age who have a normal physical examination, no symptoms, and no major coronary risk factors can exercise without any restrictions. In individuals 40 years of age or older with abnormal physical examination or presence of one or more risk factors who wish to exercise vigorously, a symptom-limited exercise stress test should be performed to ensure that there is no occult heart disease, and the activity should be restricted to moderate intensity or be medically supervised depending on the investigations (38).

Nonatherosclerotic causes of sudden death in joggers and marathon runners are similar to those seen in athletes playing team sports but are seen in lesser frequency. They include hypertrophic cardiomyopathy, left ventricular hypertrophy, valvular disease, and myocarditis. Other than coronary artery disease, the most common finding at autopsy is the absence of structural heart disease (11% of total cases; see Table 2). This relatively high proportion of unexplained sudden death is similar to that seen in athletes other than runners (8%; see Table 1). The true cause of death in these cases may be conditions that are difficult or impossible to diagnose at autopsy (e.g., coronary spasm, long QT interval, and preexcitation syndromes) as well as conditions that are currently unknown or poorly understood. Recently, it has been demonstrated that heat stroke may also present as cardiac arrhythmias and sudden death, especially in individuals with sickle cell trait (39). For this reason, heat stroke should also be carefully excluded as a cause of sudden death in runners who have no structural heart disease at autopsy (see subsequent discussion).

SEVERE CORONARY ATHEROSCLEROSIS

We have reviewed the Armed Forces Institute of Pathology (AFIP) files for all exercise-related sudden death that occurred in the state of Maryland referred to us during 1989 to 1996 (see Table 3). In 14 deaths occurring in individuals older than 35 years of age, severe coronary atherosclerosis was found at autopsy in seven (50%), four of whom were runners, compared to four of 48 (8%) deaths in individuals younger than 35 years of age, one of whom was a runner. These data corroborate results from previous studies demonstrating that atherosclerosis-related sudden death during exercise is more frequent in runners older than 35 years of age.

Previous studies have shown that joggers and marathon runners who die suddenly of severe coronary atherosclerosis often have underlying risk factors. In a prospective study by Jackson et al. (40) carried out over a 1-year period in Auckland, New Zealand, nine runners died suddenly (mean age 47 years); all ran over 60 minutes a week for at least 3 months, and two were marathon runners. All had un-derlying risk factors or previous atherosclerotic disease. Three of these runners were hypertensive, three had hypercholesterolemia, four were previous smokers, one was a current smoker, and one was a diabetic. Four had previously suffered from myocardial infarction, one had a history of angina, and one had had a carotid endarterectomy. Similarly, Thompson et al. (41) reported sudden coronary deaths in 12 runners from Rhode Island who had been running for at least 6 months at distances from 3 to 25 miles a day. The majority of these runners had risk factors or known heart disease, including hypertension (two), smoking (five), a family history of premature heart disease (five), documented ischemic heart disease prior to death (five), and hypercholesterolemia (six), and the majority of individuals had prodromal symptoms.

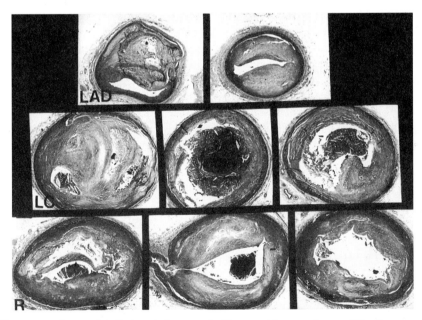

FIG. 1. Coronary atherosclerotic heart disease. A 43-year-old man who ran 50 miles per week for at least 5 years and had participated in several marathons died suddenly while running. His risk factors included a family history of coronary artery disease, and his total cholesterol was 224 mg/dL. He was nondiabetic, normotensive, and a nonsmoker. His heart weighed 600 g, and there was a transmural acute myocardial infarction of the posterolateral wall of the left ventricle and no healed infarcts were identified. The right coronary artery, the left anterior descending, and the left circumflex arteries were greater than 75% narrowed in cross-sectional area, and the left circumflex artery was totally occluded by a thrombus with underlying plaque rupture. (From Virmani R, Robinowitz M, McAllister HA Jr. Exercise and the heart. In: Sommers SC, Rosen PP, Fechner RE, eds. *Pathology annual,* Part 2. Norwalk, CT: Appleton-Century-Crofts, 1985:443, with permission.)

A study of 18 sudden deaths among joggers and runners demonstrated an increased frequency of risk factors compared to a control population, but the difference was not significant (4). The high incidence of risk factors and prodromal symptoms in runners who die suddenly of atherosclerosis warrants caution before excessive physical activity is allowed in patients with coronary heart disease or in those who are at risk for coronary artery disease.

The extent of coronary disease is well documented in most published series of exercise-related sudden coronary death (4,22,24,34,35, 41–43). In autopsies of athletes from these series (most of whom died suddenly during or immediately after running), 31 of 64 had healed infarcts (48%), 11 of 64 acute infarcts (17%), 19 of 69 (30%) had one-vessel disease, 23 of 69 (36%) two-vessel disease, and 27 of 69 (42%) three-vessel disease (Fig. 1). Eight of 32 had coronary artery thrombi, and 20 of 29 cardiomegaly. The frequency of thrombi (25%) may be a low estimate, because autopsies were performed without postmortem angiography or perfusion fixation allowing for the optimal detection of a thrombus; in such studies, the incidence of acute thrombosis is more than 50% in sudden coronary death in sedentary people (44). In contrast, the incidence of myocardial infarction in these cases of exercise-related death is similar to what has been observed in sudden coronary death victims who died without any history of exercise (44). The frequency of plaque rupture, plaque erosion, and vulnerable plaques throughout the coronary tree has not been determined in exercise-related coronary death.

HYPERTROPHIC CARDIOMYOPATHY

Among 550 athletes dying suddenly (see Table 1), 163 died of cardiomyopathies. Of these cases of cardiomyopathy, 91 were subclassified as hypertrophic cardiomyopathy, representing the second most common diagnosis following coronary artery atherosclerosis. Of the published series in Table 1, those by Maron et al. (6,24) have the highest incidence of hypertrophic cardiomyopathy as the cause

of death. In their first series in 1980 of 29 highly conditioned, competitive athletes aged 13 to 30 years, 14 (49%) had hypertrophic cardiomyopathy; in their second series, this proportion was 36%. In the more recent series, Maron et al. (6) reported that black athletes are more likely to die suddenly with hypertrophic cardiomyopathy than whites (48% versus 26%; $p = 0.01$). In our study of 24 exercise-related sudden deaths in the state of Maryland, 24% of deaths were due to hypertrophic cardiomyopathy; we also noted a predilection for blacks (35). In our more recent data from the state of Maryland (see Table 3), five of 48 (10%) exercise-related sudden cardiac deaths in individuals younger than age 35 years (and none of 14 cases older than 35 years of age) were due to hypertrophic cardiomyopathy. The reason for the lower frequency of hypertrophic cardiomyopathy in our series may be that we did not select for highly trained athletes, rather all exercise-related deaths were included. The smallest proportion of exercise-related sudden deaths is seen in the Italian series (31); a possible explanation for this low incidence is that Italian law requires prescreening electrocardiography in all young adults who wish to participate in sport.

The gross and microscopic pathologic features of hypertrophic cardiomyopathy have been described in detail (45–50). Grossly, the heart is typically enlarged to twice its normal weight. The left atrium usually demonstrates dilatation, with a small left ventricular cavity. There is left ventricular outflow tract obstruction resulting in a discrete left ventricular outflow tract plaque in approximately 50% of cases. In most hearts, there is septal asymmetry, resulting in a ventricular septum to free wall ratio of 1.3:1 or greater (Fig. 2). The most common location of septal asymmetry is the anterior septum toward the cardiac base, but the thickening may diffusely involve the septum or be isolated near the cardiac apex (so-called apical cardiomyopathy). Left ventricular outflow tract obstruction causes thickening and elongation of the anterior leaflet of the mitral valve, and mitral valve prolapse is occasionally observed. Histologically, in areas of septal

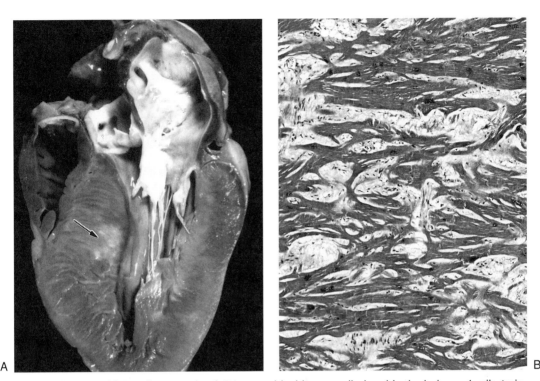

FIG. 2. Hypertrophic cardiomyopathy. A 24-year-old white man died suddenly during a 4-mile training hike. The patient had an electrocardiogram (prior to being enrolled in the ranger school), which showed presence of left ventricular hypertrophy, but the patient was cleared to attend ranger school. The heart weighed 650 g with asymmetric septal hypertrophy and focal areas of fibrosis within the area of the greatest hypertrophy (*arrow*). There was no outflow tract plaque (**A**). Sections of the ventricular septum showed marked fibromuscular disarray (**B**) and no intramyocardial coronary artery thickening.

thickening, there is myofiber disarray, characterized by disorganized, branched, whorled bundles of myocytes. Interstitial fibrosis often accompanies the myofiber disarray, and may be prominent and grossly visible. Intramural myocardial coronary artery thickening is present in approximately 80% of hearts and may be a helpful diagnostic feature.

There are unusual variants of hypertrophic cardiomyopathy. In rare cases of sudden death caused by hypertrophic cardiomyopathy, the heart may be grossly normal without an increased mass. In such cases, the diagnosis is first suspected at histologic study, which demonstrates myofiber disarray (6,51). We have rarely encountered cases of exercise-related sudden cardiac death in which there was

severe intramural myocardial arterial thickening, but significant myofiber disarray was lacking. Finally, we have encountered another entity, which we have called focal, localized hypertrophic cardiomyopathy. It is morphologically characterized by the presence of myocyte hypertrophy, fibromuscular disarray, fibrosis, and intramyocardial coronary artery thickening but no outflow tract plaque, anterior mitral leaflet thickening, or asymmetric septal hypertrophy; the islands of hypertrophied disarrayed myocytes are focally identified in the walls of all four chambers.

Patients with hypertrophic cardiomyopathy and a family history of premature sudden death have an especially high risk of sudden death, especially during exercise (52). Other clinical and pathologic variables are not useful in identifying those at risk for sudden death (53), although excessive ventricular hypertrophy may predispose to sudden death in hypertrophic cardiomyopathy (54). Recently, nonsustained ventricular tachycardia on ambulatory electrocardiogram, a prior occurrence of syncope (or cardiac arrest), and inducible supraventricular or ventricular tachycardia have been identified as risk factors for sudden death in patients with hypertrophic cardiomyopathy (55). In familial forms of the disease, certain missense mutations in the β-myosin heavy chain gene are associated with a particularly poor prognosis and sudden death (56,57).

RIGHT VENTRICULAR CARDIOMYOPATHY/DYSPLASIA

Right ventricular cardiomyopathy has received significant attention only since the late 1980s. Most of the reports of right ventricular cardiomyopathy and sudden death come from the Italian group from the region of Veneto in northeastern Italy. Thiene et al. reported their findings in 60 individuals younger than 35 years of age who died between 1979 and 1986, 12 of whom died of right ventricular cardiomyopathy (20%) (29). Ten of the 12 subjects had died during exercise, and seven had history of palpitations, syncope, or both; in five of seven patients, ventricular arrhythmias had been recorded (29). In another publication of sudden deaths from the same region from the same group from 1979 to 1989, of 22 persons who died suddenly with exercise, six (27%) had right ventricular cardiomyopathy (31).

The incidence of right ventricular cardiomyopathy in the United States is much lower than the incidence in Italy. In our series of exercise-related sudden death in individuals aged 14 to 40 years, only one of 34 (3%) died with the diagnosis of right ventricular cardiomyopathy (35). Similarly, Maron et al. (6), in their most recent publication of young competitive athletes dying suddenly, reported right ventricular cardiomyopathy was the cause of death in only four (3%) of 134 subjects aged 12 to 40 years, with a mean of 17 years of age (6). In our more recent series tabulated in Table 3, right ventricular dysplasia was only present in individuals younger than 35 years of age and was the cause of death in 9%. This increase in incidence compared to our earlier series (35) may be related to the greater awareness of right ventricular dysplasia or a true increase in the incidence.

The reason for the geographic differences in the incidence of right ventricular cardiomyopathy are largely unknown and may, in part, be due to genetic variation. Because diagnostic criteria at autopsy are not yet fully standardized, this condition may be either overdiagnosed or, in some cases, not recognized. Because fat accumulation is common in the anterior portion of the right ventricle in normal hearts, we rigorously define right ventricular cardiomyopathy to include only those cases that demonstrated fat and fibrous tissue intermingled with myocytes.

The gross pathologic features of right ventricular cardiomyopathy include extensive replacement of the right ventricle by fat with focal thinning and aneurysm formation of the right ventricle (29,58–62). The aneurysms may occur anywhere in the right ventricle, but are most frequent in the anterior outflow tract and posteroapical regions (Fig. 3). In most cases, there are foci of ventricular thinning of 1 mm or less, including the epicardial fat. Histologically, the characteristic finding is the intermixing of fat, fibrous tissue, and degenerating atrophic myocytes with a myofibrillar loss characterized by intracytoplasmic vacuoles. In 80% of cases, there are foci of myocarditis, which may or may not be associated with areas of myofibrillar loss or scarring. Corresponding to gross findings, the replacement by fat and fibrous tissue is most often seen in the posterior wall of the right ventricle and in the right ventricular outflow tract. It has recently been recognized that left ventricular involvement is common in right ventricular cardiomyopathy; this consists of subepicardial replacement by fat and fibrous tissue.

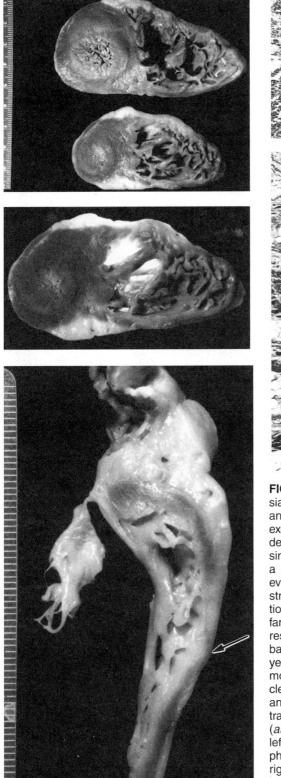

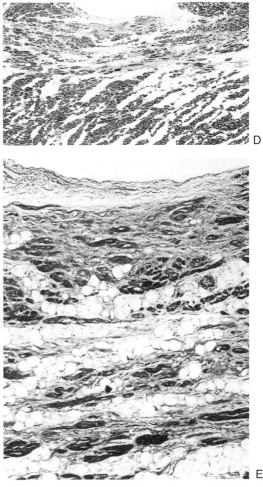

FIG. 3. Right ventricular cardiomyopathy/dysplasia. A 26-year-old man with history of syncope and atrial fibrillation collapsed during exercise; exercise stress test performed 5 months prior to death was remarkable for frequent, multifocal single premature ventricular depolarizations with a single couplet; myocardial ischemia was not evident. Subsequent Holter monitoring demonstrated rare, isolated atrial premature depolarizations conducted normally to the ventricles. His family history was significant for early cardiac arrest (father died at age 42 years while playing basketball) and "myocardial infarction" in a 28-year-old brother. The heart weighed 490 g with moderate to severe dilatation of the right ventricle (**A**). There was apical aneurysm with thinning and dilation, and the translucent area is illustrated in (**B**). The right anterior wall was thinned (*arrow*) with mild aneurysmal dilatation (**C**). The left ventricle was unremarkable without hypertrophy or dilatation. The histologic section of the right ventricle demonstrated patchy fibrosis with intermingling of fat and myocytes (**D** and **E**).

The association between right ventricular cardiomyopathy and sudden death has been well documented. In 83% of patients reported by Thiene et al. (29), death occurred during or soon after exercise. In our experience, exercise is a factor in more than 50% of deaths resulting from ventricular cardiomyopathy (63,64).

The origin of right ventricular dysplasia is poorly understood. The role of myocarditis as a primary or secondary phenomenon in the pathogenesis of the disease has long been debated (64–67). The disease has a strong familial component, with 26% of sudden deaths in our experience occurring in families with the disease, which is similar to the familial incidence in Minnesota (68). The genetic basis for the disease is unknown, but genetic loci linked to right ventricular cardiomyopathy include 14q23-q24, 1q42-q43, and 14q12-q22 (65,69).

CONCENTRIC IDIOPATHIC LEFT VENTRICULAR HYPERTROPHY

We have found a relatively high incidence of concentric left ventricular hypertrophy of unknown etiology in exercise-related sudden death, ranging from 9% in our series of individuals younger than 40 years of age (35) to seven of 48 (15%) in our more recent series of individuals younger than 35 years of age who died during exercise (see Table 3). These percentages are similar to those of Maron et al. (6), who classified 10% of cases as having an unexplained increase in cardiac mass in their recent series of 134 young competitive athletes who died suddenly. Idiopathic left ventricular hypertrophy, which is relatively poorly characterized, is an uncommon cause of sudden death in athletes older than 35 years of age (7% in our experience; see Table 3).

The true nature of idiopathic left ventricular hypertrophy remains unknown. These cases may represent occult systemic hypertension, an exaggerated form of "athlete's heart," or a variant of hypertrophic cardiomyopathy. It is possible that it may be an abnormal response to exercise or a form of hy-

pertrophic cardiomyopathy without the characteristic features of the disease as it is currently defined. Identification of mutations in contractile components of cardiac myocytes, as has been done in hypertrophic cardiomyopathy, has yet to occur in idiopathic left ventricular hypertrophy.

From a practical point of view, given the normal increase in cardiac mass that occurs as an adaptation in chronic conditions, we make the diagnosis of idiopathic concentric left ventricular hypertrophy only if at least three conditions are met, in addition to concentric hypertrophy (Fig. 4). The heart weight must exceed 95% confidence intervals for the athlete's height and weight (70), myofiber disarray must not be present in greater than 5% of septal myocardium, and intramural coronary

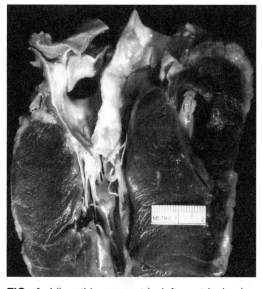

FIG. 4. Idiopathic concentric left ventricular hypertrophy. A 35-year-old white man collapsed while playing basketball. There was no history of hypertension or any other known clinical cardiovascular problems. At autopsy, his heart weighed 650 g with septum measuring 2.3 cm and the left ventricular free wall 2.1 cm and right ventricle 0.5 cm. There was no asymmetry or left ventricular outflow tract plaque. Histologic sections showed myocyte hypertrophy but failed to show any fibromuscular disarray or intramyocardial coronary artery thickening.

arterial thickening must be absent, other than in the papillary muscles.

NATURAL DEATH IN THE ABSENCE OF UNDERLYING STRUCTURAL ABNORMALITIES AND EXERTIONAL HEAT ILLNESS WITH SICKLE CELL TRAIT

The causes of exercise-related sudden death in U.S. military recruits differs greatly from those in other series of sudden death in athletes. Up to 35% of exercise-related sudden death in recruits are unexplained even after autopsy, a high percentage are heat-related illnesses, and myocarditis is a relatively frequent finding (39). The reasons for these differences include a high proportion of individuals with relatively poor cardiac conditioning, living in crowded conditions that might predispose to infectious myocarditis, and exercising in conditions with high ambient temperature and humidity.

In a prospective series of deaths among 2.08 million recruits aged 17 to 30 years who entered military basic training in the Armed Forces from 1977 to 1981 (39), exercise-related natural deaths occurred in 41 individuals (Table 4). A diagnosis of sudden death from exertional heat illness was made on the basis of high fever at presentation and nonfocal encephalopathy progressing to coma during or shortly after exercise. The exercise-related sudden cardiac death rates in recruits are 20 to 80 times higher than in unselected American population (39,71,72). Of the 41 exercise-related sudden deaths in recruits, only 12 (29%) were due to silent preexisting cardiac disease, whereas 13 (32%) were due to unexplained sudden cardiac death and 14 (34%) to exertional heat illness (heat stroke or rhabdomyolysis). These data indicate that heat illness is a significant factor in exercise-related cardiac death, a fact that previously has been little appreciated and may, in part, explain the high rate of sudden death in recruits.

The number of heat-related sudden deaths in U.S. recruits is similar in those with and without sickle cell trait (see Table 4). Because of the low rate of hemoglobin (Hb) AS in U.S. recruits (8% in African Americans versus 0.046% in other Americans), the rate of sudden death associated with sickle cell trait was 63-fold higher than the risk with Hb AA, and the attributable risk for sickle cell trait was a mortality rate of 1.75 in 1,000 person-years. The difference in heat-related death is not attributable to race alone, because exercise-related death unexplained by preexisting disease was 30 times greater among black recruits with sickle cell trait than in black recruits without Hb S (39,71).

The diagnosis of heat-related sudden death is not always straightforward, because hyper-

TABLE 4. *Comparison of exercise-related and non–exercise-related sudden death among recruits in U.S. Armed Forces Basic Training, 1977–1981*

	With Hb AS	Hb AA
Exercise-related	14	27
Deaths not due to preexisting disease	13	14
Rhabdomyolysis without heat stroke	5	1
Heat stroke with rhabdomyolysis	2	4
Heat stroke alone	0	2
Unexplained sudden cardiac death	6	7
Death attributed to preexisting diseases	1	13
Sudden death	1	11
Noncardiac	0	2
Nonexercise–related	0	3
Sudden cardiac	0	2
Noncardiac	0	1

From ref. 39, with permission.

thermia is not always evident at the time of clinical assessment. There is a wide range of presentation of severe exertional heat illness, which may be approximately subdivided into several syndromes (39). When muscle necrosis is mild or absent, the syndrome is divided into heat exhaustion (dominated by low central blood volume, high cardiac output to skin and muscle, orthostatic hypotension, and electrolyte abnormalities), heat injury, and heat stroke [characterized by delirium, combative state, obtundation, or coma, and hyperthermia (temperature greater than 105°F)]. The term *heat injury* is used for cases with intermediate levels of encephalopathy and hyperthermia between those encountered with heat exhaustion and heat stroke.

When muscle necrosis is prominent, the term *exertional rhabdomyolysis* is used.

Heavy exercise is probably required for the development of rhabdomyolysis, which can occur with or without hyperthermia. Muscle symptoms are usually absent in the first 6 to 12 hours, because muscle necrosis progresses slowly. Symptoms of heat injury and heat stroke are usually present and are often related to taking salt tablets in the field with water. Renal failure with elevated blood urea nitrogen and serum creatinine is usually seen in heat injuries, especially those with myoglobinemia and rhabdomyolysis, but may be delayed.

The interrelationship between sickle cell and heat-related illness is poorly understood, but may be related to physiologic changes (dehydration, increased body temperature, hypoxia, and acidosis) that are related to heavy exercise and that promote polymer formation

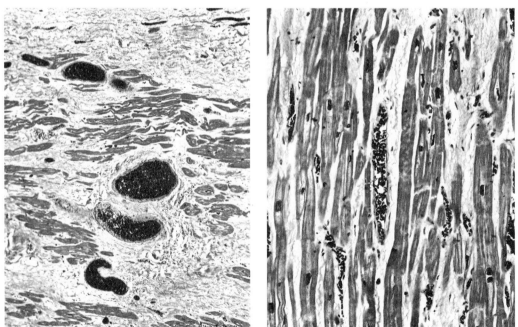

FIG. 5. Sickle cell disease. A 35-year-old black man was found dead by the roadside in jogging attire. At autopsy, the heart weighed 590 g and all four chambers were dilated. There was focal scarring of the subendocardium in the posterolateral wall of the left ventricle. Myocardial sections showed diffuse sickling of red cells in all intramyocardial arteries and veins, with organized thrombi seen focally in areas of scarring. The patient was known to have sickle cell disease and was an avid jogger. Note focal scarring in the subendocardial region (**A**) and extensive sickling of red cells (**A and B**).

by purified Hb S. Exertional heat illness usually occurs with activities that require very high metabolic rates; the activity most frequently causing sudden death associated with sickle cell trait among recruits is running 1 to 3 miles (39). The pace of these runs generally requires a metabolic rate 11 to 14 times the basal rate sustained for periods of about 5 to 30 minutes. The pathologic changes in heat-related sudden death are nonspecific and may include intravascular myocardial sickling (in patients with Hb AS) and myoglobin casts within the renal tubules (in cases with rhabdomyolysis). Postmortem sickling within the myocardial vessels is nonspecific, however, and may be seen as an agonal change in patients dying of other causes.

Sudden cardiac death with sickle cell disease has rarely been reported in patients who exercise (73). In such cases, the cause of death is not necessarily related to heat illness, but to ischemic damage to the myocardium that occurred as a result of coronary arteries obstructed by organized thrombi (Fig. 5).

In a fairly large proportion of autopsies in exercise-related sudden cardiac death, no structural abnormalities are found at autopsy. This proportion varies, but is greatest with younger-aged athletes, and is approximately 10% overall (see Tables 1, 2, and 3). The number of these cases that actually represent missed cases of heat illness in athletes with and without sickle cell trait is unknown, because autopsy findings are nonspecific, and the diagnosis must be made with clinical data (including ambient temperature and humidity at the time before exercise, rectal temperatures, and clinical course). In most investigations of recruits who die during exercise, the rectal temperature is not available to exclude exertional rhabdomyolysis. The number of exertion-related cases reported with sickle cell trait are few in Table 1 (3%), but this may reflect possible bias with more deaths reported in whites or a large number of deaths labeled unknown (8%), which may have occurred because of heat injury in men with sickle cell trait. In addition, it is important to define sudden death as onset following critical illness

within 1 hour, because, in heat-related illness, a rather lengthy period of survival on life-support may follow.

CORONARY ARTERY ANOMALIES

Coronary artery anomalies are the third most frequent cause of death among exercising individuals, the first two being coronary artery atherosclerosis and cardiomyopathies (see Table 1). Congenital anomalies of the coronary arteries are difficult to detect clinically and premortem symptoms are absent or vague. In the Veneto region of Italy, where sudden deaths in athletes are prospectively studied with clinical correlation, deaths resulting from coronary artery anomalies represented the largest group that had few if any prodromal symptoms or electrocardiographic abnormalities that would allow detection by screening (31).

The most common potentially lethal coronary artery anomaly is the anomalous left coronary artery, characterized by the left main and right coronary arteries arising from the right sinus of Valsalva (Fig. 6). A review of the literature revealed a 46% incidence of sudden death with this anomaly, over 85% of which occurred during exercise (6,24,26,74–83) (Table 5). In our files, we have studied 42 hearts with this anomaly; 25 (69%) were from autopsies of people who died suddenly, of which 65% died during exercise.

There are four pathologic variants of the anomalous left main coronary artery: (a) the left main may either arise as a first branch of the right coronary artery or arise as a separate ostium in the right sinus and pass obliquely in between the aorta and the pulmonary trunk, (b) the left main is anterior to the pulmonary trunk and then divides into the left circumflex and the left anterior descending and passes in the interventricular groove, (c) the left main courses to the right and posteriorly behind the aorta, and (d) the left main courses inferiorly and intramuscularly to the subendocardial region of the crista supraventricularis and then surfaces to the anterior interventricular groove. All subtypes have been associated with sudden death. However, the course in between the

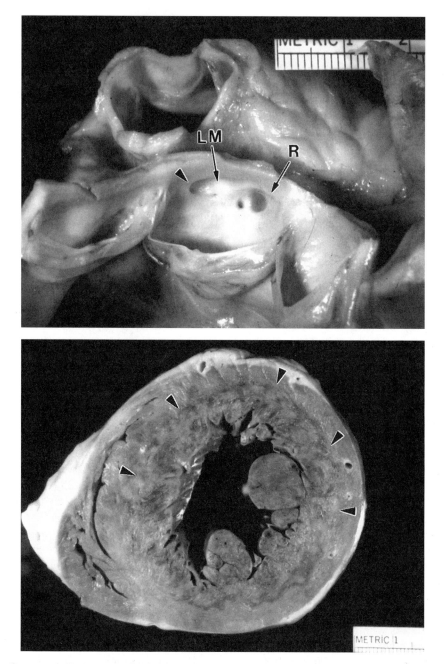

FIG. 6. Coronary artery anomaly. A 20-year-old man complained of chest pain while playing basketball. In the emergency department, hemodynamic instability, ventricular arrhythmias, significant repolarization changes on ECG, and markedly elevated creatine kinase developed. Emergency cardiac catheterization was reported as consistent with coronary artery anomaly, cardiogenic shock developed, and he died. The heart weighed 445 g with mild left ventricular dilatation and an acute subendocardial myocardial infarct (*arrowheads*) involving the septum and the anterior and lateral wall of left ventricle with involvement of both papillary muscles and relative sparing of the posterior wall of left ventricle. The left main (LM) and the right (R) coronary arteries arose from the right sinus of Valsalva (*arrow*) and the left main ostium had an ostial valve-like ridge formed by the aortic wall (*arrowhead*). The left main artery coursed anteriorly between the aorta and the pulmonary trunk.

TABLE 5. *Published reports of the frequency of sudden death among patients with left main and right coronary arteries arising from the right aortic sinus*

Author and Year	No. of Patients	Age Range, Years (Mean)	M:F	No of Sudden Deaths	No. of Sudden Deaths with Exercise
Cheitlin et al., 1974	33	13–87 (47)	32:1	9	7
Pedal, 1976	1	10	0:1	1	1
Liberthson et al., 1979	3	1–17 (3)	3:0	3	2
Maron et al., 1980	4	17–22 (18)	4:0	4	4
Lynch, 1980	2	19,20	2:0	2	2
Tsung et al., 1982	2	14,18	2:0	2	2
Betend et al., 1983	1	16	1:0	1	1
Topaz et al., 1985	1	15	0:1	1	1
Barth et al., 1986	5	13–81 (38)	3:2	3	3
Taylor et al., 1992	49	2–87 (37)	44:5	28 (57%)	18
Land et al., 1994	1	15	0:1	1	1
Janata et al., 1994	1	16	0:1	1	1
Maron et al., 1996	13	12–23 (15)	(90%,M)	13	13
Total	116	2–87	102:14	69 (59%)	56 (81%)

M, male; F, female.
From ref. 87, with permission.

aorta and the pulmonary trunk has the highest association with sudden death and exercise-related death. Of the nine cases of anomalous left main coursing between the aorta and the pulmonary trunk in our files, seven patients died during exercise.

The mechanism of sudden death resulting from an anomalous left coronary artery is unknown. The most favored theory involves compression of the artery between the aorta and the pulmonary trunk. We have reported that there is acute angle takeoff of the anomalous coronary artery, which results in an ostial slitlike opening (84). As the aorta lengthens during diastole, it causes the compression of the coronary artery, especially during exercise when there is increased oxygen demand. We have recently measured the angulation of the anomalous coronary artery origin at its takeoff and proximal intimal course, comparing cases with and without sudden death. There were no significant differences between patients with and without sudden cardiac death with respect to coronary ostial size, length of aortic intramural segment, angle of takeoff of the anomalous coronary artery, and degree of displacement from the correct coronary sinus (85). Among patients with sudden death, however, patients

with exercise-related sudden cardiac death had smaller coronary artery ostia and longer aortic intramural course, which possibly contributed to myocardial ischemia as the mechanism of death. In this study, age older than 30 years was the only variable associated with a decreased risk for exercise- or non–exercise-related sudden cardiac death (85).

A less common and less clinically significant coronary anomaly is the presence of both right and left coronary ostia in the left sinus of Valsalva. Until recently, this anomaly was not considered lethal, but it has come to be recognized as a rare cause of ischemic symptoms and even sudden death. In the initial series of this anomaly, Roberts et al. (86) reported sudden death in three of ten patients (one in an athlete playing basketball) in whom the coronary anomaly was the only significant cardiac abnormality found at autopsy. The incidence of sudden death in patients with this anomaly is far lower (25%) than in patients with both arteries arising from the right sinus (57%). Of the 52 patients with this anomaly, 13 (25%) died suddenly; of these deaths, six (11%) occurred during exercise (87). The reason for the low lethality of this condition is unclear, but it is likely related to the lesser extent of myocardium supplied by the right coronary artery as compared to the left.

An uncommon cause of sudden cardiac death is an anomalous left main or left anterior descending coronary artery arising from the pulmonary trunk. We observed this anomaly in 37 patients, 25 of whom were younger than 12 months of age (87). In clinical series, 90% of patients die before 1 year of life, because of the severe hemodynamic consequences of this condition. In our autopsy series, 14 of 37 (38%) of the deaths were sudden and, of these, death occurred during exercise in two patients (5%) over 5 years of age.

A single coronary ostium giving rise to all three major coronary arteries is a rare anomaly that results in sudden death in approximately 14% of cases. In the AFIP series of 44 patients with anomaly, (Table 6), six anomalous arteries were the cause of sudden death and three of those were exercise-related. In two of the exercise-related deaths, the single coronary ostium arose from the right and in one case the single ostium arose from the left sinus of Valsalva. Congenital absence of the right coronary artery, in which there is a single coronary ostium without an artery supplying the right ventricle and posterior cardiac wall, has been associated with exercise in a rugby player (88).

Hypoplastic coronary arteries is an uncommon coronary artery anomaly that has been associated with sudden death with exercise. The precise incidence of this entity is unknown because there are no standard criteria for diagnosis. We define hypoplastic coronary arteries as an absence of the posterior descending coronary artery, resulting in an avascular area in the posterior wall of left ventricle (i.e., neither the right nor the left coronary system extends beyond the lateral borders of the heart). Less stringent criteria, such as diffusely narrowed diameters without precise parameters (89), have been used for the diagnosis of hypoplastic coronary arteries but are difficult to adopt. We have examined the hearts of 13 patients with hypoplastic coronary arteries using our strict criteria (see Table 6); three of the patients had died suddenly during exercise. In addition, we have recently encountered an angiographically documented case of hypoplastic coronary arteries in a patient with a positive treadmill test. At autopsy, the coronary arteries were small, varying from 1 to 4 mm without atherosclerotic coronary disease,

TABLE 6. *Distribution and mode of death in 242 autopsy cases with isolated coronary artery anomalies*

	All Deaths	Sudden Deaths (%)	Nonsudden Cardiac Deaths (%)	Exercise-Related Sudden Deaths (%)
I. Anomalous origin of ≥ 1 CA from Pul. trunk				
A. LMCA or LAD from Pul. trunk	37	14 (38)	23 (62)	2 (14)
B. Both CA from Pul. trunk	3	3 (100)	0	0
C. RCA from Pul. trunk	1	0	1	0
II. Anomalous origin of ≥ 1 CA from Aorta				
A. LMCA and RCA from R Ao sinus	49	28 (57)	8 (16)	18 (64)
B. RCA and LMCA from L Ao sinus	52	13 (25)	2 (4)	6 (46)
C. LCx and RCA from R Ao sinus	21	2 (10)	6 (29)	0
D. RCA and/or LMCA from posterior Ao sinus	17	5 (29)	4 (24)	2 (40)
E. RCA and LAD from R Ao sinus	1	1 (100)	0	0
III. Single CA ostium from Aorta				
A. Single RCA ostium	22	4 (18)	5 (23)	2 (50)
B. Single LCA ostium	22	2 (9)	8 (36)	2 (50)
IV. Hypoplastic CAs	13	5 (38)	4 (31)	3 (60)
V. CA fistula	4	1 (25)	3 (75)	0
Total	242	78 (32)	64 (26)	34 (44)

Ao, aorta or aortic; CA, coronary artery; L, left; LAD, left anterior descending; LCA, left coronary artery; LCx, left circumflex coronary artery; LMCA, left main coronary artery; R, right; RCA, right coronary artery; Pul., pulmonary.
From ref. 80, with permission.

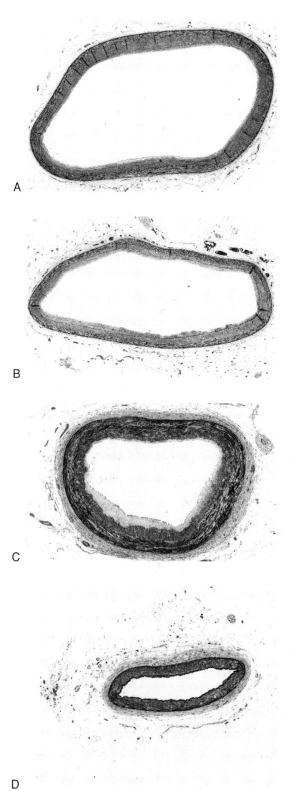

FIG. 7. Hypoplastic coronary arteries. Note the area enclosed by the internal elastic lamina in the left anterior descending and the left circumflex coronary arteries from a normal age-matched heart (**A** and **B**) as compared to the arterial size of the left anterior descending and left circumflex from a patient with hypoplastic coronary arteries (**C** and **D**). The right artery was similar to the left circumflex and neither extended to the lateral wall of the left ventricle.

and the posterior septum had a healed sub-endocardial infarct (Fig. 7).

MYOCARDITIS

In published reports of causes of death in exercising individuals, myocarditis is an uncommon cause of sudden death (see Tables 1, 2, and 3). In the study of Maron et al. (6), myocarditis was found at autopsy in 3% of athletes dying suddenly. The incidence among recruits is relatively high in comparison to studies of athletes dying suddenly (39), possibly because crowded living conditions facilitate the spread of infectious disease. In 1986, Phillips et al. (90) reported a 20-year review from 1965 to 1985 of sudden death during exercise in 1.6 million healthy young U.S. Air Force recruits in a 42-day basic military training with 30 active days (90). There were 19 sudden cardiac deaths (over half of which were cardiac-related); the most frequent anatomic cause of death in this group was myocarditis, occurring in eight recruits (42%). Of

these, four were lymphocytic myocarditis, three rheumatic myocarditis, and one vaccinia-related myocarditis. The high incidence of viral myocarditis in barracks-residing recruits is also documented in a Finnish study, which documented asymptomatic myocarditis in 126 conscripts by electrocardiographic changes or echocardiography (91,92).

There are few gross pathologic findings in hearts with myocarditis. Occasionally, the myocardium may appear soft and flabby, and there may be a slight to mild cardiac dilatation. Microscopically, the hallmarks of myocarditis are a lymphocytic infiltrate with myocyte necrosis (Fig. 8). The origin of myocarditis is often impossible to determine at autopsy, because enteroviral infections of the myocardium are often transient, resulting in negative postmortem cultures. Other viruses that may result in lymphocytic myocarditis include adenovirus, influenza virus, vaccinia, and varicella. There are no distinguishing histologic features among these different agents. Other forms of myocarditis, such as hypersensitivity

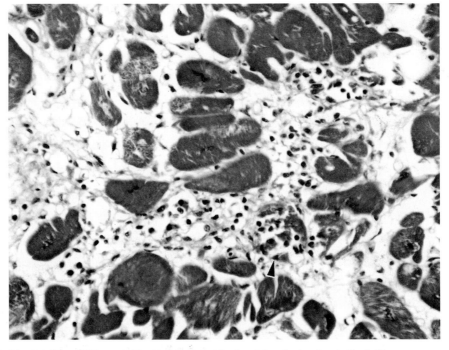

FIG. 8. Myocarditis. A 27-year-old man died suddenly while playing basketball. There was no significant medical history except for history of flulike symptoms 3 weeks prior to death. The gross examination of the heart was unremarkable. Histologic sections of the ventricles revealed lymphocytic myocarditis with myocyte necrosis (*arrowhead*).

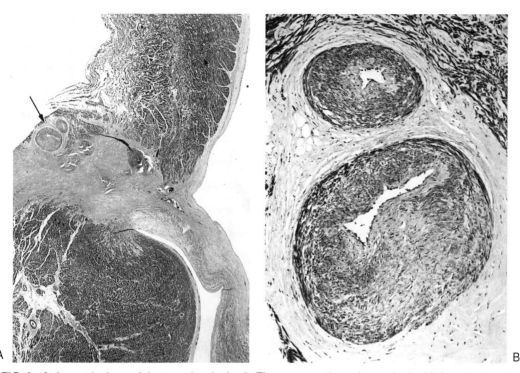

FIG. 9. Atrioventricular nodal artery dysplasia. **A:** The artery to the atrioventricular (AV) node (*arrow*) is shown in low power in the region of the approach to the AV node. **B:** High-power view of the arteries shown in (A). Note marked thickening of the arterial wall and dysplasia. This was the only abnormal finding in the heart of this young man who died suddenly.

(allergic) myocarditis, toxic myocarditis, and bacterial myocarditis are rare causes of exercise-related sudden death.

ABNORMALITIES OF THE CONDUCTION SYSTEM

There have been several abnormalities of the conduction system reported in athletes dying suddenly. Maron et al. (24) reported sclerosis of small arteries in the conduction system of two athletes who died suddenly. In one, a 24-year-old basketball player with hypertrophic cardiomyopathy, the autopsy disclosed a thickened, dysplastic artery to the sinoatrial node. In the other, a 17-year-old basketball player with idiopathic left ventricular hypertrophy, the autopsy demonstrated dysplasia of the atrioventricular nodal artery with marked luminal narrowing.

We have also reported dysplasia of the atrioventricular nodal artery in association with sudden cardiac death (Fig. 9), half of which

were exercise-related, in the absence of other cardiac findings (93). Other conduction system abnormalities that have been described in athletes dying suddenly include accessory pathways (Wolff-Parkinson-White syndrome) (94) and premature sclerosis of the conduction system (95).

REFERENCES

1. Gillum RF. Sudden coronary death in the United States. *Circulation* 1989;79:756–765.
2. Hunink MG, Goldman L, Tosteson AN, et al. The recent decline in mortality from coronary heart disease, 1980-1990. The effect of secular trends in risk factors and treatment. *JAMA* 1997;277:535–542.
3. Myerburg RJ, Castellanos AJ. Cardiac arrest and sudden cardiac death. In: Braunwald E, ed. *Heart disease: a textbook of cardiovascular medicine.* Philadelphia: WB Saunders, 1997:742–749.
4. Thompson PD, Funk EJ, Carleton RA, Sturner WQ. Incidence of death during jogging in Rhode Island from 1975 through 1980. *JAMA* 1982;247:2535–2538.
5. Siscovick DS, Weiss NS, Fletcher RH, Lasky T. The cidence of primary cardiac arrest during vigorous cise. *N Engl J Med* 1984;311:874.
6. Maron BJ, Shirani J, Poliac LC, Mathenge F WC, Mueller FO. Sudden death in young

athletes. Clinical, demographic, and pathological profiles. *JAMA* 1996;276:199–204.

7. Siscovick D, Ekelund L, Hyde J, Johnson J, Gordon D, LaRose J. Physical activity and coronary heart disease among asymptomatic hypercholesterolemic men. *Am J Public Health* 1988;78:1428–1431.

8. Slattery ML, Jacobs DE, Nichaman MZ. Leisure time physical activity and coronary heart disease death. The US Railroad Study. *Circulation* 1989;79:304–312.

9. Siscovick DS. Exercise and sudden cardiac death: is the run worth the risk? *Trans Assoc Life Insur Med Dir Am* 1990;73:37–44.

10. Friedewald VE Jr, Spence DW. Sudden cardiac death associated with exercise: the risk-benefit issue. *Am J Cardiol* 1990;66:183–188.

11. Gott PH, Roselle HA, Crampton RS. The athletic heart syndrome. Five-year cardiac evaluation of a champion athlete. *Arch Intern Med* 1968;122:340–344.

12. Maron BJ. Structural features of the athlete heart as defined by echocardiography. *J Am Coll Cardiol* 1986;7:190–203.

13. Morganroth J, Maron BJ, Henry WL, Epstein SE. Comparative left ventricular dimensions in trained athletes. *Ann Intern Med* 1975;82:521–524.

14. Ben-Ari E, Gentile R, Feigenbaum H, et al. Left ventricular dynamics during strenuous isometric exercise in marathon runners, weight lifters and healthy sedentary men: comparative echocardiographic study. *Cardiology* 1993;82:75–80.

15. Galanti G, Comeglio M, Vinci M, Cappelli B, Vono MC, Bamoshmoosh M. Echocardiographic Doppler evaluation of left ventricular diastolic function in athletes' hypertrophied hearts. *Angiology* 1993;44:341–346.

16. Missault L, Duprez D, Jordaens L, et al. Cardiac anatomy and diastolic filling in professional road cyclists. *Eur J Appl Physiol* 1993;66:405–408.

17. Wight JN, Salem D. Sudden cardiac death and the "athlete's heart." *Arch Intern Med* 1995;155:1473–1480.

18. Lavie CJ, Milani RV, Squires RW, Boykin C. Exercise and the heart. Good, benign, or evil? *Postgrad Med* 1992;91:130–134, 143–150.

19. Hull SS Jr, Evans AR, Vanoli E, et al. Heart rate variability before and after myocardial infarction in conscious dogs at high and low risk of sudden death. *J Am Coll Cardiol* 1990;16:978–985.

20. Zehender M, Meinertz T, Keul J, Just H. ECG variants and cardiac arrhythmias in athletes: clinical relevance and prognostic importance. *Am Heart J* 1990;119:1378–1391.

21. Rodriguez Reguero JJ, Iglesias Cubero G, Lopez de la Iglesia J, et al. Prevalence and upper limit of cardiac hypertrophy in professional cyclists. *Eur J Appl Physiol* 1995;70:375–378.

22. Waller B, Newhouse P, Pless J, Foster L, Wills E. Exercise-related sudden death in 27 conditioned subjects aged <30 and >30 years: coronary artery abnormalities are the culprit. *J Am Coll Cardiol* 1984;3:621(A).

23. Buddington RS, Stahl CJ, McAllister HA, Schwartz RA. Sports, death and unusual heart disease. *Am J Cardiol* 1974;33:129A.

24. Maron BJ, Roberts WC, McAllister HA, Rosing DR, Epstein SE. Sudden death in young athletes. *Circulation* 1980;62:218–229.

25. [...]ie LH. Sudden death and sport. *Lancet* 1975;1:[...]–266.

26. Tsung SH, Huang TY, Chang HH. Sudden death in athletes. *Arch Pathol Lab Med* 1982;106:168–170.

27. Kennedy HL, Whitlock JA. Sports related sudden death in young persons. *J Am Coll Cardiol* 1984;3:622A.

28. Northcote RJ, Flannigan C, Ballantyne D. Sudden death and vigorous exercise—a study of 60 deaths associated with squash. *Br Heart J* 1986;55:198–203.

29. Thiene G, Nava A, Corrado D, Rossi L, Penneli N. Right ventricular cardiomyopathy and sudden death in young people. *N Engl J Med* 1988;318:129–133.

30. Niimura I, Maki T. Sudden cardiac death in childhood. *Jpn Circ J* 1989;53:1571–1580.

31. Corrado D, Thiene G, Nava A, Rossi L, Pennelli N. Sudden death in young competitive athletes: clinicopathologic correlations in 22 cases. *Am J Med* 1990;89:588–596.

32. Burke AP, Farb A, Virmani R. Causes of sudden death in athletes. *Cardiol Clin* 1992;10:303–318.

33. Virmani R, Robinowitz M. Cardiac pathology and sports medicine. *Hum Pathol* 1987;18:493–501.

34. Virmani R, Robinowitz M, McAllister HA Jr. Exercise and the heart. *Pathol Annu* 1985;2:430–444.

35. Burke AP, Farb A, Virmani R, Goodin J, Smialek JE. Sports-related and non-sports-related sudden cardiac death in young adults. *Am Heart J* 1991;121:568–575.

36. Shotar A, Busuttil A. Myocardial bars and bridges and sudden death. *Forensic Sci Int* 1994;68:143–147.

37. McHenry PL. Role of exercise testing in predicting sudden death. *J Am Coll Cardiol* 1985;5:9B–12B.

38. Fletcher GF, Froelicher VF, Hartley LH, Haskell WL, Pollock ML. Exercise standards. A statement for health professionals from the American Heart Association. *Circulation* 1990;82:286–322.

39. Kark JA, Ward FT. Exercise and hemoglobin S. *Semin Hematol* 1994;31:181–225.

40. Jackson RT, Beaglehole R, Sharpe N. Sudden death in runners. *N Z Med J* 1983;96:289–292.

41. Thompson PD, Stern MP, Williams P, Duncan K, Haskell WL, Wood PD. Death during jogging or running. *JAMA* 1979;242:1265–1267.

42. Noakes TD, Rose AG, Opie LH. Hypertrophic cardiomyopathy associated with sudden death during marathon racing. *Br Heart J* 1979;41:624–627.

43. Virmani R, Robinowitz M, McAllister HA. Nontraumatic death in joggers. *Am J Med* 1982;72:874–881.

44. Farb A, Tang A, Burke A, Sessums L, Liang Y, Virmani R. Sudden coronary death: Frequency of active coronary lesions, inactive coronary lesions, and myocardial infarction. *Circulation* 1995;92:1701–1709.

45. Maron BJ, Roberts WC. Quantitative analysis of cardiac muscle disorganization in the ventricular septum of patients with hypertrophic cardiomyopathy. *Circulation* 1979;4:689–706.

46. Maron BJ, Bonow RO, Cannon RO, Leon MB, Epstein SE. Hypertrophic cardiomyopathy. *N Engl J Med* 1987;316:780–789.

47. Maron BJ, McIntosh CL, Klues HG, Cannon RO, Roberts WC. Morphologic basis for obstruction to right ventricular outflow in hypertrophic cardiomyopathy. *Am J Cardiol* 1993;71:1089–1094.

48. Davies MJ, McKenna WJ. Hypertrophic cardiomyopathy: an introduction to pathology and pathogenesis. *Br Heart J* 1994;72:S2–S3.

49. Shirani J, Maron BJ, Cannon RO, Shahin S, Roberts WC. Clinicopathologic features of hypertrophic cardio-

myopathy managed by cardiac transplantation. *Am J Cardiol* 1993;72:434–440.

50. Roberts WC, Ferrans VJ. Pathologic anatomy of the cardiomyopathies. Idiopathic dilated and hypertrophic types, infiltrative types, and endomyocardial disease with and without eosinophilia. *Hum Pathol* 1975;6:287–342.

51. McKenna W, Stewart J, Nihoyannopoulos P, McGinty F, Davies M. Hypertrophic cardiomyopathy without hypertrophy: two families with myocardial disarray in the absence of increased myocardial mass. *Br Heart J* 1990; 63:287–289.

52. Maron BJ, Lipson LC, Roberts WC, Savage DD, Epstein SE. Malignant hypertrophic cardiomyopathy: identification of a subgroup of families with unusually frequent premature death. *Am J Cardiol* 1978;41:1133–1140.

53. Maron BJ, Roberts WC, Epstein SE. Sudden death in hypertrophic cardiomyopathy: a profile of 78 patients. *Circulation* 1982;65:1388–1394.

54. Spirito P, Maron BJ. Relation between extent of left ventricular hypertrophy and occurrence of sudden cardiac death in hypertrophic cardiomyopathy. *J Am Coll Cardiol* 1990;15:1521–1526.

55. Maron BJ, Fananapazir L. Sudden cardiac death in hypertrophic cardiomyopathy. *Circulation* 1992;85: I57–I63.

56. Epstein MD, Cohn GM, Cyran F, Fanananpazir L. Differences in clinical expression of hypertrophic cardiomyopathy associated with two distinct mutations in the beta-myosin heavy chain gene. A 908Leu→ Val mutation and a 403Arg→ Gln mutation. *Circulation* 1992; 1992:345–352.

57. Watkins H, Rosenzweig A, Hwang DS, et al. Characteristics and prognostic implications of myosin missense mutations in familial hypertrophic cardiomyopathy. *N Engl J Med* 1992;326:1108–1114.

58. Fontaine G. Arrhythmogenic right ventricular dysplasia. *Curr Opin Cardiol* 1995;10:16–20.

59. Lobo FV, Heggtveit HA, Butany J, Silver MD, Edwards JE. Right ventricular dysplasia: morphological findings in 13 cases. *Can J Cardiol* 1992;8:261–268.

60. Marcus FI, Fontaine GH, Guiraudon G. Right ventricular dysplasia: a report of 24 adult cases. *Circulation* 1982;65:384–398.

61. Goodin JC, Farb A, Smialek JE, Field F, Virmani R. Right ventricular dysplasia associated with sudden death in young adults. *Mod Pathol* 1991;4:702–706.

62. Virmani R, Robinowitz M, Clark M, McAllister H. Sudden death and partial absence of the right ventricular myocardium: a report of three cases and a review of the literature. *Arch Pathol Lab Med* 1982;106:163–167.

63. Burke AP, Farb A, Virmani R. Arrhythmogenic right ventricular dysplasia-cardiomyopathy: a form of healing myocarditis? *J Am Coll Cardiol* 1996;27:399A.

64. Burke AP, Farb A, Virmani R. Inflammation, fibrosis, and fat in right ventricular dysplasia. *Mod Pathol* 1996; 9:28A.

65. Basso C, Thiene G, Corrado D, Angelini A, Nava A, Valente M. Arrhythmogenic right ventricular cardiomyopathy. Dysplasia, dystrophy, or myocarditis? *Circulation* 1996;94:983–991.

66. Fontaliran F, Fontaine G, Brestescher C, Labrousse J, Vilde F. Significance of lymphoplasmocytic infiltration in arrhythmogenic right ventricular dysplasia. Apropos of 3 own cases and review of the literature. *Arch Mal Coeur Vaiss* 1995;88:1021–1028.

67. Sabel KG, Blomstrom-Lundqvist C, Olsson SB, Enestrom S. Arrhythmogenic right ventricular dysplasia in brother and sister: is it related to myocarditis? *Pediatr Cardiol* 1990;11:113–116.

68. Kullo IJ, Edwards WD, Seward JB. Right ventricular dysplasia: the Mayo Clinic experience. *Mayo Clin Proc* 1995;70:541–548.

69. Rampazzo A, Nava A, Erne P, et al. A new locus for arrhythmogenic right ventricular cardiomyopathy (ARVD2) maps to chromosome 1q42-q43. *Hum Mol Genet* 1995;4:2151–2154.

70. Kitzman D, Scholz D, Hagen P, Ilstrup D, Edwards W. Age-related changes in normal human hearts during the first 10 decades of life. Part II (Maturity). A quantitative anatomic study of 765 specimens from subjects 20 to 99 years old. *Mayo Clin Proc* 1988;63:137–146.

71. Kark JA. Sickle-cell trait as an age-dependent risk factor for sudden death in physical training. *N Engl J Med* 1987;317:781–787.

72. Kark JA, Martin SK, Canik JJ. Sickle-cell trait as an age-dependent risk factor for sudden death in basic training. *Ann N Y Acad Sci* 1989;565:407–408.

73. Martin CR, Johnson CS, Cobb C, Tatter D, Haywood LJ. Myocardial infarction in sickle cell disease. *J Natl Med Assoc* 1996;88:428–432.

74. Cheitlin MD, DeCastro CM, McAllister HA. Sudden death as a complication of anomalous left coronary origin from the anterior sinus of Valsalva. A not so minor congenital anomaly. *Circulation* 1974;50:780–787.

75. Pedal I. Aortale Ursprungsanomalie einer koronarterie. *Dtsch Med Wochenschr* 1976;101:1601–1604.

76. Liberthson RR, Dinsmore RE, Zuberbuhler JR, Bahnson HT. Anomalous aortic origin of coronary arteries. *Circulation* 1979;59:748–754.

77. Lynch P. Soldiers, sport and sudden death. *Lancet* 1980; 1:1235–1237.

78. Topaz O, Edwards JE. Pathologic features of sudden death in children, adolescents, and young adults. *Chest* 1985;87:476–482.

79. Barth CW, Roberts WC. Left main coronary artery originating from the right sinus of Valsalva and coursing between aorta and pulmonary trunk. *J Am Coll Cardiol* 1986;7:366–373.

80. Taylor A, Rogan KM, Virmani R. Sudden cardiac death associated with isolated congenital coronary artery anomalies. *J Am Coll Cardiol* 1992;20:640–647.

81. Land RN, Hamilton AY, Fuchs PC. Sudden death in a young athlete due to an anomalous commissural origin of the left coronary artery, and focal intimal proliferation of aortic valve leaflet at the adjacent commissure. *Arch Pathol Lab Med* 1994;118:931–933.

82. Janata K, Regele H, Bankier AA, et al. Sudden cardiac death of a teenage girl [see comments]. *Resuscitation* 1994;28:37–42.

83. Betend B, Gillet P, Moreau P, David L. Origine aortique anormale de l'arterie coronaire gauche. A propos de la mort subite d'un adolescent. *Arch Fr Pediatr* 1983;40: 479–481.

84. Virmani R, Chun P, Goldstein R, Robinowitz M, McAllister H. Acute takeoffs of the coronary arteries along the aortic wall and congenital coronary ostial valve-like ridges: association with sudden death. *J Am Coll Cardiol* 1984;3:766–771.

85. Taylor AJ, Byers JP, Cheitlin MP, Virmani R. Variations in the coronary artery artery course do not correlate

with occurrence of sudden cardiac death in anomalous right or left coronary artery from the contralateral coronary sinus. *Am Heart J* 1997;133:428–435.

86. Roberts WC, Siegel RJ, Zipes DP. Origin of the right coronary artery from the left sinus of Valsalva and its functional consequences: analysis of 10 necropsy patients. *Am J Cardiol* 1982;49:863–868.

87. Virmani R, Rogan K, Cheitlin M. Congenital coronary artery anomalies: Pathologic aspects. In: Virmani R, Forman M, eds. *Non-atherosclerotic ischemic heart disease.* New York: Raven Press, 1989:153–183.

88. Yoshida K, Ogura Y, Wakasugi C. Sudden death case of single coronary artery with special reference to the effect of ischemia on actomyosin. *Nippon Hoigaku Zasshi* 1990;44:481–488.

89. Zugibe FT, Zugibe FT Jr, Costello JT, Breithaupt MK. Hypoplastic coronary artery disease within the spectrum of sudden unexpected death in young and middle age adults. *Am J Forensic Med Pathol* 1993;14:276–283.

90. Phillips M, Robinowitz M, Higgins JR, Boran K, Reed T, Virmani R. Sudden cardiac death in Air Force recruits. *JAMA* 1986;256:2696–2699.

91. Karjalainen J, Nieminen MS, Heikkila J. Influenza A1 myocarditis in conscripts. *Acta Med Scand* 1980;207:27–30.

92. Karjalainen J, Heikkila J, Nieminen MS. Etiology of mild acute infectious myocarditis. *Acta Med Scand* 1983;1978:65–73.

93. Burke A, Subramanian R, Virmani R, Smialek J. Non-atherosclerotic narrowing of atrioventricular nodal artery and sudden death. *J Am Coll Cardiol* 1993;21:117–122.

94. Thiene G, Pennelli N, Rossi L. Cardiac conduction system abnormalities as a possible cause of sudden death in young athletes. *Hum Pathol* 1983;14:704–709.

95. Bharati S, Bauernfeind R, Miller L, Lev M. Sudden death in three teenagers: conduction system studies. *J Am Coll Cardiol* 1983;1:879–885.

The Athlete and Heart Disease:
Diagnosis, Evaluation & Management,
edited by R. A. Williams.
Lippincott Williams & Wilkins, Philadelphia © 1999.

16

Cardiovascular Preparticipation Screening of Competitive Athletes[1]

Barry J. Maron

Cardiovascular Research Division, Minneapolis Heart Institute Foundation,
Minneapolis, Minnesota 55407

Sudden deaths of competitive athletes are personal tragedies with great impact on the lay and medical communities (1); they are usually due to a variety of previously unsuspected cardiovascular diseases (2–19). Such events often assume a high public profile because of the generally held perception that trained athletes constitute the healthiest segment of society, with the deaths of well-known elite athletes often exaggerating this visibility (1,20,21). These athletic field catastrophes inevitably raise a number of practical and ethical issues.

This chapter discusses (a) the benefits and limitations of preparticipation screening for early detection of cardiovascular abnormalities in competitive athletes, (b) cost-efficiency and feasibility issues as well as the medicolegal implications of screening, and (c) consensus recommendations and guidelines for the most prudent, practical, and effective screening procedures and strategies, based on a recent American Heart Association consensus panel (22). It is particularly relevant to reproduce those concepts in the present format, given the large number of competitive athletes in this country and the recent public health initiatives on physical activity and exercise.

DEFINITIONS AND BACKGROUND

The present considerations focus on the competitive athlete, previously described as one who participates in an organized team or individual sport requiring systematic training and regular competition against others, while placing a high premium on athletic excellence and achievement (20). The purpose of screening, as described here, is to provide medical clearance for participation in competitive sports through routine and systematic evaluations intended to identify clinically relevant and preexisting cardiovascular abnormalities and thereby reduce the risks associated with organized sports. Raising the possibility of a cardiovascular abnormality on a standard screening examination is, however, only the first tier of recognition after which referral to a specialist for further diagnostic investigation will probably be required. When a definitive cardiovascular diagnosis is made, the consensus panel guidelines of the 26th Bethesda Conference (23) should be used to formulate recommendations for continued participation or disqualification from competitive sports.

The American Heart Association guidelines (22) reproduced herein focus primarily

---

[1]The present text is adapted from the American Heart Association Medical/Scientific Statement, "Cardiovascular Preparticipation Screening of Competitive Athletes" (Maron BJ, Thompson PD, Puffer JC, McGrew CA, Strong WB, Douglas PS, Clark LT, Mitten MJ, Crawford MH, Atkins DL, Driscoll DJ, Epstein AE. *Circulation* 1996;94:850–856), with permission of the American Heart Association.

on the potential for population-based screening of high school and collegiate student-athletes rather than individual clinical assessments of athletes, and are designed to apply to competitors of all ages and both genders. These recommendations may also be extrapolated to athletes in youth, middle school, masters or professional sports, and in some instances to participants in intense recreational sporting activities. It is also recognized that overall preparticipation screening goes well beyond the considerations described herein, which are limited to the cardiovascular system, and involves many other organ systems and medical issues, particularly skeletal and orthopedic problems.

Screening recommendations are predicated on the probability that intense athletic training is likely to increase the risk for sudden cardiac death (or disease progression) in trained athletes with clinically important underlying structural heart disease, although presently it is not possible to quantify that risk. Certainly, the vast majority of young athletes who die suddenly do so during athletic training or competition, although a minority of deaths occur independent of exercise (3,5). These observations suggest that physical exertion is an important trigger for sudden death, given the presence of certain underlying cardiovascular diseases. Finally, the early detection of clinically significant cardiovascular disease through preparticipation screening will, in many instances, permit timely therapeutic interventions that may prolong life.

CAUSES OF SUDDEN DEATH IN ATHLETES

A variety of cardiovascular abnormalities represent the most common cause of sudden death in competitive athletes (2–19). The precise lesions responsible for athletic field catastrophes differ considerably with regard to age. For example, in youthful athletes (younger than about 35 years of age), most deaths are due to a variety of largely congenital cardiac malformations (Fig. 1) (3–5). Virtually any disease capable of causing sudden death in young people potentially may do so in young competitive athletes. Although these cardiovascular diseases may be relatively common in young athletes who die suddenly, each is uncommon in the general population. Also, the lesions responsible for sudden death do not occur with the same frequency, with most being responsible for less than or equal to 5% of all deaths (see Fig. 1).

The single most common cardiovascular abnormality among the causes of sudden death in young athletes is hypertrophic cardiomyopathy, usually in the nonobstructive form (2–5,24–29) and with a prevalence in the range of 35% (see Fig. 1). Hypertrophic cardiomyopathy is a primary and familial cardiac malformation with heterogeneous expression, complex pathophysiology, and diverse clinical course for which several disease-causing mutations in genes encoding proteins of the cardiac sarcomere have been reported (27, 30–34), including β-myosin heavy chain, cardiac troponin T, troponin I, α-tropomyosin, and myosin-binding protein C. Within the general population, hypertrophic cardiomyopathy is a relatively uncommon malformation occurring in about 0.2% (35).

The next most frequent cause is a variety of congenital coronary anomalies, particularly anomalous origin of the left main coronary artery from the right (anterior) sinus of Valsalva (36–40). Less common causes are myocarditis, dilated cardiomyopathy, Marfan syndrome with aortic rupture, arrhythmogenic right ventricular dysplasia, sarcoidosis, mitral valve prolapse, aortic valve stenosis, atherosclerotic coronary artery disease, long QT syndrome, and possibly intramural (tunneled) coronary arteries (2–5,41–44). Such deaths occur most commonly in intense team sports such as basketball and football, which also have the highest levels of participation.

Occasionally, athletes dying suddenly demonstrate no evidence of structural cardiovascular disease, even after careful gross and microscopic examination of the heart. In such instances (approximately 2% of our series) (3), it may not be possible to exclude noncardiac factors with certainty (e.g., drug abuse)

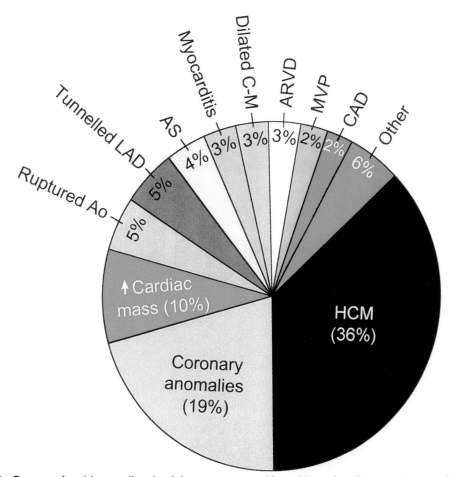

FIG. 1. Causes of sudden cardiac death in young competitive athletes (median age, 17 years) based on systematic tracking of 158 athletes in the United States, primarily 1985–1995. Ao = aorta; ARVD = arrhythmogenic right ventricular dysplasia; AS = aortic stenosis; CAD = coronary artery disease; C–M = cardiomyopathy; LAD = left anterior descending coronary artery; MVP = mitral valve prolapse; HCM = hypertrophic cardiomyopathy; ↑ = increased. (Adapted from ref. 22, with permission of the American Heart Association.)

as responsible for the catastrophe, or to know whether careful inspection of the specialized conducting system and associated vasculature with serial sectioning (which is not part of the standard medical examiners' protocol) would have revealed occult but clinically relevant abnormalities (9,45,46). Although one can only speculate on the potential causes of such deaths, it is possible that some are due to a primary arrhythmia in the absence of cardiac morphologic abnormalities (47), previously unidentified Wolff-Parkinson-White syndrome, rare diseases in which structural abnormalities of the heart are characteristically lacking at necropsy [e.g., long QT syndrome (41–43)], or possibly exercise-induced coronary spasm, or undetected segmental right ventricular dysplasia (7).

Athletes older than approximately age 35 years represent a different athletic population because they do not participate primarily in organized team sports, but rather focus on individual endeavors such as long-distance running. Furthermore, most deaths in middle-aged athletes are due to atherosclerotic coronary artery disease (16–19,48–50), and only rarely to congenital cardiovascular diseases such as hypertrophic cardiomyopathy or coronary artery anomalies.

This discussion focuses on the cardiovascular evaluation of athletes; other related medical problems that may occasionally cause sudden death in the young, such as cerebral aneurysm, sickle cell trait (51), nonpenetrating blunt chest impact (52), or bronchial asthma, are excluded. Neither are issues related to drug screening a part of this discussion, although the ingestion of agents such as cocaine are known to have important adverse cardiovascular consequences (53–55). Screening for systemic hypertension is addressed, although this disease is not regarded as an important cause of sudden unexpected death in young athletes (56).

PREVALENCE AND SCOPE OF THE PROBLEM

Relevant to the design of any screening strategy is the fact that sudden cardiac death in athletes is a devastating but rather infrequent event, and only a small proportion of participants in organized sports in the United States are at risk (48,57). Indeed, each of the lesions known to be responsible for sudden death in young athletes occur infrequently in the general population, ranging from the relatively common hypertrophic cardiomyopathy to the apparently very rare (e.g., coronary artery anomalies, arrhythmogenic right ventricular dysplasia, long QT syndrome, or Marfan syndrome), for which reliable estimates of frequency are lacking. It is reasonable to estimate that congenital malformations relevant to athletic screening may account for a combined prevalence of only less than or equal to 0.3% in general athletic populations.

The large reservoir of competitive athletes in the United States constitutes a major obstacle to screening strategies (4,22). At present, there are approximately 5 million competitive athletes at the high school level (grades 9 to 12), in addition to lesser numbers of collegiate (500,000) and professional (5,000) athletes. This does not include an unspecified number of youth, middle school, and masters level competitors for which reliable numbers are not available. Therefore, the total number of trained athletes in the United States every year is probably in the range of 7 to 8 million.

On a national scope, the prevalence of athletic field deaths owing to cardiovascular disease is not known with certainty, but it appears to be in the approximate range of 1:200,000 athletes of high school age (57). For older athletes, estimates (17,22,48) suggest that the frequency of sudden cardiac death, principally resulting from coronary artery disease (1:15,000 joggers and 1:50,000 marathon runners), may exceed the occurrence of these deaths in younger athletes. Considering such a relatively low prevalence, the heightened awareness and intense interest concerning sudden deaths in athletes, often fueled by the news media, is perhaps disproportionate to their actual numerical impact as a public health problem.

ETHICAL CONSIDERATIONS IN SCREENING

There is a general consensus that within a benevolent society, a responsibility exists on the part of physicians to initiate prudent efforts for the identification of life-threatening diseases in athletes, for the purpose of minimizing the cardiovascular risks associated with sport and protecting the health of such individuals (1,20,22,23,58,59). Specifically, there would also appear to be an implicit ethical (and possibly legal) obligation on the part of educational institutions (e.g., high schools and colleges) to implement cost-effective strategies to ensure that student-athletes are not subject to unacceptable and unavoidable medical risks (22). The libertarian view that high school and college-aged athletes should be permitted to assume any cardiovascular risk associated with sport as part of the overall risk of living is not ascribed to here. Despite sufficient financial resources, it is recognized that in professional sports a high motivation to implement cardiovascular screening may not exist because of the economic pressures inherent in such a sports environment for which athletic participation represents a vocation and remuneration for services that is often substantial.

The extent to which preparticipation screening efforts can be supported at any level of competitive athletics is mitigated by cost-efficiency considerations, practical limitations, and the awareness that it is not possible to achieve a "zero-risk" circumstance in competitive sports (59). Indeed, there is often implied acceptance of risk on the part of athletes; society permits or condones many athletic activities known to have intrinsic risks that cannot be controlled absolutely—for example, automobile racing or mountain climbing, as well as more traditional competitive sports such as football in which the possibility of serious traumatic injury exists.

It is also important to clearly acknowledge the limitations currently associated with preparticipation screening. Only in this way can an informed public be created that may otherwise harbor important misconceptions regarding the principles and efficacy of athletic screening. Italy has had a longstanding systematic national program over the past 25 years for the detection of cardiovascular disease in competitive athletes (58). This program is designed to disqualify those athletes with potentially lethal lesions from subsequent training and competition. In a sense, this national effort in Italy appears to place a particular priority on the health and welfare of athletes, relative to that of other citizens.

LEGAL CONSIDERATIONS

Although educational institutions and professional teams are required to use reasonable care in conducting their athletic programs, there is no clear legal precedent regarding their duty to conduct preparticipation screening of athletes for the purpose of detecting medically significant abnormalities (59,60). Indeed, no lawsuits have apparently been brought forward alleging negligence in the failure to either perform cardiovascular screening or diagnose cardiac disease in young competitive athletes as part of a screening program. In the absence of binding requirements established by state law or athletic governing bodies, most institutions and teams rely on the team physician to determine the appropriate medical screening procedures.

A physician who has medically cleared an athlete to participate in competitive sports is not necessarily legally liable for an injury or death caused by an undetected cardiovascular condition. Malpractice liability for failure to discover a latent, asymptomatic cardiovascular condition requires proof that a physician deviated from customary or accepted medical practice in his (or her) specialty in performing preparticipation screening of athletes and that the use of established diagnostic criteria and techniques would have disclosed the medical condition.

The medical profession is allowed to establish the appropriate nature and scope of preparticipation screening of athletes based on the exercise of its collective medical judgment. This necessarily involves the development of reliable diagnostic procedures in light of cost-benefit and feasibility factors. The

American Heart Association recommendations for cardiovascular preparticipation screening of athletes described herein (22) represent evidence of the proper medical standard of care; these guidelines will establish the legal standard of care if generally accepted or customarily followed by physicians, or if relied upon by courts in determining the nature and scope of the legal responsibility borne by sponsors of competitive athletes (59–61).

CURRENT CUSTOMARY PRACTICE

Currently, there are no universally accepted standards for the screening of high school and college athletes, nor are there approved certification procedures for the health care professionals who perform such screening examinations. Some form of medical clearance by a physician or other trained health care worker, usually consisting of a history and physical examination, presently appears most customary for high school athletes. Standards may be mandated by state legislative action or be the responsibility of individual state high school athletic associations or school districts. However, there is no uniform agreement among the states as to the precise format of preparticipation medical evaluations; in fact, not all states even require this process or have a recommended standard medical form. Some of the available forms (that represent guidelines for the examiner) are reasonably specific, whereas others require only the signature of a physician to provide clearance for the athlete to compete in organized sports. In a substantial minority of states, nonphysician health care workers are sanctioned to perform preparticipation screening, including chiropractors (in 11 states) and advanced nurse practitioners or physician assistants (in 16 states).

EXPECTATIONS OF STANDARD SCREENING PROCEDURES

Preparticipation screening by history and physical examination alone (without noninvasive testing) does not have sufficient power to guarantee detection of many critical cardiovascular abnormalities in large populations of

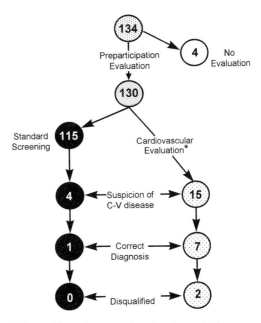

FIG. 2. Flow-diagram showing impact of preparticipation medical history and physical examinations on the detection of structural cardiovascular disease (and causes of sudden death) in high school and college athletes. *Asterisk* indicates cardiovascular evaluation with testing (independent of standard school or institutional preparticipation screening) performed in 15 athletes because of symptoms, family history, cardiac murmur, or physical findings suggestive of heart disease. (From ref. 3, with permission of the American Medical Association.)

young trained athletes. Indeed, hemodynamically significant congenital aortic valve stenosis is probably the lesion most likely to be reliably detected during routine screening because of its characteristically loud heart murmur. Detection of hypertrophic cardiomyopathy by the standard screening history or physical examination is unreliable because most patients have the nonobstructive form of this disease, characteristically expressed by no or only a soft heart murmur (22,24–26). Furthermore, most athletes with hypertrophic cardiomyopathy do not experience syncope or have a family history of premature sudden death; therefore, this disease is also not easily detected by the preparticipation personal history (22,24–26).

When symptoms such as chest pain or impaired consciousness are involved, the standard personal history conveys a generally low specificity for the detection of many cardiovascular abnormalities that lead to sudden cardiac death in young athletes. One retrospective study showed that potentially lethal cardiovascular abnormalities, including hypertrophic cardiomyopathy, were suspected by preparticipation history and physical in only 3% of high school and collegiate athletes who ultimately died suddenly of such diseases (Fig. 2) (3). In older athletes, however, a personal history of coronary risk factors (and a family history of premature ischemic heart disease) can be useful for identifying at-risk individuals.

EFFECTIVENESS AND LIMITATIONS OF NONINVASIVE SCREENING TESTS

The addition of noninvasive diagnostic tests to the screening process clearly has the potential to enhance the detection of certain cardiovascular defects in young athletes. For example, the two-dimensional echocardiogram is the principal diagnostic tool for clinical recognition of hypertrophic cardiomyopathy by virtue of demonstrating otherwise unexplained asymmetric left ventricular wall thickening, the sine qua non of this disease (24–26,28,62). Comprehensive and routine screening for hypertrophic cardiomyopathy by genetic testing for a variety of known disease-causing mutations is not yet practical or feasible for large populations, given the substantial genetic heterogeneity of the disease, and the expensive and time-intensive methodologies involved (30–34).

Echocardiography could also be expected to detect other relevant abnormalities associated with sudden death in young athletes such as valvular heart disease (e.g., mitral valve prolapse and aortic valvular stenosis), aortic root dilatation, and left ventricular dysfunction (caused by myocarditis or dilated cardiomyopathy). However, even such diagnostic testing cannot itself guarantee identification of all important lesions, and some relevant cardio-

vascular diseases may be beyond detection with any screening methodology. For example, identification of many congenital coronary artery anomalies usually requires sophisticated laboratory testing such as coronary arteriography, although it is possible in selected young athletes to raise a strong suspicion (or even identify) important anomalies such as left main coronary artery from the right sinus of Valsalva with echocardiography (38–40). Arrhythmogenic right ventricular dysplasia usually cannot be reliably diagnosed solely with echocardiography and electrocardiography (ECG); the best available noninvasive test for this disease is probably magnetic resonance imaging, which is both expensive and not universally available (44,63).

Cost-efficiency issues are important when assessing the feasibility of applying expensive noninvasive testing to the screening of large athletic populations (64–68); in most instances, adequate financial and personnel resources are lacking for such endeavors. If the full (i.e., unreduced) expense of testing would be the responsibility of administrative bodies such as a school, university, or team, the costs are probably prohibitive, ranging from about $400 to $1,000 per echocardiographic study (average about $600). For example, if the occurrence of hypertrophic cardiomyopathy in a young athletic population is assumed to be 1:500 (35), even at $500 per study it would theoretically cost $250,000 to detect even one previously undiagnosed case.

Screening protocols that incorporate noninvasive testing at greatly reduced cost have been described (64,66,67); however, these efforts have been in unique circumstances in which equipment was donated and professional expenses were waived for all but technician-related costs. Also, some investigators have suggested an inexpensive shortened-format echocardiogram for population screening (limited to parasternal views; about 2 minutes in duration) (64,67). Although such individual initiatives are lauded, it should also be noted that public service projects based largely on volunteerism usually cannot be sustained on a consistent basis because priorities for the use of available resources often change; therefore, such efforts are unlikely to be implemented on a scale necessary to provide effective screening to all high school and collegiate athletes.

Another important limitation of preparticipation screening with two-dimensional echocardiography is the potential for false-positive or false-negative test results. False-positive results arise from the assignment of borderline values for left ventricular wall thicknesses (or particularly enlarged cavity size), which require formulation of a differential diagnosis between normal but extreme physiologic adaptations of athlete's heart (69–72) and pathologic conditions such as hypertrophic cardiomyopathy or other cardiomyopathies (73). Indeed, such clinical dilemmas (which may not always be definitively resolvable in individual athletes) generate emotional, financial, and medical burdens for the athlete, family, team, and institution by virtue of the uncertainty created and the requirement for additional testing. False-negative screening results may occur when encountering athletes with hypertrophic cardiomyopathy at a point of incomplete phenotypic expression during adolescence (74). In athletes with hypertrophic cardiomyopathy who are younger than approximately 13 to 15 years old, left ventricular hypertrophy is often absent or mild, and therefore the echocardiographic findings may not yet be diagnostic at the time of preparticipation screening.

The 12-lead ECG has been proposed as a more practical and cost-efficient alternative to routine echocardiography for population-based screening (75–77). The ECG is abnormal in about 95% of patients with hypertrophic cardiomyopathy (78), and usually identifies the important (but uncommon) long QT syndrome (41–43). However, a certain proportion of genetically affected relatives in families with long QT syndrome may have little or no phenotypic expression on the ECG (41).

As a primary screening test, the ECG suffers in comparison to the echocardiogram by its lack of imaging capability for recognition of structural cardiovascular malformations.

Also, the ECG has relatively low specificity as a screening test in athletic populations because of the high frequency with which ECG alterations occur in association with the normal physiologic adaptations to training of the athlete's heart (79). Such false-positive test results substantially complicate efforts at using the 12-lead ECG as a primary screening tool in athletic populations. In the context of preparticipation screening, it can be anticipated that approximately 20% to 25% of athletes examined will have ECG patterns that ultimately stimulate echocardiographic study (77). Finally, elite athletes not infrequently demonstrate distinctly abnormal ECG patterns consistent with pathologic conditions (79), even in the absence of structural heart disease and without evidence of a morphologic adaptation to training. In older trained athletes, the routine application of exercise testing to detect coronary artery disease in large populations is limited by its low specificity and pretest probability (80).

To date, there have been relatively few published reports of cardiovascular screening efforts in large athletic populations (64,65,67, 68,77). Most of these studies have implemented noninvasive testing (i.e., conventional or limited echocardiographic examination or 12-lead ECG) in young high school or collegiate athletes. The populations subjected to screening ranged in size from 250 to 2,000 athletes, usually studied over a 1-year period. In general, these reports are consistent by virtue of describing the detection of very few definitive examples of potentially lethal cardiovascular disease.

PERSPECTIVES ON RACE AND GENDER

Hypertrophic cardiomyopathy is an important cause of sudden death in young black athletes and such catastrophes may even be more common in black athletes compared to their white counterparts (3,81). The substantial occurrence of hypertrophic cardiomyopathy-related sudden death in young black male athletes contrasts sharply with the very infrequent reporting of black patients with hypertrophic cardiomyopathy in hospital-based populations from tertiary centers (24–29). Therefore, in blacks, hypertrophic cardiomyopathy is most frequently encountered when it results in sudden and unexpected death during competitive athletics. These data emphasize the disproportionate access to subspecialty health care between the black and white communities in the United States that makes it less likely for young black male athletes to receive a relatively sophisticated cardiovascular diagnosis such as hypertrophic cardiomyopathy. Consequently, black athletes with hypertrophic cardiomyopathy are less likely to be identified or disqualified from competition, in accordance with the recommendations of 26th Bethesda Conference (23), to reduce their risk for sudden death.

Sudden death on the athletic field is uncommon in young women (3) (comprising about 10% of all such deaths), which may be explained on the basis of lower participation rates or less severe training demands and cardiac adaptation (72) in some instances, but also because hypertrophic cardiomyopathy is less commonly recognized clinically in women (24–26,28); this observation also suggests the possibility that a measure of protection from sudden death is attributable in some physiologic fashion to gender itself. Nevertheless, the available data do not provide a compelling justification to construct specific screening algorithms, based on gender, race, or demographic subgrouping.

AMERICAN HEART ASSOCIATION RECOMMENDATIONS FOR PREPARTICIPATION SCREENING

Advisability

The 1996 American Heart Association consensus panel recommendations state that some form of preparticipation cardiovascular screening for high school and college student-athletes is justifiable and compelling based on ethical, legal and medical grounds

(22). Noninvasive testing can enhance the diagnostic power of the standard history and physical examination; however, it is not prudent to recommend the routine use of tests such as 12-lead ECG, echocardiography, or graded exercise testing for the detection of cardiovascular disease in large populations of youthful or older athletes. This recommendation is based on both practical and cost-efficiency considerations, given the large number of competitive athletes in the United States, the relatively low frequency with which the cardiovascular lesions responsible for these deaths occur, and the low rate of sudden cardiac death in the athletic community. This viewpoint is not, however, intended to actively discourage all efforts at population screening that may be proposed by individual investigators. Nevertheless, there is concern that the widespread application of noninvasive testing to athletic populations could result in many false-positive results, creating unnecessary anxiety among substantial numbers of athletes and their families, as well as unjustified exclusion from competition. Indeed, in such a circumstance with a low incidence of disease in the community, a great likelihood exists that the number of false-positive results would exceed that of true positives (77).

Consequently, it appears that a complete and careful personal and family history and physical examination designed to identify (or raise suspicion of) those cardiovascular lesions known to cause sudden death or disease progression in young athletes is the best available and most practical approach to screening populations of competitive sports participants regardless of age. Such cardiovascular screening is an obtainable objective and should be mandatory for all athletes. It is recommended that both a history and physical examination be performed before the initial engagement in organized high school (grades 9 through 12) and collegiate sports, and that these be subsequently repeated every 2 years. In intervening years, an interim history should be obtained. Indeed, this recommendation is consistent with those procedures that are customary for most high school and college athletes in the United States.

However, official recommendations or requirements by athletic governing bodies regarding the nature and scope of preparticipation medical evaluations of athletes are not standardized among the states, nor can they necessarily be viewed as medically sufficient in many instances. Therefore, because of this heterogeneity in the design and content of preparticipation examinations, it is recommended that a systematic national standard for preparticipation medical evaluations be developed. Adherence to uniformly applicable guidelines would impact substantially on the health of student-athletes in a cost-effective manner by enhancing the safety of their athletic activities.

For athletes older than 35 years of age, despite the limitations of the history and physical examination in detecting coronary artery disease, a personal history of coronary risk factors or familial occurrence of premature ischemic heart disease may be useful for identification of that disease in a screening setting, and therefore should be performed before initiating competitive exercise. In addition, it is prudent to selectively perform medically supervised exercise stress testing in men older than age 40 years (women older than age 50 years) who wish to engage in habitual physical training and competitive sports if the examining physician suspects occult coronary artery disease on the basis of at least two risk factors (other than age and gender) or of one markedly abnormal finding. Older athletes should also be warned specifically about prodromal cardiovascular symptoms such a exertional chest pain.

The present guidelines should not promulgate a false sense of security on the part of medical practitioners or the general public, because the standard history and physical examination intrinsically lacks the power to reliably identify many potentially lethal cardiovascular abnormalities. Indeed, it is an unrealistic expectation that large-scale standard athletic screening examinations can reliably exclude most important cardiac lesions.

Methodology

Preparticipation sports examinations are presently performed by a variety of individuals, including paid or volunteer physicians or nonphysician health care workers with variable training and experience. Examiners may be associated with, or administratively independent of, the concerned institution, school, or team.

Consequently, athletic screening should be performed by an appropriately trained health care worker with the requisite training, medical skills, and background to reliably perform a detailed cardiovascular history and physical examination and to recognize heart disease. Even though it is preferable that such an individual be a licensed physician, this may not always be feasible, and it may be acceptable for an appropriately trained registered nurse or physician assistant to perform the screening examination. In those states in which nonphysician health care workers (including chiropractors) are permitted to perform preparticipation screening, it will be necessary to establish a formal certification process to demonstrate expertise in cardiovascular examinations.

Specifically, athletic screening evaluations should comprise a complete medical history and physical examination including brachial artery blood pressure measurement. This examination should be conducted in a physical environment conducive to optimal cardiac auscultation, whether performed individually in a private office or in a station-format as part of a school program. The evaluation should also emphasize certain elements critical to the detection of those cardiovascular diseases known to be associated with morbidity or sudden cardiac death in athletes.

The cardiovascular *history* should include key questions designed to determine (a) prior occurrence of exertional chest pain and discomfort or syncope (or near-syncope) as well as excessive, unexpected, and unexplained shortness of breath or fatigue associated with exercise; (b) past recognition of a heart murmur or increased systemic blood pressure;

and (c) family history of premature death (sudden or otherwise), morbidity from cardiovascular disease in close relatives younger than age 50 years, or the occurrence of certain conditions in family members (e.g., hypertrophic cardiomyopathy, dilated cardiomyopathy, long QT syndrome, Marfan syndrome, or clinically important arrhythmias). The accuracy of some responses elicited from young athletes may depend on their level of compliance and historical knowledge. Indeed, parents should be responsible for completing the history form of high school athletes.

The *physical examination* should emphasize (but not necessarily be limited to) (a) precordial auscultation in both the supine and standing positions to identify, in particular, those heart murmurs consistent with left ventricular outflow obstruction, (b) assessment of the femoral artery pulses to exclude coarctation of the aorta, (c) recognition of the physical stigmata of Marfan syndrome, and (d) brachial blood pressure measurement in the sitting position.

Eligibility Criteria

When a previously unsuspected cardiovascular abnormality is identified in a competitive athlete, whether by standard screening or other means, the following considerations arise: (a) the magnitude of risk for sudden cardiac death associated with continued participation in competitive sports and (b) the criteria to be implemented for determining whether that athlete would benefit from disqualification from athletics. In this regard, the 26th Bethesda Conference sponsored by the American College of Cardiology (23) offers prospective and consensus recommendations for athletic eligibility or disqualification, taking into account the severity of the cardiovascular abnormality as well as the nature of sports training and competition. The 26th Bethesda Conference recommendations are predicated on the likelihood that intense athletic training will increase the risk for sudden cardiac death (or disease progression) in trained athletes with clinically important

structural heart disease, although it is not possible to quantify that risk precisely for individual participants. Nevertheless, it is presumed that the temporary or permanent withdrawal of selected athletes from participation in certain sports is prudent and likely to diminish their perceived risk.

REFERENCES

1. Maron BJ. Sudden death in young athletes: lessons from the Hank Gathers affair. *N Engl J Med* 1993;329:55–57.
2. Burke AP, Farb V, Virmani R, Goodin J, Smialek JE. Sports-related and non–sports-related sudden cardiac death in young adults. *Am Heart J* 1991;121:568–575.
3. Maron BJ, Shirani J, Poliac LC, Mathenge R, Roberts WC, Mueller FO. Sudden death in young competitive athletes: clinical, demographic and pathological profiles. *JAMA* 1996;276:199–204.
4. van Camp SP, Bloor CM, Mueller FO, Cantu RC, Olson HG. Nontraumatic sports death in high school and college athletes. *Med Sci Sports Exerc* 1995;27:641–647.
5. Maron BJ, Roberts WC, McAllister HA, Rosing DR, Epstein SE. Sudden death in young athletes. *Circulation* 1980;62:218–229.
6. Corrado D, Thiene G, Nava A, Rossi L, Pennelli N. Sudden death in young competitive athletes: clinicopathologic correlations in 22 cases. *Am J Med* 1990;89:588–596.
7. Thiene G, Nava A, Corrado D, Rossi L, Penelli N. Right ventricular cardiomyopathy and sudden death in young people. *N Engl J Med* 1988;318:129–133.
8. Tsung SH, Huang TY, Chang HH. Sudden death in young athletes. *Arch Pathol Lab Med* 1982;106:168–170.
9. James TN, Froggatt P, Marshall TK. Sudden death in young athletes. *Ann Intern Med* 1967;67:1013–1021.
10. Furlanello F, Bettini R, Cozzi F, et al. Ventricular arrhythmias and sudden death in athletes. *Ann N Y Acad Sci* 1984;427:253–279.
11. Maron BJ, Epstein SE, Roberts WC. Causes of sudden death in competitive athletes. *J Am Coll Cardiol* 1986;7:204–214.
12. Drory Y, Turetz Y, Hiss Y, et al. Sudden unexpected death in persons < 40 years of age. *Am J Cardiol* 1991;68:1388–1392.
13. Topaz O, Edwards JE. Pathologic features of sudden death in children, adolescents and young adults. *Chest* 1985;87:476–482.
14. Liberthson RR. Sudden death from cardiac causes in children and young adults. *N Engl J Med* 1996;334:1039–1044.
15. McCaffrey FM, Braden DS, Strong WB. Sudden cardiac death in young athletes: a review. *Am J Dis Child* 1991;145:177–183.
16. Thompson PD, Stern MP, Williams P, Duncan K, Haskell WL, Wood PD. Death during jogging or running. A study of 18 cases. *JAMA* 1979;242:1265–1267.
17. Thompson PD, Funk EJ, Carleton RA, Sturner WQ. Incidence of death during jogging in Rhode Island from 1975 through 1980. *JAMA* 1982;247:2535–2538.
18. Waller BF, Roberts WC. Sudden death while running in

conditioned runners aged 40 years or over. *Am J Cardiol* 1980;45:1292–1300.

19. Virmani R, Robinowitz M, McAllister HA Jr. Nontraumatic death in joggers: a series of 30 patients at autopsy. *Am J Med* 1982;72:874–882.

20. Maron BJ, Mitchell JH. Revised eligibility recommendations for competitive athletes with cardiovascular abnormalities. [Introduction to Bethesda Conference #26]. *J Am Coll Cardiol* 1994;24:848–850.

21. Maron BJ, Garson A. Arrhythmias and sudden cardiac death in elite athletes [Zipes D, ed]. *Cardiol Rev* 1994; 2(1):26–32.

22. Maron BJ, Thompson PD, Puffer JC, et al. Cardiovascular preparticipation screening of competitive athletes. *Circulation* 1996;94:850–856.

23. Maron BJ, Mitchell JH. 26th Bethesda Conference. Recommendations for determining eligibility for competition in athletes with cardiovascular abnormalities. *J Am Coll Cardiol* 1994;24:845–899.

24. Wigle ED, Sasson Z, Henderson MA, et al. Hypertrophic cardiomyopathy. The importance of the site and extent of hypertrophy—a review. *Prog Cardiovasc Dis* 1985;28:1–83.

25. Maron BJ, Bonow RO, Cannon RO, Leon MB, Epstein SE. Hypertrophic cardiomyopathy: interrelation of clinical manifestations, pathophysiology, and therapy. *N Engl J Med* 1987;316:780–789 and 844–852.

26. Louie EK, Edwards LC. Hypertrophic cardiomyopathy. *Prog Cardiovasc Dis* 1994;36:275–308.

27. Spirito P, Seidman CE, McKenna WJ, Maron BJ. The management of hypertrophic cardiomyopathy. *N Engl J Med* 1997;336:775–785.

28. Klues HG, Schiffers A, Maron BJ. Phenotypic spectrum and patterns of left ventricular hypertrophy in hypertrophic cardiomyopathy: morphologic observations and significance as assessed by two-dimensional echocardiography in 600 patients. *J Am Coll Cardiol* 1995;26: 1699–1708.

29. Maron BJ, Klues HG. Surviving competitive athletics with hypertrophic cardiomyopathy. *Am J Cardiol* 1994; 73:1098–1104.

30. Geisterfer-Lowrance AAT, Kass S, Tanigawa G, et al. A molecular basis for familial hypertrophic cardiomyopathy: a β-cardiac myosin heavy chain gene missense mutation. *Cell* 1990;62:999–1006.

31. Thierfelder L, Watkins H, MacRae C, et al. α-Tropomyosin and cardiac troponin T mutations cause familial hypertrophic cardiomyopathy: a disease of the sarcomere. *Cell* 1994;77:701–712.

32. Watkins H, Conner D, Thierfelder L, et al. Mutations in the cardiac myosin binding protein-C gene on chromosome 11 cause familial hypertrophic cardiomyopathy. *Nat Genet* 1995;11:434–437.

33. Schwartz K, Carrier L, Guicheney P, Komajda M. Molecular basis of familial cardiomyopathies. *Circulation* 1995;91:532–540.

34. Marian AJ, Roberts R. Recent advances in the molecular genetics of hypertrophic cardiomyopathy. *Circulation* 1995;91:532–540.

35. Maron BJ, Gardin JM, Flack JM, Gidding SS, Bild D. Assessment of the prevalence of hypertrophic cardiomyopathy in a general population of young adults: echocardiographic analysis of 4111 subjects in the CARDIA Study. *Circulation* 1995;92:785–789.

36. Roberts WC. Congenital coronary arterial anomalies unassociated with major anomalies of the heart or great vessels. In: *Adult congenital heart disease.* Philadelphia: FA Davis Co, 1987:583.

37. Cheitlin MD, De Castro CM, McAllister HA. Sudden death as a complication of anomalous left coronary origin from the anterior sinus of Valsalva. A not-so-minor congenital anomaly. *Circulation* 1974;50:780–787.

38. Gaither NS, Rogan KM, Stajduhar K, et al. Anomalous origin and course of coronary arteries in adults: identification and improved imaging utilizing transesophageal echocardiography. *Am Heart J* 1991;122: 69–75.

39. Maron BJ, Leon BJ, Swain JA, Cannon RO III, Pelliccia A. Prospective identification by two-dimensional echocardiography of anomalous origin of the left main coronary artery from the right sinus of Valsalva. *Am J Cardiol* 1991;68:140–142.

40. Jureidini SB, Eaton C, Williams J, Nouri S, Appleton RS. Transthoracic two-dimensional and color flow echocardiographic diagnosis of aberrant left coronary artery. *Am Heart J* 1994;127:438–440.

41. Vincent GM, Timothy KW, Leppert M, Keating M. The spectrum of symptoms and QT intervals in carriers of the gene for the long-QT syndrome. *N Engl J Med* 1992;327:846–852.

42. Moss AJ, Schwartz PJ, Crampton RS, et al. The long QT syndrome: prospective longitudinal study of 328 families. *Circulation* 1991;84:1136–1144.

43. Roden DM, Lazzara R, Rosen M, Schwartz PJ, Towbin J, Vincent GM. Multiple mechanisms in the long-QT syndrome: current knowledge, gaps, and future directions. *Circulation* 1996;94:1996–2012.

44. McKenna WJ, Thiene G, Nava A, et al. On behalf of the Task Force of the Working Group Myocardial and Pericardial Disease of the European Society of Cardiology and of the Scientific Council on Cardiomyopathies of the International Society and Federation of Cardiology: diagnosis of arrhythmogenic right ventricular dysplasia/cardiomyopathy. *Br Heart J* 1994;71: 215–218.

45. Bharti S, Lev M. Congenital abnormalities of the conduction system in sudden death in young adults. *J Am Coll Cardiol* 1986;8:1096–1104.

46. Thiene G, Pennelli N, Rossi L. Cardiac conduction system abnormalities as a possible cause of sudden death in young athletes. *Human Pathol* 1983;14:706–709.

47. Benson DW, Benditt DG, Anderson RW, et al. Cardiac arrest in young, ostensibly healthy patients: clinical, hemodynamic and electrophysiologic findings. *Am J Cardiol* 1983;52:65–69.

48. Maron BJ, Poliac JC, Roberts WO. Risk for sudden cardiac death associated with marathon running. *J Am Coll Cardiol* 1996;28:428–431.

49. Noakes TD, Opie LH, Rose AG, Kleynhans PHT. Autopsy-proved coronary atherosclerosis in marathon runners. *N Engl J Med* 1979;301:86–89.

50. Northcote RJ, Evans ADB, Ballantyne D. Sudden death in squash players. *Lancet* 1984;21:148–151.

51. Kark JA, Posey DM, Schumacher HR, Ruehle CJ. Sickle-cell as a risk factor for sudden death in physical training. *N Engl J Med* 1987;317:781–787.

52. Maron BJ, Poliac L, Kaplan JA, Mueller FO. Blunt impact to the chest leading to sudden death from cardiac arrest during sports activities. *N Engl J Med* 1995;333: 337–342.

53. Virmani R, Robinowitz M, Smialek JE, Smyth DF. Cardiovascular effects of cocaine. An autopsy study of 40 patients. *Am Heart J* 1988;115:1068–1076.

54. Isner JM, Estes NAM III, Thompson PD, et al. Acute cardiac events temporally related to cocaine abuse. *N Engl J Med* 1986;315:1438–1443.

55. Kloner RA, Hale S, Alkekr K, Rezkalla S. The effects of acute and chronic cocaine use on the heart. *Circulation* 1992;85:407–419.

56. Kaplan NM, Deveraux RB, Miller HS Jr. Systemic hypertension. Task Force 4. In: Maron BJ, Mitchell JH, eds. Recommendations for determining eligibility for competition in athletes with cardiovascular abnormalities. *J Am Coll Cardiol* 1994;24:885–888.

57. Maron BJ, Stead D, Gohman TE, Aeppli D. Prevalence of sudden cardiac death during competitive sports activities in Minnesota high school athletes. *J Am Coll Cardiol* 1996;94:I–388(abst).

58. Pelliccia A, Maron BJ. Preparticipation cardiovascular evaluation of the competitive athlete: perspectives from the 30 year Italian experience. *Am J Cardiol* 1995;75:827–831.

59. Maron BJ, Brown RW, McGrew CA, Mitten MJ Jr, Caplan AL, Hutter AM Jr. Ethical, legal and practical considerations affecting medical decision-making in competitive athletes. In: Maron BJ, Mitchell JH, eds. Recommendations for determining eligibility for competition in athletes with cardiovascular abnormalities. 26th Bethesda Conference. *J Am Coll Cardiol* 1994;24:854–860.

60. Mitten MJ. Team physicians and competitive athletes. Allocating legal responsibility for athletic injuries. *U Pitt L Rev* 1993;55:129–169.

61. Knapp v. Northwestern University, 101 F.3d 473 (7th Circuit 1996).

62. Maron BJ, Epstein SE. Hypertrophic cardiomyopathy: a discussion of nomenclature. *Am J Cardiol* 1979;43:1242–1244.

63. Ricci C, Longo R, Pagnan L, et al. Magnetic resonance imaging in right ventricular dysplasia. *Am J Cardiol* 1992;70:1589–1595.

64. Weidenbener EJ, Krauss MD, Waller BF, Taliercio CP. Incorporation of screening echocardiography in the preparticipation exam. *Clin J Sport Med* 1995;5:86–89.

65. Feinstein RA, Colvin E, Oh MK. Echocardiographic screening as part of a preparticipation examination. *Clin J Sport Med* 1993;3:149–152.

66. Risser WL, Hoffman HM, Gordon BG Jr, Green LW. A cost-benefit analysis of preparticipation sports examination of adolescent athletes. *J School Health* 1985;55:270–273.

67. Murry PM, Cantwell JD, Heith DL, Shoop J. The role of limited echocardiography in screening athletes. *Am J Cardiol* 1995;76:849–850.

68. Lewis JF, Maron BJ, Diggs JA, Spencer JE, Mehrotra PP, Curry CL. Preparticipation echocardiographic screening for cardiovascular disease in a large, predominantly black population of collegiate athletes. *Am J Cardiol* 1989;64:1029–1033.

69. Huston TP, Puffer JC, Rodney McW. The athlete heart syndrome. *N Engl J Med* 1985;4:24–32.

70. Maron BJ. Structural features of the athlete heart as defined by echocardiography. *J Am Coll Cardiol* 1986;7:190–203.

71. Pelliccia A, Maron BJ, Spataro A, Proschan MA, Spirito P. The upper limit of physiologic cardiac hypertrophy in highly trained elite athletes. *N Engl J Med* 1991;324:295–301.

72. Pelliccia A, Maron BJ, Culasso F, Spataro A, Caselli G. Athlete's heart in women: echocardiographic characterization of highly trained elite female athletes. *JAMA* 1996;276:211–215.

73. Maron BJ, Pelliccia A, Spirito P. Cardiac disease in young trained athletes. Insights into methods for distinguishing athlete's heart from structural heart disease with particular emphasis on hypertrophic cardiomyopathy. *Circulation* 1995;91:1596–1601.

74. Maron BJ, Spirito P, Wesley YE, Arce J. Development and progression of left ventricular hypertrophy in children with hypertrophic cardiomyopathy. *N Engl J Med* 1986;315:610–614.

75. Zehender M, Meinertz T, Keul J, Just H. ECG variants and cardiac arrhythmias in athletes: clinical relevance and prognostic importance. *Am Heart J* 1990;119:1378–1391.

76. LaCorte MA, Boxer RA, Gottesfeld IB, Singh S, Strong M, Mandell L. EKG screening program for school athletes. *Clin Cardiol* 1989;12:41–44.

77. Maron BJ, Bodison SA, Wesley YE, Tucker E, Green KJ. Results of screening a large group of intercollegiate competitive athletes for cardiovascular disease. *J Am Coll Cardiol* 1987;10:1214–1221.

78. Maron BJ, Wolfson JK, Ciró E, Spirito P. Relation of electrocardiographic abnormalities and patterns of left ventricular hypertrophy identified by two-dimensional echocardiography in patients with hypertrophic cardiomyopathy. *Am J Cardiol* 1983;51:189–194.

79. Pelliccia A, Cullasso F, Di Paolo FM, et al. Clinical significance of abnormal electrocardiographic patterns in elite athletes: the impact of gender and cardiac morphologic adaptations to training. *Circulation* 1996;94:I–326(abst).

80. Diamond GA, Forrester JS. Analysis of probability as an aid in the clinical diagnosis of coronary artery disease. *N Engl J Med* 1979;300:1350–1358.

81. Maron BJ, Poliac LC, Mathenge R. Hypertrophic cardiomyopathy as an important cause of sudden cardiac death on the athletic field in African-American athletes. *J Am Coll Cardiol* 1997;29(Suppl A):462A(abst).

The Athlete and Heart Disease:
Diagnosis, Evaluation & Management,
edited by R. A. Williams.
Lippincott Williams & Wilkins, Philadelphia © 1999.

17

Race and Gender Considerations in Sudden Death in the Athlete

Richard Allen Williams

Department of Medicine, UCLA School of Medicine, Los Angeles, California 90024;
Minority Health Institute, Inc., Beverly Hills, California 90211

Are the race and the sex of the competitive athlete important factors to consider in looking at sudden cardiac death (SCD)? Are there significant differences in incidence of SCD between black and white athletes? Why is there such a great disparity between male and female athletes in the occurrence of this phenomenon? Is there enough evidence to establish black race and male sex as risk factors for SCD in competitive athletes?

These questions and others regarding race and gender are addressed in this chapter. It is important to attempt to find answers to these questions in order to provide direction for future initiatives and to give some guidance and perspective to the clinician who examines an athlete either during a preparticipation physical or after an acute event has occurred. Toward these ends, information obtained from a comprehensive literature review is analyzed, as are accounts gathered from newspaper reports, investigations conducted by myself, and reports from the Armed Forces Institute of Pathology and the National Center for Catastrophic Sports Injury Research (NCCSIR). The focus in this chapter is on SCD in the athlete younger than 30 years of age who participates in organized sports at the high school, college, and professional levels.

BACKGROUND OF SUDDEN CARDIAC DEATH IN BLACKS

It is well recognized that there is a different disease profile in blacks than in whites (1) and that the race of a patient must be taken into account when the clinician attempts to evaluate and treat various medical conditions. It is known, for instance, that certain diseases tend to predominate in blacks whereas others are more commonly found in whites. Cardiovascular conditions seen more frequently in blacks and resulting in sudden death include left ventricular hypertrophy (2), sarcoidosis (3), and coronary disease (4–8). Left ventricular hypertrophy is found primarily in association with hypertension and has been determined to be a risk factor for SCD (9,10). This must be distinguished from a condition described by Topol (11), which he terms hypertensive hypertrophic cardiomyopathy; the latter is seen principally in elderly black females and may involve sudden death. SCD is the most common form of death in patients with cardiac sarcoidosis, about two-thirds of whom are black (12). Coronary artery disease presents an interesting situation in which the prevalence of the condition is greater in whites but the incidence of SCD is higher in blacks (13). For instance, in a 1984 study involving 2,275 subjects in Charleston, SC, Keil and associates (14) found that the rate of SCD in black male subjects was three times higher than in white male subjects. Other studies that have demonstrated what appears to be a paradox include the 1971 Hagstrom study (15) in Nashville, TN, and the Oalmann investigation (16) in New Orleans (1971); the latter report showed a fivefold higher rate of SCD in black as opposed to white male subjects in the 30- to 44-year age category, and there was a 47% higher rate in black as opposed to white male subjects in those who were 45 to 64 years of age, despite a higher proportion of deaths being assigned to coronary heart disease.

Another entity that deserves consideration but is not thought of as a cardiac condition is sickle cell trait. There are several studies (17–22) of death during exertion of individuals with sickle cell trait, and isolated instances of sudden death in athletes with this disorder have been reported. It is thought that the mechanism of death in cases related to heavy physical effort such as in the athletes and in military recruits involves dehydration and low oxygen tension, leading to sickling of erythrocytes, as well as to exertional rhabdomyolysis. One report contained seven cases of the latter condition found in nontraumatic sports deaths; all seven individuals were African Americans with sickle cell trait (23). This disorder, therefore, must be considered when the risk for death among athletes is discussed, particularly in regard to black athletes. However, there must be thousands of individuals with sickle cell trait who participate in competitive sports who never have become ill from this disorder, and it seems wise not to create special screening or precautionary measures for athletes who may have sickle cell trait.

SUDDEN CARDIAC DEATH IN BLACK ATHLETES

SCD in black athletes is an area that has not been well investigated because SCD has not been regarded as having an inordinate or different representation in the African American population, although, as discussed previously,

several studies indicate a higher incidence of SCD in blacks. No demographic evidence exists that blacks in general have a higher prevalence of conditions that have been found to predispose to SCD in young athletes, such as hypertrophic cardiomyopathy (HCM) and coronary artery anomalies. Additionally, there is no indication that a genetic predilection exists in blacks for these conditions. However, information is beginning to evolve that strongly suggests that black athletes do indeed suffer a disproportionate amount of the SCD that occurs in competitive sports. It has been shown that about 30% to 40% of athletes succumbing to SCD are African American, and 36% to 48% of the deaths in black athletes are associated with HCM. These are staggering statistics that strongly suggest that black athletes are experiencing a disproportionate amount of SCD, especially caused by HCM, given that blacks constitute only 12% of the U.S. population but suffer about three times as many athletic SCDs.

Case Reports of SCD in Black Athletes

Media reports of SCD episodes provided an early suggestion that black athletes were dying in a disproportionate manner. Between 1975 and 1990, I noted the appearance of a string of SCD reports in small black newspapers in the Los Angeles area, and I collected, reviewed, and analyzed clinical and autopsy data on 24 black athletes (24) who had died under various circumstances; other cases were added to the list later to a total of 30 (Table 1). The distribution of deaths showed 15 basketball fatalities, 11 football deaths, three in track athletes, and one in volleyball. Most of the autopsies showed the presence of HCM; other diseases represented were coronary artery anomalies, Marfan syndrome with aortic rupture, and idiopathic concentric left ventricular hypertrophy. All except two were male, the age range was 13 to 31 years (average age 17 years), and all died either during vigorous physical activity or immediately thereafter. Toxicologic studies were performed in all cases and showed no evidence of illicit or performance-enhancing drugs. An example of the cases

TABLE 1. *Media-reported deaths of young black athletes*

Name of Athlete	Age	Year	Sport
Edward D. Bell	16	1975	Football
George W. Stewart	20	1975	Football
Stanley Neal	16	1979	Football
Isam Maynard		1979	Football
James Barber	16	1979	Football
Jim O'Brien	17	1979	Football
J. V. Cain	28	1979	Football
Hayward Harris		1980	Football
Greg Pratt	20	1983	Football
Paul Cunningham		1983	Football
Kevin Copeland	17	1989	Football
Ellis Files	19	1974	Basketball
Owen Brown	22	1976	Basketball
Eddie Brooks	13	1976	Basketball
Antonio Britt		1981	Basketball
Leon Richardson		1981	Basketball
Arturo Brown		1982	Basketball
Hank Gathers	23	1990	Basketball
Tony Penny	23	1990	Basketball
Weston Hatch	17	1990	Basketball
Ron Copeland	28	1975	Track
Freeman Miller	21	1980	Track

cited is that of Ron Copeland, Sr., who had competed in organized sports at high school, college, and professional levels. He had been a track and football standout at UCLA who was the NCAA champion in the 120-yard high hurdles in 1966 and subsequently played with the Chicago Bears as a split end in 1969. However, he was unable to continue his sports career because of hypertension. He subsequently became a physical education instructor at a junior college, and while running wind sprints with his track students, he suddenly collapsed and died in 1975 at the age of 28. (Coincidentally, Ron's father, Harold Copeland, had died just a week earlier of heart disease.) Autopsy revealed a huge heart, weighing 630 g, which demonstrated hypertrophy of the lower third of the intraventricular septum. Microscopic analysis showed severe, diffuse myocardial fibrosis. Fourteen years later, Ron's 17-year-old son, Kevin, a stand-out high school football star in Los Angeles, collapsed and died during a football game in which he was participating, on October 6, 1989. Postmortem examination revealed HCM, despite the fact that he had been asymptomatic and had no physical stigmata of HCM. His two brothers, Ron, Jr., 21, and Kyle, 16, both outstanding athletes who wanted to continue competing, also showed no signs of the disease when I had the opportunity to examine them in 1990. Their echocardiograms and other noninvasive parameters were normal. On the urging of their mother, backed by my advice, they decided to retire from competitive sports. They were further advised to continue receiving regular medical attention from cardiologists.

Two other cases of SCD involving prominent African American athletes were the deaths of Hank Gathers and Reggie Lewis, who were both outstanding basketball players. Gathers, 23 years old, was the starting power forward on the Loyola Marymount University basketball team in the Los Angeles area. Standing 6 feet 7 inches and weighing 220 pounds, he seemed completely healthy, and in his junior year in 1988, he had led the nation in both scoring and rebounding, only the second person ever to accomplish this difficult double. It appeared that he was headed for a successful career in the National Basketball Association. However, on December 9, 1989, while standing at the foul line shooting a free throw, he noticed that his heart was racing; this was a sensation that he had experienced previously. He later admitted to feeling tired and disoriented while standing at the line. He missed the first shot and then, without warning, he collapsed and fell to the floor. He was down for only a few seconds, then jumped back up. After receiving emergency treatment, he was taken to a local hospital and underwent a battery of heart tests over the next 2 days. It was determined that he had a cardiac arrhythmia, allegedly ventricular tachycardia, and he then underwent electrophysiologic testing, after which he was told that he had an irregular heartbeat; treatment was begun with propranolol, 80 mg three times a day, and he was told not to play basketball. However, on the day after Christmas 1989, 17 days after his syncopal episode, he returned to practice wearing a Holter monitor, apparently with a letter from his doctors allegedly granting him permission to play. He returned to the starting lineup 4 days later while remaining under medical attention and as cardiac testing continued.

Sometime after January 4, 1990, his antiarrhythmic medication was reduced under unclear circumstances. His level of play improved, and he became a major factor again in his team's performance. Two months later, on March 4, after playing vigorously in a game against Portland State, he suddenly collapsed and generalized seizures ensued (Fig. 1). Resuscitation attempts were unsuccessful; Hank Eric Gathers, who had called himself the strongest man in America, was pronounced dead 2 hours later, and 3 months and 5 days after his initial syncopal attack. Postmortem examination revealed the presence of cardiomyopathy with areas of patchy fibrosis; toxicologic tests found no illegal or performance-enhancing drugs.

The case of Reggie Lewis was equally tragic, and was perhaps even more complex than that of Hank Gathers. It was the first truly high-profile episode of SCD involving a superstar in professional sports. Lewis, who was co-captain of the Boston Celtics basketball team, had had a history of dizzy spells before his first syncopal attack during a playoff game on April 12, 1993 (Fig. 2). Following this attack, he was

admitted to New England Baptist Hospital in Boston where he underwent a battery of cardiac tests. Although his coronary arteries were found to be normal, a large apical defect was noted, and a group of 14 expert cardiologists, led by Mark Josephson and dubbed the "dream team," consulted on the problem but allegedly never saw the patient. Based on the results of the cardiac tests and the clinical history, they concluded that Lewis was in imminent danger of SCD, especially in view of the runs of nonsustained ventricular tachycardia, which were noted during his workup. They recommended that he stop playing basketball entirely and advised the implantation of an automatic implantable cardiac defibrillator (AICD). However, a decision was made to seek another opinion, and to do so in a surreptitious manner. It is unclear who made the call for the next move—was it the Celtics management, who stood to lose a superstar player, his family, which was in anguish, or other doctors who disagreed with the diagnosis and severe recommendations? In any event, Lewis was secretly moved by private ambulance late at night from New England Baptist Hospital to Peter Bent Brigham Hospital, also in Boston, where a new workup was initiated under Gilbert Mudge and his associates. After achieving a positive result on a tilt test, which was interpreted as indicative of vasodepressor syncope, he was given this new diagnosis, which was announced at a press conference. Lewis was told that he should not play competitively at that time and that his progress would be monitored while he underwent treatment with a betablocker medication. Apparently his family was comforted enough to think that Lewis might be able to play basketball again, but Lewis was still uncertain and he sought a third opinion from cardiologists at UCLA headed by William Stevenson, an electrophysiologist. After his visit to UCLA, however, he was still uncertain as to what course to take. He returned to Boston and while shooting baskets at Brandeis University in nearby Waltham, he had a cardiac arrest on July 27, 1993, and could not be revived. Postmortem examination showed areas of patchy fibrosis in the heart. Toxico-

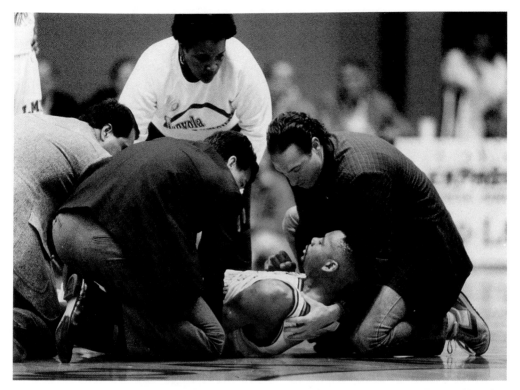

FIG. 1. Hank Gathers being attended to during his final, fatal syncopal episode resulting from ventricular fibrillation. Cardiopulmonary resuscitation attempts were unsuccessful. Los Angeles, March 5, 1990. (From *The Los Angeles Times*, Los Angeles, CA, 1990, by permission.)

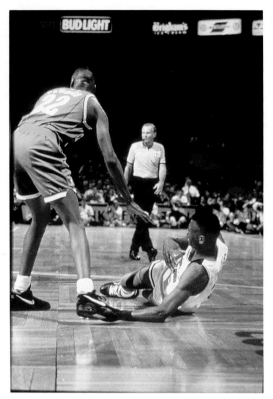

FIG. 2. Boston Celtics star Reggie Lewis collapses during a basketball game. He was admitted to a hospital and underwent cardiac tests soon thereafter. He died about 3 months later after collapsing again. (From *Sports Illustrated*, by permission.)

logic studies showed no abnormal substances. The family has filed a lawsuit against several parties, which is still pending.

The cases detailed herein are representative of SCD occurring on the high school, college, and professional levels of athletic competition. Moreover, all of the individuals were black males who showed no signs of heart disease at the beginning of their athletic careers. They serve to illustrate, through their case histories, the unusual risk that characterizes the black athlete.

Studies of Sudden Cardiac Death in Black Athletes

In 1980, Maron et al. (25) published a report on sudden death in young athletes, citing HCM as the most common cause. In that retrospective study, approximately 30% of the decedents were African American, but no speculation was entertained about the apparent disproportionate representation of blacks in this group. In 1988, the first article in the medical literature to suggest that there may be a special problem in blacks related to SCD and HCM appeared as a three-part special report by Lubell (26). Hypertensive left ventricular hypertrophy was also cited as a cause of SCD in blacks who engage in vigorous exercise. A following report in 1990 in the same journal, *The Physician and Sportsmedicine,* by Thomas and Cantwell (27), contained a series of case reports on SCD occurring in basketball players. Of the four subjects described, three were

black male athletes. Two had HCM and the third died of an ischemia-related arrhythmia caused by an anomalous coronary artery. The one white athlete died of arrhythmias associated with severe aortic stenosis and moderately advanced coronary atherosclerosis. The next study of sports-related SCD was performed as a retrospective analysis of 34 young athletes (mean age 24 years) by Burke et al. (28) in 1991. In this group in which individuals were matched for age, sex, and race with a non–sports-related cohort, African Americans had a greater likelihood of dying from HCM than did whites. In the eight cases of HCM, six athletes were black and two were white (Table 2).

Overall, of the 34 exercise-related SCDs, 15 were in blacks and 19 were in whites; three individuals were female, only one of whom, a swimmer, had HCM. In this study, the blacks whose deaths were exercise-related were younger than the whites (mean ages 23.5 years versus 27.2 years, respectively), and the incidence of HCM was higher in the exercising blacks, although the incidence of HCM in those blacks and whites whose deaths were non–sports-related was similar. This information regarding the differences in SCD between blacks and whites with HCM is important; inasmuch as approximately one-half of the cases of SCD in athletes younger than age 30 years that are due to HCM should be genetically influenced in an autosomal dominant manner, equal racial distribution of deaths would be expected. Such a result occurred in the sedentary individuals in this

TABLE 2. *Exercise-related deaths: distribution of race/sports*

Cause of Death (n)	Black	White	Sport
Severe atherosclerosis (9)	1	9	Running (5) Other (4)
Hypertrophic cardiomyopthy (8)	6	2	Basketball (7) Swimming (1)
Anomalous coronary arteries (4)	2	2	Basketball (2) Basketball (1) Soccer (1)
Others (13)	6	7	Basketball (5) Running (4) Other (4)

From ref. 28, with permission.

TABLE 3. *Characteristics of 136 high school and college athletes experiencing nontraumatic sports death, July 1983–June 1993*

Characteristic	Total	Male	Female
Number of Athletes	136	124	12
Race, number (%)			
Caucasian	78 (57.4%)	69 (55.6%)	9 (75%)
African American	52 (38%)	49 (39.5%)	3 (25%)
Hispanic	3 (2.2%)	3 (2.4%)	0
Asian	1 (0.7%)	1 (0.8%)	0
Puerto Rican	1 (0.7%)	1 (0.8%)	0
Native American	1 (0.7%)	1 (0.8%)	0
Activity at time of collapse-no. (%)			
Practice	83 (61%)		
Competition	53 (39%)		

From ref. 30, with permission.

study, but as was observed, the racial distribution was skewed in the exercising group, which showed more blacks dying of HCM. Does vigorous exercise serve more as a trigger for SCD in blacks with HCM than in whites? Although the numbers of cases in this study are small, the data pose this intriguing question and indicate an area that merits future investigation.

Another study, on sudden death in young competitive athletes by Maron et al. (29) in 1996 indicated a higher prevalence of HCM in African Americans than in whites. In an analysis of clinical, demographic, and pathologic profiles involving a total of 134 sudden deaths resulting from cardiovascular causes, HCM, the most common cause of SCD, was found to predominate in blacks (48%) over whites (26%). Furthermore, of the 14 individuals with possible HCM (hearts with some morphologic features consistent with but not diagnostic of HCM), the 17 persons with anomalous origin of the coronary arteries, and the six athletes with ruptured aortic aneurysm, most of the decedents were black. No deaths were reported in blacks from aortic valve stenosis or arrhythmogenic right ventricular dysplasia (ARVD). This study may be considered pivotal for two reasons: First, it is the first one involving a sizable number of cases to show a grossly disproportionate incidence of SCD in black athletes compared to whites, and second, it suggests that the three principal causes of SCD in young athletes (HCM,

anomalous coronary arteries, and aortic rupture) occur more commonly in blacks.

Mueller et al. (30) have conducted a similar investigation of 160 nontraumatic deaths in high school and college athletes based on data collected by the National Center for Catastrophic Sports Injury Research (NCCSIR). These data showed that, of 136 athletes whose cause of death could be determined, 78 (57.4%) were white and 53 (38%) were black. The racial breakdown for those with HCM roughly paralleled these figures: of 56 athletes with HCM, 33 (59%) were white and 20 (36%) were black (Table 3). Although the disparity between the two racial groups regarding HCM and SCD is not as great as in the Maron study, there is still a disproportionate representation of black individuals.

SUDDEN CARDIAC DEATH IN FEMALE ATHLETES

As stated previously, HCM should be equally distributed among male and female subjects. In the subpopulation of athletes younger than age 30 years dying of this disorder, male athletes have been found to predominate in overwhelming numbers in all studies conducted thus far in which the genders of the individuals analyzed have been reported. As an example, the study by Burke examined 34 individuals; only three (9%) were women, and only one of these had HCM (Table 4). In the 1995 report by Van Camp et al. (23) in which

TABLE 4. *Causes Of death, sports-versus non–sports-related*

	Sports-Related		Non–sports-Related	
n	34	(5%)	656	(95%)
Age (yr, mean)	26		32	
Sex				
Male	31	(91%)	501	(76%)
Female	3	(9%)	155	(24%)
Race				
White	19	(56%)	368	(56%)
Black	15	(44%)	281	(43%)
Asian			7	(1%)
Cause of death	*n*	Percent	*n*	Percent
Severe atherosclerosis (CHD)	9	26	307	47†
Hypertrophic cardiomyopathy	8	24*	20	3.0
Idipathic LV hypertrophy	3	9	42	6.4
Unknown (tunnel)	6 (2)	18	104 (7)	16
Anomalous coronary artery	4	12	8	1.2
Myocarditis	2	6	31	4.5
Right ventricular dysplasia	1	3	0	0
SH with LV hypertrophy	0	0	31	4.7
Aortic dissection	0	0	17	2.6
Cardiac sarcoidosis	0	0	13	2.0
Aortic stenosis	0	0	12	1.8
Floppy mitral valve	0	0	11	1.7
Other	1	3	60	9.1

*Statistically significant increase over total and age- and sex-matched control whites.

†Statistically significant increase over total blacks, but not with age- and sex-matched controls. Other differences were not statistically significant.

CDH, coronary heart disease; LV, left ventricular; SH, systemic hypertension.

From ref. 28, with permission.

160 nontraumatic deaths in college and high school athletes occurring between 1983 and 1993 were analyzed, there were 146 male athletes (90%) and 14 female athletes (10%). The authors also derived an estimated death rate for male and female athletes involved in nontraumatic sports fatalities and determined that the death rate for high school and college male athletes was 7.47 per million athletes per year versus 1.44 for female athletes—a more than fivefold higher rate of nontraumatic sports deaths for male athletes ($p<0.0001$). Football was the principal sport involved in the male deaths (67 cases) followed by basketball (37), track (ten), and wrestling (nine) (Table 5). For female sports, basketball was the main sport (five cases) followed by swimming (three) (Table 6).

Cardiovascular causes of death were determined for 100 of the 160 individuals; HCM was the most frequently found cause (51 cases, 51%) (Table 7). Of those with HCM,

50 were male (98%) and only one was female (2%). Five additional cases, all male athletes, were classified as probable HCM because they did not meet the strict criteria for this disorder. In the study by Maron (29) on 134 young competitive athletes with SCD, there were 14 female subjects (10%); only two had HCM. In the 24 aforementioned cases, which were collected and analyzed by myself, only two were female subjects (10%).

These data concerning the frequency of SCD in women indicate that the death rate for female athletes is about 10% of all cases, and the incidence of HCM in those who die during competitive sports is 2% to 5%. This shows a vast difference between the sexes in the outcomes of vigorous physical activity.

There has been speculation that perhaps female athletes are somehow protected from SCD during intense physical exertion. Pelliccia et al. (31) have shown that elite female

TABLE 5. *Nontraumatic sports deaths in male high school and college athletes, July 1983–June 1993*

		Total Deaths	Estimated Athletes Participating*	Estimated Death Rates per Million Athletes per Year
Fall Sports				
Cross country	High school	3	1,552,413	1.93
	College	1	138,873	7.2
Field hockey	High school	0	290	0
	College	0	0	0
Football	High school	53	9,449,220	5.61
	College	14	690,219	20.28
Soccer	High school	6	2,108,958	2.85
	College	1	246,085	40.6
Water polo	High school	0	92,055	0
	College	1	16,175	61.82
Winter Sports				
Basketball	High school	28	5,112,448	5.48
	College	9	259,364	34.7
Gymnastics	High school	0	50,286	0
	College	0	8,007	0
Ice hockey	High school	1	229,655	4.35
	College	1	43,823	22.82
Swimming	High school	0	832,919	0
	College	1	98,797	10.2
Volleyball	High school	0	140,384	0
	College	0	9,747	0
Wrestling	High school	9	2,397,129	3.75
	College	0	102,388	0
Spring Sports				
Baseball	High school	5	4,107,505	1.22
	College	2	389,339	5.14
Golf	High school	0	1,196,635	0
	College	0	112,722	0
Lacrosse	High school	0	180,393	0
	College	1	54,478	18.36
Tennis	High school	1	1,336,764	0.75
	College	0	123,737	0
Track	High school	9	4,296,343	2.09
	College	1	272,263	3.67
Total	High school	115	33,083,397	1.9[†]
			17,412,314	6.60
	College	31	2,566,017	1.2[†]
			2,138,348	14.50
	High school and college	146	19,550,662	7.47

*Athletes counted once for every year of participation and for each sport in which they participated.

[†]Estimation of the total number of athletes participating in high school and college sports requires division by estimated number of participated in by athletes per year (1.9 for high school athletes and 1.2 for college athletes). This estimate is then used to calculate the estimated death rates for the high school, college, and combined high school and college groups.

From ref. 23, with permission.

athletes do not demonstrate significant increases of left ventricular wall thickness, which was found to be within normal limits in their echocardiographic study of 600 highly trained Italian female athletes who were preparing for the Olympic games between 1986 and 1993. In addition, when the measurement for left ventricular cavity dimension and wall thickness in these athletes was compared to those for 738 male athletes, the cavity size and thickness were significantly less in the women than in the men (11% less for

TABLE 6. *Nontraumatic sports deaths in female high school and college athletes, July 1983–June 1993*

		Total Deaths	Estimated Athletes Participating*	Estimated Death Rates per Million Athletes per Year
Fall Sports				
Cross country	High school	1	1,023,646	0.98
	College	0	105,953	0
Field hockey	High school	0	491,274	0
	College	0	51,991	0
Football	High school	0	844	0
	College	0	0	0
Soccer	High school	1	1,052,873	0.95
	College	1	84,530	11.83
Water polo	High school	0	9,006	0
	College	0	0	0
Winter Sports				
Basketball	High school	4	3,907,849	1.02
	College	1	213,010	4.69
Gymnastics	High school	0	288,506	0
	College	0	17,043	0
Ice hockey	High school	0	698	0
	College	0	0	0
Swimming	High school	3	852,480	3.52
	College	0	95,277	0
Volleyball	High school	0	2,884,819	0
	College	0	186,317	0
Wrestling	High school	0	1,494	0
	College	0	0	0
Spring Sports				
Golf	High school	0	323,767	0
	College	0	12,547	0
Lacrosse	High school	0	87,167	0
	College	0	29,466	0
Softball	High school	0	2,500,642	0
	College	0	199,629	0
Tennis	High school	0	1,264,627	0
	College	1	108,913	9.18
Track	High school	2	3,312,021	0.60
	College	0	175,321	0
Total	High school	11	18,001,713	
			1.9[†]	
			9,474,586	1.16
	College	3	1,281,997	
			1.2[†]	
			1,068,331	2.81
	High school and College	14	10,542,917	1.33

*Athletes counted once for every year and participation and for each sport in which they participated.
[†]Estimation of the total number of athletes participating in high school and college sports requires division by estimated number of participated in by athletes per year (1.9 for high school athletes and 1.2 for college athletes). From ref. 23, with permission.

the cavity dimensions and 23% less for the wall thickness measurements). It was also noted that left ventricular wall thickness in women athletes was only 6 to 12 mm and thus offered no confusion with the measurements usually seen in HCM. It is therefore easier to differentiate the female athlete's heart, with its physiologic adaptations, from that of an in-dividual with HCM. This is not always the case with male athletes, in whom there may be overlap in measurement and blurring of distinctions on the echocardiogram.

Some studies have also suggested that the male-female difference in cardiac response to physical training may be a result of androgen-mediated changes in cardiac protein synthesis

TABLE 7. *Causes of nontraumatic sports deaths in high school and college ahletes*

Nontraumatic Sports Deaths	Total (n = 136)	Male (n = 124)	Female (n = 12)
Athletes with cardiovascular conditions	100[a,b]	92[a,b]	8
Hypertrophic cardiomyopathy	51[c,d]	50[c,d]	1
Probable hypertrophic cardiomyopathy	5	5	0
Coronary artery anomaly	16[a,d]	14[a,d]	2
Myocarditis	7[e]	7[e]	0
Aortic stenosis	6	6	0
Dilated cardiomyopathy	5	5	0
Atherosclerotic coronary artery disease	3	2	1
Aortic rupture	2	2	0
Cardiomyopathy—nonspecific	2[e]	2[e]	0
Tunnel subaortic stenosis	2[f]	2[f]	0
Coronary artery aneurysm	1	0	1
Mitral valve prolapse	1	1	0
Right ventricular cardiomyopathy	1	0	1
Ruptured cerebellar arteriovenous malformation	1	0	1
Subarachnoid hemorrhage	1	0	1
Wolff-Parkinson-White syndrome	1[a]	1[c]	0
Athletes with noncardiovascular conditions	30[a]	27[a]	3
Hyperthermia	13	12	1
Rhabdomyolysis and sickle cell trait	7[a]	6[a]	1
Status asthmaticus	4	3	1
Electrocution from lightning	3	3	0
Arnold-Chiari II malformation	1	1	0
Aspiration—blood-GI bleed	1	1	0
Exercise-induced anaphylaxis	1	1	0
Athletes with cause of death undetermined	7	6	1

[a]One male athlete had a cardiovascular condition (coronary artery anomaly) and a noncardiovascular condition (rhabdomyolysis and sickle cell trait).
[b]Five male athletes had multiple cardiovascular conditions.
[c]One male athlete had hypertrophic cardiomyopathy and Wolff-Parkinson-White syndrome.
[d]Three male athletes had hypertrophic cardiomyopathy and a coronary artery anomaly.
[e]One male athlete had myocarditis and a nonspecific cardiomyopathy.
[f]One male athlete had hypoplasia of the aortic arch associated with tunnel subaortic stenosis.
From ref. 23, with permission.

that affects males (32). Research in rodents has demonstrated a cardiac sexual dimorphism presumably resulting from testosterone (33).

Furthermore, women athletes may have lower death rates because they are less exposed as a group to intense physical exercise and are less involved in competitive sports; this may therefore create a bias in favor of fewer deaths in women as compared to men. Even so, there is a vast gender difference in SCD rates, and the reasons for this difference are not completely known.

CONCLUSION

In regard to young African American athletes, the data presented herein indicate that they are at increased risk of SCD, especially from HCM. This fact should be taken fully into consideration in all deliberations on the subject of SCD in athletes. Although it is true that not enough is known about the denominators, that is, how many black individuals in the general population and in the subset of black athletes are at risk, and although there seems to be a preponderance of black athletes involved in certain competitive sports such as basketball and football in which the highest number of deaths occur, nevertheless, the evidence shows that there is a disproportionate impact of SCD upon the subgroup of African American athletes. More data collection will help to clarify this situation, and further research focused on the African American athlete should help to explain why this increased risk exists. There is also the perception that blacks are, in large part, missed or under-counted, and that perhaps many individuals who suffer SCD do not share equal access to health care or are not appropriately evaluated in the best medical centers. Further research focused upon the African American athlete should be conducted to explain the racial disparity that exists.

While the differences in expression of SCD along racial and gender lines are considered, it must also be questioned whether some of the disparity phenomenon is due to different rates of participation in various sports by blacks and whites and women and men. Is there a participation bias? In the years since Jackie Robinson broke the color barrier in professional sports and since college coaches such as Adolph Rupp at the University of Kentucky and Paul Bear Bryant at the University of Alabama began recruiting black players for their teams, there has been a dramatic increase in the numbers of blacks competing at the collegiate and professional levels. Seventeen percent of professional baseball players, 67% of professional football players, and 80% of professional basketball players are black. Although this quantum leap in black participation may be responsible for some of the increased rate of SCD observed in black athletes, it is not the cause of the entire amount. The remainder is due to the operation of a real cardiac disease process most commonly identified as HCM. The participation bias and the disease mechanism seem to work as separate but codependent variables leading to a heightened incidence of SCD. Proper collection of pertinent data should result in more exact data that will allow determination of whether black race should be considered a risk factor for SCD in sports.

Future iterations of the Bethesda Conference on Cardiovascular Abnormalities in the Athlete (34,35) and of the recommendations from the American Heart Association concerning cardiovascular preparticipation screening of competitive athletes (36) should place greater emphasis on the unusual profile of the black athlete and devise more focused methods of pursuing this mystery. Establishment of a federal registry of SCD by the National Heart, Lung, and Blood Institute is also a goal worthy of pursuit.

Regarding gender differences in SCD prevalence, important lessons can be learned through a search for the putative protective mechanism that appears to lower the risk for women of dying from athletic participation. As more is learned about how female athletes avoid SCD, perhaps we will be inclined to reverse the question that Professor Henry Higgins posed in *My Fair Lady*: "Why can't a woman be more like a man?"

REFERENCES

1. Williams RA, ed. *Textbook of black-related diseases.* New York, McGraw-Hill, 1975:381.
2. Gordon T, Kannel WB. Premature mortality from coronary heart disease. The Framingham Study. *JAMA* 1971; 215:1617.
3. Roberts WC, McAllister HA, Ferrans VJ. Sarcoidosis of the heart: a clinicopathologic study of 35 necropsy patients (group I) and review of 78 previously described necropsy patients (group II). *Am J Med* 1977;63:38.
4. Friedman M, Manwaring JH, Rosenman, et al. Instantaneous and sudden deaths. Clinical and pathological differentiation in coronary artery disease. *JAMA* 1973; 225:1319.
5. Gillum RF. Coronary artery disease in black populations: mortality and morbidity. *Am Heart J* 1982;104: 839–851.
6. Williams RA. Coronary artery disease in blacks. In: Hall WD, Saunders E, Shulman NB, eds. *Hypertension in blacks: epidemiology, pathophysiology and treatment.* Chicago: Year Book Medical Publishers, 1985:71–82.
7. Shapiro S, Weinblatt E, Frank CW, et al. Incidence of coronary heart disease in a population insured for medical care (HIP). *Am J Public Health* 1969;59[Suppl 2]: 1–101.
8. Gillum RF, Liu KC. Coronary heart disease mortality in United States blacks, 1940–1978: trends and unanswered questions. *Am Heart J* 1984;108:728–732.
9. Savage DD, Garreson RJ, Castellli WP, et al. Echocardiographic left ventricular hypertrophy in the general population is associated with increased 2-year mortality, independent of standard coronary risk factors—the Framingham study. *AHA Council Cardiovasc Epidemiol Newslett* 1985;37:33.
10. McLenachan JM, Henderson E, Morris KI, et al. Ventricular arrythmias in patients with hypertensive left ventricular hypertrophy. *N Engl J Med* 1987;317:787.
11. Topol EJ, Traill TA, Fortuin NJ. Hypertensive hypertrophic cardiomyopathy of the elderly. *N Engl J Med* 1985;312:277.
12. Porter GH. Sarcoid heart disease. *N Engl J Med* 1960; 263:1350.
13. Kuller L, Lillienfield A, Fisher R. Epidemiological study of sudden and unexpected deaths due to arteriosclerotic heart disease. *Circulation* 1966;1056–1068.

14. Keil JE, Loadholt CB, Weinrich MC, et al. Incidence of coronary heart disease in blacks in Charleston, South Carolina. *Am Heart J* 1984;108:779–786.

15. Hagstrom RM, Federspiel CF, Ho YC. Incidence of myocardial infarction and sudden death from coronary heart disease in Nashville, Tennessee. *Circulation* 1971; 44:884–890.

16. Oalmann MC, McGill HL, Strong JP. Cardiovascular mortality in a community: result of a survey in New Orleans. *Am J Epidemiol* 1971;94:546.

17. Kark JA, Posey DM, Schumacher HR, et al. Sickle-cell trait as risk factor for sudden death in physical training. *N Engl J Med* 1987;317:781–787.

18. Koppes GM, Daley JJ, Coltman CA, et al. Exertion-induced rhabdomyolysis with acute renal failure and disseminated intravascular coagulation in sickle cell trait. *Am J Med* 1977;63:313.

19. Phillips M, Robinovits M, Higgins JR, et al. Sudden cardiac death in Air Force recruits: a 20-year review. *JAMA* 1986;256:2696.

20. Jones SR, Binder RA, Nonowho EM Jr. Sudden death in sickle cell trait. *N Engl J Med* 1970;282:323.

21. Diggs LW. The sickle cell trait in relation to the training and assignment of duties in the Armed Forces. III. Hyposthenuria, hematuria, sudden death, rhabdomyolysis, and acute tubular necrosis. *Aviat Space Environ Med* 1984;55:358.

22. Death of an athlete with sickle cell trait. *Med World News* 1974;15:44.

23. Van Camp SP, Bloor CM, Mueller FO, et al. Nontraumatic sports death in high school and college athletes. *Med Sci Sports Exerc* 1995;27:641–647.

24. Williams RA. Sudden cardiac death in blacks, including black athletes. In: Saunders E, ed. *Cardiovascular diseases in blacks.* Philadelphia: FA Davis Co, 1991:309.

25. Maron BJ, Roberts WC, McAllister HA, et al. Sudden death in young athletes. *Circulation* 1980;62:218–229.

26. Lubell A. Special report: blacks and exercise. *Physician Sportsmed* 1988;16:162.

27. Thomas RJ, Cantwell JD. Sudden death during basketball games. *Physician Sportsmed* 1990;19:75.

28. Burke AP, Farb V, Virmani R, et al. Sports-related and non-sports-related sudden cardiac death in young adults. *Am Heart J* 1991;121:568–575.

29. Maron BJ, Shirani J, Poliac LC, et al. Sudden death in young competitive athletes: clinical, demographic, and pathological profiles. *JAMA* 1996;276:199–204.

30. Mueller FO, Cantu RC, Van Camp SP. Catastrophic injuries in high school and college sports. Unpublished monograph, with permission.

31. Pelliccia A, Maron BJ, Calasso F, et al. Athlete's heart in women. Echocardiographic characterization of highly trained elite female athletes. *JAMA* 1996;276:211–215.

32. McGill HC, Anselmo VC, Buchanan JM, et al. The heart is a target for androgen. *Science* 1980;207: 775–777.

33. Koenig H, Goldstone, A, Lu CY. Testosterone-mediated sexual dimorphism of the rodent heart. *Circ Res* 1982; 50:782–787.

34. Mitchell JH, Maron BJ, Epstein SE. 16th Bethesda Conference: Cardiovascular abnormalities in the athlete: recommendations regarding eligibility for competition. *J Am Coll Cardiol* 1985;6(6):1186–1232.

35. Maron BJ, Mitchell JH. 26th Bethesda Conference: Recommendations for determining eligibility for competition in athletes with cardiovascular abnormalities. *J Am Coll Cardiol* 1994;24(4):845–899.

36. Maron BJ, Thompson PD, Puffer JC, et al. Cardiovascular preparticipation screening of competitive athletes. A statement for health professionals from the Sudden Death Committee (Clinical Cardiology) and Congenital Cardiac Defects Committee (Cardiovascular Disease in the Young), American Heart Association. *Circulation* 1996;94:850–856.

The Athlete and Heart Disease:
Diagnosis, Evaluation & Management,
edited by R. A. Williams.
Lippincott Williams & Wilkins, Philadelphia © 1999.

18

Ethical and Economic Issues Regarding Athletes with Heart Disease

*B. Waine Kong, †Richard Allen Williams, and ‡Stephanie H. Kong

*Association of Black Cardiologists, Atlanta, Georgia 30303; †Department of Medicine,
UCLA School of Medicine, Los Angeles, California 90024; Minority Health Institute, Inc.,
Beverly Hills, California 90211;
‡Coopers and Lybrand L.L.P., Atlanta, Georgia 30309

In recent years, there have been several cases of high-profile college athletes who have been diagnosed with serious, life-threatening cardiovascular conditions who have decided nevertheless to continue to compete in sports at the risk of injury or even death. To many people, such decisions seem based on poor judgment, greed, inadequate information, or lack of "common sense." Physicians, in particular, are inclined to become disturbed when their advice is challenged or ignored by endangered athletes. Many physicians wonder why any sane, rational person would still participate in sports despite knowing that competing may result in sudden death. Controversy and conflicting viewpoints are commonplace regarding what is the correct thing to do in these situations. Physicians, trainers, coaches, school officials, parents, and college athletes themselves differ on these issues. There is a need therefore to analyze the various factors that motivate an athlete to compete under life-threatening circumstances.

In this chapter, an attempt is made to explore not only the reasons why such apparently paradoxical decisions are made, but also some of the ethical and economic considerations that go into the choices. The legal ramifications are explored in Chapter 19. However, some medicolegal considerations are unavoidable in exploring this particular set of issues. The principal objective in this chapter is to provide physicians, and cardiologists in particular, the information they need to make these agonizing decisions. Health educators, parents, coaches, trainers, college administrators, sports executives, and anyone who might have an impact on the athlete's decision making may find the information useful as well. There is no intent here to instruct the reader as to how a particular case should be dealt with, nor to recapitulate recommendations regarding competition for athletes with cardiovascular conditions that were promulgated by the 26th Bethesda Conference. Rather, the purpose here is to go beyond the purely physical aspects of the problem and to examine the more abstract, less tangible but nonetheless very significant factors that cause an athlete to "play hurt." In this expository process, a few cases and studies are presented as examples of what can result when the desire to compete seems to overwhelm logic, subdue reason, and repudiate wisdom.

Although parents would not ordinarily allow their progeny to play while injured, college athletes may believe it is perfectly sensible to sacrifice their bodies for the glory of sports. Athletes, as talented as they may be, are nonetheless young adults whose judgment may be impaired because they are in an age range in which vulnerability and their own mortality are not considered. "Machismo," pride, and the joy of playing can mask severe injury, even when it is cardiovascular in nature. The nature of cardiovascular disease compounds the problem. Its symptoms, being short of breath, having a rapid pulse, or even having chest pain and pressure, are also the signs of extreme exertion. Although athletes may feel the pain, one suggests that they would rather play with the risk than suffer the emotional pain and the economic consequences of not playing (1).

One memorable scene from the Monty Python movie "Quest of the Holy Grail" depicts the duel between King Arthur and the black knight. After one of the black knight's arms is severed, he forges ahead and proclaims that it is only a flesh wound. After the second arm is amputated by another cut of King Arthur's sword, the black knight proclaims that he can still kick. After his legs are severed and King Arthur leaves him to die, he loudly protests "Come back and fight, you coward, I can still spit." This is not unlike the conduct of some college athletes. Thirteen percent of injuries to college athletes are reinjuries (2). To some, to stop playing because of heart disease would be unthinkable simply because heart disease is thought by many to be a disease of advanced age. Without proper screening and diagnosis, the athlete may overlook serious signs and symptoms of cardiovascular disease because he or she may not be able to distinguish between the symptoms of fatigue and heart disease. While the athlete's heart may be impaired, athletic performance is not. But even those who are diagnosed correctly and advised to reduce their exertion still insist on playing the game.

It is a familiar pattern. Athletes are diagnosed with potentially life-threatening cardiovascular-related disorders (high blood pressure, mitral valve prolapse, ventricular tachycardia, ventricular hypertrophy, hypertrophic cardiomyopathy) and advised by a cardiologist to discontinue the extreme exertion that is required for peak performance. Most heed this medical advice, but others do not. Although men may take more risks with their health than women, this decision has not been conclusively shown to be related to family income or race. While some, like world heavyweight boxing champion Evander Holyfield, fight the good fight with heart disease and survive to enjoy their substantial bounty, others, like Hank Gathers, who played for Loyola Marymount College, collapse and die suddenly during competition. At the time of his death (March 4, 1990), Hank Gathers was both the leading scorer and rebounder in college basketball. He was also one of many college athletes who die engaging in sports because of a serious preexisting cardiovascular disease. Among other reasons, these athletes gamble with their lives for the glory of playing professional sports. This may be a culturally and environmentally influenced situation.

Shortly after Hank Gathers' death, Joseph Rhett, a basketball star at the University of North Carolina, passed out several times after exertion, was diagnosed with an irregular heart rhythm (atrial fibrillation), and was advised not to continue in sports. He continued to play with a pacemaker with the blessing of the university and even his mother, who said, "We can't live our life in fear. Nobody's life is tragedy-free; none of us is promised tomorrow, or this afternoon. You've got to have courage, otherwise you just sit around in life and just exist" (3). While this point of view may be valid, it does raise important issues regarding the rights of athletes and their families to continue to engage in life-limiting behaviors when diagnosed with a potentially lethal cardiovascular disease. (Eventually Rhett did discontinue playing basketball.)

On the other hand, Terry Cummings, who played for the San Antonio Spurs and who as an adult signed a waiver and continued to play despite heart disease, feels strongly that colleges should protect student athletes from themselves. He points out that no young adult athlete should be placed in a position of being Solomon; that is, does the athlete disappoint his or her team members and forego celebrity status to remain healthy or does the athlete place his or her life on the line? Cummings contends that the college athlete is not likely to support a decision that will limit his or her earning potential, regardless of the consequences. College athletes will always want to play (4).

Although performance pressures are applicable to all athletes, it may be instructive to look at the circumstances of the male college athlete. Given that athletes are usually durable and persevering, it is not surprising that they persist when common sense may dictate otherwise. Some of the heroes from recent Olympic games include a gymnast who vaulted with a fractured ankle and a Japanese star who completed his routine on the high bars with a broken leg. In short, an athlete is expected to compete even at the risk of dying. Living on the edge is certainly what speed racers, boxers, and "real men" do. Additionally, the rewards are wonderful for athletes who survive the risk. They are adored, admired, and handsomely paid. In some societies, those who fail are subjected to ridicule, scorn, and ostracism.

THE SPORTS CARDIOLOGIST

Whereas team physicians and other physicians who practice sports medicine are usually not cardiologists, cardiologists are often called in as consultants to evaluate and give advice about the future participation of athletes with suspected cardiovascular diseases. What the cardiologist should immediately realize is that, because the economic stakes are so high, this is not business as usual. These are not competent adults seeking medical diagnosis and treatment; these are young adults and their families looking for evidence that the major bread earner will be able to compete. Even though in a normal medical practice, patient autonomy and self-determination are sacred, this is not the norm in college sports. Even though college athletes may be legally adults, according to case law, they are not presently trusted with decisions relating to the amount of risk they take. Whether the cardiologist believes that colleges should protect athletes despite themselves will determine whether it is appropriate merely to provide information and advice or whether a decision is required from the

cardiologist as to whether an athlete should participate or not.

When called upon to consult, the cardiologist is judged by degree of clinical skill and expertise. Liability, in these cases, can ensue not only from misdiagnoses but also from negligent false-positive diagnosis and from inappropriate treatment.

In the usual clinical setting, the prevailing standard of care for physicians determines how much information is given to patients as evidenced by *Canterbury v. Spence* (5). This case states that all material information available to make an informed decision should be explained in clear, uncomplicated language. The patient should understand the information. If the patient speaks only Spanish, it must be explained in Spanish. The burden of responsibility for effective communication lies with the physician. In a standard physician-patient relationship, the physical examination determines whether the patient-athlete is fit to withstand the physical challenges of the sport. It also documents the health status of the patient-athlete before competition. The physician is also expected to provide appropriate medical advice to promote optimal health and fitness, counsel the atypical candidate as to the sports or modification of sports, which, for him or her, would provide suitable activity, and restrict from participation those whose physical limitations present undue risk (6).

The usual patient seeking medical care seeks cures and accepts the physician's diagnosis and treatment in the best interest of his or her overall life interests. For emotional and economic concerns, some athletes refuse the physician's recommendations and are willing to assume the risks associated with the diagnosis. If the athlete is not able to persuade the physicians to let him or her play, then the athlete may seek second, third, or fourth opinions. Richard Kehoe, the physician who treated Terry Cummings' heart condition so he could successfully pursue a professional basketball career, would also have cleared Hank Gathers. In the absence of absolutely overwhelming compelling evidence, Dr. Kehoe believes these athletes should have been allowed to use their one-in-a-million basketball talent (7).

The reasons most cited for not affording student athletes autonomy to decide whether they should participate in sports are (a) the student is too immature to make life and death decisions, (b) the student may have misguided feelings of immortality and invincibility, which are common among young adults, (c) the student may have pressures from family, friends, teammates, alumni, coaches, and others to perform at peak levels and win, (d) the student may lack the ability to understand either the medical diagnosis or its implications, and (e) the student may hold on to an obsession of big professional contracts and subsequent hero worship from a sports obsessed society.

The consultant physician/cardiologist must make an individualized evaluation of the medical risks of participation for each athlete. After examining the student athlete, the physician may exercise several options: (a) advise the school to consult another physician/cardiologist if the school fails to support the physician's recommendation, (b) disqualify the student from further participation if evidence of cardiovascular disease is found, and (c) allow participation while treating and monitoring the problem. Each option is potentially fraught with the danger of angry responses and potential lawsuits. For example, upon obtaining a history of exertional chest pain, Dr. Milton Sands did not clear Tony Penny of Connecticut State University to play basketball. A diagnosis of hypertrophic cardiomyopathy was made. Two other cardiologists concurred. Nevertheless, Dr. Sands was sued for $1,000,000 for disrupting Penny's athletic career. Penny later died playing professional basketball in Europe (8).

The lawsuit brought by the Gathers family after his tragic death claimed that cardiologist Vernon T. Hattori should not have cleared him to play (9). It was also alleged that the Gathers family was not told of the potential fatal consequences of the athlete's playing basketball. The cardiologist settled with the family out of court for $1,000,000.

What should a physician do when a patient is not only a patient but a commodity? Should not cardiologists only be negligent if they withhold material information or perform substandard diagnostic and therapeutic procedures? Physicians who care for athletes are also under extreme pressure to clear talented athletes with cardiovascular complications to play or to return to play. Additionally, physicians may fall prey to being star struck and therefore may be possessed with a passion for the team's success, which may compromise their decisions.

The issues of malfeasance and malpractice centers on who is party to the contract, that is, in the athlete-physician relationship, is the contract between the student and the physician or between the school and the physician? For whom does the physician work? To whom is the physician answerable? Does the physician have divided loyalties? In all occasions, the physician is being paid by the college. Does the physician then have a duty to the college or to the student? The standard of care may play a role in defining the boundaries of the contract in that a contract is usually viewed as being executed when a physician renders services to a patient and the patient allows the physician to perform the evaluation. In all cases, the party that will pay for the services is not material, because, in most situations in the United States, the college is considered a third-party payer. That being the case, the physician who delivers services to a student has established a professional relationship with the student and the student's family.

Both the athlete and the college may have powerful incentives to keep information from the physician. It goes without saying that the physician must be able to obtain a reliable medical history, perform a thorough diagnostic workup, and be completely candid in his communication to the student and the college about the student's health status. The physician should always obtain a release from the student to share his medical records with the college lest the physician breach his or her fiduciary obligations.

In most instances, the team physician is an independent contractor who does physical examinations, attends games to take care of injuries, and follows up with athletes who are on medication and need continuing care. Even in this situation, the team physician may not know the athletes well enough to fully appreciate the motivating factors that keep an "at-risk" athlete playing despite physical infirmities.

With emerging case law, there may be some risks that the college may not be able to delegate to an independent contractor. While there is no uniform policy before college athletes can participate in competitive sports, their health status must be evaluated (10). According to National Collegiate Athletic Association (NCAA) guidelines, it is recommended that the athlete's cardiac function, heartbeat, and blood pressure be screened. If the athlete is found to have an irregular heartbeat or other preexisting cardiac conditions, a complete cardiac workup is required.

In the final analysis, the athlete must understand his or her condition, the proposed treatment, the consequences of the proposed treatment, and the alternatives before he or she can legally immunize the college from liability for injury resulting from related injuries. Athletes are also entitled to know and comprehend the risks, benefits, and alternatives to treatment. Although unnecessary exclusion of a gifted athlete is not justified, exclusion of athletes with various cardiac conditions appears to be rational if none of the physicians examining the patients clears that athlete for participation because the risks are unreasonable—regardless of how motivated the athletes may be. However, the physician's primary responsibility is to provide accurate information and recommendations so that the athletes have the basis for making informed judgments.

WHY NOT PATIENT AUTONOMY FOR COLLEGE ATHLETES?

Patient autonomy and self-determination are *au courant* in medicine. As long as in-formed consent is obtained before any procedure is done and before any treatment, teenagers can independently agree to an abortion, 12-year-olds can independently consent to receive treatment for venereal disease, drug addiction, alcoholism, and short-term acute care in most states. Many other decisions can be made by minors. The presumption in these situations is that a minor can appreciate the consequences of his or her decision and exercise adult judgment. Why are college athletes unable to make decisions relating to their participation in sports? Are they not competent adult patients seeking medical treatment and advice? After a patient is examined and he or she is told that there is a substantial risk of sudden death, who should decide? The optional decision makers are the student, the coach, the university administration, parents, or some other surrogate. Do attorneys have a role? Should not college athletes be afforded the same rights and responsibilities as other competent adults in society? This question is complicated by the fact that both constitutional contract and tort law apply.

Although colleges have an affirmative obligation to make and enforce reasonable regulations designed to protect order and promote the educational process, modern college students claim the right to define and regulate their own lives. The days of one's alma mater acting "in loco parentis" (substitute parents) are long gone for college students but not for college athletes who continue to be viewed as incompetent adults. After being apprised of the risks, why should not college athletes assume the risk and determine whether they should participate or not? Why should not a waiver of liability be effective if the athlete is appropriately informed about the risks posed by their conditions and by their continued participation? An athlete who has been diagnosed with a heart condition that poses a clear and present danger to his or her health if the athlete continues to participate in competitive sports should still be afforded the right to make a knowing and voluntary decision to continue playing—if he or she wants to.

THE COLLEGE MAY BE
LIABLE ANYWAY

In *Moore v. Student Affairs Committee of Troy State University* (11), the court determined that colleges have an obligation to keep students safe from serious harm no matter what the source. College students who sign waivers and are injured could probably claim that college officials (coaches) encouraged previously injured athletes to return to play with the knowledge they would be injured. The fact that the college provided the medical care just so the athlete could be returned to play knowing that there was a high probability of injury. In tort law, however, an athlete voluntarily assumes the risk of harm from negligent or reckless conduct, having no one to blame but himself or herself (12). For this to be true, however, the athlete must have known of the risk and appreciated its imminence (13).

The NCAA readily recognizes that competitive sports are dangerous and presumes that the risks are shared between the athlete and the college. The institutions should provide the safest possible environment and equipment, coaches should warn the athletes about the risks they are undertaking, and students must follow the rules and not take unnecessary chances. On occasion, courts have found the college liable even when the risks were thoroughly explained and the student expressly consented to relieve the college of liability. Colleges may find themselves liable if they allowed an athlete to chance injury from a known risk even when the athlete insisted on playing. The theory is that colleges may have an absolute duty to keep the athlete from returning to play even if the risk of sudden death is remote.

Just as one is allowed to contract with minors, there are some things that public policy will not allow individuals to contract for. For example, one cannot legally contract to become someone else's slave or agree to be battered.

Even if a person is willing to assume the risk, he or she must not only know that the risk exists but also appreciate how unreasonable it is. The questions is whether a college athlete, in his or her invincible state of mind, can appreciate how unreasonable the risk is (14). Even if all the elements are answered in favor of the college, the college cannot escape liability for the tortuous (harmful to others) conduct of one of its agents. What if it could be shown that the coach played his star center (who signed a waiver) for an entire basketball game, because it was a big game that the coach wanted to win at all costs, while the coach knew that the chances of injury were greatly enhanced. The college would most likely be liable, regardless of the voluntary waiver the student signed. In this case, the tortuous conduct would have been created by the coach. Elements in determining whether the conduct was tortuous include the "importance of the interest, right, or privilege which the plaintiff is seeking to advance or protect, the probability and gravity of each of the alternative risks, the difficulty or inconvenience of one course of conduct" (15). Even though it may be difficult to overcome the presumption that college athletes feel too invincible to appreciate the risks involved in their sport, there are ways to enhance the information to make it understandable and realistic. The physician should take the time to explain the dangers and options as fully as possible. The athlete could obtain the services of a lawyer at the school's expense to monitor the proceedings and to ascertain the credibility of the process. Whatever method is used, demonstrating that the athlete understood the information presented will help the defense.

Other than the connection with a college, athletes are usually afforded the right to contract and engage in all other adult activities with the consent of parents or other adults. They may vote, enlist in the army, consume alcohol, agree to an abortion, and own property. Why are they not afforded the right to participate in college sports at their own peril? If a college experience is to teach students that they must assume responsibility for their decisions and conduct as responsible citizens, coddling adversely impacts on this lesson. For students older than 21 years of age, no adult concurrence should be required. For those younger than 21 years of age, a lawyer and a physician selected by the student and paid by the college should aid the parents and the student to make this decision. This was the decision in *Wright v. Columbia University* (16). Only by giving them this right will the students assume adult responsibilities and make decisions about the most important issues affecting their lives. The only caveat would be if the student made a truly informed and voluntary decision. These are the difficult elements of the student's consent.

Colleges have great incentive to persuade their talented students to continue playing even with heart disease. Coaches want to win. Revenues for successful athletic programs are enormous. In the end, the relationship between the player and the coach is so powerful that even a hint in one direction or the other may be too much influence. These incentives and opportunities potentially rob the student of volition. Nevertheless, in *Wright v. Columbia University*, the court supported a decision by the student to engage in competitive football even if he only had vision in one eye. After assurance that the student had seriously considered the gravity of his decision and the risk of injury, the student was allowed to sign a waiver and continue to participate in sports. Assurances can be solidified by audiotaping or videotaping the explanation to the student by the coach or physician or taking the extra step of having the student actually pass a test on the information presented. This information is admissible evidence in court and communicates the sincerity of the parties regardless of the Monday-morning quarterbacking about what "I really meant." Although there are no guarantees that a jury will find the information persuasive, this is as much as can be done to ensure that the athlete knows and understands all the information necessary to decide whether he or she should return to play with a potentially devastating cardiovascular disease.

Both Section 504 of the Rehabilitation Act (17) and the Americans with Disabilities Act of 1990 (18) protect people with handicaps and others who may be denied the benefits of, or be subjected to discrimination under, any college-offered program or activity. No qualified person may be restricted from participation in competitive sports because of his or her handicap. An individual with handicaps is defined under Section 706(8)(B) of the act as any person who has a physical or mental impairment that substantially limits one or more of such person's activities. Colleges therefore may not deny a qualified handicapped person the opportunity to participate in sports but must be afforded equal opportunity. An athlete with serious heart disease is an individual with a handicap as defined in Section 504—an otherwise qualified person who is able to meet all of a program's requirements despite his handicap (19). Therefore, an athlete who has been diagnosed with heart disease who insists on playing *must* be afforded the opportunity to play. A college's refusal to allow a college athlete to return to play would appear to constitute a violation of the student's right under Section 504, even if "reasonable" accommodation must be made by the college (20).

From a history of colleges being too conservative to allow handicapped students to participate fully in college life, the ruling in *Alexander v. Choate* sends the message that colleges are prohibited from paternalism—prohibiting them from deciding what is too risky for a student with a handicap. "Life has risks" (21). Handicapped individuals have a right to live their lives as fully as they and their parents decide. On the positive side, as a result of these laws, the achievements of individuals with handicaps, cardiovascular or otherwise, have been astounding in practically every field of endeavor. To a great extent, the objectives of these laws are being realized. Congress was right—except for the few times such as in the Hank Gathers case, when Congress, the court, the individual, and the college were all wrong.

If the college is to assert "direct threat" or potential harm to prohibit a student's participation in sports, safety requirements must be based on actual risks and not on speculation, stereotypes, or generalizations about individuals with disabilities (22). Colleges do not have the right to prevent certain athletes from exacerbating their preexisting conditions. Generalized fears about risks cannot be used by a college to disqualify an athlete with heart disease.

The issue of a college student returning to play after a diagnosis with cardiovascular disease is perplexing because there are no bright lines to follow and because the issue is suspended somewhere between constitutional law, tort law, contract law, and the Rehabilitation Act of 1979. Tort law holds individuals responsible for acts of negligence such as subjecting another to danger; contract law dictates that parties may make agreements as they see fit; the Americans with Disabilities Act gives permission to disabled athletes to play if they desire to. All this is complicated by NCAA rules, traditions, how things might look, other federal statutes (23), and case law, all of which contradict each other. There are case laws on the books supporting every kind of position that one may want to assert under the circumstances.

Because athletes must pass a physical examination before being cleared to play, colleges may argue that a student with heart disease does not qualify. In this case, the physical examination would be considered a "technical standard...essential to participation" (24). This is a reasonable argument but not a winning one. Courts will most likely view physical examinations as they relate to cardiovascular disease as required for full participation in the sport rather than a disqualification event. The physician's liability will turn on the reasons the athlete returned to play. To help win the big game is one scenario, and the student deciding to assume the risk is quite another. If the physician and the college act without negligence, the athlete should not be able to hold anyone but himself or herself responsible for a bad outcome. The final caveat is that the institution must continue to provide good medical care, provide the best equipment, and be as vigilant as they would with any of their students to protect them from un-

necessary harm. As long as the college takes reasonable steps to prevent foreseeable injury, there should be no liability.

If a college athlete with heart disease is able to show that (a) he or she is handicapped, (b) he or she is otherwise qualified, (c) he or she is being excluded because of the handicap, and (d) the college receives federal funds (25) (they all do), the athlete cannot be refused the opportunity to participate in competitive sports—regardless of how dangerous the college may believe the sport to be for that student. Students can claim that exclusion from sports because of heart disease denies them equal protection of the law while colleges can claim that handicapped persons do not have a constitutionally protected right to participate in sports because they are not a suspect class of citizens justifying a heightened scrutiny of alleged discrimination. There is no property interest in playing college sports. However, if the student is on scholarship, he or she may invoke the protections of due process before the college can take away the scholarship benefits (26). In addition, a potential professional career may form the basis for a claim. In *Poole v. South Plainfield Board of Education*, the court held that a handicapped athlete can recover damages for unlawful restriction from a sport (27). It would appear that "substantial" justification would be needed before a student with heart disease could be justifiably restricted from participation. Such a justification was found in *Larkin v. Archdiocese of Cincinnati* (28).

In the case of 17-year-old Stephen Larkin, brother of Cincinnati Reds baseball star Barry Larkin, a diagnosis of hypertrophic cardiomyopathy was made in this talented athlete after he had two syncopal attacks during workouts. A review of his family history revealed that Stephen's father and an older brother, Byron, had the same condition. Stephen desperately wanted to pursue a career in sports so he sued the college for the right to play despite his diagnosis and against the unanimous recommendations of medical experts. Even though he found no remedy in court, the college agreed that he could play if he and his parents signed a waiver and he had a pacemaker implanted. The principal legal point is that Larkin could not find a medical expert to agree with him.

It is possible that a significant risk or a substantial likelihood of harm remains even after reasonable accommodations are made. Could this justify the college's refusal to allow an athlete on the field? This was the opinion in *Doe v. New York University* (29). If the risk cannot be substantially reduced and harm to the individual and to others is likely, the college has a right to restrict participation. In the heart disease scenario, however, this will not likely be the case without circumventing the Rehabilitation Act. There has been no ruling on the long-term risk of harm.

In the final analysis, it appears that, for a student with heart disease, the decision to return to play is one for the student and the student's parents or guardians to make (30). Under no circumstances should the college, the physician, or the coach make this decision for the athlete. The worst case would be for the physician to refuse to clear the athlete for fear of being sued "in case something happens." The presumption is that the physicians and the college have been candid and forthright in their sharing, disclosing, and divulging information in clear, understandable language. Perhaps little can be done to undo the lure of professional contracts and the pressures to excel and win. Life has risks and is often unfair. For those who want the college to continue their paternalistic decision making and overrule a college athlete's decision to return to play, the anticipation is that "something will happen." For those who want the student to make an autonomous decision, the anticipation is that the student will go on to glory, wealth, and power in the face of his or her handicap.

Whereas the student athlete should be guaranteed that he or she will receive a scholarship regardless of his or her decision and that psychological support will be available to help him or her deal with the "bad news" about the student's health, after being appraised of the risks, the student and his or her parents should exercise the same rights and responsibilities of any other competent adult to decide whether to participate. Informed consent is possible. Whereas Hank Gathers died with his sneakers on, Terry Cummings not only played basketball in college but went on to an illustrious career in professional sports with medication, close monitoring, and protective equipment (31).

The present rule appears to be that, as long as an athlete can find at least one physician to sign off on his participation, the decision to participate shifts to the student and his parents. In other words, if competent physicians differ, it is no longer a decision for the college. The athlete is then obliged to consider carefully whether the benefits of participation outweigh the risks of permanent injury or even death. There are good arguments on both sides.

SUMMARY

A number of considerations and examples have been presented from several sports venues regarding the factors that may influence an athlete's decision to compete despite having cardiovascular disease. This chapter has explored the approaches that may be and have been used by a spectrum of cardiologists, colleges, coaches, and courts. We have raised the questions of the physician's responsibility to render an expert opinion, the college's authority to require athletes with cardiac conditions to follow certain regulations, and the athlete's rights to make autonomous decisions regarding his or her health and activities that may adversely affect his or her health. It is clear that the physician has an obligation first to understand the patient athlete's total situation from an ethical, economic, social, legal and physical perspective. The physician is obliged to make the individual comprehend the dangers of competing. How the college should handle these situations is less clear because there are so many competing interests to consider, but the college must use its best judgment in the interest of the student athlete as well as other students in deciding whether to allow an individual with cardiac disease to participate and compete. Finally, the student athlete has a responsibility to self, family, and even to society not to put himself or herself at such great risk, even in the face of the incentives and temptations. In brief, he or she may have to opt for a less exciting and pedestrian lifestyle. On the other hand, in a free society, people have the option of parachuting out of airplanes, climbing mountains, bungee jumping, and participating in boxing and kick boxing at their own peril. To what extent society can protect people from themselves is an ongoing question for politicians. These are not easy choices and they require a great deal of thought and counseling.

REFERENCES

1. Thornton JS. Playing in pain: when should an athlete stop? *Phys Sports Med* Sept. 1990 at 138.
2. Eskienazi G. Athletes and health: many at risk. *The New York Times*, March 11, 1990, Sports section at 2.
3. Rhoden WC. One player's victory over fear. *The New York Times,* December 29, 1990, Sports section at 41.
4. Eskenazi G. Athletes and health: many at risk. *The New York Times,* March 11, 1990, Sports section at 1.
5. 464 F.2d at 784.
6. Committee on the Medical Aspects of Sports, American Medical Association. A guide for medical evaluation of candidates for school sports I (1972).
7. Ritter M. Gathers' death points up tough medical choices, doctors say. Associated Press, March 6, 1990.
8. Altman LK. An athlete's health and a doctor's warning. *The New York Times,* March 13, 1990, at C3.
9. Altman LK. Suit calls coach and doctors negligent in Gathers' death. *The New York Times,* April 21, 1990, at 43.
10. *NCAA Sports Medicine Handbook.*
11. Moore v. Student Affairs Committee of Troy State University, 284 F. Supp. 725 (M.D. Ala. 1968).
12. Restatement (Second) of Tort, Section 496A, 1965.
13. Kirk v. Washington State University, 746 P.2d 285.
14. Rutter v. Northwestern Beaver County School District, 437 A.2d 1198 (Pa. 1981).
15. Restatement (Second) of Torts, Section 496E(2), comment d, 1965.
16. 520 F. Supp. 789 (E.D. Pa 1981).
17. Rehabilitation Act of 1973, 29 U.S.C. 794 (West Supp. 1991).
18. 42 U.S.C.A. Sections 12101-12213 (West Supp. 1991).
19. Southeastern Community College v. Davis, 442 U.S. 397 (1979).
20. Alexander v. Choate, 469 U.S. 287 (1985).
21. Poole v. South Plainfield Board of Education, 490 F. Supp. 948 (D.N.J. 1980).
22. 56 Fed. Reg. 35,564 (1991).
23. Rehabilitation Act and the Americans with Disability Act of 1990.
24. 34 C.F.R. Section 1044.3(k)(3) (1990).
25. Strathie v. Department of Transportation, 716 F.2d 227, (3d Cir. 1983).
26. Rutledge v. Arizona Board of Regents, 660 F.2d 1345 (9th Cir. 1981).
27. Poole v. South Plainfield Board of Education, 490 F. Supp. 948 (D.N.J. 1980).
28. Larkin v. Archdiocese of Cincinnati, Njo. C-1-90-619 (S.D. Ohio, filed Aug. 31, 1990).
29. 666 F.2d 761 (2d Cir. 1981).
30. George W. Schubert et al., Sports Law 256 (1986).
31. Ritter M. Gathers' death points up tough medical choices, doctors say. March 6, 1990.

The Athlete and Heart Disease:
Diagnosis, Evaluation & Management,
edited by R. A. Williams.
Lippincott Williams & Wilkins, Philadelphia © 1999.

19

Medicolegal Issues

Matthew J. Mitten

South Texas College of Law, affiliated with Texas A & M University, Houston, Texas 77002

This chapter identifies important legal issues arising in connection with diagnosing, evaluating, and treating athletes with heart disease or cardiovascular abnormalities and determining their medical eligibility for athletic competition. There currently is very little precedent in the form of case law or statutes establishing the legal duties of a physician in providing cardiovascular care and treatment to athletes. Although there have been several recent lawsuits alleging physician malpractice in connection with medical treatment rendered to athletes, virtually all of them have been settled by the involved parties before judicial resolution of their merits and establishment of legal precedent for resolving future similar disputes. Along with general legal principles regulating the physician-patient relationship, this chapter discusses the developing body of law concerning the provision of sports medicine care to athletes that governs the provision of cardiovascular care to athletes (1).

NATURE OF PHYSICIAN-ATHLETE RELATIONSHIP

The nature of the physician-athlete relationship is unique in many respects and differs from the ordinary physician-patient relationship. Athletes generally are highly motivated to participate in their chosen sports and are reluctant to spend time on the sideline because of an injury or illness. Both a typical patient and an athlete want a cure or treatment for a specific physical malady, but an athlete usually also seeks the quickest possible return to competition. Competitive athletes often feel invincible, have a strong desire to play a sport for psychological or economic reasons, and may be willing to sacrifice their bodies to accomplish an athletic objective. For these reasons, athletes may not readily accept physician medical recommendations that delay a return to play or advise against further participation in a desired activity.

Sports medicine physicians may encounter the sometimes conflicting objectives of protecting an athlete's health while minimizing the time spent away from athletic competition. Like many aspects of sports medicine, cardiovascular sports medicine is evolving and often lacks definitive scientific data on which a physician can rely in providing care and treatment to athletes. In addition to facing medical uncertainty, a physician may be subjected to extreme pressure from an athlete with a cardiovascular abnormality or from team officials to provide medical clearance or treatment necessary for the athlete to play. Moreover, the playing season and team's need for a player's services continue while the athlete's medical condition is being evaluated and treated, thereby creating an environment that is not optimal for making well-considered and medically sound judgments that protect the athlete's health.

A physician has special knowledge, training, and skill in diagnosing and treating diseases and injuries that a patient such as an athlete lacks, which is the primary reason that patients seek medical services from physicians. Because athletes entrust their physical well-being to their physicians and rely on the physician to protect their health in providing sports medicine care and treatment, the physician-athlete relationship is characterized as fiduciary in nature. This means that a physician has a legal obligation to act primarily for the athlete's benefit in connection with medical matters.

Even the physician who is selected or paid by an institution must provide medical care, treatment, and advice consistent with an individual athlete's best health interests because there is a physician-patient relationship with the athlete. If an athlete seeks an evaluation or care of his or her cardiovascular condition and a physician undertakes to provide such services, the physician owes the athlete a legal duty of care, even if the team selects or pays the physician or benefits from the medical care rendered to the athlete. It is important for physicians to be aware of this potential conflict of interest and not to place their own economic interests or the team's needs before an athlete's medical best interests. Although one of a sports medicine physician's objectives is to avoid the unnecessary restriction of athletic activity, the paramount responsibility is to protect the athlete's health, and the physician's judgment should be governed only by medical considerations rather than economic or psychological factors.

PHYSICIAN'S GENERAL LEGAL DUTY OF CARE

While providing medical care to a patient, a physician has a legal obligation to have and use the knowledge, skill, and care ordinarily possessed and used by members of his or her specialty in good standing, considering the state of medical science at the time such care is rendered. The law generally permits the medical profession to establish the parameters of appropriate medical care as well as to designate any specific medical practices or treatment that a physician should follow within

those boundaries. Thus, the medical standard of care, which must be established by physician expert testimony, becomes the legal standard of care for malpractice purposes. Malpractice liability for harm caused to an athlete may arise if a physician deviates from reasonable or accepted practices within his or her area of specialty in providing medical care, but the physician will not be liable for failing to use the highest degree of medical care, skill, and judgment exercised by physicians within his specialty.

In resolving malpractice claims involving medical specialists, the trend among courts is to apply a uniform national standard of care within a particular specialty because national specialty certification boards, standardized training, and certification procedures exist. In treating cardiovascular conditions in athletes, a cardiologist will be held to the standard of a reasonably competent cardiologist, and may be held to an even higher standard if the cardiologist holds himself or herself out as having specialized expertise in cardiovascular sports medicine. A physician without specialized training in cardiovascular care may incur potential liability for not promptly referring a symptomatic athlete to a cardiologist for evaluation and treatment, or for otherwise negligently providing cardiovascular care to an athlete. A physician has a legal duty to inform an athlete of the medical risks of failing to see a cardiologist or other specialist for recommended evaluation and treatment of a cardiovascular condition.

During recent years, consensus guidelines concerning the cardiovascular care of athletes have been promulgated. In 1994, the 26th Bethesda Conference formulated guidelines for medically clearing or excluding competitive athletes with cardiovascular abnormalities from sports participation (2). In 1996, the American Heart Association developed recommendations for cardiovascular preparticipation screening of competitive athletes (3). These guidelines are intended to enhance the quality of cardiovascular care provided to athletes and improve self-regulation of the medical profession. Guidelines have the beneficial effect of pooling medical knowledge, distilling research and clinical experience, and enabling physicians to provide cardiovascular care to athletes on something other than their own background and experience.

Standing alone, consensus guidelines do not conclusively establish the legal standard of care that physicians must comply with. The legal standard of care is reasonable or accepted practice within a physician's specialty, but current medical guidelines are relevant in judicially resolving this issue. Under current law, consensus guidelines established by medical organizations and societies that are based on the present medical state-of-the-art are admissible evidence of what constitutes good medical practice in malpractice litigation. For example, a monograph on preparticipation physical evaluations of young athletes developed by five organizations of family physicians, pediatricians, orthopedic surgeons, and sports medicine physicians recommends that medical clearance of athletes with cardiovascular abnormalities conform to the 26th Bethesda Conference guidelines (4). The monograph's endorsement of these guidelines evidences that adherence to them constitutes reasonable or acceptable medical practice in providing cardiovascular medical clearance.

A physician's deviation from authoritative consensus guidelines regarding cardiovascular care of athletes may create malpractice liability. However, failing to follow such guidelines does not necessarily mean that a physician did not satisfy the proper medical and legal standard of care in treating an athlete. Deviations from guidelines are legally justifiable if they are medically acceptable and necessary in a specific situation. A physician should carefully document the medical basis for not following authoritative guidelines at the time cardiovascular care is provided to an athlete.

To summarize, in providing cardiovascular care to athletes, physicians must comply with the legal standard of care by following good medical practice within their respective specialties as determined by reasonable or accepted practices and state-of-the-art consensus guidelines. The most likely potential areas of malpractice liability are (a) failing to conduct appropriate screening or diagnostic tests, (b) misinterpreting test results to determine cardiovascular fitness, (c) providing improper treatment of a particular identified cardiovascular condition, (d) improperly clearing an athlete to play with a known cardiovascular abnormality and/or incomplete disclosure of the medical risks of doing so, or (e) failing to follow generally accepted guidelines for sports medicine cardiovascular care of athletes. These topics are discussed in more detail in the following sections of this chapter.

SCREENING AND SCOPE OF CARDIOVASCULAR EXAMINATION

The law relies upon the collective judgment of the medical profession to establish the appropriate nature and scope of a screening examination or preparticipation evaluation to discover cardiovascular abnormalities and potentially life-threatening conditions in athletes. This necessarily involves the development of reliable diagnostic procedures considering cost-benefit and feasibility factors as well as the current state of medical science. To further this objective, the American Heart Association recently developed consensus recommendations and guidelines for cardiovascular preparticipation screening of competitive athletes (3). A consortium of five medical organizations whose members practice sports medicine also has developed a monograph, which includes guidelines for the recommended scope of a preparticipation cardiovascular evaluation (4). As more fully discussed in the preceding section, such guidelines are some evidence of a physician's legal duty of care in screening athletes for cardiovascular conditions. The medical and legal acceptability or reasonableness of the comprehensiveness of a cardiovascular evaluation appears dependent upon the individual athlete's level of competition, physical demands of the particular sport, and economic ability of the team, athletic sponsoring organization, or athlete to pay for an extensive examination.

There is little judicial precedent regarding the legally required scope of a preparticipation physical examination. In *Ivey v. Providence Hospital* (5), the estate of a former Catholic University football player who died from respiratory distress during an asthma attack after football practice sued a physician for alleged negligence in conducting a preparticipation physical examination. The complaint asserted that the physician failed to conduct a proper and sufficient examination to determine whether the decedent could physically withstand the stress that intercollegiate football would place on his respiratory system. More specifically, the estate asserted that the physician did not obtain an adequate medical history of the player's respiratory condition and properly evaluate the effects that vigorous exercise placed on his condition. This case was settled by the parties before its judicial resolution. To establish the physician's legal liability for the player's death, the estate would have been required to prove by expert medical testimony or applicable guidelines that the physician did not follow reasonable or accepted medical practice in obtaining an athlete's full medical history or otherwise evaluating his fitness to play intercollegiate football.

A physician is not necessarily legally liable for failing to discover a latent cardiovascular condition during screening or evaluation of an athlete. Potential liability arises only if the examining physician deviates from accepted or reasonable medical practice, the use of which would have led to detection of the subject condition in the athlete. In *Rosensweig v. State* (6), the court ruled that a physician was not liable for failing to discover a boxer's preexisting brain injury from a previous fight. The court found that the physician had conducted a standard examination (without discussing its nature and scope), which did not reveal a prior brain injury. The court also observed that the boxer's medical history indicated no symptoms of concussions or brain injury and that the physician had relied upon the opinions of other physicians who had examined the boxer after his prior fight without finding any indications of a brain injury. Similarly, in *Classen v. State* (7), the court found that a physician had conducted an extensive physical and neurologic examination of a boxer in accordance with accepted medical practice and was not liable for malpractice in medically clearing the boxer to fight. It is important to recognize that a "standard examination" must conform to the medical state-of-the-art and may not alone be sufficient for certain individual athletes.

An athlete's malpractice claim arising out of alleged negligence in connection with preparticipation screening or evaluation must be encompassed within the scope of the physician's understood duty to provide medical care or advice to the athlete. In *Murphy v. Blum* (8), the court held that a physician hired by the National Basketball Association (NBA) solely to advise it whether a referee would be physically capable of performing his duties did not have a physician-patient relationship with the referee that could form the basis of a malpractice claim. The NBA physician had informed an NBA official of the abnormal results of the referee's stress test who then forwarded these results to the referee's personal physician. The NBA physician did not directly advise the referee of the abnormal test results and did not recommend or provide any treatment for his heart condition. After suffering a heart attack that prevented him from continuing to referee, the referee sued the NBA physician for malpractice in a suit that the court dismissed because of the lack of a physician-patient relationship between the parties.

The Murphy case suggests that a physician who conducts preparticipation examinations solely for the benefit of an athletic team is not legally required to directly inform an athlete of discovered cardiovascular abnormalities. Nevertheless, to minimize any potential legal liability, it is advisable for an examining physician to directly inform both the athlete and the athlete's personal physician of any such abnormalities in writing. Even if a physician who merely provides routine mass screening for certain medical conditions has no legal duty to provide follow-up cardiovascular care, it is strongly recommended that the physician inform all athletes of the limited nature of the medical services being provided in conducting preparticipation examinations and promptly refer symptomatic athletes to cardiovascular specialists for fuller evaluation.

TESTING AND DIAGNOSIS OF CARDIOVASCULAR CONDITION

A physician may incur malpractice liability for not conducting appropriate diagnostic tests to determine the nature of an athlete's cardiovascular condition that are required by the exercise of reasonable or accepted medical practice. In *Goldman v. St. Francis Hospital of Port Jervis* (9), the court upheld a jury's finding that a thoracic surgeon deviated from good and accepted medical practice by not performing a stress test to determine the cardiovascular condition of a patient who had received a pacemaker and subsequently died while playing recreational basketball. Expert testimony indicated that performing a stress test would have disclosed that the patient had an arterial blockage and that strenuous exercise was contraindicated. It also was proven that the patient's death was related to the exercise he was doing at the time. The physician's failure to utilize proper diagnostic tests resulted in a misdiagnosis of the patient's condition and an erroneous failure to give cautionary instructions regarding appropriate exercise, culminating in his death from ventricular fibrillation caused by circulatory failure. Based on this evidence, the jury found the physician liable for his patient's death.

In the well-publicized death of former Boston Celtics basketball player Reggie Lewis, medical experts were sharply divided regarding their diagnosis of his cardiovascular condition and evaluation of the risks associated with continuing to play professional basketball. After collapsing during a Celtics game, Lewis was examined by numerous cardiologists. A team of 12 cardiologists assembled by the Celtics team physician diagnosed cardiomyopathy in Lewis and concluded that this condition probably would prevent him from resuming his basketball career. A second medical opinion, rendered by other cardiologists at Lewis' request, concluded that Lewis had a relatively benign neurologic condition that affected his heartbeat, but that he had the normal heart of an athlete. A third medical opinion found evidence to support both opinions. Lewis died during a medically unsupervised workout, and autopsy results showed his heart to be abnormal, with ventricular cavity enlargement and extensive scarring, a finding consistent with healed myocarditis.

In April 1996, Lewis' spouse filed a pending lawsuit against the physicians who concluded that Lewis did not have a potentially life-threatening heart condition (10). Without asserting any specific acts of negligence, she broadly alleges that these physicians failed to care for and treat Lewis in accordance with the standard of care and skill ordinarily exercised by qualified cardiologists. This case probably will not be finally judicially resolved for several years but may establish important legal precedent regarding the cardiovascular care of athletes.

A physician generally does not guarantee the correctness of a diagnosis, and a doctor is not liable for a mere honest mistake of judgment if he or she performed appropriate tests and the proper diagnosis or interpretation of test results is in reasonable doubt. However, a physician may be liable for malpractice if he or she does not use the requisite degree of care and skill ordinarily possessed by those within the physician's specialty in interpreting test results and determining a patient's need for treatment. In *Gardner v. Holifield* (11), a basketball player's surviving mother alleged that a cardiologist misinterpreted two echocardiograms ordered to confirm an initial diagnosis during a routine physical examination that the player had Marfan syndrome. As a result, proper follow-up care, including the probable need for cardiovascular surgery, was not provided, and the athlete died 6 months after initially being evaluated by the cardiologist. Medical experts testified that a proper confirming diagnosis and treatment would have prevented the athlete's death and given him a normal life expectancy. This testimony created a factual issue regarding the physician's alleged malpractice for resolution by the jury.

MEDICAL TREATMENT OF AN ATHLETE'S KNOWN CARDIOVASCULAR CONDITION

A physician has a legal duty to either provide appropriate care or ensure that an athlete with a known cardiovascular condition receives medically necessary treatment in a timely manner. In *Dailey v. Winston* (12), expert medical testimony that a surgeon negligently failed to immediately hospitalize a basketball player for an arteriogram after discovering he had an arterial blockage and not informing him of the seriousness of his condition created an issue of malpractice liability for resolution by a jury.

Two recent lawsuits alleged that the deaths of Hank Gathers and Earnest Killum were caused, at least in part, by the reduction of medication prescribed to treat the players' respective cardiovascular conditions below a therapeutic dosage to enable them to continue playing college basketball at a highly skilled level. In *Gathers v. Loyola Marymount University* (13), the Gathers heirs asserted, along with claims of other negligent medical treatment, that Gathers was given a nontherapeutic dosage of heart medication to enable him to perform well in upcoming intercollegiate basketball tournament games. This action allegedly contributed to Gathers' collapse and death during a March 1990 basketball game at Loyola Marymount University.

In *Lillard v. State of Oregon* (14), Killum's mother alleged that his non–playing-field death was caused by physician malpractice. Killum had a history of two strokes and then experienced numbness and slurred speech during a recreational basketball game; tests determined that he had peripheral vascular disease. Physicians prescribed anticoagulant agents, and he was initially advised to withdraw from competitive basketball. Thereafter,

his medications were reduced, and he was cleared to resume playing college basketball despite recommendations to the contrary by a consultant. He died one month later, apparently of a massive cerebral infarction. A nontherapeutic dosage of medication to enable him to continue his intercollegiate career allegedly caused his death.

The Gathers and Lillard lawsuits raised important medical and legal issues concerning the appropriate care of an athlete with a known cardiovascular abnormality. Because both cases were settled out of court, these issues were not judicially resolved, and no legal precedent was established. However, permitting nonmedical factors to interfere with the exercise of a physician's medical judgment breaches a physician's paramount responsibility to protect the athlete's health and would constitute malpractice. A court may allow a jury to award punitive damages against a physician to deter and punish this breach of the trust relationship between an athlete and the physician responsible for that athlete's medical care.

On the other hand, a physician is not legally liable merely because an athlete under his or her care with an adverse cardiovascular condition experiences a tragedy or undesirable result from treatment. Physicians generally do not guarantee that the effects of medical treatment will be favorable, and liability ordinarily will not result unless a particular result has been promised or the physician's care is outside medically acceptable norms. Physicians have a legal obligation to keep abreast of new developments and advances in cardiovascular treatment, and they may be liable for using outdated treatment methods that no longer have a sound medical basis or do not currently constitute appropriate care.

The law permits the use of innovative cardiovascular care of athletes if it is within the bounds of reasonable or accepted medical practice under the circumstances. A physician may exercise his or her judgment and choose between medically recognized alternative methods of appropriate cardiovascular treatment. If competent and well-respected medical authority is divided over the appropriate method of cardiovascular treatment for an athlete, a physician will not be held legally responsible for adverse consequences that are caused by the exercise of his or her medical best judgment. Harm to an athlete that results from the physician's good faith choice of one proper treatment method over another does not constitute malpractice.

INFORMED CONSENT REQUIREMENTS AND MEDICAL CLEARANCE RECOMMENDATIONS

A physician must have an athlete's informed consent before providing medical treatment. The informed consent doctrine is based on the principle of individual autonomy, namely that a competent adult has the legal right to determine what to do with his or her body. This autonomy includes the right to accept or refuse medical treatment. A competent adult athlete has the legal capacity to consent to medical care, but consent for treatment of athletes who are minors generally must be obtained from the athlete's parents or guardian.

For an athlete's consent to be legally valid, it must be the product of an informed decision regarding the proposed medical treatment. The average person has little understanding of medicine and relies upon his or her physician to provide the information necessary to make a responsible decision regarding treatment. The extent of a physician's duty to disclose medical information to a patient traditionally has been determined by prevailing practices in the medical profession. Physician custom or what a reasonable physician would disclose under the circumstances has been the controlling legal standard. The recent judicial trend, however, is to focus on the patient and require physicians to disclose all material information to enable the patient to make an informed decision. A risk is material when a reasonable person, in what the physician knows or should know to be the patient's position, would be likely to attach significance to the risk or cluster of risks in deciding whether or not to forego the proposed therapy (15). Thus, a physician should ask himself or herself what information regarding the athlete's cardiovascular condition and treatment would the athlete want and need to know, and then the physician should disclose this medical information to the athlete in a timely manner.

A physician should fully disclose to an athlete the material medical risks of playing with the subject cardiovascular illness or abnormality and the potential health consequences of using or foregoing a given medication or treatment. The availability and pros and cons of accepted alternative methods of treatment need to be considered and discussed with the athlete. All material short- and long-term medical risks of continued athletic participation and treatment, including any potentially life-threatening or permanently disabling health consequences, must be disclosed.

Treating physicians have a duty to disclose material medical risks to an athlete in plain and simple language. Information concerning the athlete's medical condition, proposed treatment and alternatives, probability of future injury and severity of harm from continued athletic participation, and potential long-term health effects should be preferably in writing or tape recorded when given verbally. It also is advisable to discuss any conflicting second opinions regarding appropriate cardiovascular care of the athlete, but not to downplay other physicians' conclusions about the athlete's medical condition and potential consequences of playing. A physician would be prudent to take affirmative steps to ensure that an athlete understands the available treatment options, side effects, and the potential consequences of engaging in athletics with a cardiovascular condition, which might include questioning the athlete or asking the athlete to write down his or her understanding of what has been said.

A failure to provide an athlete with full disclosure of material information about playing with a medical condition or the potential consequences of proposed treatment may create physician liability for negligence or fraud. In *Krueger v. San Francisco Forty Niners* (16), the court held that the conscious failure to inform a player that he risked a permanent knee injury by continuing to play was fraudulent concealment of a material fact in connection with his medical treatment. The court found that Charley Krueger was not informed by his physicians of the true nature and extent of his knee injuries, the consequences of steroid injection treatment, or the long-term dangers associated with playing professional football with his medical condition. The court also found that the purpose of this nondisclosure was to induce Krueger to continue playing football despite his injuries. The jury accepted Krueger's testimony that he would have rejected the proposed treatment and discontinued playing football, thereby preventing his subsequent permanent harm from occurring. The jury awarded Krueger $2.366 million in damages.

The *Krueger* case illustrates that a physician may incur legal liability for not fully disclosing material information about an athlete's cardiovascular condition which is necessary to enable the athlete to determine whether to accept proposed medical treatment or to continue playing a sport. To prevail in litigation against a physician for negligent or fraudulent nondisclosure of medical information, an athlete must prove that he or she would not have played or undergone the cardiovascular treatment that caused the athlete's harm if he or she had been properly informed of the material risks of doing so. Physicians providing cardiovascular care to athletes can minimize potential liability and comply with the legal requirements of the informed consent doctrine by communicating openly and honestly with their patients.

Physicians should provide all material information about an athlete's cardiovascular condition directly to the athlete and obtain permission, preferably in writing, before communicating any medical information about the athlete to team officials. Ethically, a physician is prohibited from disclosing a patient's medical condition to others without patient consent or legal requirement. Unauthorized disclosure of information about an

athlete's medical condition to third parties may create legal liability. In *Chuy v. Philadelphia Eagles Football Club* (17), a federal appellate court affirmed a jury finding that the Philadelphia Eagles team physician intentionally inflicted emotional distress on a professional football player by falsely informing the press that the player suffered from a fatal blood disease. The physician's statement was found to be intolerable professional conduct because he knew that the player did not have the reported condition. Moreover, physicians' unauthorized disclosure of even accurate information about an athlete's medical condition creates potential legal liability for invasion of the athlete's privacy.

Even if an athlete's illness or condition has been properly diagnosed and the athlete has been warned of the potential health consequences of continued play, a physician may be liable for making a negligent medical clearance recommendation. In *Mikkelson v. Haslam* (18), a patient alleged that a physician negligently provided her with medical clearance to snow ski after undergoing hip replacement surgery. The jury found the physician negligent based on undisputed testimony that advising a total hip replacement patient that skiing is permissible is a departure from orthopedic medical profession standards.

The *Gathers* (13) and *Lillard* (14) litigation both involved unresolved allegations that physicians improperly cleared a college athlete to continue playing basketball with a serious cardiovascular abnormality. The Gathers lawsuit claimed that Hank Gathers was not fully informed of the seriousness of having ventricular tachycardia and should not have been medically cleared to play college basketball with this condition. This action, which was filed in 1990, asserted that physicians providing such clearance acted negligently because the 16th Bethesda Conference guidelines (19) (which were in effect at that time) recommended that persons with ventricular tachycardia should not participate in any competitive sports. The Gathers heirs contended that Gathers was sacrificed on the altar of college basketball in Loyola Marymount University's quest for basketball success, notoriety, and economic gain.

In the *Lillard* case, Earnest Killum's mother alleged that her son's physicians did not inform him of the material medical risks of playing college basketball with an impaired vascular condition caused by two prior strokes. She also claimed that these physicians negligently cleared her son to return to competition although doing so subjected him to an increased risk of death or serious injury. She further contended that the physicians breached their duty to (a) refuse to provide medical clearance to avoid allowing an athlete to expose himself or herself to an enhanced risk of death or serious harm and (b) not compromise an athlete's medical care in order to advance a university's economic interests.

Both the *Gathers* and *Lillard* lawsuits were settled before their judicial resolution established legal precedent regarding medical clearance recommendations. These cases, however, illustrate the need for physicians to consider carefully the parameters of the acceptable medical risks of athletic participation with known cardiovascular abnormalities and always to adhere to their paramount obligation to protect an athlete's health. It is a serious violation of a physician's ethical and legal duties owed to an athlete to allow nonmedical factors to impair the exercise of medical best judgment in making clearance recommendations or not to fully inform an athlete of the health risks of athletic participation with the athlete's condition. A physician should refuse to clear an athlete to participate if he or she believes there is a significant medical risk of harm from sports participation, regardless of the team's need for the player or the player's strong psychological or economic motivation to play and willingness to risk his health.

In formulating a participation recommendation, a physician should only consider the athlete's medical best interest. The following factors may be appropriately considered: the athlete's unique physiology, the intensity and physical demands of the subject sport, whether the athlete has previously participated in the sport with his or her physical condition, available clinical evidence, medical organization and society guidelines, the probability and severity of harm from athletic participation with the athlete's condition, and whether medication, monitoring, or protective devices will minimize potential health risks and enable safe athletic participation. In cases in which there is an uncertain potential for life-threatening or permanently disabling harm to an athlete with a cardiovascular condition, it is advisable to err on the side of caution and recommend against athletic participation.

Consensus guidelines regarding participation recommendations for athletes with cardiovascular abnormalities such as those established by the 26th Bethesda Conference (2) provide a source of objective and collective guidance to physicians that may ultimately establish both the medical and legal standard of care in making medical clearance recommendations. As the *Gathers* case (13) demonstrates, it is likely that, in litigation, noncompliance with such guidelines will be alleged to constitute malpractice.

There has been one case in which an athlete sued a physician for refusing to medically clear him to play a sport with a cardiovascular condition. In *Penny v. Sands* (20), Anthony Penny filed a malpractice suit against a cardiologist who diagnosed him as having cardiomyopathy and recommended against his continued participation in intercollegiate basketball. Two other cardiologists concurred with this opinion, and Central Connecticut State University refused to allow Penny to engage in its basketball program for 2 years. Penny ultimately obtained medical clearance to play competitive sports from two other cardiologists. He alleged that Dr. Sands' negligence caused economic harm to his anticipated professional basketball career because of his involuntary 2-year exclusion from college basketball. Penny voluntarily dismissed his malpractice suit before he collapsed and died while playing in a 1990 professional basketball game in England.

Although Penny's allegations were not judicially resolved, it is unlikely that a court would permit an athlete to recover any economic loss because team officials accepted a physician's recommendation against permitting the athlete to participate in a sport with a properly diagnosed cardiovascular abnormality. Legal recognition of such claims would unduly impair a physician's medical judgment and may cause him or her to place greater weight on legal rather than medical considerations. This also would create the paradoxical and undesirable situation of imposing legal liability on a physician for complying with his primary obligation to protect an athlete's health.

ATHLETE'S RESPONSIBILITY TO PROTECT OWN HEALTH

An athlete has a legal duty to reasonably protect his or her own health. One court has defined a patient's duties regarding the receipt of medical care as follows:

> A patient is required to cooperate in a reasonable manner with his treatment. This means that a patient has a duty to listen to his doctor, truthfully provide information to his doctor upon request, follow reasonable advice given by his doctor, and cooperate in a reasonable manner with his treatment. A patient also has a duty to disclose material and significant information about his condition or habits when requested to do so by his physician (21).

An athlete must satisfy these obligations to comply with his or her duty to reasonably protect his or her health. Otherwise, the athlete may be found to be contributorily negligent for exposing himself or herself to an unreasonable risk of harm.

Physicians and patients have corresponding legal obligations to facilitate the provision of quality medical care. A physician has a duty to obtain a complete and accurate medical history from an athlete. In turn, an athlete must exercise due care for his or her own safety by truthfully relating his or her medical history to the physician. Although an athlete has no general duty to diagnose his or her own condition or volunteer information, the athlete should disclose known information about his or her cardiovascular condition that may expose him or her to a risk of future harm if

the athlete knows the physician has failed to ascertain these facts while taking the medical history. For example, an athlete would not be exercising reasonable care for his or her own safety if the athlete minimizes his or her heart symptoms to avoid medical restriction of athletic activities.

An athlete generally may rely upon the recommendations of his or her treating physicians without seeking a second medical opinion. It ordinarily is reasonable for an athlete to rely on his or her physician's recommendations concerning cardiovascular care and treatment because of the physician's superior knowledge and expertise. In *Mikkelson v. Haslam* (18), the court found that a patient was not contributorily negligent for following her physician's advice that she could snow ski after total hip replacement surgery without seeking a second opinion from other physicians. She did not assume the risk of her permanently disabling injury, which occurred while skiing, because her physician had not informed her of this potential risk and it was not an obvious risk to a lay person. Under *Mikkelson*, an athlete with a cardiovascular condition that does not expose him or her to an obvious risk of injury while engaging in athletics is not contributorily negligent for participating in an athletic activity with physician medical clearance, even if the athlete does not consult with other physicians.

Courts have held that an athlete's failure to use reasonable care to protect his or her own health may totally bar or reduce the recoverable damages in a malpractice suit against the treating physicians. In *Gillespie v. Southern Utah State College* (22), a college basketball player was found to be solely responsible for aggravating an ankle injury by not following physician instructions. He iced his ankle for longer than the physician's prescribed period of time, causing thrombophlebitis and frostbite, requiring amputation of his toe and other foot tissue.

If an athlete fails to take prescribed medication in the required dosage to treat his or her heart condition or deliberately takes steps to reduce the therapeutic effectiveness of the drug, such conduct would be an unreasonable disregard for the athlete's own safety. Similarly, disobeying physician restrictions on athletic activity by an athlete with a cardiovascular condition would constitute contributory negligence.

LEGAL ENFORCEABILITY OF LIABILITY WAIVERS

Under certain circumstances, the law permits an adult to whom a legal duty of care is owed to waive, by contractual agreement among the parties, his or her right to recover damages in litigation for harm caused by another's breach of this duty. A waiver of legal rights signed by a minor usually is not enforceable, even if it also is signed by the minor's parents or guardian or entered into with their approval because minors have only a limited legal capacity to enter into binding contracts. In general, an adult may prospectively agree to knowingly and voluntarily waive his or her legal right to recover for future harm attributable to another's wrongful conduct unless such an agreement violates public policy. In some instances, courts may uphold waivers of liability from future negligence but not more culpable conduct such as intentional, reckless, or grossly negligent torts.

As more fully discussed in the section titled "Physician's General Legal Duty of Care," a physician providing cardiovascular care to an athlete has a legal duty to comply with reasonable or accepted medical practice and may be liable for malpractice for breach of this obligation. Courts generally will not enforce waivers purporting to release physicians from liability for negligent medical care of their patients. Such waivers have been held to violate public policy because medical services are essential public services; the patient places himself or herself under the physician's control but remains subject to the risks of the physician's negligence, and the physician may have the bargaining power to require a release from negligence liability as a condition of providing medical treatment.

Although a court may not enforce a waiver signed by an athlete in which he or she agrees not to hold a physician liable for providing negligent cardiovascular care that causes injury, a physician will incur malpractice liability only if he or she deviates from the appropriate medical standard of care or fails to comply with the requirements of the informed consent doctrine. It is important to recognize that merely informing an athlete about the risks of participation with his or her condition does not discharge a physician's legal duty of care in providing cardiovascular care and providing medical clearance recommendations. For example, advising an athlete that he should not play a sport with his or her cardiovascular condition but then medically clearing him or her to play in exchange for a waiver of liability probably will not protect a physician from malpractice liability if the physician acted negligently. Conforming to current standards of cardiovascular sports medicine practice and fully apprising the athlete of all material information about his or her condition are the best means by which a physician can avoid legal liability.

IMMUNITY FROM MALPRACTICE LIABILITY

In some instances, physicians may be immune from legal liability for malpractice claims brought by athletes. Several states have enacted so-called "Good Samaritan" statutes protecting licensed physicians from negligence liability for emergency medical care rendered to athletes in good faith and without compensation. These statutes apply when a physician provides emergency treatment to an athlete suffering from a cardiovascular problem. Immunity generally is not provided for emergency medical treatment found to be grossly negligent, reckless, or willful or wanton. Preparticipation physical exams, general nonemergency medical care rendered to athletes, and physician medical clearance recommendations are not normally subject to immunity.

In some jurisdictions, state law immunizes physicians employed by public educational institutions from malpractice liability in suits brought by athletes. In *Gardner v. Holifield* (11), the court ruled that alleged negligent medical care provided to a college basketball player by a physician is encompassed within the scope of tort immunity under Florida law if he was acting in his capacity as director of a public university's student health center when such treatment was rendered. Florida state employees, including physicians, are immune from liability for negligence committed within the scope and course of their employment.

Similarly, in *Sorey v. Kellett* (23), a federal court held that a public university's team physician was immune from a negligence suit by the mother of a deceased football player. The player collapsed during a football practice and was given medical treatment by the team physician, but he died while being transported to the hospital. The court ruled that public employees have a qualified immunity from tort claims based on their discretionary acts. Finding that the physician was performing a discretionary function in administering emergency medical care to the decedent, the court dismissed the lawsuit.

A professional athlete's claim against a physician for negligent medical care may be barred by a state workmen's compensation statute prohibiting actions against coemployees for injuries caused to fellow employees when acting within the scope of their employment. If so, the athlete's legal remedy is limited to receipt of the statutorily determined workmen's compensation benefits under state law. In *Hendy v. Losse* (24), the court dismissed a professional football player's suit against a team physician for negligently diagnosing and treating his knee injury and medically clearing him to continue playing football. The court held that California's workmen's compensation law bars tort suits between coemployees for injuries caused within the scope of employment. The player's malpractice claim was dismissed because both he and the physician were employed by the San Diego Chargers team, and the physi-

cian acted within the scope of his employment in treating the player's knee injury. However, the court stated that a physician who is an employee of a professional team is subject to malpractice liability for improper medical services provided to athletes that are outside of the scope of the services the physician agrees to provide to players pursuant to an employment agreement with the team.

In most instances in which cardiologists provide nonemergency medical care to athletes, there will not be immunity for malpractice liability. There will be no immunity for providing negligent cardiovascular care to an athlete unless a physician both is an employee of a public educational institution or professional team and is acting within the designated scope of his or her employment at the time treatment is rendered. Physicians serving as independent consultants rather than team employees do not satisfy these requirements.

JUDICIAL RESOLUTION OF ATHLETIC PARTICIPATION DISPUTES

Ideally, whether an athlete will participate in a sport with a particular cardiovascular abnormality should be the product of mutual agreement between the team physician and consulting cardiologists, team or school officials, and the athlete and family. However, it is not uncommon for physicians to disagree in their medical clearance recommendations, or for highly motivated athletes at all levels of competition to be reluctant to accept a medical recommendation not to continue playing a sport. Disagreements regarding the propriety of participation in athletics with a cardiovascular abnormality will be judicially resolved on a case-by-case basis under federal or state laws prohibiting discrimination against persons with physical impairments.

Both the Americans with Disabilities Act of 1990 (ADA) (25) and the Rehabilitation Act of 1973 (26) prohibit unjustified discrimination against athletes who have cardiovascular abnormalities or impairments. These federal laws apply to virtually all professional teams and intercollegiate or interscholastic sports programs, but do not appear to render a physician personally liable for determining that an athlete is medically ineligible to participate in a sport. State education, human rights, and employment laws also may prohibit medically unwarranted discrimination against athletes with physical impairments.

Federal law requires that an athlete with the physical capabilities and skills necessary to play a sport despite a cardiovascular abnormality is entitled to have his or her condition individually evaluated in light of current medical evidence. Exclusion from an athletic team or event must be based on reasonable medical judgments by physicians, given the state of medical knowledge. The ADA and Rehabilitation Act require a careful balancing of an impaired athlete's right to participate in athletic activities within his or her physical abilities, physician evaluation of the medical risks of athletic participation, and the team's interests in conducting a safe athletics program (27).

Exclusion of an athlete because his or her cardiovascular condition increases the risk of personal injury to others or to the athlete while engaging in athletic activity must be based on reasonable medical judgments given the state of medical knowledge (28). Relevant medical factors include the nature, duration, probability, and severity of harm from athletic participation as well as whether the risk of injury can be effectively reduced by medication, monitoring or protective devices, or other reasonable accommodations to enable athletic participation.

An athlete may be legally excluded from an athletic event or competition if his or her participation exposes others to significant health and safety risks. In *Myers v. Hose* (29), a federal court held that a county transit authority's determination that a person with chronic heart disease, hypertension, and uncontrolled diabetes was not qualified for employment as a bus driver did not violate the ADA. He failed to pass a medical examination establishing certain minimum health requirements to operate county vehicles. The court found that his poor cardiovascular condition prevented him

from operating a bus in a responsible fashion that does not threaten the safety of his passengers or of other motorists. Under *Myers*, a team or entity sponsoring an athletic competition may exclude an athlete with a cardiovascular abnormality from participation if doing so is medically necessary to prevent a significant risk of harm to others.

Even if such participation does not expose others to significant harm, developing judicial precedent holds that a college or high school athlete with a cardiovascular condition may be excluded from a sport to prevent exposing himself or herself to a significant risk of injury. To date, there have not been any cases in which professional athletes have asserted a legal right to play a sport with a cardiovascular abnormality. Although the medical issues may be the same, courts may develop a different legal framework for resolving participation disputes involving professional athletes because sports is the athlete's livelihood rather than an extracurricular activity that is merely a component of a high school or college education (30).

In *Larkin v. Archdiocese of Cincinnati* (31), a federal court held that a high school could exclude Stephen Larkin from its football team because he was diagnosed with structural heart disease. Larkin and his family were informed of the medical risks of future athletic competition and were willing to waive any future legal claims against the school if he were permitted to play football. Because examining cardiologists unanimously recommended against Larkin's continued participation in competitive interscholastic sports and Larkin was unable to satisfy an Ohio high school athletic association bylaw requiring physician medical clearance, the court held that the school's decision did not violate the Rehabilitation Act.

In *Knapp v. Northwestern University* (32), a federal appellate court held that Northwestern University did not violate the Rehabilitation Act in following its team physician's recommendation that an athlete with idiopathic ventricular fibrillation not play intercollegiate basketball. As a high school senior, Nicholas Knapp suffered sudden cardiac arrest while playing recreational basketball, which required cardiopulmonary resuscitation and defibrillation to restart his heart. Thereafter, he had an internal cardioverter-defibrillator implanted in his abdomen. He subsequently has played competitive recreational basketball without any incidents of cardiac arrest and received medical clearance to play college basketball from three cardiologists who examined him.

Northwestern agreed to honor its commitment to provide Knapp with an athletic scholarship, although it adhered to its team physician's medical disqualification from intercollegiate basketball. This recommendation was based on Knapp's medical records and history, the 26th Bethesda Conference (2) guidelines for athletic participation with cardiovascular abnormalities, and opinions of two consulting cardiologists who concluded that Knapp would expose himself to a significant risk of ventricular fibrilla-tion or cardiac arrest during competitive athletics.

All medical experts agreed that (a) Knapp had suffered sudden cardiac death due to ventricular fibrillation, (b) even with the internal defibrillator, playing college basketball would place Knapp at a higher risk for suffering another event of sudden cardiac death compared to other male college basketball players, (c) the internal defibrillator has never been tested under the conditions of intercollegiate basketball, and (d) no person currently plays or has ever played college or professional basketball after suffering sudden cardiac death and having a defibrillator implanted.

The court held that a university legally may establish legitimate physical qualifications that an individual must satisfy to participate in its athletic program. An athlete can be disqualified from athletics if necessary to avoid a significant risk of personal physical injury to himself or herself that cannot be eliminated through the use of reasonable medical accommodations. The court explained that Knapp's exclusion from Northwestern's basketball team was legally justified:

> We disagree with the district court's legal determination that such decisions are to be made by the courts and believe instead that medical de-

terminations of this sort are best left to team doctors and universities as long as they are made with reason and rationality and with full regard to possible and reasonable accommodations. In cases such as ours, where Northwestern has examined both Knapp and his medical records, has considered his medical history and the relation between his prior sudden cardiac death and the possibility of future occurrences, has considered the severity of the potential injury, and has rationally and reasonably reviewed consensus medical opinions or recommendations in the pertinent field—regardless whether conflicting medical opinions exist—the university has the right to determine that an individual is not otherwise medically qualified to play without violating the Rehabilitation Act. The place of the court in such cases is to make sure that the decision-maker has reasonably considered and relied upon sufficient evidence specific to the individual and the potential injury, not to determine on its own which evidence it believes is more persuasive.

> We do not believe that, in cases where medical experts disagree in their assessment of the extent of a real risk of serious harm or death, Congress intended that the courts—neutral arbiters but generally less skilled in medicine than the experts involved—should make the final medical decision. Instead, in the midst of conflicting expert testimony regarding the degree of serious risk of harm or death, the court's place is to ensure that the exclusion or disqualification of an individual was individualized, reasonably made, and based upon competent medical evidence. So long as these factors exist, it will be the rare case regarding participation in athletics where a court may substitute its judgment for that of the school's team physicians.

> In closing, we wish to make clear that we are *not* saying Northwestern's decision necessarily is the right decision. We say only that it is not an illegal one under the Rehabilitation Act. On the same facts, another team physician at another university, reviewing the same medical history, physical evaluation, and medical recommendations, might reasonably decide that Knapp met the physical qualifications for playing on an intercollegiate basketball team. Simply put, all universities need not evaluate risk the same way. What we say in this case is that if substantial evidence supports the decision-maker—here Northwestern—that decision must be respected.

It is important to note that the Knapp case holds that it is legally appropriate for physicians to follow consensus medical opinions such as those established by the 26th Bethesda

Conference (2) in making participation recommendations for athletes with cardiovascular abnormalities. This view is consistent with the essential requirement of both the ADA and Rehabilitation Act that there be a reasonable medical basis for excluding an athlete from a sport. Thus, consensus guidelines and recommendations probably will play an important role in future participation disputes involving athletes with cardiovascular conditions, both in preventing and resolving litigation.

REFERENCES

1. Mitten MJ. Team physicians and competitive athletes: allocating legal responsibility for athletic injuries. *U Pitt L Rev* 1993;55(1):129–169.
2. 26th Bethesda Conference: Recommendations for determining eligibility for competition in athletes with cardiovascular abnormalities. *J Am Coll Cardiol* 1994; 24(4):845–899.
3. Mason BJ, Thompson PD, Puffer JC, et al. Cardiovascular preparticipation screening of competitive athletes. *Circulation* 1996;94:850–856.
4. American Academy of Family Physicians, American Academy of Pediatrics, American Medical Society for Sports Medicine, American Orthopaedic Society for Sports Medicine, American Osteopathic Academy of Sports Medicine 1997. *Preparticipation physical evaluation 2d*, Minneapolis: McGraw Hill.
5. Civil Action No. 93-010-330 (Dist. Col. Sup. Ct., filed Sept. 10, 1993).
6. 171 N.Y.S.2d 912 (N.Y. App. 3d Dept. 1958), *aff'd*, 185 N.Y.S.2d 521 (N.Y. 1958).
7. 500 N.Y.S.2d 460 (N.Y. Ct. Cl. 1985).
8. 554 N.Y.S.2d 640 (N.Y. App. 2d Dept. 1990).
9. No. 80 CIV 1729 (CBM) (WDNY Aug. 31, 1981) (slip opinion available on LEXIS).
10. Lewis v Mudge, No. 96-2349-F (Mass. Super. Ct., filed April 30, 1996).
11. 639 So. 2d 656 (Fla. App. 1994).
12. 1986 WL 12063 (Tenn. App. 1986).
13. No. C 795027 (Los Angeles, CA Super. Ct., filed April 20, 1990).
14. No. BC 2941 (Los Angeles, CA Super. Ct., filed Jan. 19, 1993).
15. Canterbury v Spence, 464 F.2d 772, 787 (D.C. 1972), *cert. denied*, 409 U.S. 1064 (1972).
16. 234 Cal. Rptr. 579 (Cal. Ct. App. 1987).
17. 595 F.2d 1265 (3d Cir. 1979).
18. 764 P.2d 1384 (Utah Ct. App. 1988).
19. Mitchell JH, Maron BJ, Epstein SJ. 16th Bethesda Conference: Cardiovascular abnormalities in the athlete: recommendations regarding eligibility for competition. *J Am Coll Cardiol* 1985;6:1186–1232.
20. No. H89-280 (D. Conn., filed May 3, 1989).
21. Benedict v. St. Luke's Hospital, 365 N.W.2d 499, 505 (ND 1985).
22. 669 P.2d 861 (Utah 1983).
23. 849 F.2d 960 (5th Cir. 1988).
24. 819 P.2d 1 (Cal. 1991).
25. 42 USCA §12101-12213 (West 1995 and 1996 Supp.).
26. 29 USCA §701-796 (West 1995).
27. Mitten MJ. Amateur athletes with handicaps or physical abnormalities: who makes the participation decision? *Neb L Rev* 1992;71:987–1032.
28. School Board of Nassau County, Florida v Arline, 480 U.S. 273 (1987).
29. 50 F.3d 278 (4th Cir. 1995).
30. Mitten MJ. Enhanced risk of harm to one's self as a justification for exclusion from athletics. *Marq Sport L J* 1998;8(2):189–223.
31. No. C-90-619 (SD Ohio, Aug. 31, 1990) (oral findings of fact and conclusions of law supporting denial of injunctive relief and dismissal of complaint) (Partial Transcript of Proceedings).
32. 101 F.3d 473 (7th Cir. 1996).

Subject Index